# Handbook of Human Development for Health Care Professionals

**Kathleen Thies, PhD, RN**
Associate Professor, Graduate School of Nursing
University of Massachusetts Medical School
Worcester, MA

**John Travers, EdD**
Professor, Lynch School of Education
Boston College
Chestnut Hill, MA

**JONES AND BARTLETT PUBLISHERS**
*Sudbury, Massachusetts*
BOSTON    TORONTO    LONDON    SINGAPORE

**World Headquarters**
Jones and Bartlett Publishers
40 Tall Pine Drive
Sudbury, MA 01776
978-443-5000
info@jbpub.com
www.jbpub.com

Jones and Bartlett Publishers Canada
6339 Ormindale Way
Mississauga, Ontario L5V 1J2
CANADA

Jones and Bartlett Publishers International
Barb House, Barb Mews
London W6 7PA
UK

Jones and Bartlett's books and products are available through most bookstores and online booksellers. To contact Jones and Bartlett Publishers directly, call 800-832-0034, fax 978-443-8000, or visit our website www.jbpub.com.

Substantial discounts on bulk quantities of Jones and Bartlett's publications are available to corporations, professional associations, and other qualified organizations. For details and specific discount information, contact the special sales department at Jones and Bartlett via the above contact information or send an email to specialsales@jbpub.com.

**Production Credits**
Acquisitions Editor: Kevin Sullivan
Production Director: Amy Rose
Associate Production Editor: Tracey Chapman
Associate Editor: Amy Sibley
Marketing Manager: Emily Ekle
Manufacturing & Inventory Coordinator: Amy Bocus
Cover Design: Anne Spencer
Printing and Binding: Malloy
Cover Printing: Malloy

**Library of Congress Cataloging-in-Publication Data**
Thies, Kathleen M.
  Handbook of human development for health care professionals / Kathleen M. Thies, John F. Travers.
    p. ; cm.
  Includes bibliographical references and index.
  ISBN 0-7637-3614-7 (pbk.)
  1. Child development—Handbooks, manuals, etc.   2. Developmental biology—Handbooks, manuals, etc.   3. Developmental psychobiology—Handbooks, manuals, etc.   4. Developmental disabilities—Handbooks, manuals, etc.
    [DNLM: 1. Human Development.   2. Developmental Disabilities. ]   I. Travers, John F.   II. Title.
  RJ131.T554 2005
  618.92—dc22
                                                                                          2005004204

Printed in the United States of America
09  08  07  06  05    10 9 8 7 6 5 4 3 2 1

*For my children Evan and Julia, who taught me most of what I know about human development.*

*—Kathleen Thies*

*To my children Elizabeth, Ellen, John, and Jane who have been a source of inspiration, love, and happiness through the years.*

*—John Travers*

# Contributors

**Ori Ashman**
Murdoch University
School of Psychology

**Jamie Barrett, MA**
Lynch School of Education, Counseling
  Psychology Department
Boston College

**Yvette Blanchard**
Associate Professor of Physical Therapy
University of Hartford
Faculty NBAs lead trainer, NBO trainer
Brazelton Institute, Children's Hospital

**Mary Brabeck, PhD**
Dean, School of Education
New York University

**Paul D. Connor, MD**
Acting Instructor
Psychiatry & Behavioral Sciences/Fetal Alcohol
  and Drug Unit
University of Washington

**John Dacey, PhD**
Professor, Boston College
Lynch School of Education

**Philip DiMattia, PhD**
Adjunct Professor, Boston College
Lynch School of Education

**Jean Eckrich, PhD**
Department of Exercise and Sports Science
Colby-Sawyer College

**Lisa Fiori**
Assistant Professor, Lesley University

**James Gips**
Professor, Boston College
Fulton Hall

**Dr. Kathleen Gorman**
Associate Professor Department of Psychology
University of Rhode Island

**Penny Hauser-Cram, PhD**
Professor, Boston College
Lynch School of Education

**Janet Huggins**
Professional Staff
University of Washington
Project Director
Psychiatry & Behavioral Sciences/Fetal Alcohol and
  Drug Unit
University of Washington

**Ronald J. Iannotti, PhD**
Prevention Research Branch
Division of Epidemiology, Statistics, & Prevention
  Research
National Institute of Child Health and Human
  Development

**Mary Kazanowski**

**George Ladd, PhD**
Assistant Professor, Department of Psychiatry
University of Connecticut Medical School

**Jacqueline Lerner**
Editorial Board, Child Development
Professor, Boston College
Lynch School of Education

**Deborah Margolis, PhD**
Assistant Professor, Merrimack College

**Kathleen McCartney, PhD**
Department of Human Development and Psychology
Harvard University, Graduate School of Education

**Elizabeth Metallinos-Katsaras**
Assistant Professor, Nutrition Department,
  School for Health Studies
Simmons College

**Tonja Nansel, BSN, PhD**
Investigator, Prevention Research Branch
Division of Epidemiology, Statistics, and
  Prevention Research
National Institute of Child Health Development

**J. Kevin Nugent, PhD**
Professor, University of Massachusetts
Director, Brazelton Institute
Children's Hospital

**Erin O'Connor, Doctoral Student**
Department of Human Development and Psychology
Harvard University, Graduate School of Education

**David Scanlon, PhD**
Boston College
Lynch School of Education

**Caryn Sheehan**

**George H. Singer, PhD**
Professor of Education, Gevritz Graduate School of
  Education
University of California at Santa Barbara

**Scott Strohmeyer**
Professor, Health and Human Performance
Central Missouri State University

**Kathleen Thies, PhD, RN**
Chair, Department of Nursing
Colby-Sawyer College

**John Travers, EdD**
Professor, Boston College
Lynch School of Education

**Mary Walsh, PhD**
Professor, Boston College
Lynch School of Education

# Table of Contents

# Introduction

In recent years, health care has seen a shift in focus from curing acute illness to managing chronic illness and disability, from institution-based care to community-based care, and from care that is provider and disease oriented to care that is individual and family centered. People are surviving diseases that once would have killed them and are living longer with chronic health issues. In these emerging models of care, the health professional is a partner, a resource, a guide. We do not so much "do to" our patients as "do with" them. Being a health professional means entering into a relationship with patients that is designed for their benefit.

Traditionally, physicians, nurse practitioners, nurses, physical therapists, occupational therapists, and nutritionists have focused on the diagnosis and treatment of disease and illness, on human response to disease and illness, on restoring health, and more recently, on preventing future occurrences of poor health as well as facilitating a peaceful death. We have conveniently divided growth, development, and behavior into the normal and abnormal, as if they are two distinctly different paths; the former seems to occur naturally and thus does not require our attention, whereas the latter presents as a problem requiring our expertise. We have been content to know surprisingly little about "normal" because it is not a problem for us to solve.

A developmental perspective shows us that the difference between "normal" and "abnormal" is not so clear and that even normal development cannot occur without an appropriate relationship with the environment. A developmental perspective tells us that human development occurs in the context of the relationship between the individual and his/her environment and within the context of historical time for that individual. Health professionals are players in the environment of the people we see as patients. Because we are part of the relationship with the environment, we contribute to human development and are able to influence people's life trajectories in ways both positive and negative. Because the relationship is for their benefit, we must become stewards of our influence. We must learn more about developmental processes so that we can help people to manage their own health in the context of their lives and promote optimal development as a condition for optimal health.

The *Handbook of Human Development for Health Care Professionals* is intended to provide health care professionals with a current and practical overview of human development. In writing this book, the most critical question we faced was: *What is the most efficient way to provide access to the vast amount of developmental theory and research now available?* We knew we could not produce a comprehensive review in one volume. *Where to begin?*

First, we needed to establish a theoretical perspective on human development. Given the emphasis on pathology in most of health care, we wanted to focus on normative developmental processes. We chose exemplars of those processes based on a survey of colleagues.

Second, a theoretical perspective would allow us to address some alternative routes along the developmental path in the context of normative processes rather than as pathologies in and of themselves. For example, anxiety and aggression are normative and even healthy aspects of human development that can become pathological under certain conditions. In another example, different ways of learning are a problem only if the environment cannot support them.

Third, we wanted to cover issues that are of concern or interest to health professionals but that are usually not addressed in depth in the health-related literature. For example, there is a large collection of literature on aging directed toward health professionals, but there is less focus on middle adulthood. We chose authors who work within a developmental perspective but are not necessarily health care providers, and asked them to review the literature with an eye toward applications for health care.

Finally, and most importantly, a developmental perspective provides a theoretical framework within which to study human development and the implications for health that goes beyond the age-related stages approach.

# Organization of the Handbook

Most books on human development are textbooks that are organized sequentially, birth to old age. For the novice, the lifespan approach is easy to learn because of its familiarity: development appears to occur in predictable stages, one after the other. In this approach to studying human development, age is the organizing factor.

We assume that our readers are no longer novices. Your professional education and clinical experience tells you that age-related stages are not a sufficient explanation for human growth, development, and behavior. You know how to think in systems and processes related to the human body—everything is interconnected. For example, you know that diabetes isn't simply a lack of insulin that can be corrected with injections. Its effects are pervasive and complex, and they tend to worsen with time even with optimal management. As a complex systems thinker, you are ready to move beyond a more concrete stage-and-age approach to development and begin to think like a developmentalist.

We believe the present volume will be a rich source of developmental knowledge for those professionals who wish to enhance their expertise as they seek to improve the health and welfare of their clients.

## Introduction to Part One: Theoretical Foundations in Development

In Chapter One, Travers, who is the author of several textbooks on human development, reviews the major theories in developmental psychology. Many are familiar to you, such as Piaget, but he also introduces some of the more recent literature that both supports and challenges traditionally held notions about development. In Chapter Two, Margolis—who writes on women's issues—points out that although gender is genetic, it is also a social construction. How different are males and females, and how much of that difference is inherent in what the individual brings to his/her relationship with the environment and how much in the environment? She reviews the major theories of gender development—social learning, gender schema, and role socialization, as well as the all-pervasive psychoanalytic approach—and discusses the possible implications for health care.

In Chapter Three, Lerner—known for her work on the influences of culture and society on development—and Ashman discuss culture in Bronfenbrenner's biopsychosocial framework of development. The relationship between children and parents is embedded in broader social systems. Culture is not so much a factor in human development as the very context for it. In Chapter Four, Thies—a developmentalist and a nurse who has written on the development of children with chronic illness—addresses the question, *Are children naturally resilient?* She uses the developmental perspective to demonstrate that resilience is a product of the relationship between a child and—usually—her environment. The child is able to take advantage of intrapersonal and interpersonal resources to stay the developmental path in circumstances that common wisdom suggest would lead to less optimal outcomes.

## Introduction to Part Two: Normative Processes of Development

Development is not a matter of passing through age-related stages; it is an integrative process across the lifespan. We chose some physical and social exemplars of normative developmental processes: responding, relating, thinking, eating, moving, reproducing, and maturing.

Chapters Five and Six lay the early foundations for later development. In Chapter Five, Nugent—a developmental psychologist well known for his work with the Brazelton Newborn Assessment Scale—and Blanchard explain that human behavior is organized from birth and that it can be assessed objectively to identify potentially problematic patterns in its organization. Organization of behavior is key to understanding the process of attachment in human relationships, addressed in Chapter Six. McCartney—a Harvard researcher widely acclaimed for her work on the implications of nonmaternal child care for healthy attachment between mother and child—and O'Connor review the literature on this fundamental process in human development. The quality of the early attachment relationship shapes the developmental trajectory for other relationships later in life.

In Chapter Seven, Travers reviews theories of cognitive development, including recent developments in Piagetian stage theories as well as theories that focus on information processing. In Chapter Eight, our nutrition experts—Metallinos-Katsaras and Gorman—remind us that we are what we eat. Or maybe not. Although most health care providers are familiar with concerns about obesity, the authors look at the relationship between behavior and food in children. Is there such a thing as a "sugar high"? It is not so simple. In keeping with the developmental perspective, exercise physiologists Eckrich and Strohmeyer remind us in Chapter Nine that physical development is hierarchically organized over time, with more variation among adults and elders than among children. In Chapter Ten, Dacey and Margolis look at how sexual identity and expression emerge during adolescence in ways that reflect earlier patterns of relationships and sense of self. The choices adolescents make during this time can have a dramatic and lasting affect on their developmental trajectory. Finally, in Chapter Eleven, Dacey—who has authored several books on adult development—and Fiori address the common developmental tasks of mature adulthood.

## Introduction to Part Three: Alternative Routes Along the Development Path

Sometimes the developmental path is not typical. The normative processes associated with thinking, feeling, and relating are organized differently, yielding a clinical picture that can be construed as simply different or as problematic. In Chapter 12, Connor and Huggins demonstrate that when the prenatal uterine environment contains alcohol, the developmental trajectory of the fetus is altered irrevocably throughout the lifespan. In Chapter 13, Singer presents the philosophy that developmental disabilities are differences in the organization of development rather than medical diagnoses. In Chapter 14, Hauser-Cram—a researcher in early intervention—makes the case for the role of the early educational environment in keeping children who learn differently on the developmental path. As Scanlon points out in Chapter 15, not everyone who learns differently is a youngster in school. He looks at the implications of learning disabilities for generative development in adulthood. In Chapter 16, Ladd reminds us that anxiety shapes our awareness of our relationship with the environment in ways that are normal and healthy, but that can also undermine our ability to form effective relationships. Similarly, Walsh and Barrett make the point in Chapter 17 that normal aggression and violent behavior have common roots in physiology and in relationships, but are organized toward very different ends.

## Introduction to Part Four: Toward Developmentally Appropriate Care

In this section, we take the next step: applying developmental theory to health-related interventions. In Chapter 18, Thies makes the case that if development is not simply a matter of age-related stages, then health care providers cannot use age-specific care as a theoretical framework for what is appropriate for the individual. She reviews the literature on the normative development of thinking, feeling, relating, and sense of self through adolescence, and poses implications for the developmental trajectory of children with chronic illness. In Chapter 19, Nansel—a researcher with the National Institute of Child Health Development—presents a developmental model of adherence to health care regimens that includes cognitive development, self-knowledge, and appraisal of environmental challenges. In Chapter 20, DiMattia and Gips demonstrate that technology can enable individuals who require assistance with communication to stay the developmental path. Finally, Kazanowski and Sheehan examine the experience of pain across the lifespan in Chapter 21.

## Introduction to Part Five: Philosophical Perspectives on Human Development

Our last chapter takes us outside of the realm of theories of human development and their application to health care and to a more philosophical plane. Whereas most developmental textbooks end with chapters on death and dying—topics broadly covered in the health care literature—we chose to focus instead on the uniquely human condition called hope. Brabeck challenges us to look at the human condition as hopeful, not in spite of our problems or differences but because of them.

# About the Editors

**Kathleen M. Thies, PhD, RN**

Dr. Thies is a clinical specialist in mental/health psychiatric nursing, with a PhD in developmental psychology from Boston College. She has taught both nursing and psychology full-time and did a post-doctoral fellowship in developmental disabilities in a joint program at the University of New Hampshire Institute on Disabilities and Dartmouth Medical School. She is a developmentalist and writes on developmental issues in children with chronic illness as well as on models of nursing education. She is currently an Associate Professor in the Graduate School of Nursing in the University of Massachusetts Medical School, Worcester, Massachusetts.

**John Travers, EdD**

Dr. Travers is an educational psychologist and a senior member of the faculty at the Lynch School of Education at Boston College. He has authored many books on human development, cognitive development, and educational psychology. His textbooks include *Human Development* with John Dacey of Boston College (for McGraw-Hill) and *Growth and Development Through the Lifespan* with Kathleen Thies (for SLACK).

# Part One

# THEORETICAL FOUNDATIONS IN DEVELOPMENT

# Chapter 1

# Current Views of Life Span Development

John Travers

## Introduction

In preparing the first of what is hoped will be many editions of a handbook intended for health care professionals, we addressed several important and interesting issues, among which were the following:

1. We asked our authors, all acknowledged specialists in their fields, to focus on the latest theory and research and how it supports or challenges present data, and to draw relevant and constructive conclusions for health care professionals.

2. We emphasized that developmental psychology is experiencing significant changes in its theoretical structure—changes that have unavoidable implications for understanding the psychological mechanisms that underlie the behavior of your clients.

3. We attempted to present developmental theories and research, which are general by nature, in a context that simultaneously retains the concept of individuality. Two clients presenting with similar symptoms may have totally different reactions de-

pending on cognitive level, emotions, and social support.

4. Finally, we have been guided by one principle: health care professionals who possess knowledge of human development—the characteristics, problems, and needs of people of various ages—can utilize this knowledge and their personal expertise to bring comfort to their clients.

## Our Point of View

As readers of this text you have every right to know the perspective from which this book is written. We are NOT advocating an overly simplistic interaction model between heredity and environment, but one that recognizes the complexity of a multilayered organism interacting with multilayered environmental systems. (For an excellent discussion of this topic, see Rutter 2002 and Pinker 2002.)

The following two quotations reflect the enormous power of heredity and environment as they act in concert to shape the direction of human development. The first quotation that follows (Dacey & Travers 2005, p. 66) addresses the impact of our inheritance.

*On a sparkling June day, 2000, Dr. Francis Collins (Director of the National Human Genome Research Institute) and Dr. J. Craig Venter (President of Celera Genomics) announced at a White House ceremony that they had completed a "rough draft of the human genome." Today we are more fully aware of the enormity of the task. The Human Genome Project has been nothing less than an attempt to identify and map the 30,000 to 50,000 genes that are our genetic endowment.*

*Much remains to be done: sequencing the genome (determining the exact order of the 3 billion chemical letters), finding the specific location of the genes and determining their functions, correcting disease-causing genes, etc. In the process, HGP is revolutionizing biology, medicine, and pharmacology, to say nothing of its ethical, legal, and social ramifications. Despite controversy and some disappointing results, gene therapy continues to offer promise for treating a wide range of problems.*

In this next quotation (Dacey & Travers 2005, p. 3), we see the power of the environment on human behavior.

*It all began in 1955. During those 365 days, the psychologists Emmy Werner and Ruth Smith began to collect data on the 837 children born on the island of Kauai, a part of the Hawaiian chain. Amazingly, Werner and Smith studied 505 of these children from their prenatal days until they were in their early thirties. Differences in the number of children studied was due to some of the children dying, some moving to other islands, and some moving to the U.S. mainland.*

*Of these 505 children, one in three was born with the threat of serious developmental difficulties, such as the effects of a difficult birth or an environment that triggered formidable challenges. Poverty, parental divorce, desertion, alcoholism, or mental illness were only some of the problems they faced. Two out of three children in this vulnerable group were exposed to four or more of these risk factors. And yet, one in three of these high-risk children developed into a confident, competent young adult.*

*How can we explain this phenomenon? What developmental forces were at work that enabled certain children to overcome dramatically difficult obstacles, and yet permitted others to succumb? In a sense, the children of Kauai provide us with a window through which we can view the events that shape the lifespan, the biological, psychological, and environmental interactions that make us what we are.*

We hope that this emphasis on the heredity–environment interaction will help you to evaluate your clients in a manner that recognizes the multilayered and complex causes of their behavior. As a result, your work with them should be even more insightful and helpful. Let's turn now to several key ideas about the meaning of development itself.

# What Is Development?

*Development is about change* and is the key to understanding the relationship between you and your clients. But development, as interpreted by today's psychiatrists and psychologists, is seen as a much different process than the developmental pathways traced by Freud, Piaget, or Kohlberg. Before discussing these changes, however, here are several ideas that convey the depth and richness of recent developmental research.

- *Development can't be explained by age alone.* Age may give a rough estimate of when behavior appears, but it tells us nothing about *why* a particular behavior appears at a specific time (Rutter 2002). Although no one denies the importance of age in development, age alone isn't the answer because by itself age cannot explain changes in psychological functioning. The answers still remain hidden in the interactions among the various developmental forces acting on a person. We discuss this insightful new approach to analyzing development in the coming sections.

- *The timing of experiences exerts an important influence on development.* Infants who experience the separation of parents don't suffer negative effects as severely as children of early childhood. They haven't developed the emotional attachments of older children, nor do they possess the cognitive capacity to assign blame, often to themselves, as older children do. An unwanted teen-age pregnancy is likely to produce a different parenting style than a planned, wanted pregnancy in early adulthood. Most adolescents who carry their babies to term are not married (Moore & Brooks-Gunn 2002) and depend on family and peer support systems. (For an excellent discussion of the role of timing in development, see Rutter & Rutter 1993.)

- *Development includes behaviors that change in form but result from the same process.* Attention in infancy, for example, appears different from problem-solving ability in later years, but there's a significant link between the two.

- *Reciprocal interactions are at the heart of development.* We realize today that human beings are not born as passive sponges; they immediately seek stimulation from their environment and *instantly interpret, and react to, how they are being treated,* a process called *reciprocal interactions.* Think of it this way: You react to me in a particular manner and I change. As a result of the changes that occur in me, you change. Back and forth, on and on it goes, constantly changing the relationships you have with your clients.

  For example, as we develop cognitively, we attempt to make sense of our world; we "tune into" the social and emotional atmosphere around us and immediately begin to shape our relationships with others. Thinking about and analyzing the interactions you have with your clients helps you to realize how they change as a result of your behavior and how you change as a re-

sult of their reactions. In other words, both partners in the relationship exercise some control over the interactions. These *reciprocal interactions* demonstrate continuity over your time with a client and are a powerful force in developing positive relationships.

Do you respond to all of your clients in the same manner? Of course not. You react to something in their appearance, behavior, attitude, and so on, which structures your approach to their problem. "How can I best get this person to respond to what's needed?" Your answer to this question depends on circumstances such as age, anxiety, and intelligence. Thus, these initial interactions establish the nature of the relationship, giving it a particular tone or style.

- *Development demands careful examination of cause-and-effect relationships.* For example, a Swedish study (Stattin & Magnusson 1990) reported that girls who reached puberty at an early age (under 11 years of age) showed a significantly higher rate of misconduct (drinking, taking drugs, etc.) at age 14 than later-maturing girls or those who followed a more typical pattern. Early puberty (a physical cause) seemed to be the reason for the misbehavior. But more detailed analysis showed that the early-maturing girls became friends with chronologically older girls, a social cause.

  Here again we note how the interactions among various aspects of development—biological, psychological, social *(biopsychosocial)*—combine to produce a specific behavior (Lerner 2002). As a result of recent findings, today's developmental psychologists have turned to an analysis of biopsychosocial interactions in their efforts to understand development.

With these ideas in mind, it became clear that we should approach our subject using a cohesive model of development. Consequently, our rationale proceeds as follows.

## The Importance of Biopsychosocial Interactions

Viewing development as the product of the interaction of biological, psychological, and social forces helps you to better understand and appreciate the complexity of development. For example, emerging *genetic* evidence clearly illustrates the significance of *nongenetic* influences. Even with those traits most powerfully influenced by genetic forces, environmental effects are far from trivial (Rutter 2002, p. 3).

As you think about the interactions that occur among the three categories—biological, psychological, social—keep in mind how these interactions affect development. To give a simple example, genetic damage (biological) may negatively affect cognitive development (psychological) and lead to poor relationships (social). Figure 1.1 illustrates these processes.

Note in Figure 1.1 the "top-down, bottom-up" nature of the constant interactions that occur within a child (Gottlieb 1997). It's no longer correct to state that once the genes initiate developmental activity, their job is done. The environment can influence genetic impact, which in turn affects behavior and the environment. (Developmental psychologists refer to this type of action as *bidirectional interactions.*)

For example, consider language development. With regard to genetic activity, it's safe to say that genes propel children into a language world, their brains assume direction of the process, but—and this is a major warning—it's children's experiences that shape the final outcome. Children exposed to a more stimulating environment will develop a richer network of brain connections than children whose experiences are more limited. As human beings, infants are programmed to receive verbal stimulation, which then enhances their language ability (Dacey & Travers 2005). The bidirectional nature of these interactions remains throughout their lives.

Finally, if you examine Figure 1.1 carefully, you can better understand how it is no longer possible to talk about cognitive development or language development or personality development as separate issues. Long lists of developmental characteristics tell us nothing about how or why these behaviors have appeared or become integrated. We believe that by recognizing the significance of biopsychosocial interactions, you will better understand the complexity of development and use it as a guide in helping your clients.

*Figure 1.1*    The Interactive Nature of Developmental Influences

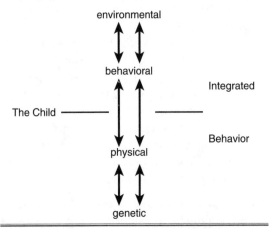

# Developmental Theory: Current Status, Future Direction

As you can well imagine, today's developmental theorists argue that traditional developmental theories cannot cope with exploding and pertinent knowledge from varied sources (biological, social, cultural, psychological). The world of developmental theory is changing as you read these words, and we want you to be aware of the latest thinking of today's theorists.

Current criticism of such traditional theorists as Piaget and Freud is that they are simply too unidimensional to explain the complexity of development. That is, they focus on only one aspect of development. For example, Piaget was consumed by the lure of cognitive development, and Freud spent his lifetime delving into the secrets of personality development. But as Lerner noted (1998), in current developmental theories, the person is not simply "biologized, psychologized, or sociologized."

## Theories of Development

In spite of the previous comments, these theorists continue to offer guidance along particular developmental paths. For example, the importance Freud placed on the initial years of development earned him a lasting place in developmental psychology. Erikson's sensitive understanding of psychosocial crises provides cogent clues to the identity problems many adolescents face. Piaget remains a trusted guide for unlocking many of the enigmas of cognitive development.

With gratitude, then, we use their insights when they seem appropriate in interpreting the various themes of development. Consequently, let's briefly review the basic ideas of some of the major theorists of past years by focusing on those features that will most help you in analyzing development and the implications for understanding your clients.

### PSYCHOANALYTIC THEORY

Strictly speaking, Sigmund Freud (1856–1939) was not a developmental psychologist, but his ideas and his insistence that the early years were decisive in development demand recognition in any analysis of developmental theory. Also, his views on the unconscious have come under close scrutiny as current neuroscientific research reveals secrets of our memories. Freud may have been right for the wrong reasons. For example, recent memory studies point to an obscure and difficult-to-analyze type of memory called *implicit memory* that involves the cerebellum, the amygdala, and the motor cortex.

Implicit memory acts to improve task performance by using previous experiences that are not consciously recollected (Sternberg 2003). Think about learning to ride a bike and retaining that memory. We really *don't* think about it. When we require the information needed to perform this kind of task (riding a bike), we are not aware of consciously searching for specific steps that will help us to remember. We may have taken a long time to acquire the skill, but, once mastered, it doesn't demand any effort to be retrieved. (This sort of memory is called *implicit, nondeclarative, memory without record,* or *knowing how.*) We don't recall where, when, and how we learned it.

Implicit memory may also have a powerful emotional accompaniment, which explains the involvement of the amygdala. We know today that the storage of memories can be colored by the emotions and circumstances surrounding the original experience. A good example of this emotional involvement is the anxiety or panic attack. Individuals who have had vivid and disturbing events in their lives (war, accident) may have frightening flashbacks called *posttraumatic stress disorders.* For no plausible reason, they suddenly have feelings that range from intense physical reactions (pounding heart, soaked in sweat) to a sense of impending death. In these cases the amygdala is involved, explaining the emotional feelings that accompany the flashback.

What does this have to do with Freud? As Larry Squire and the Nobel prize winner Eric Kandel (2000) note, it provides biological evidence that unconscious mental processes actually exist. Although implicit memory exists, a neuroscientific explanation is far different from Freud's interpretation. As these authors state, implicit memory may be unconscious, but not for the reasons Freud stated: conflict or sexual urges. Yet, because of the importance he placed on the early years of development and his insights into human behavior, knowledge of psychoanalytic theory can only add to the depth of your understanding of your clients.

**Personality Structure.** Freud divided personality into three components: the *id,* the *ego,* and the *superego,* which appear at different stages of a child's development. Each of these components has distinct characteristics. The id contains all of our basic instincts, such as the need for food, drink, sex, and so on. It exists simply to secure pleasure and as such often clashes with society's norms and rules, thus leading to conflict. ("I don't care what happens; I'm going to get what I want now.") As it does, the ego emerges from this battle and attempts to reconcile the id's drives with society's expectations. The ego is the central part of our personality, the (usually) rational part that does all the planning and keeps in touch with reality. ("Of course I have to finish this paper now; the party will have to wait.")

Freud believed that the stronger the ego becomes, the more realistic, and usually the more successful, a person is likely to be (Lerner 2002). The superego, the moral component of personality, is the arbiter of right and wrong—our conscience. ("I feel so badly about this.") Now begins the ceaseless battle between the desires of the id and the demands of the superego, with the ego struggling mightily for compromises between these two powerful forces.

**Stages of Development.** For Freud, personality development means moving through five stages at specific ages. Each stage is distinct from the others and has a major function, which is based on a pleasure center. Unless this pleasure center is stimulated appropriately (not too much, not too little), the person becomes fixated (stuck at that stage) and is unable to become a fully mature person (Kahn 2002). Here are the five stages.

- *The oral stage* is Freud's initial stage. The mouth is the main source of pleasure from birth to 1½ years old.

- *The anal stage,* Freud's second stage, extends from 1½ to 3 years old. The anus is the pleasure center, and the major function of this stage is successful toilet training.

- *The phallic stage,* from 3 to 5 years of age, is Freud's third stage of development. The glands of the penis and the clitoris are the pleasure centers in this stage and in the two remaining stages. The major function of this stage is the healthy development of sexual interest, which is achieved through masturbation and unconscious sexual desire for the parent of the opposite sex. Resolution of the conflicts caused by this desire (called the Oedipal conflict in males and the Electra conflict in females) is the goal.

- *The latency stage,* from 5 to 12 years old, is the fourth stage. During this stage, sexual desire is repressed, which is especially true for males. Boys may refuse to kiss or hug their mothers and treat female age-mates with disdain. Because our society is more tolerant of the daughter's attraction to her father, the Electra complex is less resolved and girls' sexual feelings may be less repressed during this stage.

- Finally, *the genital stage,* 12 years old and older, sees the surge of sexual hormones for both genders, which brings about an unconscious recurrence of the phallic stage. Normally, however, youths have learned that desire for one's parents is taboo, and so they set about establishing relationships with members of the opposite sex who are their own age. If fixation occurs at any stage, anxiety results, and defense mechanisms will be used to deal with it.

Freud's influence has waned as the influence of culture has become more central to today's analyses of development. Currently, we recognize the difference between modern society and the sexual restrictions of a 19th century Victorian society and the variations such differences produce in development. Also, the lack of empirical evidence and the scarcity of application of Freudian thought to development raise serious doubts as to its general applicability to children.

## PSYCHOSOCIAL THEORY

Erik Erikson (1902–1994), born in Frankfurt, Germany early in his life came under the influence of Freud and his daughter Anna. Although his theoretical orientation was strongly psychoanalytic, he became sharply critical of Freud's emphasis on biologically based psychosexual stages. Consequently, Erikson (1950) became a leading proponent of a psychosocial theory of development. He believed that children interact with an ever-widening circle of individuals, beginning with their mothers and ending with humanity (Thies & Travers 2001).

Another distinctive aspect of Erikson's theory was his belief that as individuals pass through each of the following eight stages of development, they experience a crisis that challenges their emotional equilibrium. How these crises are resolved determines continuing healthy psychological development.

**Erikson's Eight Psychosocial Stages.** Erikson's psychosocial stages can be quite helpful to health care professionals and their relationships with their clients. Here is a brief description of Erikson's stages.

1. *Basic trust versus mistrust (birth to 1½ years old).* In the first stage, infants derive security and comfort from warm relations with their parents, which leads to a strengthening of the attachment process. The crisis to be resolved at this stage is between basic trust and mistrust, which, in Eriksonian theory actively engages infants with their environment. Although infants never develop complete trust or mistrust, those who develop more trust than mistrust are on the road to healthy psychosocial development.

2. *Autonomy versus shame and doubt (1½ to 3 years old).* At about 1½ years old, children face the crisis of autonomy versus shame and doubt. They begin to gain control over their bodies, and toilet training usually begins during these years. Erikson agreed with other psychoanalysts about the importance of toilet training and believed that the sources of generosity and creativity lie in this experience. Toilet training, however, is only one manifestation of a child's continual struggle to acquire self-control. Their rapidly developing physical skills and gradually emerging cognitive ability should be the source of their learning to act in a controlled manner. Failure to do so produces feelings of shame and doubt.

3. *Initiative versus guilt* (the preschool years). The third crisis, initiative versus guilt, begins when children are about 3 years old. Building on the ability to control themselves, children now demonstrate responsibility and a sense of purpose as they begin to acquire the ability to master such tasks as learning to read. As Erikson noted (Erikson 1950, p. 235):

   *There is in every child at every stage a new miracle of vigorous unfolding, which constitutes a new hope and a new responsibility for all. Such is the sense and the pervading quality of initiative.*

   In other words, children need to move away from constant parental guidance and, using their newly acquired skills, interact with their world in a responsible controlled manner.

4. *Industry versus inferiority* (the elementary school years). Children of these years are immersed in the task of acquiring the needed information and skills of their culture. They expand their horizons beyond the family and begin to explore the neighborhood and develop new relationships. As

children go off to school to expand on the skills they acquired at home, they commence the journey toward becoming adult members of their society. Mastering these skills lead to feelings of industry and a sense of confidence that they will become competent and functioning members of their society.

5. *Identity versus identity confusion* (adolescence). As children begin the adolescent years, the main task is to achieve a state of identity. Uncertainty produces identity confusion, and a bewildered youth may withdraw, run away, or turn to drugs. The challenges are new; the tasks are difficult; the alternatives are often bewildering. Needless to say, adolescents require considerable patience and understanding, especially during the initial years of the period.

   It's a time of increased sexual sensitivity, but Erikson looked beyond the sheer physical drive and included the psychosocial implications of these changes. As Lerner (2002) notes, if a child's development has proceeded successfully to this stage, he or she will have developed more trust than mistrust, more autonomy than shame or doubt, more initiative than guilt, and more industry than inferiority.

   Lerner (2002, p. 422) goes on to suggest that the question *Who am I?* is essentially a search for self-definition produced by the emergence of new feelings and capabilities coupled with the demands that any society places on its adolescents. In other words, personal changes (physical, cognitive, psychosocial) collide with changing societal demands placed on its "almost-adult" youth. From this collision comes a sense of identity if adolescents can balance these conflicting forces.

6. *Intimacy versus isolation.* The years of young adulthood bring a new set of challenges.

Referring to this stage, Erikson moves far beyond the concept of sexual intimacy. If adolescents successfully acquire a positive sense of identity, they possess the ability to form meaningful relationships with others in the truest sense of reciprocal interactions. In forming these relationships, however, Erikson issues a far-reaching warning: You can't find your own identity. As he often stated, less than two identities will never equal two identities. What materializes from such a relationship is not identity, but, sadly, isolation.

7. *Generativity versus stagnation.* At this stage, society expects its members to be competent, productive individuals, leading to a personal sense of self-fulfillment. Erikson (1950, p. 231) summarized the compelling goal of this stage by stating that generativity is primarily the interest in establishing and guiding the next generation. Those who achieve this sense of generativity are dedicated to making the world a better and safer place for young people in general and their own children in particular. If individuals fail in this pursuit, they begin to stagnate, to become bored and self-indulgent, and to experience feelings of interpersonal impoverishment.

8. *Integrity versus despair.* To the extent that individuals have been successful in resolving the first seven crises, they achieve a sense of personal integrity. Adults who have a sense of integrity accept their lives as having been well spent. They feel a kinship with people of other cultures and of previous and future generations. They have a sense of having helped to create a more dignified life for humankind. They have gained wisdom. Consequently, Erikson believes that these individuals are childlike in their enthusiasm and joy as they face the final years of their lives.

If, however, people look back over their lives and feel they have made the wrong decisions, or more commonly, that they have too frequently failed to make any decision at all, they see life as lacking integration. They feel despair at the impossibility of "having just one more chance to make things right." They often hide their terror of death by appearing contemptuous of humanity in general and of those of their own religion or race in particular. They feel disgust for themselves.

Understanding Erikson's ideas should provide you with deeper insights into the attitudes your clients bring to their relationships with you. Leaving the world of personality development and examining explanations of cognitive development takes us to the ideas of Jean Piaget.

## PIAGET'S THEORY OF COGNITIVE DEVELOPMENT

Jean Piaget, born in Neuchatel, Switzerland in 1896, began his scholarly career at the age of 10(!) and published numerous papers on birds, shellfish, and other topics of natural history. Based on these publications, he was offered the curator's position at the prestigious Geneva Natural History Museum. Realizing that the museum officials didn't know his age, Piaget rejected the offer and went on to finish secondary school, complete his Ph.D. in biology, and write more than 50 influential books during his lifetime (Dacey & Travers 2005).

**Critical Influences on Piaget.** Of all the intellectual threads that weave throughout Piaget's work, three stand out for their impact on his thinking: 1) Development proceeds by a series of stages; 2) biology is linked to philosophy by developmental psychology; and 3) changing cognitive structures are the mechanisms that drive cognitive development. Let's briefly examine each of these.

1. Stage theorists believe that all individuals pass through a series of qualitatively distinct stages in a predetermined sequence. (For Piaget, these are the sensorimotor, preoperational, concrete operational, and formal operational stages.) Each of these stages represents a unique network of cognitive structures. There is probably no better way to envision the meaning of these structures than by asking a famous question originally proposed by John Flavell (1971): If you were to take a psychological x-ray of each stage, what would you see? If this were possible, all of the cognitive elements that constitute a stage and their relationships to each other would be revealed. In a sense, this was what Piaget attempted to do. By a judicious combination of biological and philosophical principles applied to changing cognitive accomplishments, Piaget searched for clues that would lead to a greater understanding of cognitive development.

2. Piaget the philosopher was engaged in a lifelong pursuit of knowledge. To penetrate the secrets of how knowledge is acquired, Piaget turned to an analysis of development using the tools and content of developmental psychology. The techniques to be used in unraveling the mysteries of cognition and knowledge can be traced to his biological heritage. To understand knowledge, we must turn to development; to analyze development, we must turn to biology.

3. To justify the existence of cognitive structures, Piaget once again turned to biology. Beginning with his belief that intelligence is a special form of adaptation, he argued that as the physical structures of the body enable us to adapt to our environment, so also the cognitive structures of the mind enable us to adapt. The manner by which we adapt using our physical structures (reading this page, taking notes, etc. all involve your use of physical structures) is quite logical and thus subject to analysis. The same is true of our cognitive structures, and thus they can be analyzed.

**Key Concepts in Piaget's Theory.** Piaget believed that children develop increasingly effective *cognitive structures* that enable them to organize and adapt to their world. Cognitive development occurs as children form more sophisticated mental structures as they pass through four stages: the *sensorimotor stage* (birth to 2 years old); the *preoperational stage* (2 to 7 years old); the *concrete operational stage* (7 to 11 years old); and the *formal operational stage* (11 years old and up). Piaget's stages of cognitive development are illustrated in Table 1.1.

How does Piaget's theory actually "work"? He believed that stimuli come from the environment and are filtered through adaptation and organization. Adaptation and organization use the stimuli to form new structures or change existing structures. For example, you may have had your own idea of what intelligence is, but now you change your structures relating to intelligence because of your new knowledge about Piaget. Your behavior changes because of the changes in your cognitive structures. The process is as follows.

**Environment**
(filtered through)
**Adaptation and Organization**
(produces)
**Cognitive Structures**

Developmental psychologists have grown increasingly skeptical about some of Piaget's ideas, such as the nature of stages and children's ability to reach levels of cognitive competence earlier than he realized. Nevertheless, his monumental contributions forever changed the way in which we look at children.

Here are several ideas based on Piaget's work that you'll find helpful in working with your clients.

- Preschool children are still cognitively egocentric, which may well affect how they react to the problems they face. For example, still highly egocentric, they may blame themselves for becoming ill, which may influence how they respond to treatment.

- When children reach the stage of concrete operations, it is tempting to assume that they fully comprehend your explanations and instructions. Although they may understand the more obvious aspects of what's happening to them, other, more abstract issues may elude them. They have the ability to internally manipulate objects they can see and touch but remain uncertain about knowledge based on verbal information alone.

- Although you may believe that people should be functioning at the formal operational level, their thought processes may lack the network of cognitive structures characteristic of this period. There are many reasons for this: a dearth of vital environ-

*Table 1.1*    Piaget's Stages of Cognitive Development

| Stage | Age | Major Features |
|---|---|---|
| Sensorimotor | Birth to 2 years | Infants use their bodies to form cognitive structures (they grasp their blanket and learn that it's soft) |
| Preoperational | 2 to 7 years | Tremendous language growth and manipulation of symbols |
| Concrete operational | 7 to 11 years | Begins to think abstractly |
| Formal operational | 11+ years | Abstract thinking leads to reasoning with symbols and solving problems |

mental stimulation, few mentors to guide them by the process of social transmission, delayed maturation, and many others.

We return to the developmental aspects of Piaget's theory in Chapter 9.

## THE INFLUENCE OF CULTURE

As practicing and successful health care professionals, you are undoubtedly aware how cultural and language differences affect the relationships between you and your clients. Adopting a cultural perspective will help you to realize that different people have different worldviews that decisively influence their thinking and behavior (Stigler et al. 1990). Members of any one group (Irish American, Italian American, African American) often use standards from their own culture to judge people from other cultures, a simplistic, even dangerous, way of thinking

**The Cultural Framework.** As Jerome Bruner, a long-time icon in American psychology, has stated (Bruner 1996, p. 4):

*Culture, then, though itself man-made, both forms and makes possible the workings of a distinctively human mind. On this view, learning and thinking are always situated in a cultural setting and always dependent upon the utilization of cultural resources. Even individual variation in the nature and use of mind can be attributed to the varied opportunities that different cultural settings provide, though these are not the only source of variation in mental functioning.*

As an example of culture's importance, consider the following experience. When several American psychologists went to Rwanda to help with the massive psychological problems caused by the savagery and violence the people had experienced (Seppa 1996), they found that traditional Western therapeutic methods, such as individualized therapy, were useless. Cultural values do change, but slowly (Harrison 2000). Successful programs in Africa are those that help restore social supports and relationships. They also discovered that urging patients to "talk it out" simply did not work. Using song, dance, and storytelling, which their patients found natural and comforting, proved to be more successful.

**Lev Vygotsky.** The Russian psychologist Lev Vygotsky (1896–1934) made a remarkable contribution to our thinking about the influence of culture on development. His belief that social and cultural processes are major forces shaping the path of development has been one of the main influences responsible for keeping the heredity–environment interaction in balance. For Vygotsky, the clues to understanding mental development are in children's social processes; that is, cognitive growth depends on children's interactions with those around them. The adults around children interact with them in a way that emphasizes those things that a culture values.

Tragically, tuberculosis claimed Vygotsky in 1934. His work today, because of its cultural emphasis, is more popular than it was when he died. In contrast to Piaget, who believed that children function as "little scientists," Vygotsky turned to social interactions to explain children's cognitive development. One of Vygotsky's most famous ideas, the notion of the *zone of proximal development,* is an excellent example of his creative thinking about development.

**The Zone of Proximal Development.** Vygotsky (1978) argued forcefully that learning must be matched with a pupil's developmental level, which is too frequently identified by an intelligence test score. He stated that we cannot be content with the results of intelligence testing, which only identifies a student's developmental level at the time of testing.

For example, after administering a Stanford-Binet Intelligence Test, we find that a child's IQ on this test is 110, which would be that student's current level of mental development. We then assume that the child can only work at this level. Vygotsky argued, however, that with a little help, children might be able to do work that they could not do on their own.

We know that people who have the same IQ are quite different in other respects. Motivation, interest, health, and a host of other conditions produce different achievement levels. For example, a person with an IQ of 110 when working alone may be able to do only addition problems, but may be able to solve subtraction problems with some help.

To explain this phenomenon, Vygotsky introduced his notion of the *zone of proximal development.* He defined the zone of proximal development as the distance between a person's actual developmental level, as determined by independent problem solving, and the higher level of potential development as determined by problem solving under adult guidance or in collaboration with more capable peers. In other words, it's the difference between what children can achieve with guidance and what they can achieve through individual effort.

Remember, *the zone of proximal development is not something within a person.* It's a characteristic of activity within a specific social environment (Steward 1995). Vygotsky's ideas on what constitutes the kind of assistance to be given were general—demonstration, leading questions, introducing the beginning elements of the solution, and so on (Vygotsky 1978).

**Cultures and Scaffolding.**   Piaget or Vygotsky? Vygotsky or Piaget? From your reading, you have learned that Piaget and Vygotsky disagreed on the emphasis they placed on the basic processes of cognitive development. Piaget believed that children act as scientific investigators, acquiring knowledge as they build more and richer cognitive structures. Although it's unfair to state that Piaget ignored social and cultural influences on development, he did, however, focus on the independent, self-reliant path that children take in constructing their world.

Vygotsky turned to a child's culture and stressed social interactions as the driving force in cognitive development. If social exchanges with adults are lacking or inadequate, children's opportunities to reach, or even approach, their cognitive potential are sharply limited. Scaffolding—offering appropriate support to children as they attempt to learn—is an example of specific social interactions.

Analyzing Vygotsky's interpretation of the zone of proximal development and the notion of scaffolding, Greenfield (1999) raised an interesting possibility. She argued that those societies encouraging scaffolding are stable and in a tradition-maintaining state. Dynamic and more innovative societies, however, encourage independent, trial-and-error experimental behavior in their citizens.

It's an intriguing idea. Think about a country with which you are familiar (other countries as well as the United States). Do you agree with Greenfield's conclusion? Can a society shift from one mode to another? If you would like to have a more informed view on this issue, you may want to read one or more of the articles referenced in this chapter (e.g., Greenfield 1999).

Finally, Table 1.2 identifies the most significant differences between Vygotsky and Piaget.

## DEVELOPMENTAL CONTEXTUALISM

We know today that heredity and environment produce their results in a complex, interactive manner that reflects the role of reciprocal interactions. By stressing the complexity of developmental analysis, those adhering to a reciprocal interaction perspective have made it clear that there are no simple cause-and-effect explanations of development. All of us—children, adolescents, and adults—experience a constant state of reorganization as we move through the life cycle (Lerner et al. 2000).

**Developmental contextualism,** popularized by Richard Lerner (1991, 1998, 2002), is the current version of a perspective that begins with the idea that all of our characteristics, psychological as well as biological, function by reciprocal interactions with the environment (often referred to as

*Table 1.2*    Key Differences Between Piaget and Vygotsky

|  | **Piaget** | **Vygotsky** |
| --- | --- | --- |
| Perspective | Individual child constructs view of world by forming cognitive structures ("the little scientist") | Child's cognitive development progresses by social interactions with others ("social origins of mind") |
| Basic psychological mechanism | Equilibration—child acts to regain equilibrium between current level of cognitive structures and external stimuli | Social interaction, which encourages development through the guidance of skillful adults |
| Language | Emerges as cognitive structures develop | Language begins as preintellectual speech and gradually develops into a sophisticated form of inner speech; one of the main forces responsible for cognitive development |
| Learning | Assimilation and accommodation lead to equilibration | Learning results from the interaction of two processes: biological elementary processes (such as brain development), plus sociocultural interactions |
| Problem solving | Child independently searches for data needed to change cognitive structures, thus enabling child to reach solution | Two aspects of problem solving: 1) key role of speech to guide "planful" behavior; 2) joint efforts with others |

the *context*). In this way, developmental contextualism leads to the belief that we *construct* our view of the surrounding world.

Lerner (2002, p. 222) has emphasized that developmental contextualism requires three levels of analysis.

1. Knowledge of the characteristics of those being studied;

2. an understanding of a person's context and a justification for why this portion of the context is significant for the analysis; and

3. a conceptualization of the relationship between the individual characteristics and the contextual feature.

Exchanges between individuals and the multiple levels of their contexts are the basic change processes in development (Lerner 1998). Consequently, the crucial element in our development is the changing relationship between our complexity and a multilayered context. If you think about this deceptively simple statement,

you can appreciate the need to study development, not from any single perspective like biology or environment, but from a more sophisticated analytical appraisal. *No single level of organization is seen as the primary or the ultimate causal influence on behavior and development* (Dixon & Lerner 1999).

For example, consider what happens when you interact with your environment. Your genes provide a blueprint that is passed on to the cells, tissues, and organs of your body, influencing the growth of such widely divergent features as your brain development and temperament (to name only two). On the other hand, the intricate and involved layers of the context, ranging from your family to your peers to your wider social sphere, simultaneously weave their networks of influence. Simple explanations? Hardly. What is needed is a developmental perspective equally as intricate as the behavior it attempts to clarify.

## EVOLUTIONARY DEVELOPMENTAL PSYCHOLOGY

Although we have used developmental contextualism as an example of the changes taking place in the search for developmental explanations, other ideas continue to emerge. For example, Bjorklund and Pellegrini (2002, p. 4) argue that the basic principle of *evolutionary psychology* is that the human mind has been prepared by natural selection for life in a human group. Within the evolutionary framework, *evolutionary developmental psychology* is seen as an explanation of development that assumes our physiological and psychological systems resulted from evolution by selection.

In 1859 Charles Darwin published his *On the Origin of Species* in which he concluded that natural selection was the basic principle of change. Ongoing selection processes depend on gene action and provide the basis for evolutionary events to occur (Plotkin 1997). It's the study of how our genes are expressed during development and how the context of development influences the expression of genetic action (Geary & Bjorklund 2000, Gottlieb 2000).

Evolutionary ideas had little impact on psychological thought until approximately 1959, which was the centennial year of the publication of *On the Origin of Species*. Conferences and publications devoted to Darwin's work sparked renewed interest in his ideas and encouraged theorists and researchers to search for obscure biological causes of behavior.

At about the same time, this impetus received support from an unrelated and unexpected source: the cognitive revolution. Widely and wildly popular with psychologists, studies of cognition provided respectability to explanations of behavior that were not immediately visible (Plotkin 1997, Geary & Bjorklund 2000). In tracing the roots of evolutionary psychology, Pinker (1997) stated that evolutionary psychology brings together two scientific revolutions. One is the cognitive revolution that began in the 1950s and 1960s, which helped us to understand why we have the kind of mind that we currently possess.

The second scientific revolution identified by Pinker is the change in evolutionary biology that explained the ability of living things to adapt by selection. Thus the physiological and psychological mechanisms needed for healthy development are those that survive the process of natural selection. Conversely, developmental psychologists have expressed reservations lest the notion that "biology is destiny" becomes too easily accepted, thus diminishing the environmental input into development (Geary & Bjorklund 2000, Gottlieb 2000).

In their excellent overview of *evolutionary developmental psychology*, Bjorklund and Pellegrini (2002, p. 4) make a sharp distinction between evolutionary psychology and evolutionary developmental psychology. They define evolutionary developmental psychology as the application of the basic principles of Darwinian evolution, particularly natural selection, to explain contemporary human development. Thus evolutionary developmental psychology becomes a search for genetic and environmental mechanisms. The interactions between them become the driving forces for the appearance of social and cognitive competencies.

Yet the differences between evolutionary psychology and evolutionary developmental psychology are not simply a matter of application procedures. Including a developmental perspective implies that different types of questions emerge from the basic evolutionary framework: how to determine gene–environment interactions under specific conditions; how domain-general mechanisms such as the different aspects of memory (immediate, working, etc.) help to explain behavior; what the role and significance of individual differences is; what the role of evolutionary principles to explain cognitive processes is.

Other distinguishing features of evolutionary developmental psychology include the following.

- Evolutionary developmental psychology adopts a developmental systems model to explain how evolved genetic programs interact with specific environments.

- Domain-general mechanisms such as working memory help to explain human adaptation in any environment.

- Evolutionary developmental psychology recognizes the function of individual differences in explaining how individuals adapt to the specific demands of their environments.

These new ideas emerging from evolutionary thinking are slowly making an impact on developmental psychology and, as they do, will affect practice in many allied fields.

As we conclude this introductory chapter you may well ask "Why this book?" Perhaps paraphrasing a statement from an earlier work of the authors (Thies & Travers 2001) best answers this question.

*A major task for all health care professionals is to understand human development—the characteristics, problems, and needs of various ages—so that they can utilize their knowledge and expertise as fully as possible in bringing comfort to their clients.*

# References

Bjorklund, D., and A. Pellegrini (2002). *The origins of human nature.* Washington, DC: American Psychological Association.

Bruner, J. (1996). *The culture of education.* Cambridge, MA: Harvard University Press.

Dacey, J., and J. Travers (2005). *Human development across the lifespan,* 6th ed. New York: McGraw-Hill.

Dixon, R., and R. Lerner (1999). A history of systems in developmental psychology. In: M. Bornstein and M. Lamb, eds. *Developmental psychology: an advanced textbook.* Mahwah, NJ: Erlbaum.

Elder, G. (1998). Theories of human development: contemporary perspectives. In: R. M. Lerner, ed. *Handbook of child psychology: Volume 1. Theoretical models of human development.* New York: John Wiley.

Erikson, E. (1950). *Childhood and society,* 2nd ed. New York: Norton.

Erikson, E. (1958). *Young man Luther: a study in psychoanalysis and history.* New York: Norton.

Erikson, E. (1968). *Identity: youth and crisis.* New York: Norton.

Erikson, E. (1975). *Life, history, and the historical movement.* New York: Norton.

Ferris, P. (1997). *Dr. Freud: a life.* Washington, DC: Counterpoint.

Flavell, J. (1971). Stage related properties of cognitive development. *Cognitive Psychology* 2:421–453.

Freud, S. (1966). *The complete introductory lectures on psychoanalysis.* Translated and edited by James Strachey. New York: Norton.

Geary, D., and D. Bjorklund (2000). Evolutionary developmental psychology. *Child Development* 71:57–65.

Gottlieb, G. (1997). *Synthesizing nature–nurture.* Mahwah, NJ: Erlbaum.

Gottlieb, G. (2000). Environmental and behavioral influences on gene activity. *Current Directions in Psychological Science* 9:93–102.

Greenfield, J. (1999). Cultural change and human development. In: E. Turiel, ed. *Development and cultural change: reciprocal processes.* San Francisco, CA: Jossey-Bass.

Harrison, L. (2000). Why culture matters. In: L. Harrison and S. Huntington, eds. *Culture Matters.* New York: Basic Books.

Kahn, M. (2002). *Basic Freud.* New York: Basic Books.

Lerner, R. (1991). Changing organism–context relations as the basic process of development: a developmental contextual perspective. *Developmental Psychology* 27:27–32.

Lerner, R. (1998). Theories of human development: contemporary perspectives. In: R. M. Lerner, ed. *Handbook of child psychology: Volume 1. Theoretical models of human development.* New York: John Wiley.

Lerner, R., C. Fisher, and R. Weinberg (2000). Toward a science for and of the people: promoting civil society through the application of developmental science. *Child Development* 71:11–20.

Lerner, R. (2002). *Concepts and theories of human development.* Mahwah, NJ: Ertlbaum.

Moore, M., and J. Brooks-Gunn (2002). Adolescent parenthood. In: M. Bornstein, ed. *Handbook of parenting,* 2nd ed. Mahwah, NJ: Lawrence Erlbaum.

Piaget, J. (1952). *The origins of intelligence in children.* New York: International Universities Press.

Piaget, J. (1966). *Psychology of intelligence.* Totowa, NJ: Littlefield, Adams, & Co.

Pinker, S. (1997). *How the mind works.* New York: W. W. Norton.

Pinker, S. (2002). *The blank slate.* New York: Viking.

Plotkin, H. (1997). *Evolution in mind: an introduction to evolutionary psychology.* Cambridge, MA: Harvard University Press.

Rogoff, B. (1990). Apprenticeship in thinking: cognitive development in social context. New York: Oxford University Press.

Rutter, Michael. (2002). Nature, nurture and development: from Evangelism through science toward policy and practice. *Child Development* 73:1–21.

Rutter, M., and M. Rutter. (1993). *Developing minds: challenge and continuity across the life span.* New York: Basic Books.

Seppa, N. (1996). Rwanda starts its long healing process. *The APA Monitor* August, p. 14.

Squire, L., and E. Kandel (2000). *Memory: from mind to molecule.* New York: Scientific American Press.

Stattin, H., and D. Magnusson (1990). *Pubertal maturation in female development.* Mahwah, NJ: Erlbaum.

Sternberg, R. (2003). Cognitive psychology. Belmont, CA: Wadsworth.

Stewart, E. (1995). *Beginning writers in the zone of proximal development.* Hillsdale, NJ. Erlbaum.

Stigler, J., R. Shweder, and G. Herdt (1990). *Cultural psychology.* New York: Cambridge University Press.

Thies, K., and J. Travers (2001). *Quick look nursing: human growth and development through the lifespan.* Thorofare, NJ: Slack Incorporated.

U.S. Bureau of the Census. (1996). *Statistical abstract of the United States.* Washington, DC: U.S. Government Printing Office.

Vygotsky, L. S. (1962). *Thought and language.* Cambridge, MA: MIT Press.

Vygotsky, L. S. (1978). *Mind in society.* Cambridge, MA: Harvard University Press.

Wertsch, J., and P. Tulviste (1992). L. S. Vygotsky and contemporary developmental psychology. *Developmental Psychology* 28:548–557.

# Chapter 2

# Gender Development

Deborah Margolis

Questions of gender and sex arise frequently in our society. In both our casual conversation and our scholarly research, there tends to be more focus on gender differences than gender similarities, even though it seems clear that there are likely more gender similarities than differences.

From birth and now often prenatally, the sex of a child is of great interest to parents. When not known to parents before birth, the sex of the child is perhaps the first thing announced to the parents in the delivery room immediately after birth. The gender of a child is also one of the first things we try to determine when, even as strangers, we see a child. In fact, gender is one of the first things that we try to identify about a person, and we find ourselves confused when we cannot make an immediate identification based on expected social norms. Caregivers dress infants in what are considered gender-appropriate colors and clothing in part so they can be properly identified by gender. All of this focus on gender should raise questions for us about the societal and cultural importance placed on gender.

Why, we should wonder, is it so important to us to accurately identify the gender of a stranger, someone we may have never seen before and who we will likely not see again? Furthermore, we should also ask ourselves what cues are used to make gender identifications because these cues are important evidence of the degree of entrenchment of traditional gender norms in our society.

To illustrate this entrenchment, I offer a personal example. My son, from a very young age, had beautiful, thick, black hair and a cherubic face. We thought his hair was so beautiful that did not want to cut it and so he continued to have beautiful, LONG black hair. No matter where we went, and despite the fact that he was always dressed in "boy clothes," people would comment on the beautiful baby girl. On more than one occasion, when we responded that the baby was a boy, the stranger would argue that it was not possible because the baby was too pretty. When we would go one step further and explain that he was a boy with long hair we were regularly told that it was not the hair but rather the "pretty face." However, subsequent to an unseasonable hot day in April when we finally gave in and got his hair cut, he was never again referred to as a girl.

This example raises a number of issues. First and foremost, it raises issues about the judgments made based on appearance and expectations. It also raises personal issues for me as a psychologist with a professional interest in gender issues. I would have liked to think that it would not have been important to me to correct a stranger about gender, and yet I did it over and over again.

# Prominent Schools of Thought

There are many theories that attempt to explain gender development. The following section includes a brief overview of some prominent theories and schools of thought.

## The Psychoanalytic View of Gender

Freud's view of the development of gender is of interest mostly from an historical perspective. Though Freud wrote extensively about his ideas, he did not do empirical work to support his theories. Nevertheless, Freud's ideas influenced much of modern psychology and are therefore worthy of note. Freud believed that "biology is destiny" and that our psychological development is determined in large part by our being female or male. In addition, Freud believed that there is strong identification between a child and a parent of the same gender. It is important to keep in mind that Freud thought of the male as being whole or complete and the female as a lesser being in that females lack a penis. Freud suggested that during the period of development that he labeled the phallic period (between ages 3 and 6), children discover the difference between having a penis and not having one. Freud further suggested that girls during this phallic period develop penis envy and feel resentment over not having a penis (Freud 1923/1960).

For Freud, the Oedipus and Electra complexes also play a role in gender development. The Oedipus complex suggests that young boys develop a desire to have an exclusive relationship with their mothers. Seeing their fathers as intrud-

ing on this relationship but fearing punishment from fathers, boys repress these feelings and the repression helps to strengthen the identification with the father. According to Freud, girls develop a similar though less intense desire for an exclusive relationship with their fathers, which is repressed, thus strengthening the identification of girls with their mothers. Freud used this identification with the same-gender parent to explain gender development.

## Learning Theories and Gender Development

Social-learning theories suggest that through modeling, children learn about gender behavior that is considered socially acceptable through a variety of experiences (Bussey & Bandura 1999). According to social-learning theorists, one of the primary ways that children learn is through observational learning. Observational learning theory suggests that we learn by watching others. In other words, children watch the behavior (and consequences of behavior) of others and thus learn about socially desirable behaviors. In thinking about gender, observational learning becomes a highly potent learning tool.

Children are surrounded by models of gender behavior: peers and adults in their lives as well as media models. According to Maccoby (1998), children spend much more time playing with same-sex peers, and Shell and Eisenberg (1990) found that preschool-aged boys were more likely to approach toys being played with by other boys while staying away from toys being played with by girls. This finding would suggest that children watch others to try to determine what is socially acceptable behavior. Many, though not all, children have highly gendered observational experiences. For example, many children see a female as the person who prepares food in the home and is a nurse in the doctor's office and a preschool and/or elementary school teacher. Conversely, many children see a male as the person who does yard and repair work, watches sports on television, and is an administrator at school.

While observational learning accounts for much learning about gender according to social-learning theory, direct instruction also accounts for some of what we come to know about gender. Boys are often told quite directly that "boys don't cry" and girls are reminded to "act like a lady." Gender-appropriate toys are also a form of both direct and indirect instruction. Some research suggests that parents are more supportive of children's play and more likely to engage in play with children when it is considered gender appropriate (Fagot & Hagan 1991, Lytton & Romney 1991). This too would be a direct means of instructing children about what is considered appropriate and acceptable. Even theorists who believe that children's preferences for toys and types of play may be related to biological differences between females and males suggest that peer and adult behavior further reinforces these preferences.

There certainly seems to be plenty of evidence that social interactions do play a role in the reinforcement of gender roles. Health care providers should be aware of the power of such messages. When working with children it is important not to fall into the trap of reinforcing these gendered messages. For example, when giving children shots it would be important not to suggest that a boy be brave and not cry. Furthermore, it is important to recognize that girls typically get more practice talking about their feelings than boys do. As a result, girls may be better able to talk about their feelings when asked. When working with children we must constantly remind ourselves that both girls and boys have feelings and need to have license, opportunity, and practice expressing these feelings.

## Gender Schema Theory

Gender schema theory suggests that children develop gender schemas that help to construct their understanding of gender (Bem 1981, Martin 1993). Gender schemas are evolving mental representations or internalized understandings of beliefs, stereotypes, experiences, and messages about gender. Gender schemas are not static, and over time and with increased or changed information, gender schemas evolve to fit what the individual currently believes (Ruble & Martin 1998).

The gender schemas of young children begin as a type of classification: "similar to me" versus "not similar to me." Research has demonstrated that children seem to prefer that which they consider to be more like themselves. According to Martin and colleagues (1995), when shown gender-neutral objects (e.g., board games) that were labeled either "for boys" or "for girls," girls reported liking the items labeled "for girls" and boys preferred the items labeled "for boys." In an earlier similar study, Bradbard and colleagues (1986) found that when gender-neutral items were described as "girl" or "boy" things, the children spent more time looking at items labeled for their gender and remembered more about those items a week later. Studies also suggest that children tend to remember more details about stories in which characters behave in gender-typical ways and confuse details from stories in which characters have less traditional gender roles (Liben & Signorella 1993).

Gender schemas may develop as a result of observation of adults or peers, exposure to media, and direct instruction. For example, young children may believe that only girls have long hair, and therefore when seeing someone with long hair they assume the person to be female. Or (despite reality) that only men are doctors and only women are nurses and therefore any man in a health care setting is a doctor and any woman is a nurse. Over time and with exposure to more people in different situations, these schemas can evolve and change.

## Ecological Theories and Gender

Bronfenbrenner's ecological model of development (1979, 1993; Bronfenbrenner & Morris 1998) can also help us understand gender development.

Bronfenbrenner's ecological model comprises the microsystem (home, school), mesosystem (interaction between elements of microsystem), exosystem (society and culture to which individuals are exposed beyond microsystem—like parents jobs), and macrosystem (broader culture). Children begin to learn about gender at home, and this learning is further reinforced in school. Stereotypical messages about the likes and dislikes or strengths and weaknesses of boys and girls are often entrenched in the ways in which we teach and interact with children. Both home and school are often reflections of broader culture replete with gender messages and stereotypes. Children see the roles that adults play. They also see the kinds of jobs and careers that adults have; this too makes a contribution to gender understanding—and gender stereotypes for that matter.

Providing children with the maximum number of opportunities and role models can help all children develop into whole people less constrained by traditional gender stereotypes. Although health care is a profession replete with traditional gender stereotypes, health care professionals can help bring about change by challenging their own views and stereotypes. Health care professionals can also encourage parents of young children to think more broadly about gender-related issues.

## Biological Theories

Theories of gender development that are biologically based tend to focus on the influence of genes, hormones, and brain structure. According to these theories, the developing fetus is exposed to hormones (androgen in particular), and this exposure has an impact on prenatal as well as postnatal development. These theories further suggest that this exposure, rather than later social experience, impacts gender development. Though much of the research looking at prenatal exposure to hormones has been done with animals and thus can be difficult to generalize to humans (Fausto-

Sterling 1993), recent human research suggests that women who had more testosterone in their bloodstream during pregnancy were more likely to have daughters, who at preschool age showed a preference for stereotypically "boy" activities (Hines et al. and ALSPAC study team 2002).

## Evolutionary Psychology and Gender

Generally speaking, evolutionary psychology, reflecting evolutionary theory, suggests that genes create a predisposition toward certain behaviors in individuals, and when such behaviors are adaptive these genes become increasingly prevalent through natural selection and continue to represent the original adaptive behaviors (Geary 1999). Because evolutionary psychology focuses on the passing of genes from one generation to the next, parenting is of special interest. Evolutionary psychologists have also proposed the parental-investment theory, suggesting an evolutionary explanation for the care parents take of their children (Bjorklund & Shackelford 1999). Parental-investment theory suggests that despite the enormous cost both emotional and financial, parents expend tremendous time, energy, and financial resources to care for their children in order to maintain the gene pool. This theory is not without its difficulties and criticisms. For example, this theory would not explain the commitment of nonbiological parents to their children. However, the theory is still interesting to explore when thinking about gender.

Evolutionary psychologists believe that gender differences in behavior are the result of genetic predispositions not social constructions. Geary (1999) believes that gender differences in children's play reflects evolved tendencies in adaptive behavior. For example, whereas other theorists might suggest that girls engage in doll play and other nurturing activities (sometimes referred to as play parenting) because they are socialized to do so, evolutionary theorists would posit that girls engage in play parenting because they are genetically predisposed to do so. They would argue that child care was characteristically a female activity, and infants and children survived only if properly cared for by females; thus, nurturing behavior was adaptive. According to Geary (1999), this play behavior remains adaptive. While many questions both substantive and empirical remain about this evolutionary theory, it raises interesting issues when thinking about the nature of gender development.

## Integrative Theories of Gender

Eleanor Maccoby (1988, 1998, 2000, 2002; Maccoby & Jacklin 1987) is one of the most widely recognized theorists and researchers in the study of gender and behavior. In recent work (e.g., 1998, 2002) Maccoby has suggested that various theories explaining gender development can be integrated to provide a more complete understanding. Maccoby uses the term *gender segregation* to describe children's propensity to seek out and play with children of their own gender and to avoid play with other children of the other gender. Maccoby believes that we begin to see gender segregation in preschool age children. This segregation becomes more deeply entrenched in elementary school–aged children and slowly declines with the beginning of adolescence. Other theorists have suggested that gender segregation is not limited to American or other Western cultures and is found quite universally (Ruble & Martin 1998; Whiting & Edwards 1988). Maccoby and others believe that gender segregation is motivated primarily by the children themselves. She suggests that children learn early on that boys and girls have different styles of play and are therefore more comfortable sticking with others who share their style.

Perhaps the more interesting and by far more elusive question involves where and how these differences originate. Maccoby believes that various factors contribute to the differences in play style and suggests that the interaction of evolu-

tionary, physiological, cognitive, and sociocultural factors probably provides the most complete explanation of these differences. Based on similar sex differences in play that have been observed in some primates, Maccoby concurs that there may be an evolutionary component to gender differences in style in which boys engage in more physical, large-group, dominance-gaining activities, and that girls are more likely to engage in smaller groups or with an individual, avoiding direct confrontation and expressing any hostility indirectly. However, for Maccoby, physiological factors also seem to be important in the male fetal exposure to androgen.

Finally, Maccoby believes that cognitive and social factors play a part. Cognitive understanding of one's gender and the gender of others as well as socialization based on gender have an impact on gendered behavior. Children who attempt to cross gender lines are often teased by peers and may be subjected to ridicule by adults. If and when this is the case, it is hard to tease apart biologically driven tendencies from deeply entrenched social norms. It is crucial for health care providers to understand that issues of gender are complex and worthy of study.

# Gender Development: Terminology

The preceding review of prominent theories and schools of thought can provide ideas about theoretical frameworks employed to attempt to explain gender development. The following section is a brief overview of some of the common terminology used when discussing gender development.

## Gender Identity

Gender identity, the realization that one is either a boy or a girl, is developed sometime between 2 and 3 years of age (Fagot & Leinbach 1989, 1993). Interestingly, however, at this point children do not yet necessarily understand that gender is stable over time. In other words, at this stage children recognize themselves as being a girl or a boy but still believe that a boy could grow up to be a woman or a girl to be a man.

## Gender Stability

With gender stability, which usually develops between 3 and 4 years of age, children come to understand that gender is stable over time and thus girls grow up to be women and boys to be men. It is important to note that for young children, even those with a sense of gender stability, determinations about the gender of another are based on external, appearance-related characteristics. So, for example, a child with long hair or a child in a dress would be seen as a girl.

## Gender Constancy

Between ages 5 and 7 children typically develop a sense of gender constancy. Gender constancy suggests an understanding that gender is stable across the life span but also constant from one situation to the next regardless of external appearance. Although it may be true in theory that children develop an ability to see gender as constant regardless of external appearance, we tend in our culture to be very dependent upon external markers of appearances when we make (at times inaccurate) judgments about gender (my experience with my long-haired son is a good example). It is crucial for health care providers to understand the concepts of gender identity, stability, and constancy because anxious parents of young children often have many questions about what they consider gender-appropriate behavior and need to be reassured about the play of their young children. In addition, for children to grow up in the most supportive environments possible we must continue to question the constraints of "gender-appropriate behavior" so that neither girls nor boys are trapped in societally prescribed roles that are too constricting.

## Gender Stereotypes

The notion of "gender-appropriate behavior" is based largely on what is generally referred to as gender stereotypes or gender role stereotypes. Like other stereotypes, gender stereotypes are culturally based beliefs about appropriate, typical, or characteristic behaviors for females and males. These stereotypes tend to be steeped in long histories and may have some of their roots in religious traditions. These stereotypes also tend to be deeply entrenched and woven into the fabric of our society, so we may find ourselves acting in accordance with these stereotypes without even realizing that they are at play. Perfect examples of gender role stereotypes can be found in everyday life. We expect women to be nurturing and emotional, and we expect men to be strong and less emotionally expressive. This expectation is communicated early on to children.

## Gender Stereotypes: Toys

Though there is much debate about the nature of children's choice of toys, most people are very careful to give what are considered "gender-appropriate" toys as gifts. Boys get trucks and building materials, and girls get dolls and crafts. In a fascinating study of young children, Serbin and colleagues (2001) showed pictures of gender-stereotyped toys (dolls and vehicles) to 12-, 18-and 23-month-old children. They measured interest based on amount of time that the children looked at the different pictures. The researchers found little difference at 12 months, but by 18 months girls looked at pictures of the dolls for much longer than the boys and the boys looked at the pictures of the vehicles for much longer than the girls. By 23 months, the boys hardly looked at the pictures of the dolls at all and spent much more time looking at the vehicles, and girls looked at both the pictures of the dolls and vehicles.

Although this study relies on a preverbal measure of preference, it does suggest that interest in or preference for toys is determined even before children have developed a sense of gender identity and certainly before there is stability or constancy. It also suggests that gender role stereotyping begins early and is tremendously powerful. While it is potentially problematic to draw far-reaching conclusions from one study, the findings of Serbin and colleagues (2001) might also suggest that the effect of stereotyping or the constraints of stereotyping may be even stronger for boys than for girls, as the 23-month-old girls continued to look at both pictures though they had shown a definite preference for the dolls at 18 months.

The trend of harsher stereotyping for boys and men can be seen throughout development in that it is still more acceptable for girls to play with toys and materials that have been traditionally labeled "boy toys" than it is for boys to play with toys and materials traditionally labeled "girl toys." The logical extension of this stereotyping can be seen in the workplace where it remains more common for women to enter traditional male fields than for men to enter traditional female fields (with nursing as a prime example).

## Gender Role Socialization

Gender role socialization is the process through which we are socialized—or taught through words and actions—and we socialize—or teach others—about gender roles. Gender role socialization begins at birth (and some may argue even before birth), and the messages are loud and clear. Newborns are wrapped in pink or blue. From the earliest moments of infancy most children are dressed in clothing that is considered gender appropriate. Home nurseries are decorated accordingly, and gifts are purchased based on the gender of the child. According to Ruble and Martin (1998), by the time children are in preschool they associate certain toys, games, occupations, and clothing with one gender. For young children these associations tend to be rigid. For example, a young child might insist that girls cannot be firefighters.

# Documented Gender Differences

It is important to note that much of the discussion focuses on gender differences. In fact, despite biological differences, from a developmental and psychological standpoint, there are many more commonalities between females and males than there are differences. The stereotypes about differences far exceed the actual differences that have been documented, and even when documented the differences tend to be rather small.

## Physical Differences

There are some clear and obvious differences between females and males in terms of physical characteristics. Hormones, chromosomes, and genitalia all differ. Female infants tend to be more mature at birth and walk and talk earlier than male babies. Males tend to be more physically active and engage in more rough and tumble play as youngsters. Females reach puberty earlier and males gain more muscle mass, height, and strength (Maccoby & Jacklin 1987, Pellegrini & Smith 1998).

## Social Behavior

Despite extensive reviews of available research, most studies of social behavior conclude that there are few statistically significant gender differences in social behavior (Feingold 1994, Maccoby & Jacklin 1987). However, from an early age, males have consistently been found to be more physically aggressive than females. This difference has been found to be most prominent during the preschool years (Loeber & Hay 1997, Eagly & Steffen 1986, Hyde 1984). Girls, on the other hand, have been found to be more relationally aggressive (verbally manipulating and/or excluding others) beginning at preschool age (Bjorkquist 1994, Crick et al. 1997, Crick & Grotpeter 1995). Other researchers suggest that boys and girls differ in play style, with boys being more directive and girls engaging in more back-and-forth conversation (Carli & Bukatko 2000, Strough & Berg 2000).

## Emotion

Casey (1993) suggests that girls tend to display more of a range of emotions, both positive and negative, whereas boys tend to express only anger more frequently than girls. Cross-culturally, girls and women have been found to be more accurate when identifying the emotions through labeling facial expressions (Hall 1978).

## Mental Abilities

There are many questions about whether or not there are gender differences in mental abilities. Although general intelligence is very similar for girls and boys and women and men, there do seem to be some differences in specific areas of ability. Whereas some theorists suggest that these differences are biologically driven, many other theorists believe that it is impossible to tease out the environmental impact on these differences. The following are some examples of differences.

On the whole, girls tend to develop language skills earlier than boys. They talk earlier and have larger vocabularies earlier, although boys quickly catch up. Some suggest that girls' language develops earlier because, generally speaking, girls develop faster than boys. The left hemisphere of the brain is known to be involved in language development, and the left hemisphere of female humans and animals is slightly larger and more developed than males (Diamond et al. 1983). Although this study suggests a biological explanation, it is important not to underestimate the power of experience. Research suggests that adults talk more to female toddlers than to male toddlers.

In addition, according to Hedges and Nowell (1995) children label reading as a feminine subject, and parents believe that daughters are better readers than sons. So it is certainly possible that girls develop better and earlier language skills because they have more practice.

Interestingly, the discrepancy in reading and writing achievement continues through the elementary school years. During this time girls are also less likely than boys to be referred to remedial reading programs (Campbell et al. 2000, Halpern 2000). Beyond the elementary years this discrepancy diminishes.

Differences in mathematical ability between academically talented students and less talented students tend to emerge by the second grade. However, it is not until adolescence that a gender difference in mathematical ability emerges clearly (Bielinski & Davidson 1998). Although the overall gender difference is rather small, there is a greater gender difference in ability when only academically talented students are considered. What is especially interesting is that gender differences only emerge on certain mathematical tasks, while there are few or no differences for other tasks. Girls and boys do equally well with basic math facts, and girls tend to better with computational skills, whereas boys do slightly better with abstract reasoning and shapes. It is certainly possible that in this case too there is an experience and practice effect. Furthermore, research has suggested that gender bias tends to promote and thus intensify these discrepancies. Traditionally, boys were encouraged to do more math-related activities and take more advanced math courses that even academically talented girls were not encouraged to take. Boys also consider themselves better at math than girls, even when their grades are not as good as girls' grades (Eccles et al. 1993). After much focus on this problem there has been recent positive change—the gender gap is closing, and both boys and girls are taking advanced math courses (Campbell et al. 2000).

# Gender: Implications for Health Care Providers

Thus far in this chapter you have read a review of prominent theories and a discussion of typical gender development. The following section will address implications of gender-related issues for health care providers.

## Gender Identity Disorder

A current debate that could be of importance to health care providers surrounds the question of gender identity disorder. Gender identity disorder has been diagnosed when a child expresses a strong desire to be the opposite sex and may insist on dressing in clothing and engaging in behavior deemed more "appropriate" for the opposite sex (Zucker & Bradley 2000). According to Zucker and Bradley (2000), these children may also have significant difficulties at home or school and are especially susceptible to depression and behavior problems. Despite the possibility of this diagnosis based on the Diagnostic and Statistical Manual of Mental Disorders-IV (DSM-IV), there is some controversy about whether or not the gender development of "cross-gender" children should be considered disordered. The unhappiness experienced by these children may not be because of their desire to identify with the opposite gender but rather because of the negative reaction that they receive from peers and adults. In other words, it is possible that the children are quite happy with themselves but are made uncomfortable by others. Thus, the child would be suffering as a result of a disordered response of a surrounding society rather than a disorder of the individual. Health care providers should be sensitive to these issues both in terms of meeting the needs of the children and giving reasonable support and direction to parents to minimize the risk of mental health issues for the children.

## Eating Disorders and Disordered Eating

We live in a society obsessed with thinness. Despite our national obsession with thinness, we are also frequently reminded that we have a growing problem of obesity in our culture. It seems fairly clear that many Americans struggle with issues of proper nutrition and healthful eating habits. It also seems clear that there are individuals who suffer from eating disorders that fit clinical diagnostic criteria and many others who, though not clinically diagnosed (or even diagnosable), struggle with issues of eating and food. Issues with food and dieting are surfacing at an increasingly young age.

Young people are surrounded by media messages that suggest that happiness and popularity are linked to being thin. Though often thought of as a problem restricted to women and girls, men and boys also struggle with eating disorders. Krowchuck and colleagues (1998) found that almost 10% of sixth- through eighth-grade girls and 4% of sixth- through eighth-grade boys reported that they had vomited or used laxatives as a way to control weight. This is a startling and frightening finding that suggests an immediate need for intervention around issues of weight and proper nutrition for both boys and girls.

## Depression and Suicide

A major concern for health care providers is teen suicide. According to the National Institute of Mental Health (2002), suicide is the third leading cause of death among individuals age 15 to 24 and the fourth leading cause of death in children age 10 to 14. These are alarming statistics and speak to the urgent need for better detection and intervention services for young people at risk. A major suicide risk factor is depression. Although both boys and girls may suffer from depression, most research suggests that girls suffer from depression at a higher rate than boys (Ge et al. 1994, Petersen et al. 1993, Wichstrom 1999).

In the United States, beginning in adolescence, depression occurs twice as frequently in females as it does in males, and if left untreated can have profound effects on short- and long-term functioning (Nolen-Hoeksema 2001). Although females suffer from depression more frequently than males, it is important to note that males *do* suffer from depression. Thus, health care providers must be vigilant to be sure that the signs of depression are detected in any patient regardless of gender. Avoiding the typical gender stereotype that only women suffer from emotional distress can be helpful in reaching male patients who may be reluctant to share symptoms that are stereotyped as being female. Furthermore, if men ask for help less often and do not express emotion as readily as women, depression in male patients may be easily missed, leading to serious consequences.

The discrepancy in rates of depression has been explained both environmentally (Garber et al. 1995) and biologically (Ciccheti & Toth 1993). Children of depressed parents have a higher incidence of depression, which might suggest a genetic component but can also indicate that living in an environment with someone suffering from depression can increase risk of depression. Depression in parents may also impair emotional responsiveness and other parenting skills (Garber et al. 1995). This gender discrepancy in rates of depression is not universal. Rates of depression in developing countries tend to be more similar for males and females, and in some cases even higher for males (Culbertson 1997). This finding would certainly support the notion of a cultural component contributing to depression.

Many researchers currently believe that depression rates in the United States are related to a complex interaction of environmental and biological factors (Nolen-Hoeksema 2001). Young and Korzun (1999) believe that as teenage girls faced with stressful life events tend to place the needs of others before their own needs, they also develop an exaggerated physiological stress response. Therefore, when faced with additional or continued stressors, they become easily overwhelmed and display poor coping strategies. This pattern creates a cycle that continues unless interrupted by intervention, once again speaking to the importance of diagnosis and treatment by health care providers. Although much is still not known, it is clear that there is great need for prevention programs as well as screening programs so that intervention can be done promptly with those individuals at risk.

## Self-Harming Behavior

Deliberate self-harming behavior, which involves physical injury to the self without suicidal intent (cutting, burning, hair pulling), is behavior under increasing scrutiny (Favazza 1998). Self-harming behavior has traditionally been considered more common among adolescent girls and women than among adolescent boys and men. In a surprising finding in a recent study, Gratz and Conrad (2002) found that the college-aged men and women that they studied engaged in self-harming behaviors at similar rates. Though this finding certainly needs to be researched further, it is an important finding because so much of the prior research on self-harming behavior focused on female participants. Thus, self-harming behavior in males may not be recognized as readily. Health care providers should be aware that self-harming behavior exists and that it potentially exists among both female and male patients.

## Emotional Expression

According to recent work by Geary (1998) that reinforces many previous studies, with the exception of anger, females express emotions more freely and intensely than males. This finding has important implications for health care professionals because there are many times that it may be important for a health care professional to try to develop a sense of the emotional state of an individual. This may be easier to do when working with female patients, except when the emotion being judged is anger. In addition, patients are often asked how they feel about something, and this research suggests that females may be more willing or able to share their actual feelings than male patients.

Interestingly, some research (e.g., Hall 1978) has suggested that even very young females are slightly better than male counterparts at judging the emotional state of others. This too could have important implications for health care professionals because accurately judging the emotional state of others is an important task of a health care provider. Cultural expectations that girls and women be nurturing and supportive and boys and men be strong and self-reliant seem largely responsible for these differences. However, regardless of the source of the difference, it is important to address both with health care providers and patients so that needs of both male and female patients can be met appropriately and adequately.

## Compliance

Beginning early in life, females are more compliant than males to the demands of peers as well as authority figures. Furthermore, females seek more help and information from others and tend to score higher on personality tests that measure dependence on others (Feingold 1994). Although most experts agree that these behaviors are learned and not biologically programmed, they are nonetheless deeply entrenched. These findings about compliance suggest that female patients may be more likely to seek medical attention because they may be more likely to look to others for help in any situation. In addition, female patients may well be more compliant with medical instruction given—especially if the health care provider is seen as an authority figure. The findings lead to the following question: If females are generally more compliant (Feingold 1994) and yet do not freely express anger (Geary 1998), are female patients less likely than male counterparts to question health care providers and to advocate for their own best care? Providing avenues for patients to ask questions without feeling that they are being noncompliant is an important commitment on the part of health care providers. Also, if males are somewhat less likely to ask others for assistance, perhaps it is important to find additional ways to encourage men to access the health care system and seek medical attention.

## Substance Use and Abuse

Gender as it relates to addiction and dependence is another important issue for health care providers. Frone and colleagues (1994) suggest that it is fairly well documented that substance use is a coping strategy employed by both men and women. Generally speaking, men are more likely to use alcohol and illicit drugs, whereas women are more likely to use psychotherapeutic drugs (both as prescribed and not as prescribed). Both men and women are equally likely to smoke cigarettes and, aside from small nonstatistically significant differences, were equally successful or unsuccessful when it came to smoking cessation programs (Killen et al. 2002).

There are a variety of explanations given for these gender differences in specific substance use, among which are access to substances based on peer group and substances considered "socially acceptable" based on gender norms. For health care providers attempting to make accurate assessments and provide treatment and intervention to patients struggling with addictions, it is important to note that many studies of substance use and addiction are performed using self-report measures. Caution must be used when interpreting findings based on measures of self-report because such measures are highly subject to inaccuracy. Individuals may underreport use and may be wary of terms like "addiction." Individuals may also be sensitive to gender stereotypes in terms of what is believed to be socially acceptable use. Furthermore, consideration of the mental health factors that increase the risk of substance use and addiction may help health care providers to better meet the needs of patients.

## Gambling

According to statistics cited by Ladd and Petry (2002), women account for 32% of problem gamblers in the United States. And yet very little attention has been paid to gender issues as far as gambling is concerned. These researchers suggest that gender norms likely impact gambling behaviors in women and men. Women were found to demonstrate more problem gambling with slot machines, and men had more difficulties with table games and sporting events. Men were more likely to begin gambling for the excitement, and women were more likely to begin gambling for relief from stressful personal situations. Amongst problem gamblers seeking treatment, Ladd and Petry (2002) found that women were less likely than men to have alcohol-related difficulties (which relates to the previous section—although the present study did not look at psychotherapeutic drugs, which, given documented gender differences in type of substances used, might be an interesting angle for future study). Additionally, these researchers found that female gamblers had fewer legal problems than their male counterparts.

Although there are documented gender differences in gambling behaviors, there are also many gender similarities, not the least of which is that both women and men can develop pathological gambling behaviors that require treatment. These behaviors are not likely to decline in the near future with the increase in legalized gambling and the struggling economy. Health care providers and organizations can provide an important service by helping those struggling with addictions.

## Health Care Knowledge and Access

The knowledge that patients have about health care should be an important consideration for health care providers. Health care knowledge can be understood as how much an individual knows and understands about health care–related issues. Health care knowledge can certainly have a positive impact on the access an individual has to health care in that the more that is understood, the better an individual is able to ask questions. Gender differences have been found in health care knowledge. These differences in interaction with

some of the other gender-related behaviors that we discussed earlier (e.g, compliance and emotional expression) may ultimately have an impact on health care–related behaviors (e.g., seeking medical attention, asking for a second opinion).

Beier and Ackerman (2003) found significant gender differences in health care knowledge with women demonstrating greater knowledge in most areas of health knowledge. The gender differences were especially stark, though not surprising, around issues of reproduction and early life, but even when these topics were removed for the purpose of analysis, gender differences remained. These gender differences in health care knowledge were not found to be replicated in other knowledge areas; it was not simply a question of a more knowledgeable group of female participants. Such gender differences raise important questions and suggest the need for further research. Differences in health knowledge were also found to be related to education level and socioeconomic status of participants.

Perhaps the real question to be answered is why men have less health knowledge than women. Are men less interested in health-related issues? Are men less concerned about health-related issues than women? Perhaps, as Feingold (1994) suggests, men are less likely to seek information from others and thus have less information about health. But if this were the entire explanation, one would expect men to have less information about most topics, and this has not been demonstrated. Although it could be helpful to better understand the origin of this gender difference, it is important for current health care providers to recognize that the difference exists and act accordingly. It is clear that information must be made available for patients even if the patients do not ask for it. It is also clear that health care providers must acknowledge the fact that patients may or may not understand what they are being told and that many patients (and it seems based on the current research), male patients in particular, are less likely to ask for additional information.

# Conclusion

Our understanding of gender development in children can help us see the power of gender norms and gender stereotypes in our society. Understanding gender development can also help us to better support parents and those working with children to promote greater gender equity and break down gender stereotypes and barriers that deprive both girls and boys of opportunities to develop into whole people, encompassing all that is considered feminine and masculine in our society. Health care providers can make an important contribution to the promotion of gender equity and understanding. Health care providers should be cognizant of gender-related risk factors, as well as appropriate intervention and prevention strategies, to best meet the needs of all patients.

# References

Beier, M., & Ackerman, P. (2003). Determinants of health knowledge: an investigation of age, gender, abilities, personality and interests. *Journal of Personality and Social Psychology* 84:439–448.

Bem, S. (1981). Gender schema theory: a cognitive account of sex typing. *Psychological Review* 88:354–364.

Bielinski, J., & Davidson, M. (1998). Gender differences by item difficulty interactions in multiple choice mathematics items. *American Educational Research Journal* 35:455–476.

Bjorklund, D., & Shackelford, T. (1999). Differences in parental investment contribute to important differences between men and women. *Current Directions in Psychological Science* 8:86–89.

Bradbard, M., Martin, C., Endsley, R., & Halverston, C. (1986). Influence of sex stereotypes on children's exploration and memory: a complete versus performance distinction. *Developmental Psychology* 33:481–486.

Bronfenbrenner, U. (1979). *The ecology of human development: experiments by nature and design.* Cambridge, MA: Harvard University Press.

Bronfenbrenner, U. (1993). The ecology of cognitive development: research models and fugitive finding. In R. H. Wozniak & K. W. Fisher, Eds. *Development in context.* Hillsdale, NJ: Earlbaum, pp. 3–44.

Bronfenbrenner, U., & Morris, P. A. (1998). The ecology of developmental process. In R. M. Lerner, Ed. *Handbook of child psychology: Volume 1, Theoretical models of human development,* 5th ed. New York: Wiley, pp. 535–584.

Bussey, K., & Bandura, A. (1999). Social cognitive theory of gender development and differentiation. *Psychological Review* 106:676–713.

Campbell, J., Hombo, C., & Mazzeo, J. (2000). NAEP 1999: *trends in academic progress.* Washington, DC: U.S. Department of Education.

Carli, L., & Bukatdo, D. (2000). Gender, communication, and social influence. In: T. Eckes and H. Tráutner, *The developmental social psychology of gender,* Mahwah, NJ: Erlbaum.

Cicchetti, D., & Toth, S. (1993). *Child abuse, child development and social policy.* Norwood, NJ: Ablex.

Crick, N., and Grotpeter, J. (1995). Relational aggression, gender, and social-psychological adjustment. *Child Development* 66(3), 710–722.

Culbertson, F. (1997). Depression and gender: an international review. *American Psychologist* 52:25–51.

Diamond, M., Johnson, R., Young, R., & Singh, S. (1983). Age-related morphological differences in the rat cerebral cortex and hippocampus: male-female; right-left. *Experimental Neurology* 81:1–13.

Eagly, A., & Steffen, V. (1986). Gender stereotypes, occupational rates, and beliefs about part-time employment. *Psychology of Women Quarterly* 10(3), 252–262.

Eccles, J., Wigfield, A., Harold, R., & Blumfeld, P. (1993). Age and gender differences in children's self and task perceptions during elementary school. *Child Development* 64:830–847.

Fagot, B., & Hagan, R. (1991). Observations of parent reactions to sex-stereotyped behaviors: age and sex differences. *Child Development* 62:617–628.

Fagot, B., & Leinbach, M. (1989). The young child's gender schema: environmental input, internal organization. *Child Development* 60:663–672.

Fagot, B., & Leinbach, M. (1993). Gender-role developments in young children: from discrimination to labeling. *Developmental Review* 13:205–224.

Fausto-Sterling, A. (1993). Genetics and male sexual orientation. *Science,* Vol. 261, 1257.

Favazza, A. (1998). The coming of age of self-mutilation. *Journal of Nervous and Mental Disease* 18:259–268.

Feingold, A. (1994). Gender differences in personality: a meta-analysis. *Psychological Bulletin* 11:429–456

Freud, S. (1923/1960). *The ego and the id.* New York: W.W. Norton & Co.

Frone, M., Cooper, M. L., & Russell, M. (1994). Stressful life events, gender and substance abuse: an application of Tobit Regression. *Psychology of Addictive Behaviors* 8:59–69.

Garber, J., Braafladt, N., & Weiss, B. (1995). Affect regulation in depressed and nondepressed children and young adolescents. *Developmental Psychopathology* 7:93–115.

Ge, X., Lorenz, F., & Couger, R. (1994). Trajectories of stressful life events and depressive symptoms during adolescence. *Developmental Psychology* 30(4), 467–483.

Geary, D. (1998). *Male, female: the evolution of human sex differences.* Washington, DC: American Psychological Association.

Geary, D. (1999). Evolution and developmental sex differences. *Current Directions in Psychological Science* 8:115–120.

Geary, D., & Bjorklund, D. (2000). Evolutionary developmental psychology. *Child Development* 71:57–65.

Gratz, K., & Conrad, S. D. (2002). Risk factors for deliberate self-harm among college students. *American Journal of Orthopsychiatry* 72:128–140.

Hall, J. (1978). Gender effects in decoding nonverbal cues. *Psychological Bulletin* 85:845–857.

Halpern, D. (2000). *Sex differences in cognitive abilities,* 3rd ed. Mahwah, NJ: Erlbaum.

Hedges, I., & Nowell, A. (1995). Sex differences in mental test scores: variability and numbers of high scoring individuals. *Science* 269:41–45.

Hines, M., Golombok, S., Rust, J., Johnston, K., Avon, J. (2002). Testosterone during pregnancy and gender role behavior of preschool children. *Child Development* 73(6), 1678–1687.

Hyde, J. (1984). How large are gender differences in aggression? A developmental meta-analysis. *Developmental Psychology* 20(4), 722–736.

Killen, J., Fortmann, S., Varady, A., & Kraemer, H. (2002). Do men outperform women in smoking cessation trials? Maybe, but not by much. *Experimental and Clinical Psychopharmacology* 10:295–301.

Ladd, G. T., & Petry, N. (2002). Gender differences among pathological gamblers seeking treatment. *Experimental and Clinical Psychopharmacology* 10:302–309.

Liben, L., & Signorella, M. (1993). Gender-schematic processing in children: the role of initial interpretation of stimuli. *Developmental Psychology* 29:141–149.

Loeber, R., and Hay, D. (1997). Key issues in the development of aggression and violence from childhood to early adulthood. *Annual Review of Psychology* 48, 371–410.

Lytton, H., & Romney, D. (1991). Parents' differential socialization of boys and girls: a meta-analysis. *Psychological Bulletin* 109:267–296.

Maccoby, E. (1988). Gender as a social category. *Developmental Psychology* 24:755–765.

Maccoby, E. (1998). *The two sexes: growing up apart, coming together.* Cambridge, MA: Harvard University Press.

Maccoby, E. (2000). Perspectives on gender development. *International Journal of Behavioral Development* 24:398–496.

Maccoby, E. (2002). Gender and group process: a development perspective. *Current Directions in Psychological Science* 11:54–58.

Maccoby, E., & Jacklin, C. (1987). Gender segregation. In H. W. Reese, Ed. *Advances in child development and behavior,* Volume 20. Orlando, FL: Academic Press.

Martin, C. (1993). New directions of investigating children's gender knowledge. *Developmental Review* 13:184–204.

Martin, C., Eisenbud, L., & Rose, H. (1995). Children's gender based reasoning about toys. *Child Development* 66:1453–1471.

Nolen-Hoeksema, S. (2001). Gender differences in depression. *Current Directions in Psychological Science* 10:173–176.

Pellegrini, A., and Smith, P. (1998). Physical activity play. *Child Development* 69(3), 609–610.

Petersen, A., Compas, B., Brooks-Gunn, J., Stemmier. (1993). Depression in adolescence. *American Psychologist* 48(2), 155–168.

Ruble, D., & Martin, C. (1998). Gender development. In N. Eisenberg, Ed. *Handbook of child psychology: volume 3, Social, emotional and personality development,* 5th ed. New York: Wiley, pp. 993–1016.

Serbin, L., Poulin-Dubois, D., Colburne, K., Sen, M., & Eichstedt, J. (2001). Gender stereotyping in infancy: visual preferences for and knowledge of gender-stereotyped toys in the second year. *International Journal of Behavioral Development* 25:7–15.

Shell, R., & Eisenberg, N. (1990). The role of peers' gender in children's naturally occurring interest in toys. *International Journal of Behavioral Development* 13:373–388.

Strough, J., & Berg, C. (2000). Goals as a mediator of gender differences in high-affiliation dyadia conversations. *Developmental Psychology* 36(1), 117–125.

Wichstrom, L. (1999). The emergence of gender differences in depressed mood during adolescence. *Developmental Psychology* 35(1), 232–245.

Whiting, B., & Edwards, C. (1988). *Children of different worlds: the formation of social behavior.* Cambridge, MA: Harvard University Press.

Young, E., & Korzun, A. (1999). Women, stress and depression: sex differences in hypothalamic, -pituitary-adrenal axis regulation. In E. Leibenluft, Ed. *Gender differences in mood and anxiety disorders: from bench to bedside.* Washington, DC: American Psychiatric Press, pp. 31–52.

Zucker, K., & Bradley, S. (2000). Gender identity disorder. *Handbook of infant mental health.* New York: Guilford.

# Chapter 3

# Culture and Life Span Development

Jacqueline Lerner

Ori Ashman

Any discussion of how culture may be involved in individual development across the life span should begin with an overview of the *life span developmental perspective*. The ideas advanced in this view describe the ways that culture influences development. In addition, another major perspective in human development theory—the *ecological systems perspective*—has also provided ideas about the strong role of culture in individual development. These two perspectives have dominated developmental psychology for the past several decades and have forced theorists, scientists, and practitioners to pay attention to the processes of development in context—a context that includes culture. After an introduction to these leading theories, we turn to a specific discussion of the role of culture in various aspects of development.

A consideration of all of the ways that culture influences development is beyond the scope of this chapter. We have chosen to discuss how culture affects the socializing aspects of the context, such as parenting; how culture influences the development of self-concept and identity in childhood and adolescence; how culture leads to the development of ideas about primary and secondary control; and, finally, how all of these developmental processes affect health attitudes and behaviors.

## The Life Span Developmental Perspective

The major formulators of the life span developmental perspective were Paul B. Baltes, K. Warner Schaie, John R. Nesselroade, Hayne W. Reese, and Orville G. Brim, Jr. The life span perspective emphasizes the potential for systemic change across the lifespan. It also emphasizes the power of reciprocal interactions, that is, how the environment influences people and how people influence their environments.

When it was introduced in the 1970s, the features of the life span perspective included the following ideas:

- Development occurs across the life course. It does not end with physical maturity (puberty).
- Individual development occurs in relation to social, cultural, and historical changes. It does not occur because of internal (biological, genetic) influences acting alone or by the isolated action of environmental stimuli.

33

- Across life, there are important differences between people and within individuals. Not only do people change across life, they change in ways specific to them.

- Attempts to describe, explain, and improve/optimize development across life involves understanding the connections between individuals and their contexts. If we understand development, we should be able to improve it; to improve development we need to alter the connections between people and their social and cultural worlds.

Accordingly, the life span perspective emphasizes that human behavior and development arise as a consequence of an individual's relationships with the several aspects, or levels, of his or her social context. These levels constitute the "ecology" of human development (Bronfenbrenner 1979, Bronfenbrenner & Morris 1998) and include the family, community, society, and culture. In addition, the period in history within which people live influences their development as they experience unique combinations of economic, political, and technological conditions (Elder 1998).

As a result, the life span perspective emphasizes that variability, or diversity, arises in people as a consequence of their "embeddedness in" (relationships with) particular constellations of family, community, and societal, cultural, and historical conditions. Two types of diversity are stressed in the life span perspective. First, there are important differences *among* people, for example, in their racial, ethnic, religious, gender, physical, age-related, community, and cultural characteristics. These may be associated with differing patterns of life span development. Second, there are often underappreciated differences *within* a person over the course of his or her life. Here, life span scholars stress that 1) development occurs throughout life (children differ from adolescents and adolescents differ from adults; and the way you are in childhood or adolescence does not com-

pletely determine the rest of your life), and 2) development always involves a combination of gains and losses.

For example, in infancy, gains in visual acuity are accompanied by a loss of neurons that could have been used in other potential visual pathways. In childhood, growth in fluency in one language decreases the probability of gaining similar proficiency in another language. In adolescence, commitment to one social role (e.g., becoming a computer engineer) and to its associated beliefs or ideology (e.g., a belief in the importance of technology for society) is associated with a loss of other life paths (e.g., becoming a lawyer) as potential routes to self-definition. In the adulthood and aging years, physical or cognitive losses may be compensated by gains associated with accumulating experience, expertise, or "wisdom" in a particular domain (Baltes et al. 1998, 1999).

## Developmental Systems Theory

In tandem with the life span perspective, another theoretical approach focuses on the relation between the individual and his or her contexts across development. By the end of the 1980s there was a central interest in developmental science to understand the relation across the life span between the individual and his or her specific context. This interest was focused on considering the broader developmental system within which all dimensions of individual development emerged (e.g., Ford & Lerner 1992; Gottlieb 1992, 1997; Sameroff 1983; Thelen & Smith 1994, 1998). In other words, development was conceptualized as embedded within an integrated set of variables derived from multiple levels of organization. In this perspective, development was conceptualized as deriving from the *dynamic relations*—that is, mutually influential or reciprocal relations— among the variables within this multitiered system.

Today, as a consequence, neither a purely biological, psychological, nor sociological viewpoint characterizes the study of individuals. Instead, a body of multidisciplinary literature is tapped to formulate ideas about the lives of children, adolescents, and adults and to provide information about how best to intervene when individuals are experiencing difficulties. Developmental systems theory leads to a focus on the relations between the developing individual and the changing context. In addition, it is recognized that there are multiple developmental opportunities and challenges during childhood, adolescence, and adulthood.

For example, from birth, numerous types of changes begin to occur. Internal and external physical changes, cognitive and emotional changes, and social relationship changes all take place. Thus, childhood and adolescence are periods involving changes in the biological, psychological, and social characteristics of the person. It is with these three sets of changes—biological, psychological, and social—that the person must cope if he or she is to move adaptively across the transitions of development.

## BIOLOGY AND HEALTH

First, life is a matter of biology; the child must cope with changing physical (bodily appearance) characteristics and physiological functions (e.g., the eruption of teeth, standing, walking, and beginning of the menstrual cycle or the first ejaculation). Inherited susceptibility to diseases (e.g., diabetes) as well as the "normal" ailments of childhood (e.g., chicken pox) and of life (colds and the flu) represent additional challenges for the developing child. Other biological changes such as declining health and agility must be adapted to adult life.

## PSYCHOLOGY: THINKING, FEELING, AND THE DEVELOPMENT OF SELF

There are psychological changes of cognition and emotion, and they arise because human development is a matter of psychology (Demos 1986). New characteristics of thought and emotions arise. In infancy, knowledge of objects, the ability to mentally represent objects, the beginnings of language, and social thinking emerge. In childhood, language abilities burgeon, thoughts about the self emerge, moral reasoning begins, and concrete thinking abilities and problem-solving skills take shape. In adolescence, cognition becomes abstract and more hypothetical, and emotions involve feelings of genital sexuality. In adulthood, role transitions and the development of intimate and generative relationships emerge.

## SOCIETY AND CULTURE

The psychological nature of human development blends inextricably into a third domain of challenges. Childhood, adolescence, and adulthood are also matters of society and culture—the focus of this chapter. The developing child must learn how to attain those skills required of any member of his or her given society (e.g., hunting and gathering, farming, language abilities, or math, science, and technology skills). Across childhood, young people learn the range of customs, values, activities, and roles appropriate and available in his or her social world and come to understand their importance and meaning. In turn, during adolescence the developmental task becomes one of putting together one's identity physically and psychologically—to find the right role, the correct place, a niche, in one's society. Throughout adulthood, the person is called upon to deal with the biological, psychological, and social changes that accompany aging. However, an individual must understand one's identity as a biological and psychological individual in order to fit into a social role optimally suited for one's own specific characteristics or one's particular sense of self.

# Bronfenbrenner's Model of the Ecology of Human Development

Accompanying the ideas of developmental systems theory is a model that places more focus on the context of the developing individual. This is Urie Bronfenbrenner's model of the *ecology of human development*.

Urie Bronfenbrenner (1977, 1979, 1983; Bronfenbrenner & Morris 1998) argues that human development needs to be understood as it occurs in its real-world setting or *ecology*. He believes that the ecology of human development is composed of four distinct although interrelated systems or types of settings: the microsystem, mesosystem, exosystem, and macrosystem.

The *microsystem* is composed of "the complex set of relations between the developing person and environment in an immediate setting containing the person" (Bronfenbrenner 1977, p. 515). For example, the family is the major microsystem for youth development in our society (Belsky et al. 1984). It involves interactions between the child, his or her parents, and any siblings that are present in the home. Other microsystems of youth include the school setting, involving both adolescent–teacher and adolescent–peer interactions, athletic courts or fields, malls, or other neighborhood gathering places that most often involve just adolescent–peer interactions. For adults, microsystems include the family and work setting as well as other political, social, or community groups.

A person's microsystems may be interrelated. For a child or adolescent, what occurs in school may affect what happens in the family, and vice versa. For the adult, what occurs at work and in other groups may affect functioning in the family. Bronfenbrenner notes that such microsystem interrelations constitute a second ecological stratum termed the *mesosystem*. He defines it as "the interrelations among major settings containing the developing person at a particular point in his or her life" (Bronfenbrenner 1977, p. 515).

What happens in a microsystem (e.g., in an interaction between an adolescent and a parent within the family context) may be influenced by events that occur in systems in which the adolescent takes no part. For example, an adult who is a parent also has other social roles, such as worker. The adolescent is probably not part of his or her parents' workplace interactions, but events that affect the parents at work can influence how they treat the youth. If a parent has a particularly good day at work, he or she may respond to the adolescent more positively than otherwise by choosing to spend additional time with them in the evening.

The individual lives with people who interact in and are affected by contexts other than those containing that person. The individual may be affected by settings in which he or she plays no direct role. Bronfenbrenner sees such influences as constituting a third system within the ecology of human development. He labels it the *exosystem* and defines it as "an extension of the mesosystem embracing . . . specific social structures, both formal and informal, that do not themselves contain the developing person but impinge upon or encompass the immediate setting in which the person is found, and thereby delimit, influence, or even determine what goes on there" (Bronfenbrenner 1977, p. 515).

Within the ecology of human development, there exists a fourth system, the *macrosystem.* This system is composed of cultural values and beliefs and historical events (e.g., wars, floods, famines), both of which may affect the other ecological systems. For instance, natural disasters may destroy the homes, schools, or other microsystems of a person or a group of people, and/or they may make certain necessities of life (e.g., food, fresh water) less available. Cultural values influence the developing person in many ways. In infancy, cultural beliefs about the appropriateness of breastfeeding and about when weaning from the breast should occur can affect not only the nutritional status of the infant but, because mother's milk may make some children less likely to develop allergies later in life, it can also affect their overall health status. In adolescence, childrearing values, and indeed the role of youth in society, not only affect the behaviors developed by a young person (e.g., Baumrind 1971, 1982) but can also affect whether the person survives adolescence (e.g., Taylor 1990, 1993). In adulthood, cultural norms about the value of work and relationships affect the emotions, cognitions, and behaviors of the individual.

Bronfenbrenner's model of the ecology of human development allows us to devise a means to represent the idea that the bidirectional socialization that occurs between individuals and the people in their immediate contexts is embedded in a still more complex system of social networks and of societal, cultural, and historical influences.

## Changing Relations among Individuals and Their Contexts Produce Development

It is not only that multiple levels of the context are involved in development. The relations among levels change across the course of life, and it is these changing relations that propel a person's development (Lerner 2002). For instance, across life, humans need social relationships to nurture, protect, and stimulate their development. However, the nature of these social relationships varies across infancy, childhood, adolescence, and adulthood. In infancy, the young person is enmeshed in close, emotionally critical relationships with parents or other caregivers. In childhood, and certainly predicated on healthy and positive relationships with parents, social relationships expand in several important ways.

Nonfamily adults (teachers, coaches, mentors) play an important role in enriching the lives of children and in enhancing their skills at interacting successfully in a complex social world. In addition, peers play an important developmental role. In fact, in adolescence, the amount of time spent with peers often exceeds the amount of time spent with parents, although family members continue to be important sources of support for the adolescent. In turn, by the end of the adolescent period, many youth, both in Western and non-Western cultures, establish their own families and begin the cycle of changing person–context social relations as adults with their own

children. We now turn to a fuller discussion of culture and the specific influences that it has on various aspects of development.

# The Concept of Culture

Although defined in a number of ways, *culture* embraces the symbols, meanings, values, institutions, and behavior that characterize a distinctive and identifiable human population group. The word has its own meanings and associations in different languages and intellectual traditions.

*Culture* can be viewed as the living sum of meanings, norms, habits, and social artifacts that confers to individuals: identity as members of some visible community; standards for relating to the environment, for identifying fellow members and strangers; and for deciding what is important and what is not important to them (Bodley 1994, Goulet 1994).

*Cultures* possess

- a common system of signifying and normative values (signifying values give meaning to existence in its totality; normative values supply behavioral rules as to how life should be lived);
- some shared basis—common territory, history, language, race, or ancestors—for people to identify themselves as members of a single group; and
- the will or decision to be primarily self-identified as a member of a given community.

Although we can think of culture as having many manifestations, it supplies identity, provides a meaning system, and assigns a place to its members in the total scheme of things. This connotation of culture as a "complex whole" reflects a perception that human life is experienced as a totality. Culture thus provides an organizing concept for describing a collectivity's way of life (Goulet 1994).

Culture, then, is a way of life as well as the content of libraries, museums, moral and religious codes of conduct, and so on, and has become a common term to describe social life. In sum, culture provides lenses of perception and cognition (how people view the world); motives for human behavior; criteria of evaluation (good/bad, ugly/beautiful, terrorist/freedom fighter); a basis of identity (religion, ethnicity); a mode of communication (language, arts, ideas); a basis of stratification (class, rank, gender); and a system of production and consumption (Mazrui 1997). In short, people's culture will influence their individual development and will contribute to individual differences among people.

Culture provides resources to the developing individual by way of socialization strategies; physical structures; and economic, medical, and physical technology (Baltes et al. 1998). One's need for culture increases with age, for as we age the supports from the culture—material, social, economic, and psychological—become more necessary. In a sense, in adulthood, culture is needed to compensate for biological decline. Ideas about how culture affects both normal and atypical development have changed dramatically over the course of the last century (Shweder 1991). A key feature of the discussion has been around the concept of *individualism versus collectivism*, which are the predominant ideologies that organize ideas of self and influence behavior.

## Individualism versus Collectivism

Webster defines *individuation* as "the process by which individuals in a society become differentiated from one another" (Merriam-Webster 1998). *Individuation* or *individualism* describes the extent to which people see themselves as individuals whose identity is separate from others in their social group. The United States holds individualism as one of its strongest values, but it is equally strong in many (but not all) countries with a British cultural heritage. Although involvement with family, community, and peers is highly desirable, Americans gradually discover that the individual is directly related to the society, without

the need for an intervening group. Not all Americans are highly individualistic in their behaviors and beliefs, but most who are native-born share a core set of values. For example, expressing one's self as a distinct individual is highly valued.

The other side of individualism is the concept of *collectivism.* The idea of collectivism maintains that an individual's identity is derived primarily from affiliations with multiple work or social groups. In fact, the major goal of a collectivist society is the "seamless" integration of the individual into the group. About 70% of the world's population, including countries such as Korea and Japan, can be considered to be "collectivist" in their values (Triandis 1989). These differing societal goals surely influence the context of development—for example, how parents use discipline, what behaviors they expect of their children, and the attitudes and values they imbue. We turn now to a discussion of the impact of individualistic and collectivist ideas on parenting.

## Individualism, Collectivism, and the Parenting Context

A culture's preference for individualism or collectivism is conveyed to the developing child by how that child's parents, peers, teachers, and others encourage or discourage individual behavior in such everyday tasks as taking responsibility, solving problems, responding to questions, and following directions. In cultures on the collectivist end of the individualism–collectivism dimension, individuals are socialized into viewing their relationship with society, not as an individual who has a relationship, but rather as part of a group that has such a relationship. In other words, in highly collectivist cultures the individual has little or no relationship with society EXCEPT through the groups in their life—their family, gender-based associations, perhaps their clan or ethnic group, their workgroup, and their community. Hui and Triandis (1986) note that members of collective cultures define themselves as part of several "in-groups" (family, peer, social, or work groups) and are more likely to be aware of the implications that their behaviors have on others, to share resources, to emphasize harmony, to be controlled by shame, to share both good and bad outcomes, and to feel that they are part of their in-group's life.

In Western cultures such as the United States where individualism is emphasized, individual children are socialized into developing an independent and personal sense of duty and responsibility to society, not through the group, but by voluntarily acting for the good of the group. Highly individualistic cultures tend to have strong morality-based value systems, so that the young are socialized to create a personal sense of morality that ensures social order, at least to some degree. Members of individualistic societies are more likely to share with their immediate nuclear family, are less willing to subordinate their own personal goals to those of the collective, are willing to confront members of their in-groups, feel responsible for their own successes and failures, and experience some degree of separation from their in-groups (Hui & Triandis 1986).

The values of one's culture will influence that person's development early in life. Parents and others will begin to socialize children to "fit" with the ideology of the culture. In this way, one's individuality will be affected. The ideology of collectivism and individualism is reflected in the ways in which parents from different cultures view their children and their own parenting. Choi (1987) notes that in Korea, a collectivist culture, it is the parent's responsibility to shape the child's personality in a correct manner. Mothers follow prescriptive guidelines such as *t'aekyo* (the Korean word for the traditional form of prenatal care). These guidelines encourage the mother to synchronize herself with her unborn child during the prenatal period. For example, she becomes aware of the child's movements and moods. In this way, it is believed, the mother becomes keenly aware of the relational bond between herself and her child.

This belief affects parenting and subsequent styles of interaction with the child. Korean mothers have a very lenient and indulgent style with their children, a reflection of the emotional and relational intimacy between the two. That is, Korean mothers are not discipline-oriented, they do not have rules for bedtime or mealtime, and they are inconsistent in their parenting style. David Ho (1986) explains this pattern as being a result of the mother's view that the child is not capable of understanding rules for behavior. The mother has a clear, empathic understanding of the child because of the close emotional bond; as a consequence, she truly accepts the child's behavior.

There are differences between Eastern and Western culture groups in maternal attitudes, and these attitudes influence parenting. For example, Canadian mothers, who adopt an individualistic value system, place equal weight on their own personal development and on their role as caregivers. Korean mothers, on the other hand, view their role as mother and caregiver with greater weight and believe that they should sacrifice their own personal development for the child (Choi 1987). Korean mothers are not as likely to pursue careers when their children are in school, they take the role of mother/teacher very seriously, and they involve themselves in every aspect of their child's education. The values of these Korean and Canadian mothers will no doubt become part of the child's personal story about, or "script" for, his or her own behavioral and attitudinal development. In interaction with their parents, children develop as individuals but are strongly influenced by the behaviors and values that they experience in the family. Two key aspects of an individual's development that are strongly influenced by culture are the self-concept and identity. We turn to a discussion of these next.

## Culture and Self-Concept

Individuals hold different concepts of themselves and others, depending on their culture. It is believed that one's concept of the self plays an integral role in cognitive processes, emotion, and motivation, and thus affects behavior and development (Markus & Kitayama 1991). The two main distinctions that we have outlined in this chapter are between Western and non-Western cultures. As detailed above, members of Western cultures are said to hold an *individualist* concept of the self. The individualist self stresses autonomy, independence, self-actualization, and the pursuit of personal goals. In contrast, non-Westerners maintain a *collectivist* self that emphasizes connectedness to others, interdependence, social conformity, and subordination of self-goals for the sake of maintaining group integrity (Kojima 1984, Markus & Kitayama 1991).

In terms of the development of ideas about the self, William Damon (1991, Damon & Hart 1988) notes that prior to adolescence people view themselves in terms of their bodily characteristics (e.g., their height), their actions (e.g., playing video games, skate boarding), their membership in particular groups (e.g., their school class or 4-H or scouting group), or the state of their moods at a given moment. With the transition into the beginning of adolescence and the emergence of abstract thinking, youth begin to define themselves in enduring and general terms (Damon 1991). They see themselves as possessing specific personality traits that apply across time and situations, and this continues into adult life, shaping their behaviors and interactions with others.

However, young adolescents may apply contradictory traits to themselves, for instance, labeling themselves as both "smart" and "dumb" (Harter 1998, p. 567). It is not until the latter portion of adolescence, in fact, that a systematic and integrated sense of self develops (Damon 1991, Harter 1998). Often, youth use their moral ideas to attain this integrated and coherent sense of self. In essence, a coherent sense of self is necessary for functioning productively in society (Archer & Waterman 1991, Erikson 1968). Health care professionals are urged to consider these developmental issues in self-perception because they may influence mental health challenges among children and adolescents.

Therefore, what are some essential differences in the way that different cultural groups define "self," and how do they influence behavior and development? Within the United States, for example, Asian Americans are thought to hold collectivist values and therefore place emphasis on familial obligation, the group's goals and interests, and family loyalty, which leads to higher family cohesion (Fuligni et al. 1999). These individuals traditionally de-emphasize individuality and attempt to maintain family harmony (Fuligni 1998). However, when living in the U.S. and going through the processes of acculturation, these individual differences in values and concepts of the self may diminish. This may affect how individuals view their own mental and physical health problems. People who maintain a collectivist view of self may subordinate their own problems because they do not wish to disturb the harmony of the larger group and may resist seeking health care.

Fuligni (1998) reports that although American adolescents of different ethnic and generational backgrounds hold different beliefs about individual autonomy and parental authority, data indicate they have similar relationships with their parents. It is therefore hypothesized that if specific beliefs are not supported by the social context within society, they may have little effect on the parent–child relationship and may end up proximal to the dominant host group's norms. That is, despite parents' attempts to instill certain values and concepts in their children based on their cultural background, societal norms in the current setting will have greater effect on the children (i.e., the gravity of the social setting outweighs parental influence).

In addition, when individual autonomy is valued, children begin to question parental authority and are less keen to maintain family harmony. If so, it is not unreasonable to assume that highly collectivist values would diminish, or lose robustness over generations, leading to significant changes in adolescents' view of filial duties. However, in the research of Fuligni et al. (1999), adolescents' generation in fact *did not* affect their attitudes toward family obligations, which suggests these values are deeply ingrained and do not change over time.

In terms of self-definition, Western and non-Western differences emerge in research comparing American and Japanese samples. For example, American individuals usually view themselves in unrealistically positive terms (self-enhance) while Japanese display an inverse trend (self-criticize). Furthermore, Japanese display less unrealistic optimism, self-serving attributional biases, and better-than-average effect (the tendency of individuals to view themselves as better than the average member of their group). Simply put, Japanese individuals are not as likely to employ self-enhancing techniques (Heine & Renshaw 2002).

One explanation for the divergence is that in terms of functionality, self-criticism works best for Japanese, whereas self-enhancement serves Americans. Japanese stress harmony and adjustment to others, and, therefore, an ever-changing self that is capable of catering to a myriad of situations is viewed favorably. In other words, there is always room for change and improvement.

Yet another explanation suggests that Japanese are simply better synchronized with their surroundings. Compared to Americans, Japanese are far more sensitive to how others view them and seek to "maintain face." Therefore, by paying more attention to others and their potential evaluation of the self, one does not need to self-enhance and greater accuracy is attained (Heine & Renshaw 2002).

These cultural differences can be further extended by looking at views of the stability of self-concept. For example, Japanese do not value a stable self-view because as context-dependent individuals, they adjust according to the situation at hand. That is, flexibility and accommodation are viewed as adaptive. In contrast, Americans are more disposition-dependent and view personal qualities as fixed and unique, and are in need of confirmation from others (Heine & Renshaw 2002, Choi & Nisbett 1998).

As for accuracy or agreement between self and peer assessment, Americans attempt to protect themselves from negative affect and damage to their self-esteem. Therefore, individuals are in agreement with peers as long as the traits in question are neutral. If traits are positive or negative, agreement rates drop significantly. Japanese, in contrast, do not employ self-protective measures, and agreement is unaffected by the quality of the traits (positive/negative/neutral) (Heine & Renshaw 2002).

In sum, culture defines and influences how a person thinks and develops ideas about the self. This notion is also reflected in identity development, which is discussed next.

## Culture and Identity Development

As we discussed above, the cultural context influences one's self-definition throughout development. However, this definition undergoes changes during the adolescent period of the life span. During adolescence, the combination of physical, psychological, social, and cognitive changes leads to an alteration in how one looks, how one feels, and how one thinks (see Chapter 10 on Adolescence and Sexuality). The developmental challenge involved in these alterations is to understand who one is—ones' *identity*—in the face of these changes. If this task is dealt with successfully, it will result in a new definition of the self, as a particular individual with specific competencies, a personal life plan, and a niche in the world. This revised self-definition constitutes an alteration in personality and the development of an identity.

As a consequence of their biological and psychological changes, and of society's pressure to have them make a useful contribution to the world, during adolescence young people ask themselves the crucial psychological question: "Who am I?" While trying to answer this question the adolescent may experience an *identity crisis* (Erikson 1959). This crisis occurs because, at the same time that adolescents feel unsure about who they are, society begins to ask them questions related to their self-definitions.

Identity is the "distinctive combination of personality characteristics and social style by which one defines him- or herself and by which one is recognized by others" (Grotevant 1998, p. 1119). A person's identity is the set of thoughts, feelings, values, attitudes, and behaviors that define his or her "self." It is the conception of who you are that you use to govern your present interactions with the world and navigate your life into the future. It is "one's subjective sense of coherence of personality and continuity over time" (Grotevant 1998, p. 1119). Identity means accurately knowing ones attitudes and values, how one feels about things, and how one behaves generally and in specific situations. It means knowing one's *role* in society—knowing the set of socially prescribed behaviors one will enact to contribute to society.

Society wants to know what role adolescents will adopt. A role provides a self-definition, which coordinates for the adolescent his or her biological and psychological characteristics with a set of activities deemed useful by society (Baumeister 1986, 1991; Erikson 1968). A role typically cannot be something that is self-destructive or socially disapproved (e.g., criminal behavior).

Commitment to a role entails commitment to a set of values (Erikson 1959). An identity crisis may be elicited by the emotional upheaval provoked by this strong societal and personal mandate for role adoption, if it occurs at a time in the person's life when he or she cannot find a role that fits (Baumeister 1986; Erikson 1959, 1968). To resolve this crisis and achieve a sense of identity, the adolescent must find an orientation to life that not only fulfills the changing biological and psychological attributes of the self but one that is also consistent with what society expects of a person.

In keeping with the life span theme of this chapter, research reveals that the resolution of the adolescent identity crisis has a profound influence on development during later adulthood. If the identity crisis is not resolved by the time the adolescent enters adulthood, he or she will feel a sense of *role confusion* or *identity diffusion* (Archer & Waterman 1991, Erikson 1968). Some young adults waver between roles in a prolonged *moratorium* period in which they avoid commitment (Marcia 1980). Others *foreclose* on a socially approved, easily available identity and avoid the crisis altogether (Marcia 1980). Others resolve their crises by adopting an available but socially disapproved role or *ideology.* This is called *negative identity formation* and is often associated with delinquent behavior (Erikson 1959, Kennedy 1991) and other adjustment issues.

According to Erikson (1959, 1963), each stage of life development involves a synthesis of a new ego capacity with a new type of incapacity. To achieve identity the adolescent must discover what he or she believes in and what his or her attitudes and ideals are. Along with any role, there is an ideology, or set of attitudes, beliefs, and values, that serves to define it. These factors, which can be said to define one's ideology, provide an important component of one's role. When we know who we are, we know what we do; and when we know what we do, we know our role in society. To solve one's identity crisis, one must be committed to a role, which means showing commitment toward an ideology. Erikson (1963) terms such emotional orientation *fidelity.* Erikson was not the only theorist to attend to issues of identity development. We turn now to considerations of more current theories.

## Other Theoretical Views of Identity Development

The role of culture in the development of identity is highlighted in the work of Michael Berzonsky and his colleagues (1993, 1997; Berzonsky & Neimeyer 1994). These researchers emphasize that a person's developing identity is a feature of the individual that results from past, and contributes to future, person–context relations. As such, identity is an instrument of *self-regulation.* For example, it is the feature of adolescent psychological functioning and social life that allows the individual to *select* the paths he or she will pursue in life, to find the means to attain the goals that are chosen *(optimization),* and to cope with failures or losses in the means to reach goals *(compensation).* Similarly, Baltes and Baltes (1990, Baltes et al. 1998, Freund et al. 1999) propose a general theory of development based on selection, optimization, and compensation, or SOC.

Other scholars also stress that identity development involves relations between the person and the sociocultural context (Adams & Marshall 1996, Côté 1996, Goossens & Phinney 1996) and that it involves the regulation of these relations (Adams 1997; Baumeister & Muraven 1996; Berzonsky 1997; Grotevant, 1987, 1997; Kerpelman et al. 1997). For instance, the regulation of one's relationship with the social world, through the processes of selection, optimization, and compensation (Baltes & Baltes 1990, Freund & Baltes 1998), or through other attempts to control the relationships one has with the social context (e.g., Kerpelman et al. 1997), allows one to adapt to the context. "Adaptation may be the best way to conceptualize the complex, multilateral relationship between individual identity and sociocultural context, because it recognizes the causal importance of culture yet also recognizes individual choice and change" (Baumeister & Muraven 1996, p. 405).

Several studies provide empirical support for the theoretical ideas describing the role of identity in regulating links between the adolescent and the sociocultural context. In a study of the influence of culture on adolescent coping behavior (Oláh 1995) involving male and female 17- and 18-year-olds from India, Italy, Hungary, Sweden, and Yemen, both cultural differences and similarities in regulative behavior were observed. When needing to cope with contextual stressors, youth from European countries were more likely to use cognitive assimilation as a strategy; that is, they actively engaged with members of their peer group. On the other hand, youth from India and Yemen preferred emotion-focused solutions, and they would concentrate more on the feelings they had about the stresses they were experiencing. Youth from all cultural settings, if they possessed high levels of anxiety, coped with stresses by showing avoidance behaviors. Some particular ways of coping seem to be partly a function of culture. Health care professionals should try to understand the patterns of individual differences across cultures that may impact how patients seek treatment for problems and how they think about their own mental and physical health needs.

There are also regulation-related cultural differences between youth within a geographic region. German youth prefer a more active approach to reaching the developmental goals they select than Polish youth. In addition, Polish youth extend their goals far later into their development than German adolescents (Schönpflug & Jansen 1995). There are within-nation differences as well. Younger German youth (11–16 years old) use both behavioral approaches and avoidance coping strategies, whereas older German adolescents (17–19 years old) show both behavioral and cognitive forms of approach (Kavsek & Seiffge-Krenke 1996). In a longitudinal study of Swiss adolescents, aged between 14 and 20 years, youth saw two general domains of the context over which they needed to exert control—the personal/social domain (involving their own peer relationships) and the society domain (involving the rules and standards of society) (Grob et al. 1995).

Finally, in a sample of Korean adolescents in Grade 12, whereas problem-solving and information-seeking approaches to coping were associated with lower rates of depression, physical symptoms were associated with a coping style that involved discharge of one's emotions. Thus, we see differences across culture in the process by which adolescents engage with their environments during the development of identity.

## Relations Between Context and Identity Development

Some research demonstrates a link between the social and cultural contexts and identity development. In a study of younger (13–14 years old) and older (16–17 years old) boys and girls from either urban or rural areas in Australia or Finland, the processes of identity exploration and commitment were assessed (Nurmi et al. 1996). Older youth living in Australian urban settings possessed higher levels of exploration and commitment in regard to both future occupation and education than did younger urban youth. There were no age differences among rural Australian adolescents or among the urban and rural Finnish youth (Nurmi et al. 1996). It is not clear why these rural/urban differences emerged, and more research is needed to evaluate the particular processes that may differ across contexts.

In a study comparing identity development among American late adolescent youth and Finnish youth (Nurmi et al. 1997), comparable relationships in both groups were found between identity and self-esteem. Youth with an identity style that was oriented to the acquisition of information had higher self-esteem than other individuals, whereas youth with diffuse or avoidant identity styles were most likely to be depressed (Nurmi et al. 1997).

Researchers have also found that within a culture there are also important contextual influences on identity development. These influences are associated with family, peers, school, sports/athletics, social support, neighborhood/community, and the social, political, and economic structure of a society (e.g., DuBois et al. 1996, Grotevant & Bosma 1994, Paschall & Hubbard 1998). These cultural differences lead to our next topic of discussion. That is, how does culture influence other cognitions and behaviors, aside from self-concept and identity? We use the notion of primary versus secondary control to address this issue.

## Concepts of Primary and Secondary Control

We have discussed the differences between culturally bound self-concepts in terms of individualism and collectivism. However, another useful approach to account for the divergence in self-concept is the difference between Westerners and non-Westerners in conceptualizing the self and the life-space. Because Americans tend to view themselves as independent of the environment and other people, their attempts at regulation are usually executed by exertion of power and will. In contrast, Japanese assert that one is always in an interdependent relationship with the environment and can only be defined in reference to it, and therefore they attempt to regulate between them by striving for harmony (Kojima 1984). In addition, Church (1987) reported that compared to Americans, Filipinos place greater emphasis on suppression and control of unpleasant emotions (controlling internal processes rather than controlling external events).

The concept of primary and secondary *control* is one of the most widely accepted ways of thinking about control across cultures and across the life span (Levy & Langer 1998). A distinction between the two concepts of the self (interdependent/independent) is the utilization of *control strategies.* Using control, individuals attempt to modify existing physical, social, and behavioral environments to fit their personal goals and wishes. *Primary control (PC)* is defined as efforts directed at *external* realities, attempting to alter the environment; *secondary control (SC)* attempts to minimize losses, and maintain and expand existing levels of primary control by addressing *internal* processes (Heckhausen & Schulz 1993). It is assumed that all people use both forms of control and possess a "primary-secondary ratio." However, studies have found significant differences in this ratio between Western and non-Western cultures. For example, in non-Western cultures (collectivist) where stress is placed on social and environmental orientation, secondary control is used more frequently.

In contrast, in Western cultures (individualist) such as the United States, primary control is dominant, and individuals exert control directly on the environment and others to fulfill personally oriented wishes. This difference is a result of socially accepted practices, education, tradition, and history.

Control strategies can have far-reaching implications on the regulation of cognition, behavior, and motivation and, in particular, on one's contextual responses and socialization patterns.

The inclination toward primary or secondary control is not only culturally bound but is also determined by age. According to Heckhausen & Schulz (1998), primary control increases rapidly during childhood, plateaus in middle life, and declines in old age; secondary control flourishes in adolescence and mid-life and levels off in old age. This theory is based on the following assumptions: 1) children and adolescents are unable to attain the majority of their goals due to their age and lack of autonomy and must therefore internally adjust (secondary control) their aspiration levels, denying failure and reinterpreting action goals; 2) in old age, primary control becomes restricted due to biological declines; and 3) the elderly concentrate their efforts on minimizing losses rather than establishing and achieving new goals.

Heckhausen and Schulz (1995) believe that striving for control is a human universal across history and cultural settings. That is not to say,

however, that the focus of control does not change over the life course (Schulz & Heckhausen 1999).

Others, such as Gould (1999) have questioned the validity of that statement. As an example, Gould mentions that in Japan, secondary control is the norm, while primary control is downplayed. This claim has been substantiated by several researchers including Azuma (1984), who critiqued the seminal study of Weisz, Rothbaum, & Blackburn (1984a, b) saying, "the primary-secondary dichotomy . . . presented by Weisz, et al. is in itself quite American" (p. 971). In conclusion, Gould (1999) asserts that culture mediates how control is perceived and in some cultures secondary control takes precedence over primary control, and that the life span development theory fails to consider the possibility that different societies may hold different conceptions of control.

It is quite possible that striving for control is consistent, but variance does exist across cultures in terms of the way primary and secondary control preferences are expressed publicly or the fashion in which a culture instills control strategies in its members. Heckhausen & Schulz (1998) stress the evolutionary basis of this system and explain that primary control is dominant because humans have always favored active engagement with their environment. It follows that behavior regulation stems from those early interactions and is consistent across cultures. However, in some cultures (Asian) the group strives for primary control, whereas in other cultures striving for primary control is more salient to the individual. In other words, an interdependent individual could strive for primary control just as much as the independent individual.

As for aging, Heckhausen & Schulz (1993) assert that it too is a universal phenomenon across cultures because age-graded functional declines are rooted in biology, although medical intervention may play a role as a moderator in the West due to technological advances. In conclusion, secondary control may not override primary control but could be viewed as "confederate" (p. 608) to primary control, attempting to focus motivation on primary control goals and compensate for the deleterious effects of failure.

To summarize, Westerners are assumed to hold an individualist concept of the self and use more primary control than non-Westerners who hold a collectivist concept of the self and favor secondary control. As long as we think of these concepts abstractly, we encounter no real difficulty. However, questions begin to emerge when one considers immigration and, consequently, the transplantation of collectivistic individuals into American society. In practice, these notions are anything but clear or well defined. The health care practitioner must therefore carefully consider individual differences anchored in culture and address these issues in a sensitive and understanding manner.

# Aging, Culture, and Health Behaviors

How might culture affect the ideas and values one has about aging and declining health? Over the past decades, the average life span of Americans has increased by 27 years. This dramatic increase is most often attributed to the latest developments and innovations in medical treatments. However, research in the field has shown that psychological and behavioral factors may also affect longevity (Levy et al. 2002).

The elongated life span and the aging baby-boom generation are bound to create enormous deficits in the Medicare Trust Fund. As a result, the ever-growing need for health care, technological breakthroughs, and declining funds all combine to be construed as future burdens on young taxpayers, who shall have to ultimately pay for the health care of the elderly (Callahan 1996). However, financial implications are only part of the picture. The perceived role of the elderly in society and attitudes toward them are constantly shifting. On one hand, many believe such individuals are past their prime, can no longer be productive or contributing members of society, and

deplete public funds. Consequently, these views give rise to *ageism,* that is, negative attitudes or behaviors toward individuals based on their age (Greenberg et. al. 2002). On the other hand, the elderly live longer, healthier lives, and many are still capable of working and teaching their young colleagues thanks to knowledge grounded in years of experience. Recently CNN reported that several large companies began rehiring former retired executives to help facilitate recovery. Moreover, many companies have retiree rehiring policies, and this trend seems to be on the rise (Keller 2001).

Generally, younger individuals, who are susceptible to negative stereotypes of aging, exercise ageism toward the elderly. To the young, the elderly manifest their greatest fears: declines in health, physical attractiveness, and mental capacity, and most importantly, they crystallize impending death. These fears are especially salient to young individuals in Western society in which self-esteem is predicated mainly on appearance, esthetics, and physique. To reduce anxiety provoked by these fears, individuals employ various defenses and attempt to boost their self-esteem by looking down and distancing themselves from the elderly both physically and mentally (Greenberg et. al. 2002). We should also bear in mind that ageism is cyclical and inevitable, as young individuals go through life stages and will eventually reach old age, and thus fall victim to the same negative effects of aging and ageism.

The growing elderly population in the United States has been encouraged to take control of their lives, even when they become incapacitated. As part of this movement, policy makers have encouraged people of all ages, but particularly the elderly, to fill out *advance directives* (Callahan 1996). This document is drawn while an individual is competent and describes this person's wishes should he or she become mentally or physically unable to choose between options or communicate his wishes (Luptak & Boult 1994). This communicative tool may be beneficial in several ways. First, the health care professional must listen attentively to the patient and disseminate pertinent information in a clear and precise manner; second, family members, who might bear the ultimate consequences and burden of caring for the patient, have an opportunity to participate in the decision-making process; and third, procedural and financial decisions are facilitated (Backlar 1995). However, there exists a risk that these discussions about death and serious illness will evoke negative stereotypes of aging, which in turn may affect one's will to live, defined as, "a judgment that the perceived benefits of one's life outweigh the perceived hardships" (Levy et. al. 2002, p. 266).

The main objective of advance directives is to preserve individual autonomy even in situations where it cannot be exercised directly; this type of control is termed *indirect autonomy* (Bailly & DePoy 1995). Indirect autonomy is of paramount importance when dealing with the elderly. As one ages, shifts in the conceptualization of autonomy take place; the stress shifts from the ability to act directly on decisions to ensuring decisions are implemented. This shift is an inevitable result of deterioration in health, function, and the development of dependency on others (Bailley & DePoy 1995). Although this medical document is designed to allow individuals to preserve their rights and values, several ethicists have theorized that negative stereotypes of aging, social concerns regarding health care expenditures, and familial demands all play a role in the decision-making process, and, often, the elderly will not make a choice based on their personal preferences but rather conform to the aforementioned dictates and employ self-imposed guilt (Callahan 1996, Levinsky 1996, Levy et al. 1999–2000).

While we know very little about people's beliefs and preferences regarding death and dying, even less is known about the role of culture in such decision-making processes (Carmel 2001, Waddell & McNamara 1997). For example, Goh & Shaw (1994) compared Australians to Chinese and found that the Chinese were more reluctant to complete living wills, did not support euthanasia, and did not desire truth-telling to themselves and others in case of terminal illness. Furthermore, Waddell & McNamara's (1997) findings further support the aforementioned statement. Chinese Australian participants were less likely to favor living wills (more submissive), euthanasia, and truth-telling about terminal illness when compared to Anglo-Australians. It seems the Chinese adhere to a collectivist self-concept in which loyalty to family (protecting them from the awful truth), respect for the elderly, and avoidance of discussing personal or controversial matters take precedence over personal choice and autonomy (which is of utmost importance in Western individualistic cultures). Kimmel (1988) reminds us that in collectivist cultures such as Japan, age is a measure of social status, and as age increases, so does one's status; whereas in the U.S., age is mostly viewed negatively, and the aged often are ignored unless they become a "problem."

Religion may also play a role in life and death decisions as different beliefs about life, death, and the afterlife vary across societies. For example, Judaism focuses on life, not the afterlife, and may therefore explain findings that religious Jews fear death more than nonreligious Jews (Carmel 2001). Confucianism and Buddhism influence believers in terms of collectivism and harmony with others, which encourage accommodation, the belief in cosmic powers, and acceptance of things as they are. In contrast, Christianity throughout history stressed the need to change the world, exerting primary control, often by military means (Weisz et al. 1984a, Waddle & McNamara 1997).

Further support for a relationship between ageism, culture, and advance directives is found in cross-cultural research. Considering age stereotypes and behaviors directed toward the elderly that have been reported to be more positive in Latin and Asian cultures than in the United States (Holmes & Holmes 1995, Levy & Langer 1994, Palmore 1985), it is interesting to note that a number of studies have found that elders are less likely to fill out advance directives in these cultures. For example, Chinese Australians, Japanese, and Mexican Americans have been found to be more reluctant to complete living wills when compared to Anglo-Australians, Euro-Americans, and English-speaking Japanese Americans (Waddel & McNamara 1997, Blackhall et al. 1995, Matsumura et al. 2002, Perkins et al. 2002). Several studies also suggest that ethnically diverse individuals' preferences shift and resemble those displayed by Euro-Americans as acculturation increases. Matsumura and colleagues (2002) found that when compared to nonacculturated Japanese Americans, acculturated Japanese Americans viewed advance directive planning more positively. These findings are of utmost importance to health care professionals who interact with patients on daily basis and inevitably find themselves in situations where they must offer advice and guidance. Although interactions take place in the U.S., one must remember individuals are of diverse backgrounds and may not be fully acculturated, and thus may make unsound decisions based on culturally bound "norms" rather than personal preference.

Researchers have theorized that negative stereotypes of aging, social concerns regarding health care expenditures, and familial demands could play a part in how elders fill out living wills: Instead of making this life-and-death decision based on their personal preferences, they may conform to the aforementioned dictates and employ self-imposed guilt (Callahan 1996, Levinsky 1996, Levy et al. 1999–2000). A survey found support for the prediction that societal beliefs, including the value placed on older people's lives, may influence why old older adults refuse treatment on advance directives. Survey respondents who were 65 years of age or older revealed that the reasons for refusing treatment included the expense of treatment and "younger people should be afforded more rigorous or extended interventions than elderly people, who had already lived their lives" (Bailley & DePoy 1995, p. 225). It is clear

that as individuals age, culture plays a role in how they plan the end of their lives.

## Summary

In this chapter we have attempted to outline the major theoretical approaches that lead to an understanding of the impact that culture has on life span development. We have included research from all stages of the life span to illuminate the effects of culture on the developing individual. We believe that culture serves to direct individual development in specific ways, from the way that parents discipline children to the overall sense of self that the child develops. In adolescence and adulthood, culture helps to define one's place in the world and to form ways of thinking and behaving. It is important to recognize the impact of culture on development when working with individuals in our diverse culture.

# References

Adams, G. R. (1997). Identity: A brief critique of a cybernetic model. *Journal of Adolescent Research* 12:358–362.

Adams, G. R., and S. K. Marshall (1996). A developmental social psychology of identity: understanding the person-in-context. *Journal of Adolescence* 19:429–442.

Archer, S. L., and A. S. Waterman (1991). Ego development. In: R. M. Lerner, A. C. Petersen, and J. Brooks-Gunn, eds. *Encyclopedia of adolescence,* Volume 1. New York: Garland pp. 295–300.

Azuma, H. (1984). Secondary control as a heterogeneous category. *American Psychologist* 39:970–971.

Backlar, P. (1995). The longing for order: Oregon's medical advance directive for mental health treatment. *Community Mental Health Journal* 31:103–108.

Bailly, D. J., and E. DePoy (1995). Older people's responses to education about advance directives. *Health & Social Work* 20:223–228.

Baltes, P. B., and M. M. Baltes (1990). Psychological perspectives on successful aging: the model of selective optimization with compensation. In: P. B. Baltes and M. M. Baltes, eds. *Successful aging: perspectives from the behavioral sciences.* New York: Cambridge University Press, pp. 1–34.

Baltes, P. B., U. Lindenberger, and U. M. Staudinger (1998). Lifespan theory in developmental psychology. In: W.

Damon, series ed., and R. M. Lerner, volume ed. *Handbook of child psychology: Volume 1, Theoretical models of human development,* New York: Wiley, 5th ed. pp. 1029–1144.

Baltes, P. B., U. M. Staudinger, and U. Lindenberger (1999). Lifespan psychology: theory and application to intellectual functioning. In: J. T. Spence, J. M. Darley, and D. J. Foss, eds. *Annual Review of Psychology* Volume 50, pp. 471–507. Palo Alto, CA: Annual Reviews.

Baumeister, R. F. (1986). *Identity: cultural change and the struggle for self.* New York: Oxford University Press.

Baumeister, R. F. (1991). Identity crisis. In: R. M. Lerner, A. C. Petersen, and J. Brooks-Gunn, eds. *Encyclopedia of adolescence.* New York: Garland, pp. 518–521.

Baumeister, R. F., and M. Muraven (1996). Identity as adaptation to social, cultural, and historical context. *Journal of Adolescence* 19:405–416.

Baumrind, D. (1971). Current patterns of parental authority. *Developmental Psychology Monographs* Volume 4, No. 1, Part 2.

Baumrind, D. (1982). Some thoughts about child rearing. In: U. Bronfenbrenner, ed. *Influences on human development.* Hinsdale, IL: Dryden, pp. 270–281.

Belsky, J., R. M. Lerner, and G. B. Spanier (1984). *The child in the family.* Reading, MA: Addison-Wesley.

Berzonsky, M. D. (1993). A constructivist view of identity development: people as post-positivist self-theorists. In: J. Kroger, ed. *Discussions on ego identity.* pp. 169–203. Hillsdale, NJ: Erlbaum.

Berzonsky, M. D. (1997). Identity development, control theory, and self-regulation: an individual differences perspective. *Journal of Adolescent Research* 12:374–353.

Berzonsky, M. D., and G. J. Neimeyer (1994). Ego identity status and identity processing orientation: the moderating role of commitment. *Journal of Research in Personality* 28:425–435.

Blackhall, L. J., S. T. Murphy, G. Frank, V. Michel, and S. Azen (1995). Ethnicity and attitudes toward patient autonomy. *Journal of the American Medical Association* 274:820–825.

Bodley, J. (1994). *Cultural anthropology: tribes, states, and the global systems.* Mountain View, CA: Mayfield.

Bronfenbrenner, U. (1983). The context of development and the development of context. In: R. M. Lerner, ed. *Development psychology: historical and philosophical perspectives.* Hillsdale, NJ: Erlbaum.

Bronfenbrenner, U. (1977). Toward an experimental ecology of human development. *American Psychologist* 32:513–531.

Bronfenbrenner, U. (1979). *The ecology of human development: experiments by nature and design.* Cambridge, MA: Harvard University Press.

Bronfenbrenner, U., and P. A. Morris (1998). The ecology of developmental process. In: W. Damon, series ed., and R. M. Lerner, volume ed. *Handbook of child psychology: Volume 1, Theoretical models of human development,* 5th ed. New York: Wiley, pp. 993–1028.

Callahan, D. (1996). Controlling the costs of health care for the elderly—Fair means and foul. *New England Journal of Medicine* 335:744–746.

Carmel, S. (2001). The will to live: gender differences among elderly persons. *Social Science & Medicine* 52:949–958.

Choi, J. S. (1987). *The study of Korean family system* (in Korean). Seoul: Il-Ji-Sa.

Choi, I., and R. E. Nisbett (1998). Situational salience and cultural differences in the correspondence bias and actor-observer bias. *Personality and Social Psychology Bulletin* 24:949–960.

Church, A. T. (1987). Personality research in a non-western culture: The Philippines. *Psychological Bulletin* 102:272–292.

Coté, J. E. (1996). Sociological perspectives on identity formation: the culture-identity link and identity capital. *Journal of Adolescence* 19:417–428.

Damon, W. (1991). Problems of direction in socially shared cognition. In L. B. Resnick, J. M. Levine, and S. D. Teasley, eds. *Perspectives on socially shared cognition.* pp. 384–397. Washington, DC: American Psychological Association.

Damon, W., and D. Hart (1988). *Self-understanding in childhood and adolescence.* New York: Cambridge University Press.

Demos, V. (1986). Crying in early infancy: an illustration of the motivational function of affect. In: T. B. Brazelton and M. W. Yogman, eds. *Affective development in infancy.* Norwood, NJ: Ablex Publishing, pp. 39–73.

DuBois, D. L., R. D. Felner, S. Brand, R. S. C. Phillips, and A. M. Lease (1996). Early adolescent self-esteem: a developmental-ecological framework and assessment strategy. *Journal of Marriage and the Family* 56:405–414.

Elder, G. H., Jr. (1998). The life course and human development. In: W. Damon, series ed., and R. M. Lerner, volume ed. *Handbook of child psychology: Volume 1, Theoretical models of human development,* 5th ed. New York: Wiley, pp. 939–991.

Erikson, E. (1963). *Childhood and society,* 2nd ed. New York: Norton.

Erikson, E. H. (1959). Identity and the life-cycle. *Psychological Issues* 1:18–164.

Erikson, E. H. (1968). *Identity, youth and crisis.* New York: Norton.

Ford, D. L., and R. M. Lerner (1992). *Developmental systems theory: an integrative approach.* Newbury Park, CA: Sage.

Freund, A. M., and P. B. Baltes (1998). Selection, optimization, and compensation as strategies of life-management: correlation with subjective indicators of successful aging. *Psychology and Aging* 13:513–543.

Freund, A. M., K. Z. H. Li, and P. B. Baltes (1999). The role of selection, optimization, and compensation in successful aging. In: J. Brandtstädter and R. M. Lerner, eds. *Action and self-development: theory and research through the life-span.* Thousand Oaks, CA: Sage, pp. 401–434.

Fuligni, A. J. (1998). Authority, autonomy, and parent-adolescent conflict and cohesion: a study of adolescents from Mexican, Chinese, Filipino, and European backgrounds. *Developmental Psychology* 34:782–792.

Fuligni, A. J., V. Tseng, and M. Lam (1999). Attitudes toward family obligations among American adolescents with Asian, Latin American, and European backgrounds. *Child Development* 70:1030–1044.

Goossens, L., and J. S. Phinney (1996). Commentary: identity, context, and development. *Journal of Adolescence* 19:491–496.

Gottlieb, G. (1992). *Individual development and evolution: the genesis of novel behavior.* New York: Oxford University Press.

Gottlieb, G. (1997). *Synthesizing nature-nurture: prenatal roots of instinctive behavior.* Mahwah, NJ: Erlbaum.

Gould, S. J. (1999). A critique of Heckhausen and Schulz's (1995) life-span theory of control from a cross-cultural perspective. *Psychological Review* 106:597–604.

Goulet, J. G. (1994). Ways of knowing: towards a narrative ethnography of experiences among the Dene Tha. *Journal of Anthropological Research* 50:113–139.

Greenberg, J., J. Schimel, and A. Mertens (2002). Ageism: denying the face of the future. In: T. Nelson. *Ageism: stereotyping and prejudice against older workers.* Cambridge, MA: MIT Press.

Grob, A., A. Flammer, and A. J. Wearing (1995). Adolescents' perceived control: domain specificity, expectations, and appraisal. *Journal of Adolescence* 18:403–425.

Grotevant, H. D. (1987). Toward a process model of identity formation. *Journal of Adolescent Research* 2:203–222.

Grotevant, H. D. (1997). Identity processes: integrating social psychological and developmental approaches. *Journal of Adolescent Research* 12:354–357.

Grotevant, H. D. (1998). Adolescent development in family context. In W. Damon and N. Eisenberg, eds. *Social, emotional, and personality development: Volume 3, Handbook of child psychology,* 5th ed. New York: Wiley, pp. 1097–1149.

Grotevant, H. D., and H. A. Bosma (1994). History and literature. In: H. A. Bosma, T. L. G. Graafsma, H. D. Grotevant, and D. J. deLevita, eds. *Identity and development: an interdisciplinary approach.* Thousand Oaks, CA: Sage, pp. 119–122.

Harter, S. (1998). The development of self-representations. In: W. Damon and N. Eisenberg, eds. *Social, emotional, and personality development: Volume 3, Handbook of child psychology,* 5th ed. New York: Wiley, pp. 553–618.

Heckhausen, J., and R. Schulz (1993). Optimization by selection and compensation: balancing primary and secondary control in life span development. *International Journal of Behavioral Development* 16:287–303.

Heckhausen, J., and R. Schulz (1995). A life-span theory of control. *Psychological Review,* 102:284–304.

Heckhausen, J., and R. Schulz (1998). Developmental regulation in adulthood: Selection and compensation via primary and secondary control. In: J. Heckhausen and C. S. Dweck, eds. *Motivation and self-regulation across the life span.* New York: Cambridge University Press, pp. 50–77.

Heine, S. J., and K. Renshaw (2002). Interjudge agreement, self-enhancement, and liking: cross-cultural divergences. *Personality & Social Psychology Bulletin* 28:881–906.

Ho, D. (1986). Chinese patterns of socialization: a critical review. In: Michael Bond, ed. *The psychology of the Chinese people.* London: Oxford University Press, pp. 1–37.

Ho, M. W. (1984). Environment and heredity in development and evolution. In: M. W. Ho and P. T. Saunders, eds. *Beyond neo-Darwinism: an introduction to the new evolutionary paradigm.* London: Academic Press, pp. 267–289.

Holmes, E. R., and L. D. Holmes (1995). *Other cultures, elder years.* Thousand Oaks, CA: Sage.

Hui, C. H., and H. C. Triandis (1986). Individualism-collectivism: a study of cross-cultural researchers. *Journal of Cross-Cultural Psychology* 17:225–248.

Kavsek, M. J., and I. Seiffge-Krenke (1996). The differentiation of coping traits in adolescence. *International Journal of Behavioral Development* 19:651–668.

Keller, Larry (2001, January). Coming back strong—Seniors at work: what retirement? http://www.cnn.com/2001/CAREER/trends/01/23/seniors.

Kennedy, R. E. (1991). Delinqency. In: R. M. Lerner, A. C. Petersen, and J. Brooks-Gunn, eds. *Encyclopedia of adolescence.* New York: Garland, pp. 199–206.

Kerpelman, J. F., R. R. Pittman, and L. K. Lamke (1997). Toward a microprocess perspective on adolescent identity development: an identity control theory approach. *Journal of Adolescent Research* 12:325–346.

Kimmel, D. C. (1988). Ageism, psychology, and public policy. *American Psychologist* 43:175–178.

Kojima, H. (1984). A significant stride toward the comparative study of control. *American Psychologist* 39:972–973.

Levinsky, N. G. (1996). The purpose of advance medical planning—Autonomy for patients or limitation of care? *The New England Journal of Medicine* 335:741–743.

Lerner, R. M. (2002). Concepts and theories of human development. Mahweh, NJ: Lawrence Erlbaum Associates.

Levy, B., O. Ashman, and I. Dror (1999–2000). To be or not to be: the effects of aging stereotypes on the will to live. *Omega: Journal of Death & Dying* 40:409–420.

Levy, B. R., and E. J. Langer (1994). Aging free from negative stereotypes: successful memory in China and among the American deaf. *Journal of Personality and Social Psychology* 66:989–997.

Levy, B., and E. Langer (1998). Mental control across the lifespan. In: H. Friedman, ed. *Encyclopedia of Mental Health.* San Diego, CA: Academic Press.

Levy, B. R., M. D. Slade, S. R. Kunkel, and S. V. Kasl (2002). Longevity increased by positive self-perceptions of aging. *Journal of Personality and Social Psychology* 83:261–270.

Luptak, M. K., and C. Boult (1994). A method for increasing elders' use of advance directives. *The Gerontologist* 34:409–412.

Marcia, J. E. (1980). Identity in adolescence. In: J. Adelson, ed. *Handbook of adolescent psychology.* pp. 159–187. New York: Wiley.

Markus, H. R., and S. Kitayama (1991). Culture and the self: implications for cognition, emotion, and motivation. *Psychological Review* 48:224–253.

Matsumura, S., S. Bito, H. Liu, K. Kahn, S. Fukuhara, M. Kagawa-Singer, and N. Wenger (2002). Acculturation of attitudes toward end-of-life care: a cross-cultural survey of Japanese Americans and Japanese. *Journal of General Internal Medicine* 17:531–539.

Mazrui, A. A. (1997). Islamic and western values. *Foreign Affairs* 76:118.

Merriam-Webster (1998). Merriam-Webster's collegiate dictionary, 10th ed. Springfield, MA: Merriam-Webster.

Nurmi, J. E., M. D. Berzonsky, K. Tammi, and A. Kinney (1997). Identity processing orientation, cognitive and behavioral strategies and well-being. *International Journal of Behavioral Development* 21:555–570.

Nurmi, J. E., M. E. Poole, and V. Kalakoski (1996). Age differences in adolescent identity exploration and commitment in urban and rural environments. *Journal of Adolescence* 19:443–452.

Oláh, A. (1995). Coping strategies among adolescents: a cross-cultural study. *Journal of Adolescence* 18:491–512.

Palmore, E. B., and D. Maeda (1985). *The honorable elders revisited.* Durham, NC: Duke University Press.

Paschall, M. J., and M. L. Hubbard (1998). Effects of neighborhood and family stressors on African American male adolescents' self-worth and propensity for violent behavior. *Journal of Consulting and Clinical Psychology* 66:825–831.

Sameroff, A. J. (1983). Developmental systems: contexts and evolution. In: W. Kessen, ed. *Handbook of child psychology: Volume 1, History, theory, and methods.* pp. 237–294. New York: Wiley.

Perkins, H. S., C. M. A. Geppert, A. Gonzales, J. D. Cortez, and H. P. Hazuda (2002). Cross-cultural similarities and differences in attitudes about advance care planning. *Journal of General Internal Medicine* 17:48–57.

Schönpflug, U., and X. Jansen (1995). Self-concept and coping with developmental demands in German and Polish adolescents. *International Journal of Behavioral Development* 18:385–405.

Schulz, R., and J. Heckhausen (1999). Aging, culture and control: setting a new research agenda. *Journal of Gerontology* 54:139–145.

Shweder, R. A. (1991). *Thinking through cultures: expeditions in cultural psychology.* Cambridge, MA: Harvard University Press.

Taylor, C. S. (1990). *Dangerous society.* East Lansing, MI: Michigan State University Press.

Taylor, C. S. (1993). *Girls, gangs, women, and drugs.* East Lansing, MI: Michigan State University Press.

Thelen, E., and L. B. Smith (1994). *A dynamic systems approach to the development of cognition and action.* Cambridge, MA: MIT Press.

Thelen, E., and L. B. Smith (1998). Dynamic systems theories. In: W. Damon, series ed., and R. M. Lerner, volume ed. *Handbook of child psychology: Volume 1, Theoretical models of human development,* 5th ed. New York: Wiley, pp. 563–633.

Triandis, H. (1989). Cross-cultural studies of individualism and collectivism. *Nebraska Symposium on Motivation* 37:41–133.

Waddel, C., and B. McNamara (1997). The stereotypical fallacy: A comparison of Anglo and Chinese Australians' thoughts about facing death. *Mortality* 2:149–161.

Weisz, J. R., F. M. Rothbaum, and T. C. Blackburn (1984a). Standing out and standing in. *American Psychologist* 39:955–969.

Weisz, J. R., F. M. Rothbaum, and T. C. Blackburn (1984b). Swapping recipes for control. *American Psychologist* 39:974–975.

# Chapter 4

# Resilience

Kathleen Thies

The playroom on the pediatric unit is busy. John, a 10-year-old boy in a long leg cast, is propped on crutches leaning against a video game machine, shooting down enemy planes. He has a rare soft-tissue cancer and is waiting to go home and resume yet more physical therapy after his sixth major surgery in less than two years. Emilio, 15, is lying on a stretcher, directing his younger roommate in the finer points of the game. His legs are encased in spiked metal cages, rods piercing his long bones, attached to screws that are periodically tightened to stimulate tiny fractures. As the fractures heal, they lay down new bone, lengthening his legs. Emilio has been growing his legs for years now.

Jenny, age 6 or 7, and bald from treatment for leukemia with IV bags dangling above her, is playing Chutes and Ladders with her mother. Ben, a preschooler who had emergency surgery late yesterday afternoon for testicular torsion, is literally running after a toy car he has propelled down a hallway, a heparin lock momentarily freeing him of his IV pole. The toddler Samia lays miserably in the lap of a volunteer, an advertisement for tubes and pumps. She soberly surveys the scene, taking in every movement, every sound, every person who enters and leaves.

The scene in the playroom advances the notion among health professionals that children are naturally resilient. They bounce back, even thrive, despite the adversities that ill health and invasive treatment visit upon them; they amaze and inspire the adults who care for them. Doctors, nurses, and parents alike concur that 4-year-old Ben is a special little boy if he can *run* within 24 hours of emergency removal of a testicle, surgery that would bring a grown man to his knees. The tendency to view Ben's behavior as both natural and special at the same time begs the question that is central to this chapter: Why do we expect that adversity should thwart healthy development, and why are we intrigued when it does not?

## Resilience: A Definition

Let us begin with a working definition:

*Resilience is characterized by "good outcomes in spite of serious threats to adaptation or development"* (Masten 2001, p. 228).

This definition is the culmination of years of work with children and adolescents considered to be "at risk" in the United States and in England. The purpose of this chapter is to examine the meaning of this definition in developmental theory, research, and intervention for health professionals who are not developmentalists. First, we will discuss the recent history of theoretical approaches to child development as they provide a context for the interest in resilience and how it has been studied. Findings on "good outcomes" from studies of three populations will be presented, followed by an in-depth discussion of the meaning of resilience and the implications for health care.

# History

The history of the psychology of adaptation begins with Darwin's *The Origin of the Species* (1859). Our collective interest in adaptation shifted the focus from animals to humans in short order, and to children in particular during the early to mid-20th century. Two schools of thought emerged. The mechanistic school favored the role of environment in shaping human behavior. The organismic school viewed humans as actively constructing their development. As research methods have improved, and knowledge about the role of genes has expanded, the nature–nurture debate instigated by Darwin has grown in complexity.

## Darwin and Evolution

Darwin (1859) asserted that successful organisms have adapted to fit their particular environments, and that human beings, like other animals, have evolved as a species in response to changing environmental demands and opportunities. Furthermore, he observed that although there were similarities in adaptive behaviors across species— for example, young humans and mammals vocalize to elicit parental attention—there was also considerable variation within species, such as size, appearance, and level of ability. Darwin's theory of evolution displaced divine creationism as both rationale and justification for human primacy in the natural order, turning the prevailing religious and scientific beliefs upside down.

Darwin's introduction of the two key variables of evolution—inherited characteristics and environment—ushered in the era of the scientific study of human development, and child development in particular, that emerged in England and the United States in the late 19th and early 20th centuries. Interest evolved in part due to societal disruption that accompanied the Industrial Revolution, as immigrants and rural families crowded into cities, and institutional rearing of orphaned children became synonymous with Dickensian deprivation. It was a period of major social reforms in labor laws, public health, and public education. As education emerged as a democratizing force, John Dewey (1899) and G. Stanley Hall (1891) argued for child-centered schools, while Alfred Binet (Binet & Simon 1905) began to examine the characteristics of innate intelligence. Professional advice manuals on child rearing for the lay audience became popular.

# Psychoanalytic Theory of Child Development

Sigmund Freud's (1924/1952, 1930/1961) theories of personality development set the tone for the 20th century. Influenced by Darwin's view of humans' animal heritage, Freud introduced the *id* as the seat of universal primitive drives for food, aggression, sex, and pleasure. He theorized that these drives were civilized through identification with a love object, which is the parent, promoting the emergence of a healthy *ego* and *superego*. Because of his emphasis on the primacy of the early parent–child relationship, psychologists came to believe that early experiences, especially parental loss, would determine a child's psychological course for life.

Within the context of the First and Second World Wars and worldwide economic depression, Freud's psychoanalytic theory shifted the focus of child studies from the realization of Darwinian potential to understanding the potential for and realization of disordered behavior. During the

1940s, René Spitz (1946) used the term "hospitalism" to describe the depressed affect and poor outcomes of displaced and traumatized children gathered into institutions in Europe during and after the war.

## Bowlby and Attachment

At the same time in England, Anna Freud (Freud & Burlingham 1943), Sigmund's daughter, and John Bowlby (1951) (who would later author the definitive biography of Darwin) began to study the effects on war orphans of early loss and bereavement, deprivation, and institutional care. Bowlby considered affiliative relationships with parental figures as the cornerstone of healthy development in children. Older siblings and sometimes even peers could serve as relatively effective substitutes, as stories of lost children who banded together to survive seemed to attest. Conversely, children without emotional attachments had been observed to fare poorly and to develop symptoms of pathology. Bowlby's extensive writings, published from the 1950s and into 1980, are the seminal work for theories of attachment (see Chapter 10) and the study of resilience.

## Nature–Nurture

During the 1950s and 60s, the focus of child study broadened. How could lessons learned from children whose life trajectories had been fundamentally altered by unusually adverse circumstances be applied to children living in ordinary poverty and to middle-class children as well? At the same time, research methods in psychology began to be more theory-driven and empirical. Darwin's two key variables in evolution—inherited characteristics and environment—became dichotomized into the nature–nurture debate. However, the role of the environment in human development and behavior captured more interest. Why?

One reason for the emphasis on environment may have been that it has been easy to study. As an independent variable, it could be controlled, ma-

nipulated, and quantified by investigators in laboratory-based experimental designs. John Watson (1913) and B. F. Skinner (1938) typify this mechanistic view of human behavior as passively shaped by external conditions (e.g., through reward and punishment as reinforcements of behavior).

By comparison, the study of inherited characteristics was, and still is, in its infancy. Moreover, inherited characteristics reflect both group norms and individual differences. Individual differences, such as shyness or math ability, might be considered "constitutional"; that is, attributed to a child's innate and unique makeup. Whether or how they may be genetically inherited has been beyond the reach of investigation until very recently. Group norms reveal that all healthy human beings seem genetically programmed to mature on a predictable schedule, starting with conception. For example, Andre Gesell (1948) and Jean Piaget (1950) observed the "natural unfolding" of the typically developing child.

Research on developmental norms during the 1950s, 1960s, and 1970s helped to identify the characteristics of successful, or at least normative, development. Some theorists parted with the mechanistic view of human behavior in favor of an organismic approach. That is, human beings are not acted upon by their environments, and they are not receivers of influence and knowledge; rather, they are active organisms that construct their understanding of the world through interactions with their environments. Piaget (1950), Bronfenbrenner (1979), Vygotsky (1978), and Sameroff (1983) among others began to emphasize the importance of the relationship between individuals and their environments in shaping development. That is, they argued the nature–nurture debate was artificial; however, research methods to capture such a relationship were still in development.

### THE IMPACT OF ENVIRONMENTALISM

Regardless, from the 1950s through the 1970s, the study of children was marked by "rampant environmentalism" (Rutter 2002). The importance of environmental influences, especially during early childhood, appealed to the American democratic belief that given equal opportunity, any one can and should succeed. Nurture mattered more than nature, or at the very least, nurture had the potential to either ensure healthy development or to derail it. Given the "right" environment and the "right experiences," children would thrive.

As a result, many of the social programs begun in the 1960s, such as Head Start, sought to level the playing field for disadvantaged children, a means of both optimizing developmental potential and preventing the social and psychological disorders associated with poverty. At the same time, the study of risk emerged in an effort to identify the harmful environmental factors that can undermine promise. A corollary to the risk findings was the identification of factors that seem to protect children from risk, especially those who were members of the underclass and/or had parents with serious psychopathology (e.g., Anthony 1974, Bleuler 1978, Murphy & Moriarty 1976, Rutter 1979, Werner & Smith 1982). Which children did well despite a less-than-optimal environment, and why? Some of these ground-breaking studies will be discussed in more detail later in this chapter.

There are two points to make regarding the place of this body of work in the history of the psychology of adaptation. First, resilience in the face of adversity is more common than previous theories would lead us to believe. Resilient children are not so much invincible or invulnerable as they are developmentally normal. Research tells us that children with healthy attachments to at least one parental figure, and who exhibit good social and cognitive skills, manage to avoid serious social and psychological pathology at worst and to become competent adults at best despite expectations to the contrary (Masten & Coatsworth 1998).

Second, theories of development that sought to explain the transactional relationship between na-

ture and nurture informed the design and interpretation of the later studies on resilience that have led to the first point. Consequently, while the research methods used in these later studies are more complex, they have also deepened our appreciation for the remarkable ordinariness of the phenomena known as resilience (Masten 2001).

# The Classic Studies of Resilience

Let us review our working definition: Resilience is characterized by "good outcomes in spite of serious threats to adaptation or development" (Masten 2001). Findings on "good outcomes" from studies of three populations are presented below: children of the underclass in and around London and the Isle of Wight, youth in the American urban ghetto, and poor rural children on Kuaui Island, Hawaii.

## *England: The Isle of Wight*

Michael Rutter, a noted British psychiatrist, and his colleagues conducted a series of studies of families in inner London and on the Isle of Wight near London during the late 1960s and early 1970s (Rutter 1979). The researchers sought to identify risk factors associated with an increased incidence of psychiatric disorders in youth in an effort to predict and possibly prevent such pathology. Six factors were identified:

1. Discord in the marital/parental relationship
2. Low socioeconomic status
3. A large family crowded into small quarters
4. Parental disorder (e.g., a father in jail)
5. Parental disorder (e.g., a mother with psychiatric diagnoses)
6. The intervention of government social service agencies, leading to removal of the

child from the home and placement in foster care

Rutter and his colleagues also noted two additional findings. First, the effect of these risk factors was not additive, but multiplicative. That is, having two risk factors was not twice the risk of having one; each additional factor multiplied the risk by as much as a factor of 10 (depending on the data analysis techniques used). Risk begat and compounded risk. For example, a father in jail may contribute to low socioeconomic status and/or social services interventions. Second, the researchers noted that some children did not exhibit the expected psychological and behavioral disorders given their "at-risk" status. Factors that seemed to buffer or protect children became known as the *triad of protective categories:*

1. Positive personality in the child

2. A supportive family

3. Support for the child's development from at least one community agency, such as school or church group

Furthermore, Rutter and his colleagues noted that gender played a role, with girls being either less vulnerable to risk or better protected from it than boys—or both.

## The American Urban Ghetto

During the 1970s, Garmezy (1981) conducted a literature survey to examine evidence for competence in black youth in American urban ghettos and other adverse circumstances. "Competent" youth were those who did not evidence disorder, such as criminal activity or psychological problems. Moreover, "competent" youth were psychologically and socially healthy, effectively negotiating difficult environments. The triad of categories noted by Rutter in the Isle of Wight studies appeared again, but breadth of the literature review yielded a deeper understanding of the processes underlying resilience. They were: "dispositional attributes [of the child], family cohe-

sion and warmth, and support figures available in the environment" (Garmezy 1985, p. 220).

### CHARACTERISTICS OF THE CHILD

In Garmezy's review, Rutter's resilient "positive personality" emerged as social competence. Competent children were friendly, easygoing, and had a positive sense of self. Teachers reported they exhibited good social skills with peers and adults, were cooperative and responsive, and participated in the classroom milieu. They were less aggressive and sullen, with good impulse control. They had effective intellectual functioning, had good problem-solving skills, could read well, and were thoughtful. In contrast, children who exhibited problems were uncooperative with peers and adults, were not engaged in learning, and had poor impulse control (Garmezy 1981, 1983).

### CHARACTERISTICS OF THE FAMILY

Garmezy and his colleagues found that in a "supportive family," parents were authority figures who were warm but firm. The boundary between parent and child was well drawn. Parents made expectations for behavior clear and fostered self-direction and personal responsibility in their children. The physical household was relatively neat and clean; children were expected to do chores; and day-to-day life was structured around work, school, family meals, and other activities. Parents were invested in their child's education; participated in school events; made sure homework was completed; and kept reading material in the home, such as books, newspapers and so on. A strong competent mother could compensate for the absence of a father (Garmezy 1981, 1983).

In contrast, Garmezy's review (Garmezy 1981, 1983) revealed that the family milieu for children who were not competent was far less supportive. Households lacked structure in the organization of day-to-day life. Boundaries were not clear, and thus roles, relationships, and expectations lacked clarity and direction as well. Parents were not the head of their households but related to their children as peers and/or were inconsistent in their parenting.

## CHARACTERISTICS OF THE COMMUNITY

The review by Garmezy and his research team also revealed that competent black children in the American urban ghetto were connected to some other institution in their community, most often school or church. There, these children found at least one adult outside of their families who was invested in them and whom the children could emulate. This person could be a teacher, a coach, a youth group leader, or a minister. For children without a father at home, the presence of a competent man in their lives was especially important, for girls and boys alike (Garmezy 1981, 1983).

# The Children of Kauai

Concerns about the children of Kauai, the garden island of Hawaii, initiated a public health study by psychologists Werner and Smith in collaboration with health care providers. The physical isolation and poverty of the island meant that pregnant women did not receive adequate prenatal care, which increased the incidence of premature births and subsequent special needs among infants and young children born to families already at risk. Beginning in 1955, the research team followed a cohort of 700 infants until the age of 40 (Werner & Smith 1977, 1982, 2001). The findings have fascinated researchers.

First, the same triad of protective factors emerged in the resilient children:

*"dispositional attributes of the child that elicit predominantly positive responses from the environment, such as physical robustness and vigor, an easy temperament, and intelligence; affectional ties and socialization practices within the family that encourage trust, autonomy, and initiative; and external support systems that reinforce competence and provide children with a positive set of values." (Werner 1990)*

Second, over time, it became apparent that resilience was more common than expected. Children have "self-righting tendencies that move [them] toward normal development under all but the most persistent adverse circumstances" (Werner 1990). The researchers did not mean that children are "naturally" resilient; rather, their point is that children have a tendency to draw from available resources along their developmental trajectory. For example, if a parent is not able to provide a warm caring relationship, then children will be drawn to other adults who will fulfill this need—provided such adults are available to them.

Although some of the children originally identified as "at risk" did demonstrate some deviant patterns of behavior during their teen years, many developed into relatively competent adults. In retrospect, the nature of their deviance distinguished them from those at-risk youth who did not become competent adults. As at-risk youth, the competent adults engaged in crimes against property, such as vandalism and petty theft, but they were not repeat offenders. Incompetent adults had engaged in crimes against people as at-risk youth, such as assault and battery, and recidivism rates were higher. Although teen pregnancy was not uncommon in either group, the resilient young women completed their education and had jobs—a pattern of competence they saw in their own mothers (Werner 1989).

By the age of 40, most of the troubled high-risk youth were generative adults. They had stable marriages and were active in a faith community. They had taken advantage of opportunities to develop job skills through military service and/or technical colleges. The researchers do not deny that many of the study cohort experienced the kind of difficulties that had been anticipated as a consequence of a difficult childhood. Their resilience was best recognized in retrospect: despite adversity, most were living relatively normal lives as adults (Werner & Smith 2001).

## Summary of Studies

Resilient children are often described as having a positive temperament (Rutter 1979), as friendly, cooperative, well-liked, emotionally stable (Garmezy 1983, 1985), active, socially responsive (Werner & Smith 1982), competent (Bleuler 1978), and more advanced in communication and self-help skills (Werner 1989). Adult authority figures—parents, teachers, older siblings, and so on—like these kind of children and youth and respond to them in a positive manner. This helps to create a bidirectional relationship between child and adult, characterized by warmth and support that promotes the child's development.

Table 4.1 lists the most commonly found protective factors that contribute to resilience in these and other studies. In summary, the research suggests that relationships with caring adults and effective intellectual functioning can mediate children's exposure to the risks inherent in poverty and family dysfunction. The definition of resilience as "good outcomes" despite "threats to adaptation or development" (Masten 2001) captures the obvious while underscoring the complexity of the construct. The key terms—"good outcomes," "threat," "adaptation," and "development"—have been the focus of investigation in psychology for years. A theoretical framework for how these apply to resilience is presented next.

## The Life Span Perspective

Earlier theories in psychology, such as Freud and Piaget, focused on childhood development, ending with puberty and adolescence. By comparison, the life span perspective recognizes that the potential for growth and change continues throughout life. Although most students of human development know Erikson's (1950) life stages, the life span perspective is both broader and deeper than a cursory familiarity with his sequential model can convey. (See Chapter 3 in this volume for an excellent theoretical overview.) Some key concepts of the lifespan perspective follow.

- *Human beings are active organisms* that give form to the meaning of their experience, through their interactions with the environment (White 1976); that is, they construct their understanding of themselves in the world.

- *Development occurs in the context of a person's relationship with the social ecosystem* (Bronfenbrenner 1979), which can be represented by expanding concentric rings of influence, centered around the individual: immediate family (microsystem); immediate community of peers, school, and work (mesosystem); the larger social structures of society (exosystem); and finally culture and history (macrosystem). Biology plays a role as well. Individuals bring their own unique genetic/biological makeup to their relationship with the ecosystem; the physical environment contributes air, water, food, and shelter.

- *The relationship between the individual and the ecosystem is characterized by reciprocal transactions;* that is, people shape their environments and vice versa (Lerner 1982, 1986; Sameroff 1975).

- *Development co-occurs within individuals, and between them and their ecosystems over time* (Lerner 1986). Within-individual processes of development include, but are not limited to, behavioral self-regulation; emotional, intellectual, and relational functioning; and sense of self. Between-systems processes, such as parenting, address the goodness-of-fit between individuals and systems (Chess & Thomas 1977, Lerner & Lerner 1983).

- *Time matters.* There appear to be sensitive periods for optimal development in any one individual in selected areas, such as

*Table 4.1*   Protective Factors Across Ecosystemic Levels

**INDIVIDUAL FACTORS**

Active, easy, outgoing temperament
Reflectiveness
Positive responsiveness to others
Appealing to adults
Sense of humor
High intelligence
Problem-solving skills
Emotional regulation
Verbal/communication skills
Realistic appraisal of the environment
Self-efficacy
Self-worth
Hopefulness
Recognized talents/accomplishments
Trust in people as resources
Social skills
Competence in normative roles
Empathy
Self-confidence
Strong, positive ethnic identity
Faith/religious affiliation
Religious participation
Educational aspirations/school commitment
Sense of direction or purpose

**FAMILY FACTORS**

Competent parent(s)
  Model competent behavior
  Provide access to knowledge
  Resilience
  Self-efficacy
Authoritative parenting style
Interpersonal warmth
Noncritical
Value children's accomplishments
High but realistic expectations of child

Educational attainment
Reading to children
Involved in schools
Connections to other competent adults
Family cohesion
Socioeconomic advantages
Religious faith/affiliation/participation
Marital harmony
Children have family/household duties

**COMMUNITY FACTORS**

Adequate resources for child care, nutrition, health care
Good schools
  Clear rules
  Effective curricula/teaching/counseling
  Focus on instilling self-esteem, personal responsibility, goal setting, clear communication, problem-solving
  Collaboration between family & school
  Free lunches
  Mentoring initiatives
  Rites of passage programs
Sense of community
Community well-being, stability, cohesiveness
Availability of prosocial role models, norms, values
Supportive friends, neighbors
Employment opportunities
Opportunities for belonging & meaningful involvement in prosocial school, sports, religious, community activities
Well-delineated community

**CULTURE/ETHNIC IDENTITY**

Strong, positive ethnic identity
Resistance to oppression/ethnic activism
Identification with traditional beliefs/values
Participation in traditional practices
Racial/ethnic socialization

attachment to caregivers (see Chapter 10) and language (see Chapter 9). Timing matters in the historical sense; members of cohorts born in the 1920s versus the 1950s grew up with different resources and expectations (Elder 1995). Finally, timing matters for individual development. Important transitions and events occur at points in time in a person's life, re-shaping that person's developmental trajectory and potentially the trajectory of generations to follow (Bronfenbrenner & Ceci 1994).

- *The development of any one person is best understood in terms of its organization,* given that the course of human development is actively embedded within an ecosystem of multiple levels of influence and dynamic transactions that occur concurrently within and between individuals and systems, and in the context of history and over time (Lerner et al. 1998).

In the life span perspective of human development, the individual and environment are intricately integrated with one another, forming an organized whole. Given the complexity of the whole, we can see that the influence of any one key variable within the whole is insufficient by itself to be the major contributor to development or predictor of a developmental trajectory (Wachs 2000). The important issue is how it all works together. In developmental psychology, we look to processes and systems to understand the workings of human development.

### EXAMPLE OF RECIPROCAL TRANSACTIONS

For example, consider the role of difficult temperament in child development (Chess & Thomas 1977), usually associated with irritability, resistance to being held and comforted, and irregularities in sleeping and eating. In the Isle of Wight studies, Rutter found that the difficult child is more difficult in a family stressed by poverty and is thus more likely to be a target of parental hostility, which in turn places the child at increased risk for psychiatric disorder and difficulties in school and with peers (Rutter 1985). Although it is fair to ask how much of a child's "difficultness" is inherent in the child's biological make-up and how much in the parent's appraisal of and response to the child's behavior (Sameroff et al. 1982), the issue is the consequences of the fit between them (Lerner & Lerner 1983) *in context of the organization of development across time* (Lerner et al. 1998).

The difficult child elicits different responses from adults than does the easygoing child, which in turn shapes a child's relationships with those adults and may—or may not—further foster the child's easy or difficult behavior through self-fulfilling expectations for interactions over time. When mothers and fathers learn to parent a difficult child, or the child is buffered from parental hostility by an older sibling, or a day care worker is effective in helping the child to develop self-regulation, the organization of the child's development is structured anew. The difficult child can make even competent parents feel inadequate, and, conversely, the easygoing child can make even dysfunctional parents feel successful. In the latter case, this may soothe the rough edges in a "difficult" home enough to enable the child to make good use of whatever effective parenting is available, or even contribute to more effective parenting.

### THE DEVELOPMENTAL TRAJECTORY

In any case, the life span perspective recognizes that being difficult or easy is not the point. Easygoing temperament is only one, albeit complex, variable, an apparently necessary contributor to resilience, but certainly not sufficient to explain eventual outcomes in any one child (Wachs 2000). Rather, an easygoing nature can be an indicator for an essential developmental system, that is, *relationships with others over time.* Of real interest are the potential implications of the temperamental fit between child and parent for the trajectory of the child's development, the parent's development, and the development of their relationship as a model for future relationships within and beyond the family.

## Resilience in Context over Time: Nature versus Nurture Revisited

Let us revisit our working definition of resilience in the context of the framework of developmental contextualism: "good outcomes in spite of serious threats to adaptation or development" (Masten

2001). Based on the previous discussion of the life span perspective, let us be clear what resilience is *not*.

The term "good outcomes" seems to imply an antecedent "good input." This would reduce the construct of resilience to one or the other side of the nature–nurture debate. For example, a child's "positive personality" could be attributed to either inherited characteristics of the child or to the causal affects from external agents, such as parents and/or community members. Similarly, "serious threat" implies that a discrete event results in disorder. It would be a mistake to draw such conclusions from the above definition and from the research.

## RESILIENCE IS NOT A CHARACTER TRAIT

To conclude that resilience lies within the individual implies either an innate individual difference and/or that resilient individuals are able to pull themselves up by the bootstraps. While rugged individualism appeals to the American ideology, resilience is not intrinsic hardiness (Kobasa 1987), which refers to characteristics inherent in the person that buffer stress, such as positive outlook. The research suggests that early references to children as "invulnerable" and "invincible" were misleading. The evidence does not support the belief that individual development unfolds along its own unique course untouched by events, referred to as the "ontogenetic fallacy." This fails to consider how development is shaped by reciprocal transactions with the environment over time. Moreover, it implies that the environment is something to overcome, which relieves the ecosystem of family, community, and society from responsibility for individual development (Waller 2001). Consequently, those who do not overcome may be considered failures.

## RESILIENCE IS NOT THE "RIGHT" ENVIRONMENT

To conclude that the "right environment" produces the "healthy child," or conversely the "wrong environment" produces a "disordered child," reduces development in general and resilience in particular to a linear causal model that ignores how individual differences can affect the larger ecosystem (Super & Harkness 1986) and the role of timing of events for both the individual and those in the environment (Bronfenbrenner & Ceci 1994). For example, a small cohort of easy-going cooperative and inquisitive children can have a positive affect on the classroom milieu, influencing the effectiveness of the novice teacher. A linear causal model begs the question of which came first, a positive personality in the child or a warm and supportive family, a positive classroom milieu or effective teaching (Masten & Coatsworth 1998)? Clearly, the answer is neither one nor the other, and not even simply "both." The answer is best understood *in context over time*.

## RESILIENCE IS NOT CAUSE AND EFFECT

The linear causal model of "good input" leads to "good outcomes" ignores the factors in between. These include the co-occurrence of multiple contexts, events, and influences in a child's life, which have indirect, direct, and combined effects on outcomes (Masten 2001, Rutter 2002, Waller 2001). In addition, positive connections with the community may make up for a less-than-optimal family situation (Brody et al. 2002). What happens *in the relationship* among children, parents, other adults, and peers, individually and as groups, to shape the developmental trajectory? We will discuss some key processes shortly.

## RESILIENCE IS DYNAMIC

We see that "good outcomes" are not something a person "has," or "does," or is "given." Rather, resilience is something that a person can "be" at a point in time and under certain circumstances. "Being" is dynamic and implies change over time; it is not a fixed trait. As the children of Kauai indicate, a troubled teenager can still grow up to be a resilient adult. "Point in time" and "circumstances" matter; in fact, without "threatening" circumstances, good outcomes alone would not constitute resilience.

# Good Outcomes: The Meaning of Competence

Given the possibly misleading implication that "good outcomes" could arise from "good input," and our appreciation for context and time, let us replace Masten's 2001 definition of resilience we have been using with one she proposed earlier with a colleague: Resilience *"generally refers to manifested competence in the context of significant challenges to adaptation or development"* (Masten & Coatsworth 1998). By competence, they mean

*a pattern of effective adaptation in the environment, either broadly defined in terms of reasonable success with major developmental tasks expected for a person of his or her culture, society and time, or more narrowly defined in terms of specific domains of achievement, such as academics, peer acceptance, or athletics. It carries the dual meaning that there is a track record of such achievement (competent performance) and also that the individual has the capability to perform well in the future. It refers to good adaptation and not necessarily to superb achievement (Masten & Coatsworth 1998).*

Competence, like resilience, is not a fixed trait. It develops and changes over time within several domains of development. These domains include physiological, psychological, social, and intellectual functioning across the life span. Twenty years of research by many investigators provides valuable insight for how we know that a child is "doing well" and what it means when he or she is not (Garmezy et al. 1984, Garmezy & Tellegen 1984, Masten & Garmezy 1985).

## Meeting Expectations

We say that someone has adapted well when he or she exhibits characteristics and behaviors associated with the accepted and expected norms for competent behavior in a reference group (Masten & Coatsworth 1998), such as a culture, a community, or a family. Expectations within the reference group are linked to children's achievement of developmental tasks (Havighurst 1972). For example, all cultures expect young children to develop close relationships with caregivers. However, as Lerner and Ashman point out in Chapter 3, the expectations of Western and Asian parents in this regard are different.

Differences also can be attributed to education, social and economic status, religious practices, as well as family and social history. Sometimes expectations may change within a single family in a culture at a point in historical time. For example, expectations for two sisters in Afghanistan changed after the fall of the Taliban. An older teenage sister, who had been restricted to the family home and denied schooling and socialization outside of the family, awaited an arranged marriage. She watched with some bitterness as her younger sister attended school, visited with friends, and talked about her future. The older sister had adapted to a set of norms that may no longer apply to the younger one (Dominus 2002).

The expectations for developmental tasks common among American parents include schooling, peer relationships, moral behavior, sense of self, and transitioning to adult roles (see Table 4.2). The competencies most associated with resilience are related to these tasks, including relationships with caregivers, self-regulation, social behavior, academic achievement, and sense of self. In the following discussion, we examine the developmental processes underlying these tasks.

## Attachment and Relationships with Early Caregivers

In Chapter 10, McCartney and O'Connor provide an excellent overview of the development of attachment between child and caregiver, as well as disorders of attachment. In most research, the caregiver of study has been the mother, although the evidence indicates that infants and toddlers form attachments with fathers, siblings, and others who interact with the child on a regular basis.

*Table 4.2*    Examples of Developmental Tasks

| Age Period | Task |
| --- | --- |
| Infancy to preschool | Attachment to caregiver(s) |
| | Language |
| | Differentiation of self from environment |
| | Self-control and compliance |
| Middle childhood | School adjustment (attendance, appropriate conduct) |
| | Academic achievement (e.g., learning to read, do arithmetic) |
| | Getting along with peers (acceptance, making friends) |
| | Rule-governed conduct (following rules of society for moral behavior and prosocial conduct) |
| Adolescence | Successful transition to secondary schooling |
| | Academic achievement (learning skills needed for higher education or work) |
| | Involvement in extracurricular activities (e.g., athletics, clubs) |
| | Forming close friendships within and across gender |
| | Forming a cohesive sense of self: identity |

Attachment develops during the first three or so years of life. The nature of the organization of the attachment system is remarkably robust over time and can be categorized as secure, anxious, avoidant, and disordered.

In secure attachment, children come to rely on a mother's ability to meet their needs with some consistency and effectiveness. This is referred to as "maternal sensitivity"; that is, the mother reads the child's moods, intentions, and cues and responds appropriately. Free from the anxiety that can result from unmet needs and inconsistency in interactions, children can explore the environment and learn to regulate their own behavior, with some assurance that the mother is "there" for them if needed. The attachment system creates a working model for how relationships work that has implications across the life span.

**EXAMPLES OF THE ATTACHMENT SYSTEM**

Toddlers with secure attachments have healthier relationships with peers later in middle childhood (Sroufe 1979, 1996). Securely attached mothers are more likely to raise securely attached daughters (Ricks 1985). Mothers who grow up making use of environmental and interpersonal resources make better choices in marriage and work, achieve a sense of mastery, and serve as models for their daughters (Moen & Erickson 1995). Recall in the Kauai studies of resilient children that the teenage girls who became pregnant and were later found to be resilient had competent mothers. The developmental trajectory of the daughter began in the developmental history of the mother.

## Self-Regulation

Plato noted that to be truly free, children needed to establish, with help from adults, "a constitutional government within them" (Hamilton & Cairns 1961). Freud used the term *superego* to connote the societal rules that children internalize during the preschool years, otherwise known as a conscience (Freud 1930/1961). In theories of social cognition, self-regulation refers to the ability to read social cues and adjust behavior accordingly. In cognitive development, self-regulation is a means to fulfilling innate interests in exploring the environment and problem solving (Bronson 2000).

## EXAMPLES OF THE SELF-REGULATORY SYSTEM

Infants learn to self-regulate in response to parental sensitivity in the attachment system, for example, quieting when soothed, held, or fed. Toddler's deal with negative emotions (e.g., frustration) as well as with socially sanctioned behaviors (e.g., waiting) through transactions with parents, older siblings, and others. Parents distract them with a toy, hold them to limit squirming, whisper reminders to "be quiet, we don't talk in church," and so on. Toddlers may talk to themselves as they internalize parental directives: "no no don't touch hot." Vygotsky (1978) believed that the development of language is key to self-regulation because it signifies that the child thinks and behaves in culturally appropriated ways.

As children enter the preschool years, they read verbal and nonverbal cues from authority figures and peers to regulate their behavior, as theories of social cognition suggest. Cues tell them to take turns, share, wait, be nice, calm down, and "it's OK." At the same time, prosocial behaviors emerge, when children can choose to do the "right" thing to benefit someone other than themselves. As children regulate their attention, they are able to learn (Bronson 2000).

During the school years, self-regulation is a good predictor of adjustment in the face of adversity and a moderator of risk and adaptation. Children with poor self-regulation are *more* vulnerable to multiple risks; that is, they evidence more negative emotion and behavior than do children with effective self-regulation who are exposed to the same multiple risks. For the latter children, their ability to control their behavior and emotions protects them, enabling them to behave in ways expected for their age and cohort; that is, they can adapt reasonably well (Lengua 2002).

## PARENTING AND THE SELF-REGULATORY SYSTEM

Thus far, we can see that self-regulation is a complex developmental system, which involves motivation, emotion, cognition, and prosocial behavior, as well as attachment and parenting. Parents who are warm and responsive but firm, convey clear expectations for children's self-regulating behavior, and shape that behavior through a range of verbal and nonverbal coaching and daily routines are referred to as being *authoritative*. *Authoritarian* parents, by contrast, are more controlling, less able to trust a child's self-regulatory system, but can be warm with high expectations. *Permissive* parents are inconsistent in their parenting, and *neglectful* parents are unresponsive to children's needs and development (Baumrind 1978). Whereas authoritative parenting is optimal by American standards, authoritarian parenting may be more effective in other cultures and in dangerous environments (Masten & Coatsworth 1998).

Recall that in Garmezy's studies of competent youth, the resilient children were described as responsive to adult directives at school. At home, the parents were responsive authority figures, and family life was structured around the routines of meals, school, work, and chores. In other words, these children had learned to regulate their behavior in developmentally appropriate ways. However, a supportive and structured classroom milieu can promote self-regulation in children whose family life is not optimal—an example of how community members serve a protective role for children at risk (Brody et al. 2002).

## Social Competence

How children get along with other children provides insight into how well they are doing in general. In school-aged children, social competence with peers has been associated with healthy family relationships, intellectual functioning, and academic achievement, whereas children who are rejected by peers are more likely to be disruptive, do less well academically, and have a history of poor parenting (Hartup 1983; Masten & Coatsworth 1995, 1998). Tolerance of aggressive behaviors among peers varies by intent and consequences, although aggression that arises from misreading socially accepted cues or inappropriate self-regulation is more likely to meet with rejection (Dodge 1986). Thus, healthy peer relationships and appropriate social conduct are good predictors of later competence in school and of better mental health (Masten & Coatsworth 1995).

### CHILDREN CHOOSE THEIR INFLUENCES

Children influence their development by making their own choices, and they are not always good ones. Peers tend to seek out their own kind. That is, competent children tend to be friends with other competent children, and antisocial children tend to form relationships with other antisocial children, which may reinforce mutual acceptance for negative behavior (Coie & Dodge 1998). Thus, peers may expose a child to greater risk or serve a protective function in adverse circumstances. Rule-bound behavior in school and the community serves the greater good, so that children who conduct themselves in acceptable fashion are also more likely to win approval and support from adults and to develop a sense of belonging to the larger group (Masten & Coatsworth 1998).

Although the quality of family life can predict the nature of children's friendships and role in the community, the life span perspective and developmental contextualism caution against overstating the case. As relationships with caregivers, parents, siblings, peers, the school, and community expands, and the complexity of their interrelatedness becomes hierarchically integrated over time, the range of variables that shape that child's developmental trajectory increases (Waller 2001). Families evolve and change, so that risk and protective factors can vary for different children within the same family (Patterson 2002). Even when risk and resource factors are similar, individual differences in children's intellectual ability, interests, motivation, and physical health may

cause siblings to be exposed to different people and to make different choices (Rutter 2002). Community events will affect these choices differentially as well, which is discussed later when we address how time matters.

## Academic Achievement

Doing well in school can be measured by grades, participation in extracurricular activities, appropriate conduct, and relationships with peers and teachers. Individual differences in innate cognitive ability, especially IQ, motivation, ability to regulate behavior and attention, and social skills influence how well a child does. For example, motivated adolescents from low income backgrounds who set goals for themselves are more likely to be resilient than those who do not, in part because of the focused effort working toward the goals entails (Rouse 2001). IQ is highly correlated with academic achievement, and both are related to parental contributions through genetics and environment (Neisser et al. 1996). Although IQ is a good indicator of academic aptitude, talent and interest in music, art, athletics, and related activities also engage children and adolescents in school.

### THE ROLE OF PARENTS

Parents who are themselves well educated and/or who value education are more likely to provide an enriched environment at home, through books, discussion, and involvement in their child's education (e.g., attention to homework and other school activities) (Masten & Coatsworth 1998). Maternal education in particular has been linked to better outcomes in children in the resilience studies noted earlier (e.g., Werner & Smith 1982) and in studies of children with chronic illness (e.g.,Wallander & Varni 1992). Better-educated mothers make choices in life that optimize resources for their children (Moen & Erickson 1995), and value education for their children as well.

## THE ROLE OF PEERS AND SCHOOL ENVIRONMENT

Peers may play a role as risk or protective factors in children's academic competence by influencing attitudes about and behaviors related to doing well academically. Children who do well in school are more likely to stay in school, which leads to better-paying jobs and more stability and resources. Children who do poorly are more likely to evidence behavior problems and to drop out (Masten & Coatsworth 1995). School environments that are clear about their educational mission and attend to the teaching–learning environment and student progress foster academic competence (Masten & Coatsworth 1998).

Recall that in Garmezy's work on competent black youth cited earlier (Garmezy 1981, 1983), resilient children were described by teachers as being academically bright, good readers and problem-solvers, cooperative, and engaged in learning. There were books in the home, and parents ensured homework was done. Children who are engaged in school, either through academics and/or extracurricular activities, spend time with competent well-educated adults who help young people set goals and strategies, get organized, and work hard. Sometimes a particular talent or interest may protect children from adversity by bringing them to the attention of adult mentors at school or in the community.

## *Discussion of Competence*

We can see that doing well in school, or at least being engaged in school activities, is an indicator for the organization of several developmental systems and processes, including self-regulation, parenting, social relationships, and cognitive abilities. Not surprisingly, children's performance in these areas contributes to their sense of mastery and sense of self. Self becomes more complex as children develop, integrating multiple domains of competence (e.g., intellectual, physical, and social) as children evaluate themselves against their own expectations and those of the environment (Harter 1999).

Sense of self and mastery should not be confused with self-esteem, which was once described by William James as "self-esteem = success/pretense" that is, success divided by pretense (James 1890). By success, James meant authenticity, being real. Real mastery is hard won and is undermined by superficial affectations of achievement. Self-esteem is rarely mentioned in the resilience literature. In Garmezy's work on competent youth in the American ghetto, the "positive sense of self" he found is related to competence and mastery. They had good social skills, were self-regulating, and had effective intellectual functioning that contributed to academic competence, such as problem-solving skills and reading. It could be argued that self-esteem is a result of competence and mastery and that efforts toward building self-esteem should be directed toward achievement of real results (Garmezy 1981, 1983).

Children need not be academic stars, nor do they need model parents to be considered competent. Rather, the organization of children's relationship with their environment has to be good enough that children can take advantage of emotional, intellectual, and material resources and stay the course of normal development. In the case of resilient children, "it appears that competence develops in the midst of adversity when, despite the situation at hand, fundamental systems that generally foster competence in development are operating to protect the child or counter the threats to development" (Masten & Coatsworth 1998).

What separates resilient children from those who are not, given the same highly adverse circumstances, is that resilient children are competent and have more resources. Competent children are more like each other regardless of their exposure to adversity. The difference is that those exposed to high adversity need the resources that contribute to competence more than do children who experience less adversity in their lives. The child who is high in adversity but low in resources and competence is most likely to demonstrate disordered behavior (Masten 2001).

# The Meaning of Threats to Adaptation

As noted earlier, without risk there is no resilience. Without threats to adaptive processes—such as attachment, parenting, self-regulation, cognitive abilities, and so on—children are not prompted to exercise self-righting tendencies. Over the past 20 years, our understanding of threat has evolved and become more complex, as have theories of coping and adaptation.

## Coping versus Adaptation

Early models of risk, like early models of development, were characterized by environmentalism: more stressful life events led to worse outcomes (Holmes & Rahe 1967). This causal linear presumption changed when Lazarus and Folkman (1984) defined stress as a "relationship between the person and environment that is appraised by the person as taxing or exceeding his or her resources and endangering his or her well-being." They introduced cognitive appraisal as the process by which meaning is assigned to the relationship between person and environment, and coping as the process through which the person manages stressful demands. The study of coping has been individual focused and situation dependent, which limits the temporal dimensions of the outcomes to circumscribed circumstances. That is, what works today and in this situation may not work at other times.

The relationship between coping today and adaptation over the long term, between type of coping and type of outcome, whether positive or negative, is a new area of research (Folkman & Moskowitz 2000, Somerfield & McCrae 2000). Capturing the relationship between person and environment over time has been difficult in coping research, however. Theory-based research on coping has focused almost entirely on adults and with only a few exceptions (e.g., Spirito et al. 1992, Thies & Walsh 1999) lacks a developmental perspective for change over time.

## On the Nature of Adverse Events

Adversity is not unidimensional. Theories of coping have acknowledged the importance of appraising the meaning of events for individuals, but the implications of the nature and timing of events for proximal and distal affects in development have received less notice. Concurrent events in the ecosystem matter, including family, peer cohort, and the larger society, as well as the availability of resources relative to the timing of the event (Rutter 2002, Rutter et al. 1995).

### EXAMPLE OF NATURE AND MEANING OF EVENTS

Death of a parent is a significant life event that is experienced in qualitatively different ways by 3 year olds and teenagers. The distal affects are different if the toddler is placed in successive foster homes than if she is raised by the surviving parent—unless the foster home provides more stability than the mother. The quality of the relationship between the deceased father and teenager who is about to go to college, and between the teen and surviving mother, as well as how the father died—suicide, accident, long-term debilitating illness—will shape the teen's proximal experience of the death—horror, shock, sadness with relief—as well as his transition to young adulthood. Also, the death may destabilize the family financially.

Let us take the example of the newly bereaved teenager further into the ecosystem and in social and historical time. The responsiveness of the teen's new peers to his loss will affect his assimilation into that group, either increasing risk in the face of loss or providing protection. However, as the new peers are also experiencing a life transition, their own adaptive processes and life history will temper their responsiveness. Major events in society will affect their transitions individually and collectively. For example, December 7, 1941, was a defining moment for an entire generation of young men, but it affected each of them differently.

What events are independent of or dependent on the teen's loss? Both the attack on Pearl Harbor and entering college occurred independently of the father's death, whereas family financial hardship and peer responsiveness to the teen's loss are distal consequences of it. The bereaved teenager is at greater risk for finding both the transition to college and the start of World War II more stressful than his peers because of the context of his loss (Rutter et al. 1995).

Nevertheless, his entire cohort will have their life trajectory shaped by service in World War II—for better or worse (Elder 1995, Vaillant 1977). As college students, they were more likely to become officers than peers who had entered the workforce after high school, including their own brothers before and after them. We can see there are gradients of risk to the newly bereaved teenager (Rutter 2002) and profound differences in the meaning and implications of the same event within any one cohort and family.

## Stress versus Risk and Adversity

It is apparent that in comparison to coping, adaptation is a much broader Darwinian construct, understood in the contexts of accepted and expected group norms and of the individual as a dynamic organism in the ecosystem over time. Risk and adversity also are broader in scope than stress, implying not discrete events but sustained circumstances that undermine the adaptive processes that shape growth and development over time. If lack of disorder can be characterized by competence, as suggested by Masten and Coatsworth (1998), the differences between short-term coping and ongoing adaptation may become clearer.

### EXAMPLE OF COPING VERSUS ADAPTATION IN ADVERSE CIRCUMSTANCES

Let us continue with the example of the bereaved 3 year old: her single mother has died and she is living with her grandmother who places the child in day care while she works. At separation, the child may cope by crying and clinging to the grandmother, but when the behavior continues after several weeks, we will say she has not begun to adapt as expected. To say she is "not coping well" distracts us from what the child is *not* doing: developing age-normative relationships with peers and teachers (e.g., playing cooperatively, responding positively to adult direction). The adverse circumstance is *not* attending day care (unless the day care situation is suboptimal); it is the distal implications of the mother's death on consistency in caregiving relationships for her daughter (Sameroff & Chandler 1975).

Adversity is not an acute single event. It is the accrual of multiple small interactions between a person and environment, a relationship that has both a history and a trajectory, that form a pattern of expectations regarding how the world works, a pattern that is either at odds with expectations for normative development or makes meeting normal expectations more difficult. Adversity is when psychological and social problems render caretakers inappropriately responsive to their child's needs for food, warmth, comfort, and other attachment-enhancing interactions. Adverse poverty is not simply a lack of money and resources; it is an indicator for social and psychological disorganization at odds with the developmental processes—attachment, self-regulation, parenting, and so on—that enable children to develop competence.

We need more information about the previous and current caregiving circumstances to determine how much at risk the motherless 3 year old may be. The death of a deviant mother followed by placement with a competent grandmother may place this child on a healthier developmental path, but she will still grieve for her mother. On the other hand, if the grandmother is either deviant or overwhelmed by other issues, the mother's death may compound the child's risk status.

# Individual Differences in Adaptation and Risk

Clearly, indicators of serious risk include 1) persistent family discord, especially if a child is the target of hostility; 2) inconsistent individualized caregiving over time (e.g., moving among foster homes and relatives); 3) lack of interactions with adults and peers (e.g., being isolated from conversation and play); and 4) a social milieu that promotes maladaptive behaviors (e.g., family, school, or neighborhood) (Rutter 2002). What is less clear is how risk undermines development in different individuals within the same cohort or family.

## Mediators of Individual Differences in the Meaning of Adverse Events

Work on individual differences in response to exposure to environmental risks has begun to shed light on the difference between risk as indicator (i.e., adverse condition) and risk as mechanism (i.e., process). In the previous example of parental death, the timing and circumstances of the death had implications for the child's affiliative processes with surviving parental figures and with peers. Rutter and his colleagues (Rutter et al. 1995) have suggested the following factors as mediators of individual differences in environment risk exposure.

- Geography (e.g., Does the family live in a high crime area? Rural? Urban?)

- Job (e.g., What kind of job does a parent have? How secure is it? Benefits?)

- Income (e.g., Can the family afford housing? Is it in debt?)

- Past experiences (e.g., What experiences do the parents bring to the marriage? What is the history of family and individual events? What was the timing of the same events for different individuals?)

- Family (e.g., Size of family? Mental and physical health of individual members?)

- Social network (e.g., Neighbors, friends, extended family, religious affiliation?)

- Personal (e.g., Physical and emotional problems and their consequences?)

## Example of Mediators of Individual Differences

An example from Bleuler (1978), who studied children of parents with severe mental illness such as schizophrenia, provides an interesting example. The father had left and the mother was in and out of the hospital. The family was somewhat socially isolated by the mother's illness and money was an issue. The oldest sibling, a young teenage girl, assumed the responsibility for running the household. Bleuler and his colleagues had initially felt that this hardship would place her at increased risk for disorder. Instead, she developed a sense of mastery: she was organized, had a role to play, and learned new skills. The younger children came to rely on her, but the brother only a year or so her junior had no clear family role or parental figure and did not fare as well.

This example is somewhat abbreviated, but it underscores a theme throughout this chapter: resilience is best understood in context over time. As Rutter has noted (Rutter et al. 1995), multiple factors working independently and together can make the difference in how effectively children can self-right using available resources. Being the youngest versus the oldest in a troubled family, male or female, the child targeted for hostility or the one with special needs may increase or decrease risk depending on circumstances.

## Biology as Individual Difference

As noted earlier, the role of genetic and physiological aspects of inherited characteristics in development has received less attention over the past century, perhaps because the basic science and research methods had not evolved sufficiently to address the questions. The mapping of the human genome and the field of neurobiology have begun to provide greater insight into human response mechanisms in acute and chronic stress, and into individual variations in particular. That is, some people may be "wired" differently, such as the child with the "difficult" temperament.

Furthermore, research suggests that small doses of manageable stress may exercise the adaptive responses and therefore may even be good for you (McEwen 2002). The stress response is far more sophisticated than a return to homeostasis, as proposed by Hans Selye (McEwen 2002, Selye 1976). "Allostasis" refers to the complex relationship among the brain, nervous system, hormones (especially cortisol), and immune system that allows us to get through a busy day. We need a jolt of cortisol just to get out of bed. The body experiences "allostatic load" not only when its reserves are spent trying to sustain a response to threat; allostatic load also occurs when the reserves are not banked as a matter of course. Sleep deprivation, poor diet, lack of exercise, and so on can create the allostatic load that predisposes to poor health. Chronic stress, and not acute stress, increases risk for allostatic load. That is, whereas healthy children with resources are banking reserves for future use, children faced with chronic physical and psychological stress compounded by poor health habits are drawing down their reserve just to get through the day.

The extent to which individual differences in processing physiological stress are genetically determined is still unclear. Nevertheless, gene–environment interactions can help us to appreciate individual differences in physical and personality development over time. By studying large populations, quantitative geneticists have begun to quantify the relative contribution of genetic and nongenetic factors in individual differences related to normal and abnormal physical and psychological characteristics.

For example, 20–40% of the variance in depression can be accounted for by heritability (Rutter 2002). Similarly, the central nervous system mechanisms underlying the self-regulatory processes that contribute to "difficult" versus "easy" temperament have genetic origins (Rutter 2002). Excessive secretion of cortisol and other stress hormones renders some adolescents at greater risk for depression (Goodyer et al. 2000) and yet seems to enhance performance among Special Forces in the military (Morgan et al. 2001, 2000). That the latter group is self-selected speaks to the issue of people choosing their environment. The real question is, what environmental factors mediate the expression of the gene for cortisol production (Rutter 2002)? What turns which genes on or off, individually and in combination?

Rutter (2002) points out that "adverse environments often have the least impact on those who are not genetically vulnerable and the most impact on the genetically susceptible (p. 3)." In other words, children who are difficult and/or have health or learning problems are at greater risk when the family is chronically stressed by poverty, family discord, and so on. Children who are easygoing, healthy, and intellectually capable are best equipped to draw on and replenish reserves when faced with adversity and will be more resilient.

# The Limits of Resilience and Implications for Health Care

Despite the glowing reports of resilience among children faced with adversity, issues and concerns abound about the cost of adversity to resilient youth and the limits of recovery. Resilient adolescents from high-risk inner city circumstances may do well in school, but they report high levels of anxiety and psychological distress (Luthar et al. 1993). They may be doing better than we expected, but they still have problems.

For children who were adopted into English homes from Romanian orphanages in which they experienced serious deprivation, there was a "dose-response" association between length of institutional rearing and cognitive scores at age 4. That is, those who spent the most time being deprived of early sensitive caretaking had lower scores than children placed earlier in life, and they took longer to reach them (O'Connor et al. 2000). This cohort is still young, and pronouncements about their recovery and resilience are premature. Attachment to caregivers and language are two areas in which the limits of recovery have been investigated (see Chapters 6 and 7).

## Return to the Playroom

Let us return to the playroom scene at the start of this chapter. With the possible exceptions of 15-year-old Emilio and 10-year-old John, none of the children has a long enough track record for judgments about resilience to be made. We were not given enough information about any of them to appreciate their development and adaptation in context over time. We might note that 4-year-old Ben is coping the way young children do: by *doing* something. His postoperative pain is less than the pain of testicular torsion, and he is back to business as usual.

However, the astute professional health care provider who is a student of human development will note that all but one are engaged in social, physical, and cognitive activities associated with normative developmental competence for their age: the toddler Samia. Toddlers do not naturally sit still and watch. Born prematurely to an adolescent mother, Samia has spent more time in the hospital than out. Infections have complicated her bronchopulmonary dysplasia. There is conflict between her mother and maternal grandmother about who is responsible for Samia's physical care

and early intervention therapies. We can see the risk factors piling up.

## Implications for Health Care Interventions

A small set of factors associated with resilience appears again and again in the literature: connections to competent and caring adults in the family and community; cognitive and self-regulation skills; positive views of self; and motivation to be effective in the environment. These are basic human adaptational systems at work. Resilience is about *being engaged* socially, emotionally, intellectually, and even physically; about exercising adaptational systems and processes to promote competence. The goal of intervention is to support the development of normative competence while preventing and ameliorating risk.

If threats to children are adverse circumstances that undermine normal adaptive processes and systems, then intervention efforts should focus on building and supporting these adaptive processes and systems. Resilience is multifaceted, so interventions must occur at multiple levels within the ecosystem and address multiple processes and systems of development. Masten and Coatsworth suggest three layers of strategies (1998):

- Risk-focused strategies (e.g., eliminate or prevent risks, such as prematurity)

- Resource-focused strategies (e.g., access to health care, good schools, employment opportunities)

- Process-focused strategies: development of social and cognitive competence (e.g., attachment, self-regulation, self-efficacy, parenting, problem solving)

### INTERVENTION IN THE HEALTH CARE SYSTEM

For health care providers, some of their recommendations can be incorporated into practice more easily than others. The most obvious implications for health are at the level of primary prevention for individuals, families, and communities: promotion of competence and overall wellness through prenatal care, support for parenting, well-child care, and programs to reduce specific risk, such as teen pregnancy and substance abuse. At the level of secondary prevention, we can identify those at risk early and intervene to shore up protective adaptive processes (e.g., parent education programs, counseling sexually active girls to avoid pregnancy, etc.). Once risk has been manifested at the level of tertiary prevention—the parent is not competent, the girl is already pregnant—we can try to minimize its effects and optimize functioning.

The list of prevention strategies goes on. However, the framework of developmental contextualism warns us that we cannot simply "parachute" into people's lives with the latest intervention program and expect to have any meaningful impact (Lerner et al. 1998). This narrow approach can even do more harm than good. Human development and human needs occur in context of families, communities, society, and time. Effective interventions must be based on an assessment not just of the needs and strengths of individuals, families, and communities, but also in the context of their developmental history and trajectory.

Unfortunately, our health care system does not reward contextual and process-oriented thinking. Despite efforts to enhance primary and tertiary preventive care, secondary prevention consumes most of our health care dollars and still tends to use a downstream, problem-oriented, and causal-linear framework for clinical care. Furthermore, despite rhetoric on person-centered care, models of reimbursement favor regression to the mean; that is, what is the typical hospital stay or medication dosage for this problem? As a result, the focus continues to be not only on pathology, but that the pathology rests in the disordered symptoms and characteristics of the individual at that point in time, without an appreciation for context over time (Lerner et al. 1998).

## Final Thoughts

Integrating research on resilience and adaptation with health care remains a frontier of effort. Health care has traditionally focused on the abnormal, often without appreciation for what is normal and what processes produce it under what circumstances. That children who are considered resilient are basically developing normally says more about our expectations for them than it does about their development. They have taught us to change our conceptual framework for understanding both adaptive and maladaptive behaviors. The same processes and systems are at work, but their organization over time and in context take children down different developmental paths.

# References

Anthony, E. J. (1974). The syndrome of the psychologically invulnerable child. In E. J. Anthony & C. Koupernik, Eds. *The child in his family: children at psychiatric risk.* New York: Wiley, pp. 529–545.

Baumrind, D. (1978). Parental disciplinary patterns and social competence in children. *Youth and Society* 9:229–276.

Binet, A., & Simon, T. (1905). Application of the new methods to the diagnosis of the intellectual level among normal and subnormal children in institutions and in the primary schools. *L'annee psychologique* 12:245–336.

Bleuler, M. (1978). *The schizophrenic disorders: long-term patient and family studies.* New Haven, CT: Yale University Press.

Bowlby, J. (1951). *Maternal care and mental health.* Geneva: World Health Organization.

Brody, G., Dorsey, S., Forehand, R., & Armistead, L. (2002). Unique and protective contributions of parenting and classroom processes to the adjustment of African American children living in single-parent families. *Child Development* 73:274–286.

Bronfenbrenner, U. (1979). *The ecology of human development.* Cambridge, MA: Harvard University Press.

Bronfenbrenner, U., & Ceci, S. (1994). Nature–nurture reconceptualized in developmental perspective: a bioecological model. *Psychological Review* 101:568–586.

Bronson, M. B. (2000). *Self-regulation in early childhood: nature and nurture.* New York: Guildford.

Chess, S., & Thomas, A. (1977). *Temperament and development.* New York: Bruner/Mazle Publishers.

Coie, J. D., & Dodge, K. A. (1998). Aggression and antisocial behavior. In N. Eisenberg, Ed. *Social, emotional and personality development,* Volume 3. New York: Wiley, pp. 779–862.

Darwin, C. (1859). *The origin of the species by means of natural selection.* London: John Murray.

Dewey, J. (1899). *The school and society,* Volume 1. Carbondale, IL: Southern Illinois University Press.

Dodge, K. A. (1986). A social information processing model of social competence in children. In M. Perlmutter, Ed. *Cognitive perspectives on children's social and behavioral development,* Volume 18. Hillsdale, NJ: Erlbaum, pp. 77–125.

Dominus, S. (2002) Shabana is late for school. *New York Times Magazine,* September 29, 2002.

Elder, G. H. (1995). The life course paradigm: social change and individual development. In P. Moen, G. H. Elder, & K. Luscher, Eds. *Examining lives in context: perspectives on the ecoogy of human development.* Washington, DC: American Psychological Association, pp. 101–140.

Erikson, E. H. (1950). *Childhood and society.* New York: W. W. Norton & Company.

Folkman, S., & Moskowitz, J. T. (2000). Positive affect and the other side of coping. *American Psychologist* 55:647–654.

Freud, A., & Burlingham, D. T. (1943). *War and children.* London: Medical War Books.

Freud, S. (1924/1952). *A general introduction to psychoanalysis.* (J. Riviere, Trans.). New York: Washington Square Press.

Freud, S. (1930/1961). *Civilization and its discontents.* (J. Strachey, Trans.). New York: Norton.

Garmezy, N. (1981). Children under stress: perspectives on antecedents and correlates of vulnerability and resistance to psychopathology. In A. I. Rabin, J. Aronoff, A. M. Barclay, & R. A. Zucker, Eds. *Further explorations in personality.* New York: Wiley.

Garmezy, N. (1983). Stressors of childhood. In N. Garmezy & M. Rutter, Eds. *Stress, coping and development in children.* New York: McGraw-Hill, pp. 43–84.

Garmezy, N. (1985). Stress resistant children: the search for protective factors. In J. E. Stevenson, Ed. *Recent research in developmental psychopathology.* Oxford: Pergamon Press, pp. 213–233.

Garmezy, N., Masten, A. S., & Tellegen, A. (1984). The study of stress and competence in children: a building block for developmental psychopathology. *Child Development* 55:97–111.

Garmezy, N., & Tellegen, A. (1984). Studies of stress-resistant children: methods, variables and preliminary findings. In F. J. Morrison, C. Lord, & D. P. Keating, Eds. *Applied Developmental Psychology* New York: Academic Press, pp. 231–287.

Gesell, A. (1948). *Studies in child development.* Westport, CT: Greenwood Press.

Goodyer, I. M., Herbert, J., Tamplin, A., & Altham, P. M. E. (2000). Recent life events, cortisol, dehydroepiandrosterone and the onset of major depression in high-risk adolescents. *British Journal of Psychiatry* 177:499–504.

Hall, G. S. (1891). The contents of children's mind on entering school. *Pedagogical Seminary* I:139–173.

Hamilton, E., & Cairns, H. (Eds.). (1961). *The Collected Dialogues.* New York: Pantheon Press.

Harter, S. (1999). *The construction of the self: a developmental perspective.* New York: Guilford Press.

Hartup, W. W. (1983). Peer relations. In E. M. Hetherington, Ed. *Socialization, personality and social development,* Volume 4. New York: Wiley, pp. 103–196.

Havighurst, R. J. (1972). *Developmental tasks and education,* 3rd ed. New York: David McKay.

Holmes, T. H., & Rahe, R. H. (1967). The social readjustment rating scale. *Journal of Psychosomatic Research* 11:213–218.

James, W. (1890). *The principles of psychology.* New York: Holt, Rinehart and Winston.

Kobasa, S. (1987). Stress responses and personality. In R. C. Barnett, L. Bienor, & G. K. Baruch, Eds. *Gender and stress.* New York: Free Press, pp. 308–329.

Lazarus, R. S., & Folkman, S. (1984). *Stress, appraisal and coping.* New York: Springer Publishing Company.

Lengua, L. J. (2002). The contribution of emotionality and self-regulation to the understanding of children's response to multiple risk. *Child Development* 73:144–161.

Lerner, R. M. (1982). Children and adolescents as producers of their own development. *Developmental Review* 2:342–370.

Lerner, R. M. (1986). *Concepts and theories of human development.* New York: Cambridge University Press.

Lerner, R. M., & Lerner, J. V. (1983). Temperament-intelligence reciprocities in early childhood: a contextual model. In M. Lewis, Ed. *Origins of intelligence: infancy and early childhood,* New York: Plenum, pp. 399–421.

Lerner, R. M., Walsh, M. E., & Howard, K. A. (1998). Developmental-contextual considerations: person-context relations as the bases for risk and resiliency in child and adolescent development. In T. Ollendick, Ed. *Children and adolescents: clinical formulation and treatment,* Volume 5. New York: Elsevier Science Publishers, pp. 1–24.

Luthar, S. S., Doernberger, D. H., & Zigler, E. (1993). Resilience is not a unidimensional construct: insights from a prospective study of inner-city adolescents. *Development and Psychopathology* 5:703–717.

Masten, A. S. (2001). Ordinary magic: resilience processes in development. *American Psychologist* 56:227–238.

Masten, A. S., & Coatsworth, D. J. (1995). Competence, resilience and psychopathology. In D. Cicchetti & D. Cohen, Eds. *Risk, disorder and adaptation,* Volume 2. New York: Wiley, pp. 715–752.

Masten, A. S., & Coatsworth, D. J. (1998). The development of competence in favorable and unfavorable environments: lessons from research on successful children. *American Psychologist* 53:205–220.

Masten, A. S., & Garmezy, N. (1985). Risk, vulnerability and protective factors in developmental psychopathology. In B. B. Lahey & A. E. Kazdin, Eds. *Advances in clinical child psychology,* Volume 8. New York: Plenum Press, pp. 1–52s.

McEwen, B. (2002). *The end of stress as we know it.* Washington, DC: Joseph Henry.

Moen, P., & Erickson, M. A. (1995). Linked lives: a trans-generational approach to resilience. In P. Moen, G. H. Elder, & K. Luscher, Eds. *Examining lives in context.* Washington, DC: American Psychological Association, pp. 169–210.

Morgan, C. A. I., Wang, S., Rasmusson, A., Hazlett, G., Anderson, G., & Charney, D. S. (2001). Relationship among plasma cortisol, catecholamines, neuropeptide Y and human performance during exposure to uncontrollable stress. *Psychosomatic Medicine* 63:412–422.

Morgan, C. A. I., Wang, S., Southwick, S. M., Rasmusson, A., Hazlett, G., Hauger, R. L., et al. (2000). Plasma neropeptide-Y concentrations in humans exposed to military survival training. *Biological Psychiatry* 47:902–909.

Murphy, L. B., & Moriarty, A. E. (1976). *Vulnerability, coping, and growth: from infancy to adolescence.* New Haven, CT: Yale University Press.

Neisser, U., Boodoo, G., Bouchard, T. J., Jr., Boykin, A. W., Brody, N., Ceci, S. J., et al. (1996). Intelligence: knowns and unknowns. *American Psychologist* 51:71–101.

O'Connor, T. G., Rutter, M., Beckett, C., Keaveney, L., Kreppner, J. M., & English and Romanian Adoptees Study Team. (2000). The effects of global severe privation on cognitive competence; extension and longitudinal follow-up. *Child Development* 71:376–390.

Patterson, J. M. (2002). Understanding family resilience. *Journal of Clinical Psychology* 58:233–246.

Piaget, J. (1950). *The psychology of intelligence.* London: Kegan Paul, Trench & Trubner.

Ricks, M. H. (1985). The social transmission of parental behavior. In I. Bretherton & E. Waters, Eds. *Growing points of attachment theory and research,* Volume 50. Chicago: University of Chicago Press, pp. 211–227.

Rouse, K. A. (2001). Resilient students' goals and motivation. *Journal of Adolescence* 24:461–472.

Rutter, M. (1979). Protective factors in children's responses to stress and disadvantage. In M. Kent & J. Rolf, Eds. *Primary prevention of psychopathology,* Volume 3. Hanover, NH: University Press of New England.

Rutter, M. (1985). Resilience in the face of adversity: protective factors and resistance to psychiatric disorder. *British Journal of Psychiatry* 147:598–611.

Rutter, M. (2002). Nature, nurture and development: from evangelism through science toward policy and practice. *Child Development* 73:1–21.

Rutter, M., Champion, L., Quinton, D., Maughan, B., & Pickles, A. (1995). Understanding individual differences in environmental-risk exposure. In *Examining lives in context: perspectives on the ecology of human development.* Washington, DC: American Psychological Association, pp. 61–93..

Sameroff, A. (1975). Transactional models in early social relations. *Human Development* 18:65–79.

Sameroff, A. (1983). Developmental systems: contexts and evolution. In P. H. Mussen, Ed. *Handbook of child psychology,* Volume 1. New York: Wiley, pp. 237–294.

Sameroff, A., & Chandler, M. J. (1975). Reproductive risk and the continuum of the caretaking causality. In F. D. Horowitz, M. Hetherington, S. Scarr-Salapatek, & G. Sregel, Eds. *Review of child development research,* Volume 4. Chicago: University of Chicago Press.

Sameroff, A., Seifer, R., & Elias, P. (1982). Sociocultural variability in infant temperament ratings. *Child Development* 53:164–173.

Selye, H. (1976). *The stress of life.* New York: McGraw-Hill.

Skinner, B. F. (1938). *The behavior of organisms.* New York: Appleton-Century-Croft.

Somerfield, M. R., & McCrae, R. R. (2000). Stress and coping research: methodological challenges, theoretical advances, and clinical applications. *American Psychologist* 55:620–625.

Spirito, A., Stark, L., & Knapp, L. (1992). The assessment of coping in chronically ill children: implications for clinical practice. In A. M. LaGreca, L. J. Siegel, J. L. Wallander, & C. E. Walker, Eds. *Stress and coping in child health.* New York: Guilford, pp. 327–344.

Spitz, R. A. (1946). Hospitalism: a follow-up report on investigation described in Volume I, 1945. *Psychoanalytic Study of the Child* 2:113–117.

Sroufe, L. A. (1979). The coherence of individual development: early care, attachment and subsequent developmental issues. *American Psychologist* 34:834–841.

Sroufe, L. A. (1996). *Emotional development: the organization of emotional life in the early years.* New York: Cambridge University Press.

Super, C. M., & Harkness, S. (1986). The developmental niche: a conceptualization of the interface of child and culture. *International Journal of Behavioral Development* 9:1–25.

Thies, K. M., & Walsh, M. E. (1999). A developmental analysis of cognitive appraisal of stress in children and adolescents with chronic illness. *Children's Health Care* 28:15–32.

Vaillant, G. (1977). *Adaptation to life.* Boston: Little, Brown.

Vygotsky, L. (1978). *Mind in society: the development of higher psychological processes.* Cambridge, MA: Harvard University Press.

Wachs, T. D. (2000). *Necessary but not sufficient: the respective roles of single and multiple influences of individual development.* Washington, DC: APA books.

Wallander, J. L., & Varni, J. W. (1992). Adjustment in children with chronic physical disorders: programmatic research on a disability-stress-coping mode. In A. M. LaGreca, L. J. Siegel, J. L. Wallander, & C. E. Walker, Eds. *Stress and coping in child health.* New York: Guildford Press.

Waller, M. A. (2001). Resilience in ecosystemic context: evolution of the concept. *American Journal of Orthopsychiatry* 71:290–297.

Watson, J. B. (1913). Psychology as the behaviorist views it. *Psychological Review* 20:158–177.

Werner, E. E. (1989). High risk children in young adulthood. *American Journal of Orthopsychiatriy* 59:72–81.

Werner, E. E. (1990). Protective factors and individual resilience. In S. Meisels & J. Shonkoff, Eds. *Handbook of early childhood intervention.* New York: Cambridge Press, pp. 97–116.

Werner, E. E., & Smith, R. S. (1977). *Kauai's children come of age.* Honolulu: University of Hawaii.

Werner, E. E., & Smith, R. S. (1982). *Vulnerable but invincible: a study of resilient children.* New York: McGraw-Hill.

Werner, E. E., & Smith, R. S. (2001). *Journeys from childhood to midlife: risk, resilience, and recovery.* Ithaca, NY: Cornell University Press.

White, S. H. (1976). The active organism in theoretical behaviorism. *Human Development* 19:99–107.

# Part Two

# NORMATIVE PROCESSES OF DEVELOPMENT

# Chapter 5

# Newborn Behavior and Development: Implications for Health Care Professionals

J. Kevin Nugent

Yvette Blanchard

There is a growing consensus that the period from birth to the beginning of the third month of life involves not only a major stage in the infant's behavioral adaptation to his or her new environment (Barr 1998, Rochat 1998) but also a major transformation in many neural functions (Hopkins 1998). The processes of synaptogenesis, neural differentiation, and cell migration, beginning in the prenatal period, establish the neuron's functional role during this postnatal period. The newborn period and the early months of life also constitute a critical transition stage in the development of the parent–infant relationship and in the development of the family itself (Brazelton 1995, Emde & Robinson 1979, Konner 1998, Sander et al. 1979, Stern 1995, Trevarthen1979).

In this chapter we present evidence to suggest that because of the significance of these transformations, the newborn period may well be the "teaching moment par excellence" for health care professionals. It provides a unique opportunity for the development of a therapeutic relationship between the professional and family at a time when the infant's development involves a series of dramatic transitions and when the relationship between parents and infants is also at a sensitive stage in its development. We provide the conceptual basis for this approach by describing current research on newborn behavior and development, based on our work with pre-term and full-term infants and their families. Finally, we present a model of preventative family-centered care based on the newly developed Newborn Behavioral Observations (NBO) system and present guidelines for intervention based on this infant-focused behavioral developmental approach.

## Newborn Behavior and State Organization

After three decades of intensive research on newborn behavior and development, the human newborn has proven to be both a competent and a social organism. There now exists an extensive taxonomy of newborn and infant behavior. For example, research demonstrates that the newborn can visually track (Dannemiller & Freedland 1991, Laplante et al. 1996, Slater et al. 1985), can hear and locate sounds (Muir and Field 1979), can discriminate between two vowels (Moon et al. 1993), can discriminate between unfamiliar whispered voices (Spence & Freeman 1996), and can remember speech sounds (Swain et al. 1993). There is a body of research showing that the newborn infant is a social organism, predisposed to interact with his or her caregiver from the beginning and biologically designed to elicit the kind of caregiving necessary for survival and successful adaptation. The newborn, for example, seems to prefer the mother's voice above all other stimuli, whether human or nonhuman (Clarkson & Clifton 1991, deCasper & Fifer 1980, deCasper et al. 1994, Eklund-Flores & Turkewitz, 1996), can imitate facial expressions (Field et al. 1992, Meltzoff and Moore 1989), and seems to be able to discriminate the mother's face from that of a stranger (Pascalis et al. 1995).

This body of research has yielded an impressive catalogue of newborn competencies that has transformed our scientific understanding of the human newborn, but it has also enabled a new generation of health care providers to help parents recognize that their newborn infants can see and hear and thus support the development of the parent–infant bond from the beginning (Klaus et al. 1995, Nugent & Brazelton 2000). Although the recognition of these sensory capacities is important, there is a complementary body of evidence that demonstrates that this list of discrete behaviors does not do justice to the organizational capabilities or the individuality of the human newborn. Understanding the newborn's more complex organizational capacities and the ability to describe and recognize the developmental agenda and adaptive challenges for both full-term and preterm infants over the first months of life may be even more critical in informing our clinical approach to working with parents. In this way, clinicians can provide developmentally appropriate information and individualized guidance to parents during this important life transition.

## The Importance of Newborn Behavioral States

Over 40 years ago, Peter Wolff pointed out that newborn behavior was not random and that the newborn exhibited observable patterns of behavior, which he called "behavioral states" (Wolff 1959). Wolff described five behavioral states: 1) deep (non-REM) and 2) light (REM) sleep states, 3) quiet alert and 4) active alert states, and 5) crying state. His discovery led to the important research and clinical principle that the newborn's behavioral states inevitably influence the quality of the infant's responses.

The concept of "state" can be used by health care professionals to help parents understand the infant's "language" or communication cues and gauge the appropriateness of their handling techniques or the level and quality of the stimulation they need to provide to meet the needs of their infants. It may be as simple as helping parents recognize that when the baby is in a deep non-REM state or even in a light REM sleep state, feeding cannot be successful, or that if the baby is in a sleep state, there is no possibility for interaction, no matter how ready the parent may be. Because the development of robust sleep–wake cycles is one of the key developmental tasks of the newborn infant over the first months of life, the clinician, who understands the concept of state, observes how well the infant can habituate to repeated stimuli (noise or light) by decreasing her level of responsiveness to each stimulus. With that information in hand, the clinician can help parents understand the infant's capacity for tolerating external stimulation, showing how it protects and facilitates sleep organization. On the other hand, if the infant cannot habituate to external environmental stimulation, then the clinician and parent can plan the kind of environmental support the infant may need to protect her sleep and develop a well-organized sleep–wake pattern of behavior.

## INTERPRETING STATE BEHAVIOR

The clinician can also help parents read and interpret the infant's more subtle behavioral cues. While an infant is alert and responding to her parent in the context of face-to-face interaction, for example, the infant may let her parent know she has reached her stimulation threshold by averting her eyes, by squirming, or by opening and closing her hands, as a means of signaling her need for a pause and a break from the intensity of the interaction. This understanding of "state" and the ability to read and decipher even the most subtle state behaviors can be seen, therefore, as a critical matrix, which enables clinicians and parents to assess and interpret all newborn reactions—sensory as well as motor. The baby's state behavior informs the parental response, although it is a more complex clinical task when the states are disorganized or when the infant's behavioral patterns are unpredictable or difficult to decipher, as in the case of premature or low-birthweight infants. The recognition of this simple but pivotal concept has transformed clinical practice, so that helping parents understand their infant's state behavior and state regulation is at the heart of the clinical challenge for health care professionals who work with parents in the newborn period and the first months of life.

Wolff's work on newborn behavioral states, followed by the research by T. Berry Brazelton and his colleagues based on the Neonatal Behavioral Assessment Scale (NBAS) (Brazelton 1973, 1985; Brazelton and Nugent 1995) and Heidelise Als' Synactive Model (Als 1986) based on her work with premature infants, provide clinicians with three related lenses that can contribute to a more complex understanding of newborn behavior and development over the first months of life and serve to guide clinicians in providing individualized developmental guidance to parents.

# The Process of Adaptation in Full-Term Infants

The understanding that the newborn infant has the capacity to organize discrete behaviors in order to respond to the environment in ways that become increasingly predictable over time led T. Berry Brazelton and his colleagues to develop the NBAS, in an effort to capture the full richness of the newborn infant's repertoire (Brazelton 1973, 1985; Brazelton & Nugent 1995). The model on which the NBAS is based suggests that one of the earliest developmental tasks for newborn infants is to organize their behavior, so they can play an active role in influencing their caregiving environment and elicit the support needed for successful adaptation and development. The NBAS (Brazelton 1973, 1985; Brazelton & Nugent 1995) is the most comprehensive assessment of newborn behavior. The scale describes the newborn's responses to his or her new extrauterine environment and assesses the newborn's behavioral repertoire on 28 behavioral items, each scored on a 9-point scale. The scale also includes an assessment of the infant's neurological status on 20 items, each scored on a 4-point scale. All these items can be summarized under four behavioral dimensions: *physiologic, motor, state, and attentional/interactional dimensions.*

- *Physiologic or autonomic stability* includes signs of stress related to homeostatic adjustments of the central nervous system (CNS) and records the presence or absence of tremulousness, startles, or the lability of skin color as indices of physiological organization.

- *Motor organization* is determined by the status of the infant's tone, motor maturity, activity level, the level of integrated motor movements (e.g., hand-to-mouth activities or defensive movements). The reflexes are examined as a component of the infant's motor organization and CNS status.

- *State organization* is assessed by examining the lability of states, the level of irritability, peak of excitement, capacity for shutting out negative stimuli while asleep, crying and consolability, and self-quieting capacities.

- The *quality of the infant's affective/interactive capacities* is observed in the infant's degree of alertness and his or her response to animate and inanimate visual and auditory stimuli.

## Neonatal Developmental Challenge

The task of neonatal behavioral adaptation involves the successful integration of these four behavioral dimensions and the development of the infant's capacity for self-regulation over the first months of life. From this developmental perspective, newborns are seen to face a series of hierarchically organized developmental challenges as they attempt to adapt to their new extrauterine world, both the inanimate and animate world (Brazelton 1973, 1985; Nugent & Brazelton 2000). This includes the infants' capacity to first regulate their physiological or autonomic system, then their state behavior, their motor behavior, and finally their affective interactive behavior, which develop in a stage-like epigenetic progression over the first two months of life. These developmental tasks must be successfully negotiated before the infant can develop the capacity for shared mutual engagement that constitutes the major task of the next stage of development (Adamson 1993, Brazelton et al. 1974, Stern 1995). Nevertheless, this developmental agenda and the baby's capacity to respond to her environment, including the ability to develop predictable sleep–wake states, her ability to respond to her environment, and her ability to cope with stress, can only be achieved with the support of the care-

giver. This kind of developmental information and guidance can be provided by the health care professional in the context of the administration of the Newborn Behavioral Observations (NBO) system, which is described later in the chapter.

## The Process of Behavioral Development in the Preterm Infant

The model of newborn and infant development proposed by Als (1986), in her work with preterm infants, provides a framework for the understanding of neurobehavioral functioning in the premature infant. Als' (1986) synactive model categorizes infant behaviors into interdependent subsystems consisting of the *autonomic system, the motor system,* and the *state system.* It is the integration of these subsystems that is central to early neurobehavioral functioning and adaptation. To better categorize the infant's behaviors into their respective subsystems, Als has identified behavioral channels of communication for each subsystem. The behavioral channels that are part of the autonomic system include respiration patterns, skin color, and visceral signs. Behaviors belonging to the motor system include tone, posture, and movements, whereas those of the state system include range of behavioral states, robustness and clarity of behavioral states, and transition patterns from state to state.

Attention–interaction is considered an outgrowth of the state subsystem and is observed through the infant's ability to respond and interact with animate and inanimate objects. Infants with a well-organized attention–interaction system can achieve and maintain bright-eyed alertness and well-modulated interactive periods for brief periods of time at least. A less well-organized infant may have a strained, low level of alertness, or conversely may be hyperalert and may be unable to break away from the interaction and thus may become overstimulated. For an infant with well-organized self-regulation, the subsystems are well integrated and function in smooth synchrony, supporting and facilitating the emerging differentiation and modulation of one another. An infant with less well-organized self-regulation requires more assistance from adults and the environment to achieve and maintain subsystem interaction and integration.

For each of these subsystems, Als has identified behaviors as either "approach," "self-regulatory" behaviors, or as "avoidance," "stress" behaviors. An infant is described as organized when his self-regulatory abilities are able to support the demands placed on him by the environment and approach behaviors are observed. The infant is described as disorganized when his threshold for self-regulation is exceeded and avoidance behaviors are observed. The kind and intensity of facilitation required to achieve behavioral organization becomes instructive for health care professionals and parents, and can form the basis for developing individualized developmental goals and strategies for that infant and family (Blanchard & Mouradian 2000).

## Identifying Infant Thresholds

The importance of being able to identify the infant's threshold for responding as the basis for developing individualized developmental goals for parents is demonstrated in the following clinical example. A physical therapist (PT), using the Newborn Behavioral Observations (NBO) system as part of an early intervention home visit, describes the neurobehavioral functioning of a young premature infant to her mother. Adrienne was born at 25 weeks of gestation, weighed 680 grams at birth, and this first visit took place at home 2 weeks after her due date. At the beginning of the session, Adrienne began to wake up, squirming and stretching her arms and legs, so that the PT picked her up and gently rocked her vertically to assist her transition to a more fully awake state.

When her eyes were open, Adrienne was able to follow the PT's face and voice to her right and left side. She tracked briefly, paused in her tracking by

slightly averting her gaze, but with a contingent pause by the PT, Adrienne was able to continue tracking for a few more degrees in both directions. When the PT asked her mother to call her name, once on each side, Adrienne turned her head and looked at her mother's face. Even though she responded to her mother's voice, Adrienne had more difficulty in tracking the PT's face, when no voice was offered, or to track the red ball the PT was moving in front of her. By this time, it was clear that Andrienne was tiring, as indicated by her tone and posture, which had become more floppy.

By this time, it was clear that Adrienne was tiring, as indicated by her tone and posture, which had become more floppy. She was breathing with some difficulty; her cheeks had become pale, her mouth was open and flaccid, and her breathing had become irregular. The PT decided to give her a "time-out" and placed her down on the couch for a short time before continuing with her evaluation. This provided the clinician and mother with a "teaching" opportunity to discuss Adrienne's state behavior, including her remarkable visual and auditory capabilities and her ability to respond to her mother's voice, and then to discuss the strategies she was using to reveal her threshold level. In this way, based on her observations of her infant's behavioral cues, the mother could learn how to respond to her infant in a way that would not overstimulate her and could learn to interact in a way that would support her overall development. Within this behavioral framework, therefore, infants' behaviors are seen as meaningful, communicative, and indicative of the infant's current neurodevelopmental status.

# The Newborn Period as a Formative Period in the Transition to Parenthood

These first months of life mark a major biobehavioral transition for the infant. From the parent's perspective, these first months can be considered a normative crisis—a period characterized by rapid change—as parents search for "the goodness of fit" between themselves and their new baby (Thomas & Chess 1977). In the case of mothers, Stern (1995) refers to this unique but normal psychological condition as the "motherhood constellation" and a condition or stage that every mother experiences. With the birth of a baby, a mother passes into a new and unique psychic organization, which will determine "a new set of action tendencies, sensibilities, fantasies, fears and wishes" (Stern 1995, p. 171).

This normative stage in the transition to parenthood has, therefore, its own protoclinical challenges, which will have an impact on the development of the parent–child relationship and which will in turn have a major influence on the mother's own life development. The core challenge for the new mother is to engage her baby in such a way that "fosters the baby's development and in a way that is authentic to her" (Stern 1995, p. 173). This involves her ability to nurture and care for her baby, to help her baby to grow and thrive physically, to become attached to her baby, and to provide a secure environment for her baby. Although there is a wide range of cultural variation in the role fathers play in this early stage, it should be pointed out that in most societies, both partners have a unique role to play in the socialization process of the young infant (Nugent 1991).

## The Developing Parent–Infant Relationship

The period from birth to the third month also constitutes a major transition stage in the development of the parent–infant relationship itself (Brazelton 1995, Emde & Robinson 1979, Konner 1998, Stern 1995, Trevarthen 1979). At this stage the earliest patterns of interaction are taking shape, as infant and parent are in a heightened state of readiness to exchange their first communication signals in their efforts to achieve a

mutually satisfying level of affective mutual regulation, what Stern (1985) refers to as "affective attunement." Over the first two months the infant develops the capacity for shared attentiveness (Adamson 1993), so that both parent and infant have already embarked on and are actively engaged in an interactive regulative system.

During the first weeks and months of life, the major interactive and social exchanges between parents and infant will concern the regulation of their infant's feeding, sleep–wake, and activity cycles. Infants communicate their readiness and need for feeding or sleeping through specific and predictable behaviors: infants most often cry in the first weeks of life to signal their need for food and often become fussy as they transition from an awake to sleep state. Pulling away from the bottle or breast often signals satiation. During the second month of life, babies make more sounds spontaneously and in response to their parent's vocalizations. Those episodes of regulated social behaviors still break down frequently, leading to the infant crying. Many attempts to rectify the situation by the parents are inevitable during this early life period. The quality of the exchanges between parent and infant and the "repair" that is needed in a situation of breakdown in the exchange is highly dependent on the parent's ability to understand the infant's behaviors. For example, when the infant is crying and hungry, can the mother stay calm while she prepares for his feeding? When the infant is cooing in response to his mother's singing while folding laundry, can she recognize her infant's efforts to get her attention? Can a father support his infant son's level of activity by reading his signs of readiness for play and signals for disengagement?

There are many factors that may render the parent–infant relationship vulnerable at this time, such as when the baby is admitted to the neonatal intensive care unit. As Stern stated (1995, p. 173) the core challenge for a new mother is to engage her baby in such a way that "fosters the baby's development and in a way that is authentic to her." But when faced with an infant with a prolonged stay in the hospital or with an infant who is finally home after such a stay, a new mother's ability to nurture and care for her baby becomes somewhat dependent on her ability to read and understand her baby's signals for needs of support. Many parents still do not know that young infants are already very competent in their ability to engage or disengage in their interactions with the world. Mothers of sick infants, such as Adrienne's mother, first discover their infant's abilities and challenges through an exchange with a health care provider trained in neurobehavioral assessment. Redshaw (1997) has demonstrated that the experience of separation for these mothers can be associated with the temporary loss of a sense of parental role and identity. Indeed, mothers of babies who require ventilation may feel "overwhelmed, worried" and even "panicked" when told their baby is well enough to go home and feel less confident about taking their baby home than do mothers of healthy infants. Nevertheless, a number of studies have demonstrated that during this difficult hospital time, helping parents understand their baby's behavior appears to be critical in helping them maintain their role as parents and mitigate levels of stress (Lawhon 2002, Loo et al. 2003, Redshaw 1997).

# The Newborn Period as a Formative Period in the Development of the Family

The entry of a baby into an already functioning system irrevocably changes the dynamics of family functioning because the period after birth involves a vital redefinition of roles (Belsky 1985, Minuchin 1985). After birth, all family members—mothers, fathers, siblings, grandparents—have to adjust to the presence of the new family member and renegotiate their family relationships and roles. Moreover, with the birth of a baby the family becomes an open system, so that the health

care professional also has a unique opportunity to become a part of the family support system. This kind of infant-focused intervention by the health care professional can facilitate major developmental processes by helping parents and family understand the differential effects of the infant on the family and how the infant's behavioral makeup may influence family roles and functioning (e.g., Beal 1986, Garbarino 1992, Murray & Cooper 1997, Myers 1982).

In high-risk settings, the newborn entry point can provide the clinician a unique opportunity to support the family and thereby counterbalance the risk present within the microsystem itself (Garbarino 1992, Klaus et al. 1995). With single-parent families or families who feel isolated or have no support system, the heath care professional can use the newborn assessment, especially in the context of the home visit, to serve as a bridge between the family and the broader community and increase the likelihood of informal community support for the family on the one hand and more formal family resource services in the community on the other (Anisfield & Pinkus 1978, Boger & Kornetz 1985, Brazelton 1995, Stadtler et al. 1986, Weissbourd & Kagan 1989, Wolke et al. 1994). The value of using the NBO, for example, in such situations is that it enables the clinician and parent to focus on the newborn baby, his or her strengths and needs, and draw grandparents, neighbors, and friends into the family orbit, thus building up the infant's support system from the very beginning. Infant-focused intervention sessions conducted in the home or clinic setting can not only serve to strengthen the relationship of the clinician and the family but can also be used to strengthen the relationship between the family and community support systems.

# The Role of Culture

For health care professionals working with families in today's multicultural society, the research on culture and the well-documented role of culture in shaping the beliefs, values, and child-rearing practices of parents and families throughout the world has important implications for clinical practice (Nugent 2002). Studies of newborn behavior and the study of early parent–child relations in different cultures demonstrate a wide range of variability in newborn behavior, in parent–infant interaction patterns and in child-rearing philosophies (Levine 1980; Nugent et al. 1989, 1991; Shweder et al. 1998; Whiting & Edwards 1988). These data suggest that whereas the basic organizational processes in infancy may be universal, the range and form of these adaptations are shaped by the demands of each individual culture. For clinicians who work with infants and families from different cultures, these data serve to challenge assumptions about the very nature of infant development and can also sensitize clinicians to the different trajectories of infant development and the wide range of parental child-rearing practices across cultures. It forces practitioners to revise and broaden their definitions of what they consider to be "typical" or "atypical behavior," or "appropriate" or "inappropriate parenting practices," and to reflect on their own philosophical approach to parental guidance (Nugent 1994, 2002).

## Interpreting the Role of Culture

Although describing and documenting newborn behavioral patterns may be seen as an objective process, the interpretation of these behaviors is a cultural construction, and the meaning we ascribe to behavior is mediated by our cultural value system. Whereas research demonstrates that hand-to-mouth activity in newborns, for example, can serve to reduce stress and promote the infant's state regulation, it must also be recognized that in certain cultures "thumb-sucking" is treated as an unhygienic and "ugly" habit, which must be broken even before it begins. Parents in these cultures believe they are acting as good parents when they discourage thumb-sucking in their young infants or cover their hands with mittens to prevent them from doing so. It is essential for clinicians to respect such cultural practices because each culture establishes its own expectations for infants and its own guidelines for rearing children.

In our research in Japan, for example, we found that mothers do not seem to value the self-regulating "independent" capacities of the newborn infant in the same way that parents from many Western cultures do. Because "independence," or the promotion of autonomy in infants, is not seen as a parental value in Japanese society (Doi 1991), parents tend to focus on the infant's "dependence" and immaturity because they value their own role as parents in helping their infants organize and develop. Parents cannot endure even short periods of crying in their newborn infants and see no value in letting a baby cry for any length of time. In addition, because they are more impressed by their infant's dependency needs, Japanese parents sleep with the infants because they feel that through this close extended body contact they can play a critical role in helping their infants adapt to their new extrauterine world and foster the parent–infant bond (Kawasaki et al. 1994).

In sum, working with parents who have different value systems from those we embrace should make us reexamine our own belief systems. This in turn should enable us to unmask our own cultural biases by reviewing our attitudes toward child-rearing practices. It goes without saying that without an awareness and appreciation of our own cultural value system or our own philosophy of child development, it will be extremely difficult to be sensitive to or open to the nuances of another culture and help parents make the kinds of choices that are consistent with their own cultural world view. Paradoxically, it is only through our engagement with other cultures that our understanding of our own culture is deepened and our clinical practice with parents from different cultures is simultaneously clarified and enriched.

# Preventative Intervention in the Newborn Period and the First Months of Life

There is evidence to suggest that, especially under conditions of environmental stress, early intervention can prevent the compounding of problems that occur when the caregiving environment does not adjust adequately to meet the needs of the infant (Als 1999, Bottos 1987, Brazelton & Nugent 1995, Garbarino 1992, Meisels et al. 1993, Nugent & Brazelton 2000, Sameroff 1993, Shonkoff & Phillips 2000). Planning for early intervention to assist the baby's recovery must be understood in terms of the plasticity and the potential for recovery of the nervous system and the role of a nurturing environment in supporting development (Dobbing 1990).

As infants adapt to their new extrauterine environment, their capacity for relatedness is being refined and consolidated. From this perspective, the focus on intervention in the first months of life is to support the infant's efforts to regulate and integrate his autonomic, motor, state, and affective systems. In this way, an infant consolidates his affective interactive capacities so that he is ready for the next stage, when face-to-face interaction becomes the primary developmental challenge for both infant and parent (Brazelton et al. 1974, Tronick & Cohn 1989, Weinberg & Tronick 1996).

Several studies have reported long-term effects of NBAS-based intervention procedures on developmental outcome and on the parent–child relationship. These include Gomes-Pedro and colleagues (1995), Myers (1982), Parker and colleagues (1992), Rauh and colleagues (1988), and Worobey and Belsky (1982). The success of these newborn behavior-based interventions and the established effectiveness of Gomes-Pedro's adapted version of the NBAS, in particular, led us (Nugent, Keefer, O'Brien, Johnson, & Blanchard to be published) to develop the Newborn

Behavioral Observations (NBO) system, which is an assessment developed specifically to be used with parents. In developing the NBO, our goal was to retain the conceptual richness of the NBAS and to produce a scale that was more likely to be used by doctors and nurses and allied health care professionals in clinical settings.

## The NBO: A Relationship-Building Approach for Health Care Professionals

The Newborn Behavioral Observations (NBO) system (Nugent, Keefer, O'Brien, Johnson, & Blanchard to be published) was developed especially for clinicians to be used in the care of families in hospital, clinic, or home settings up to the third month of the infant's life. The NBO is a brief neurobehavioral assessment, consisting of 18 behavioral and reflex items, designed to examine the newborn's physiological, motor, state, and social capacities (see Table 5.1: NBO recording form). It is a shared observation session, which provides a forum for parents and clinician to observe and interpret the newborn's behavior and is especially designed to help parents make informed choices about caregiving. While the NBO describes the baby's physiological, motor, state, and social-interactive behavior, it also contains items that are deemed to have an impact on parental caregiving, such as sleep behavior, feeding cues, crying and consolability, activity level, the baby's threshold for stimulation, and social-interactive capacities. The goal of the NBO is to promote a positive relationship between clinician and family and to strengthen the relationship between parents and their newborn baby.

### WORKING WITH PARENTS

The individualized nature of the NBO renders it responsive to the particular needs of individual infants and families. By eliciting, describing, and interpreting the newborn's behavior, the clinician has the opportunity to participate with parents in

*Table 5.1*   Newborn Behavioral Observations (NBO)

Name _____ Baby's Gender _____ Date of Birth _____ Date of Session _____

Gestational Age _____ Weight _____ APGAR Scores _____ Parity _____

Type of feeding _____ Setting _____ Practitioner's name _____

| Behavior | Observation Record | | | Guidance Checklist |
|---|---|---|---|---|
| | 3 | 2 | 1 | |
| | | *Habituates* | | |
| 1. Habituation to light | with ease | some difficulty | great difficulty | ___Sleep regulation |
| | | *Habituates* | | |
| 2. Habituation to sound | with ease | some difficulty | great difficulty | ‾Sleep regulation |
| | 3 | 2 | 1 | |
| 3. Tone: arms and legs | strong | fairly strong | weak | ‾Tone |
| 4. Rooting | strong | fairly strong | weak | ‾Feeding |
| 5. Sucking | strong | fairly strong | weak | ‾Feeding |
| 6. Hand grasp | strong | fairly strong | weak | ‾Strength/Contact |
| 7. Shoulder and neck tone | strong | fairly strong | weak | ‾Robustness |
| 8. Crawl | strong | fairly strong | weak | ‾Sleep positioning |
| | 3 | 2 | 1 | |
| 9. Response to face and voice | very responsive | moderate | not responsive | ‾Social interaction |
| 10. Visual response (to face) | very responsive | moderate | not responsive | ‾Social readiness |
| 11. Orientation to voice | very responsive | moderate | not responsive | ‾Voice recognition |
| 12. Orientation to sound | very responsive | moderate | not responsive | ‾Hearing |
| 13. Visual tracking | very responsive | moderate | not responsive | ‾Vision/stimulation |
| | 3 | 2 | 1 | |
| 14. Crying | very little | moderate amount | a lot | ‾Crying |
| 15. Soothability | easily consoled | moderate | with difficulty | ‾Soothability |
| | 3 | 2 | 1 | |
| 16. State regulation | well-organized | moderate | not organized | ‾Predictability |
| 17. Response to stress: color, tremors, startles | well-organized | moderate | very stressed | ‾Threshold level |
| 18. Activity level | well modulated | mixed | very high/very low | ‾Need for support |

***Behavioral Profile*** (*Strengths and Challenges*)


***Anticipatory Guidance*** (*Key Points*)


(*Source:* Nugent, Keefer, O'Brien, Johnson & Blanchard)

identifying the kinds of demands the infant will make on the environment and the kinds of caregiving techniques that can best promote the infant's organization and development. The NBO thus offers the clinician and parent a forum to observe the infant's level of functioning over the first two months and together arrive at a behavioral profile that captures the infant's individuality. Although the immediate goal of the NBO is to help reveal to parents the baby's unique adaptive and coping capacities, the long-term clinical goal is to positively influence the infant–parent relationship by developing a supportive therapeutic alliance with the family at what could be called the formative moment in the development of the family system. The NBO is thus seen as the first stage in the development of a supportive relationship between clinician and parents, which should continue beyond the newborn period.

The NBO is based on the assumption that the establishment of a relationship of trust between the clinician and family is the cornerstone for the development of the therapeutic alliance (Emde et al. 2000, Gilkerson & Shahmoon-Shanok 2000, Greenspan 1981, Stern 1995). The clinician's predominant attitude toward parents is, therefore, both respectful and supportive. The clinician must be able to listen empathically for parent's questions and observations in order to learn the "family story" (Boukydis 1986, Hirschberg 1993, MacDonough 1993, Zeanah & McDonough 1989). Moreover, listening to and searching for the authentic voices of infants and their families through the NBO is critical in making us sensitive to the unique value systems of the parents with whom we work and thus enables us to offer caregiving guidelines that are both developmentally appropriate and culturally sensitive.

The NBO is being used increasingly in early intervention home-visit settings and is integrated into the Individualized Family Service Plan (ISFP) as the blueprint for the care of the infant in the family context. Heath care professionals with a background in infant development, who have work experience with infants and families (early intervention providers; pediatric nurses; neonatal intensive care and newborn nursery nurses; pediatricians; doctors with a pediatric specialty; social workers; pediatric physical therapists, occupational therapists, speech-language pathologists; and parent educators, etc.) have been trained to use the NBO in their practices. A recent study examined the effects of the NBO on professional practice (Nugent et al. in unpublished results). In this study, 222 pediatric health care professionals, from 10 sites throughout the United States, were trained to administer the NBO. Almost half of the trainees (46%) were physicians, while the other half was made up of nurses, early intervention specialists, and allied health care professionals, representing large inner-city hospitals, and suburban and small city hospital sites. Of the total number of health care professionals who were trained, 98% of the trainees agreed that the NBO was excellent or good in helping parents learn about their newborns. The same percentage believed it could foster parents' interest in their baby, while 97% of the trainees believed that the NBO could enhance the clinician's partnership with parents. In a one-month follow-up, a subsample ($n = 78$), matching the total sample in terms of gender, age, and professional field, was asked about the effects of the NBO on their practice. Of the sample, 99% reported that parents usually or often learn new things about their baby and become better observers of their infants, and 91% felt mothers were more confident as parents as a result of the NBO. The clinicians themselves usually or often felt more "tuned in" or connected to parents as a result of the NBO (Philliber Research Associates 2001).

# Conclusions

We have attempted to operationalize a model of infant-focused family-centered care that emphasizes the transactional nature of early newborn-environment relations and the significance of the first months of life as a major transitional stage in the infant–parent relationship. We have proposed this as a conceptual basis for the use of the NBO with infants and their families in the early months of life. From this perspective, the newborn is viewed as competent and complex but also as a social organism, innately predisposed to interact with the environment to elicit from it the caregiving necessary for his survival and successful adaptation.

The focus of our approach to working with infants and parents is on the parent–infant relationship and on promoting the relationship between infant and caregiver. Our model emphasizes the role of both internal and external feedback systems in providing energy for the infant's healthy developmental progress (Brazelton 1982). The infant's own unique behavioral predispositions toward successful adaptation conspire with the powerful influences of the caregiving environment in providing the internal and external feedback that produces new levels of organization and that cannot be predicted in any linear model. Therefore, both infant and parent, as well as the family, become the focus of our intervention.

The goal becomes one of promoting infant adaptation by facilitating parent–infant interaction through the shared exploration and observation of the baby's behavioral organization. The unique characteristic of our approach to intervention is that the infant is at the center of the intervention, and it is through the infant we hope to motivate and support parents in their efforts to understand and respond to their infants. We have argued that the infant-focused but family-centered form of intervention holds promise for early screening and intervention in preventing affective disturbances in the parent–infant relationship and can thus serve as the first stage for a comprehensive follow-up program of support for infants and families.

Although not invoking the critical-period hypothesis, we have argued that the first three months could be called a unique transition stage in the infant's behavioral development and in the development of the parent–child relationship. We have presented evidence to show that it is a major transition stage in neural and behavioral development. It is a key stage in the evolution of the parent–child relationship: a time when parents and infants are in a state of heightened readiness for social exchange and a time when the earliest parent–infant interaction patterns are being laid down; a time when the family system is in a formative stage of its evolution as it prepares to accommodate the new infant into its system; a time when the family system provides a unique entree to the supportive clinician; and a time when the newborn, as she or he selectively engages her or his environment, is actively forming a sense of an emergent self, a sense of self that will remain active for the rest of the child's life (Stern 1985). The newborn period is undoubtedly a formative moment in the life of the infant, the parents, and the family, and as such presents an invaluable opportunity to the clinician to intervene in a way that has potentially long-lasting effects on the parent–child relationship.

# References

Adamson, L. B. (1993). *Communication Development During Infancy.* Madison, WI: Brown and Benchmark.

Als, H. (1986). A synactive model of neonatal behavioral organization: framework for the assessment of neurobehavioral development in the premature infant and for support of infants and parents in the neonatal intensive care unit. In J.K. Sweeney, Ed. *The high-risk neonate: developmental therapy perspectives.* New York: Haworth Press, pp. 3–53.

Als, H. (1999). Reading the premature infant. In E. Goldson, Ed. *Nurturing the Premature Infant.* New York: Oxford University Press.

Anisfeld, E., & Pincus, M. (1978). The post-partum support project: serving young mothers and older women through home visiting. *Zero to Three* 8:13–15.

Barr, R. (1998) Reflections on N-shaped curves in early infancy: regulated or re-organized development? *Infant Behavior and Development* 21:184.

Beal, J. A. (1986) The Brazelton Neonatal Behavioral Assessment: a tool to enhance parental attachment. *Journal of Pediatric Nursing* 1:170–177.

Belsky, J. (1985). Experimenting with the family in the newborn period. *Child Development* 56:407–414.

Blanchard, Y., & Mouradian, L. (2000). Integrating neurobehavioral concepts into early intervention eligibility evaluation. *Infants and Young Children* 13(2):41–50.

Boger, K., & Kurnetz, R. (1985). Perinatal positive parenting: hospital-based support for first-time parents. *Pediatric Basics* 41:4–15.

Bottos, M. (1987). *Paralisi cerebrale infantile.* Milano: Ghedini Editore.

Boukydis, C. F. Z. (Ed.) (1986). *Supports for parents and infants.* New York: Routledge & Kegan Paul.

Brazelton, T. B. (1973). *Neonatal Behavioral Assessment Scale.* Clinics in developmental medicine, No. 50, 2nd ed. Philadelphia: J. P. Lippincott.

Brazelton, T. B. (1995). Working with families: opportunities for early intervention. *Family-Focused Pediatrics* 42:1–9.

Brazelton, T. B., Koslowski, B., & Main, M. (1974). The origins of reciprocity: the early mother–infant interaction. In M. Lewis & L. Rosenblum, Eds. *The effect of the infant on its caregivers.* New York: Wiley Interscience, pp. 49–77.

Brazelton, T. B., Nugent, J. K. (1995). *The Newborn Behavioral Assessment Scale.* McKeith Press: London.

Clarkson, M. G., & Clifton, R. K. (1991). Acoustic determinants of newborn orienting. In M. J. Weiss & P. R. Zelazo, Eds. *Newborn attention: biological constraints and the influence of experience.* Norwood, NJ: Ablex.

Cramer, B. (1987). Objective and subjective aspects of parent–infant relations. In J. Osofsky, Ed. *The handbook of infant development,* 2nd ed. New York: Wiley, pp. 1037–1059.

Crockenberg, S. (1986). Professional support for adolescent mothers: who gives it, how adolescent mothers evaluate it, what they would prefer. *Infant Mental Health Journal* 7:49–58.

Dannemiller, J. L., & Freedland, R. L. (1991) Detection of relative motion by human infants. *Developmental Psychology* 27:67–78.

D'Apolito, K. (1991). What is an organized infant? *Neonatal Network* 10:23–29.

Das Eiden, R., & Reifman, A. (1996). Effects of Brazelton demonstrations on later parenting. *Journal of Pediatric Psychology* 21:857–868.

DeCasper, A. J., & Fifer, W. P. (1980). Of human bonding. *Science* 208:1174–1176.

DeCasper, A. J., Lecanuet, J. P., Busnel, M. C., Granier-Deferre, C., & Maugeais, R. (1994). Fetal reactions to recurrent maternal speech. *Infant Behavior and Development* 17:159–164.

Dobbing, J. (1990). Vulnerable periods in the developing brain. In J. Dobbing, Ed. *Brain, Behavior, and Iron in the Infant Diet.* London: Springer-Verlag.

Doi, T. (1991). *The anatomy of dependence.* Tokyo and New York: Kodansha International.

Dreher, M., Nugent, J. K., & Hudgins, R. (1994). Prenatal marijuana exposure and neonatal outcomes in Jamaica: an ethnographic study. *Pediatrics* 93:254–260.

Ecklund-Flores, L., & Turkewitz, G. (1996). Asymmetric head-turning to speech and nonspeech in human newborns. *Developmental Psychobiology* 29:205–217.

Emde, R., Korfmacher, J., & Kubricek, L. F. (2000). Towards a theory of early relationship-based intervention. In J. D. Osofsky & H. Fitzgerald, Eds. *WAIMH handbook of infant mental health.* New York: Wiley.

Emde, R. N., & Robinson, J. (1979) The first two months: recent research in developmental psychobiology and the changing view of the newborn. In J. Noshpitz, (Ed.) *Basic Handbook of Child Psychiatry.* New York: Basic Books.

Field, T, Woodson, R., Greenberg, R., & Cohen, C. (1992). Discrimination and imitation of facial expressions in newborns. *Science* 218:179–181.

Fraiberg, S. (1980). *Clinical studies in infant mental health: the first year of life.* New York: Basic.

Garbarino, J. (1992). *Children and families in the social environment.* New York: Aldine de Gruyter.

Gilkerson, L., & Shahmoon-Shanok J. (2000). Relationships for growth: cultivating reflective practice in infant, toddler and preschool programs. In J. D. Osofsky & H. E. Fitzgerald, Eds. *WAIMH handbook of infant mental health.* New York: Wiley.

Gomes-Pedro, J., de Almeida, J. B., & Costa Barbosa, A. (1984). Influence of early mother–infant contact on synaptic behavior during the first month of life. *Developmental Medicine and Child Neurology* 26:657–664.

Gomes-Pedro, J., Patricio, M., Carvalho, A., Goldschmidt, T., Torgal-Garcia, F., & Monteiro, M. B. (1995). Early intervention with Portuguese mothers: a two year follow-up. *Developmental and Behavioral Pediatrics* 16:21–28.

Greenspan, S. I. (1981). *The clinical interview of the child.* New York: McGraw-Hill.

Hirshberg, L. M. (1993). Clinical interviews with infants and their families. In C. H. Zeanah, Ed. *Handbook of infant mental health.* London/New York: The Guilford Press.

Hopkins, B. (1998) Moving into the two-month revolution: an action-based account. *Infant Behavior and Development* 21:183.

Kawasaki, C., Nugent, J. K., & Brazelton, T. B. (1994) The cultural organization of children's sleep. *Children's Environments* 11:135–141.

Klaus, M. H., Kennell, J. H., & Klaus, P. H. (1995). *Bonding.* Reading, MA: Addison-Wesley.

Konner, M. (1998). Behavioral changes around two months of age in a population of African hunter-gatherers. *Infant Behavior and Development* 21:185.

Laplante, D., Orr, R., Neville, K., Vorkapich, L., & Sasso, D. (1996) Discrimination of stimulus rotations by newborns. *Infant Behavior and Development* 19:271–279.

Lawhon, G. (2002). Facilitation of parenting the premature infant within the newborn intensive care unit. *Journal of Perinatal & Neonatal Nursing* 16:71–83.

Lester, B. M., Hoffman, J., & Brazelton, T. B. (1985). The rhythmic structure of mother–infant interaction in term and preterm infants. *Child Development* 51:15–27.

LeVine, R. A. (1980). Cross-cultural perspectives on parenting. In M. Fantini & R. Cardinas, Eds. *Parenting in a multicultural society*. New York: Longman, pp. 17–26.

Loo, K. K., Espoinosa, M., Tyler, R., & Howard, J. (2003). Using knowledge to cope with stress in the NICU: how parents integrate learning to read the physiologic and behavioral cues of the infant. *Neonatal Network* 22:31–37.

MacDonough, S. C. (1993). Interaction guidance: understanding and treating early infant caregiver disturbances. In C. Zeanah, Ed. *Handbook of infant mental health*. New York/London: The Guilford Press.

Meisels, S., Dichtelmiller, M., & Fong-Ruey L. (1993). A multidimensional analysis of early childhood intervention programs. In C. Zeanah, Ed. *Handbook of infant mental health*. New York/London: The Guilford Press.

Meltzoff, A., & Moore, K. (1989). Imitation in newborn infants. *Developmental Psychology* 25(6), 954–962.

Minuchin, B. (1985). Families and individual development: provocations from the field of family therapy. *Child Development* 59:289–302.

Moon, C., Cooper, R. P., & Fifer, W. (1993). Two-day-olds prefer their native language. *Infant Behavior and Development* 16:495–500.

Muir, D., & Field, J. (1979). Newborn infants orient to sounds. *Child Development* 50:431–436.

Murray, L., & Cooper, P. J. (1997). The role of infant and maternal factors in postpartum depression, mother–infant interactions, and infant outcomes. In L. Murray & P. J. Cooper, Eds. *Postpartum depression and child development*. New York/London: The Guilford Press.

Myers, B. J. (1982). Early intervention using Brazelton training with middle class mothers and fathers of newborns. *Child Development* 53:462–471.

Nugent, J. K. (1994). Cross-cultural studies of child development: implications for clinicians. *Zero to Three* 15(2):1–8.

Nugent, J. K. (1991). Cultural and psychological influences on the father's role in infant development. *Journal of Marriage and the Family* 53:475–485.

Nugent, J. K. (2002). The cultural context of child development: implications for research and practice in the twenty-first century. In J. Gomes-Pedro, J. K. Nugent, J. G. Young, T. B. Brazelton, Eds. *The infant and family in the twenty-first century*. New York and Hove: Brunner-Routledge.

Nugent, J. K., & Brazelton, T. B. (2000). Preventive mental health: uses of the Brazelton Scale. In J. Osofsky & H. Fitzgerald, Eds. *WAIMH handbook of infant mental health*. New York: Wiley.

Nugent, J. K., & Brazelton, T.B. (2001). *The Clinical Neonatal Behavioral Assessment Scale*. Brazelton Institute, Children's Hospital, Boston.

Nugent, J. K., Keefer, C. H., O'Brien, S., Johnson, L., & Blanchard, Y. (to be published). *The Newborn Behavioral Observations (NBO) System*. To be published.

Nugent, J. K., Lester, B. M., & Brazelton, T. B. (1989). The cultural context of infancy: biology, culture and infant development, Volume 1. Norwood, NJ: Ablex.

Nugent, J. K., Lester, B. M., & Brazelton, T. B. (1991). The cultural context of infancy: multicultural and interdisciplinary approaches to parent-child relations, Volume 2. Norwood, NJ: Ablex.

Ohgi, S., Takahashi, T., Nugent, J. K., Akiyama, T. (in press). Neonatal behavioral characteristics and later behavioral problems. *Clinical Pediatrics*.

Parker, S., Zahr, L. K., Cole, J. C. D., Braced, M. L. (1992). Outcomes after developmental intervention in the neonatal intensive care unit for mothers of preterm infants with low socioeconomic status. *Journal of Pediatrics* 120:780–785.

Pascalis, O., de Schonen, S., Morton, J., Deruelle, C., & Fabre-Grenet, M. (1995). Mother's face recognition by neonates: a replication and an extension. *Infant Behavior and Development* 18:79–85.

Philliber Research Associates (2001). *The Clinical Neonatal Behavioral Assessment Scale: training outcomes*. Accord, NY.

Rauh, V., Achenbach, T., Nurcombe, B., Howell, C., & Teti, D. (1988). Minimizing adverse effects of low birthweight: four-year results of an early intervention program. *Child Development* 59:S44–553.

Redshaw, M. E. (1997). Mothers of babies requiring special care: attitudes and experiences. *Journal of Reproductive & Infant Psychology* 15(2):109–121.

Rochat, P. (1998). The newly objectified world of 2-month-olds. *Infant Behavior and Development* 21:182.

Sameroff, A. J. (1993). Models of development and developmental risk. In C. H. Zeanah, Ed. *Handbook of infant mental health*. New York/London: The Guilford Press.

Shonkoff, J. P., & Phillips, D. A. (2000). *From neurons to neighborhoods*. Washington, DC: National Academy Press.

Shweder, R. A., Goodnow, J. J., Hatano, G., LeVine, R. A., Markus, H. R., & Miller, P. (1998). The cultural psychology of development: one mind, many mentalities. In W. Damon, Ed. *Handbook of child psychology, Volume 1: Theoretical models of human development.* New York: Wiley and Sons.

Slater, A., Morison, V., Town, C., & Rose, D. (1985). Movement perception and identity constancy in the newborn baby. *British Journal of Developmental Psychology* 3:211–220.

Spence, M. J., & Freeman. M. S. (1996). Newborn infants prefer the maternal low-pass filtered voice, but not the maternal whispered voice. *Infant Behavior and Development* 19:199–212.

Stadtler, A., O'Brien, M. A., Hornstein, H. (1986). The Touchpoints Model: building supportive alliances between parents and professionals. *Zero to Three* 15:24–28.

Stern, D. N. (1985). *The interpersonal world of the infant.* New York: Basic.

Stern, D. N. (1995). *The motherhood constellation.* New York: Basic.

Swain, I., Zealot, P., & Clifton, R. (1993). Newborn infants' memory for speech sounds retained over 24 hours. *Developmental Psychology* 29:312–323.

Thomas, A., & Chess, S. (1977). *Temperament and development.* New York: Brunner-Maze.

Trevarthen, C. (1979). Communication and cooperation in early infancy: a description of early subjectivity. In M. Bullowa, Ed. *Before speech: the beginning of interpersonal communication.* Cambridge, U.K.: Cambridge University Press.

Tronick, E. Z., & Cohn, J. F. (1989). Infant–mother face-to-face interaction: age and gender differences in coordination and occurrence of incardination. *Child Development* 60:85–92.

Weinberg, M. K., & Tronick, E. Z. (1996). Infant affective reactions to the resumption of maternal interaction after the still-face. *Child Development* 67:905–914.

Weissbourd, B., & Kagan, S. (1989). Family support programs: catalysts for change. *American Journal of Orthopsychiatry* 59:20–31.

Whiting, B., & Edwards, C. P. (1988). *Children of different worlds: the formation of social behavior.* Cambridge, MA: Harvard University Press.

Wolff, P. (1959). Observations on human infants. *Psychosomatic Medicine* 221:110–118.

Wolke, D., Gray, P., & Meyer, R. (1994). Excessive infant crying: a controlled study of mothers helping mothers. *Pediatrics* 94:322.

Worobey, J., & Belsky, J. (1982). Employing the Brazelton scale to influence mothering: an experimental comparison of three strategies. *Developmental Psychology* 18:736–743.

Zeanah, C. H., & McDonough, S. C. (1989). Clinical approaches to families in early intervention. *Seminars in Perinatology* 13:513–522.

# Chapter 6

# Psychosocial Development: Attachment in Young Children

Kathleen McCartney
Erin O'Connor

Attachment is a powerful emotional relationship that develops between children and important caregivers in their lives—caregivers who protect children during times of stress and/or danger and encourage children's independent exploration during times of safety. Children begin to develop attachment relationships with primary caregivers during their first 4 years, and individuals maintain and develop attachment relationships throughout their lives. Through these relationships, individuals develop working models that specify a view of self and others as primarily positive or negative. Because children's early attachments impact their socioemotional development, assisting children and parents in developing optimal relationships is an important task of early childhood professionals. In this chapter we review attachment theory, including the stages of attachment formation, attachment styles' influences on the formation of attachments, and the implications of attachment theory for clinical interventions.

## Attachment Theory

Attachment theory was first introduced by John Bowlby. Others have extended the theory, espe-

cially Mary Ainsworth, Inge Bretherton, and Mary Main. Attachment theory is composed of three main propositions (Belsky & Cassidy 1994; McCartney & Dearing 2002). First, infants' attachment ties are evolutionarily based. Although there is no fossil record of social behavior, theorists speculate that throughout history children who exhibited attachment behaviors were more likely to form close relationships with attachment figures and therefore more likely to survive and reproduce. In particular, children's attachment behaviors increase their proximity to primary caregivers (stereotypically mothers) who can protect and nurture them. Some attachment behaviors, such as smiling and vocalizing, are *signaling* behaviors that bring children to the attention of caregivers. Other behaviors, such as crying, are *aversive* and bring children into contact with caregivers who want to stop these behaviors. Lastly, some behaviors are active, such as approaching and following, and draw children to their caregivers.

Second, attachment is a motivational control system that organizes children's behaviors. The system regulates children's wishes to explore the environment and to maintain proximity with caregivers. In particular, when children are at a comfortable distance from their caregivers, their attachment system is deactivated and they refrain from engaging in attachment behaviors. When children are anxious about their distances from their caregivers, their attachment systems are activated and they engage in attachment behaviors to bring them closer to their caregivers. Homeostasis in the attachment system is attained when children are comfortable with their distance from their caregivers. Children's comfort levels vary as a function of age as well as context (Marvin & Britner 1999). Older children can tolerate greater distances from caregivers than can younger children. Under conditions that indicate danger or induce stress, children require close proximity to caregivers. Illness, hunger, fatigue, or pain and the environment can all activate the attachment system.

Third, attachment experiences with caregivers in early childhood guide an individual's later behaviors through internal working models (IWM). IWMs are cognitive representations of early attachments (Bowlby 1988). Early interactions within attachment relationships become internalized and shape individuals' experiences with individuals later encountered. These models exist, for the most part, outside of conscious awareness (Marvin & Britner 1999). IWMs reflect both individual's working models of self and of the self in relation to the attachment figure. A working model of the self as valued and sufficient is created when children experience attachment figures as protective and supportive of their explorations. On the other hand, children develop models of the self as incompetent and/or unvalued in relationships in which attachment figures are dismissive of children's attachment and/or exploration activities (Bretherton & Munholland 1999).

Children do not apply their IWMs to relationships until they develop recall memory, at approximately 11 months, and recognize that objects (including attachment figures) continue to exist when not seen. At this point, children's working models become operable and they use them to create and appraise uncomplicated attachment plans. They also become able to communicate their attachment needs and to predict how their attachment figures will react across a variety of contexts (Bretherton & Munholland 1999).

# The Development of Attachment Relationships

Attachment is an evoked mechanism. In other words, children are born with an innate desire to seek contact with caretaking adults. The formation of attachment relationships between children and primary caregivers, however, is a gradual process best described by four stages (see Table 6.1). From birth to 6 weeks, infants demonstrate precursor attachment behaviors, such as crying when they are hungry or scared. At this stage, infants act in the same way toward any individual who fulfills their basic needs (Berk 1997). However, as infants develop the ability to discriminate among individuals, they evidence attachment behaviors predominately to those individuals with whom they have the most contact.

By approximately 6 weeks, infants begin to respond differently to familiar and unfamiliar individuals, directing more attachment behaviors toward familiar individuals. At this point, infants enter into the second phase in the development of attachments. Infants and caregivers work to establish social synchrony, demonstrated through reciprocal vocal and affective exchanges. For example, displays of joy by mothers are met with cooing and smiling by the infant.

By 6 to 9 months, infants begin to develop "clear-cut" attachments. Children demonstrate several new attachment behaviors at this point. These behaviors include 1) following primary caregivers when they depart the room (24 weeks); 2) approaching primary caregivers when upset or

*Table 6.1*  The Development of Attachments

| Phase | Time Period | Description |
|---|---|---|
| The preattachment phase | birth to 6 weeks | Innate behaviors, such as smiling, bring the infant into contact with other humans. Infants can recognize their mothers' scent at this point but are not attached, and do not mind being left with an unfamiliar adult. |
| The "attachment-in-the-making" phase | 6 weeks to 6–8 months | Infants begin to interact with a familiar caregiver differently than an unfamiliar one. For example, babies may laugh more when held by their mothers. They also learn that their behaviors impact those around them and begin to anticipate that their caregiver will respond to them. Babies do not protest when separated from their primary caregivers. |
| The phase of "clear-cut attachment" | 6–8 months to 18 months | Attachment to the primary caretaker is evident. Children develop separation anxiety at 6 months and protest even brief separations from the primary caregiver. Separation anxiety increases until approximately 15 months. Older infants and children not only protest separation from the caregiver but also act in ways to maintain their presence. Children also begin to use the primary caregiver as a secure base, exploring the environment but then returning to the caregiver for emotional support. |
| Formation of reciprocal relationship | 18 months to 2 years and on | Children begin to understand their caregivers' needs and motives and are able to negotiate with the caregiver to alter their goals. Therefore, separation protests decline. |

*Source:* Adapted from Berk, 1997.

reunited after an absence (28 weeks); 3) burying their face when coming into contact with primary caregivers (28 weeks); 4) using primary caregivers as a secure base from which to explore (28 weeks); and 5) clinging to primary caregivers when stressed or ill (43 weeks). It is when children begin to form attachments that they demonstrate separation anxiety when their primary caregiver is not present (Marvin & Britner 1999).

Clear-cut attachment formation is also marked by developments of other behavioral systems associated with the attachment system. Specifically, exploratory, sociable, and wary systems develop at this time. These systems, like the attachment system, are motivational control systems. The exploratory system involves infants' desires to interact with their environments; the sociable system involves infants' desires to affiliate with others; and the wary system involves infants' suspicions of novel and unfamiliar events, places, and individuals (Marvin & Britner 1999). During this phase, children's behavioral systems become more coherent as they begin to engage in activities organized on the basis of goal-corrected behaviors. The synchronous workings of these systems are demonstrated in children's behaviors during the presence of unfamiliar adults. During the second half of the first year, children become increasingly wary of unfamiliar adults. If their wary system is activated by an encounter with an unfamiliar adult, children's attachment behavioral systems are activated but their sociable systems are deactivated. Children subsequently seek the primary caregiver as a secure base. The development and balance of these systems results in stable variations in the organization of children's attachment behaviors by the end of the first year. Therefore, the third phase of attachment represents a sensitive period, an optimal time for the development of these abilities, in children's social-emotional development (Marvin & Britner 1999).

The fourth and final phase in the development of attachment relationships occurs during the middle of children's second year when they develop reciprocal relationships or goal-corrected partnerships (Lamb et al. 1985). Within these partnerships, children balance their needs with those of their attachment figures. Children acquire at least five component skills by the age of four that allow them to develop goal-corrected partnerships with their attachment figures: 1) the capacity to recognize that attachment figures have their own internal thoughts, feelings, and wishes; 2) the capability to differentiate between their own and their caregivers' understandings; 3) the facility to deduce what influences caregivers; 4) the ability to evaluate the amount of concordance between their desires and those of their caregivers; and 5) the capacity to manipulate caregivers' plans in a goal-corrected fashion (Marvin 1977). With the ability to internally operate on both their own and their caregivers' perspectives, children no longer rely on physical proximity to maintain feelings of safety and security within relationships. Therefore, by 4 years of age, children tend to be minimally distressed by physical separations from primary caregivers (Marvin & Britner 1999).

# Attachment Styles

Most children, except potentially those who suffer from severe neglect, develop attachment relationships with primary caregivers; however, attachment patterns and/or styles are not uniform across children. Mary Ainsworth pioneered studies both in the field and in the laboratory that documented individual differences in attachment styles. Ainsworth and her colleagues (1978) developed the Strange Situation procedure to observe these differences. This is a structured laboratory technique designed to produce sufficient stress in infants to activate their attachment behavioral systems. The stress is produced by a series of brief separations from and reunions with the mother in the presence of a stranger.

Ainsworth and colleagues (1978) originally used the Strange Situation procedure with a small sample of American 1-year-olds. From this sample, they identified three patterns of attachment: secure, avoidant, and ambivalent (see Table 6.2). Securely attached children demonstrated minimal anxiety and explored the environment in their mothers' absence. When reunited with their mothers, they were soothed, comforted, and reassured. Infants with avoidant attachments showed little fear or anxiety about upon their mothers' departures; however, they did not explore the environment during their absences. They evaded their mothers upon reunion. Infants with ambivalent attachment styles evidenced a great deal of stress when initially separated from their mothers and did not actively explore their environments during their mothers' absences. Upon reunion, they sought out their mothers but were not quickly soothed by their presence (Carlson et al. 1989). In subsequent work with children in the Strange Situation, researchers identified numerous children that could not be classified using the original tripartite classification system. Based on these observations, Main and Solomon (1986) identified criteria for an additional insecure attachment pattern termed disorganized/disoriented.

*Table 6.2*    Strange Situation Classification Groups

| Group | Children's Behavior Strange Situation | Maternal Behavior Associated with Classification |
|---|---|---|
| Secure (B) | Infants use parents as a secure base to explore environment. Infants may cry when left with strangers but are immediately soothed when reunited with parents. | Sensitive and responsive caregiving in which parental behaviors are contingent on infants' needs. |
| Avoidant (A) | Infants appear unresponsive to parents when they are present. They are usually not distressed when left with strangers and react toward strangers similar as to parents. Upon reunion with parents they often do not seek contact. | Intrusive care and overstimulation in which parents continue to intensively engage with infants despite signals from the infants to disengage. |
| Ambivalent (C) | Before separation, infants cling to parents and do not explore their environments. Infants are very distressed when left with strangers but are not easily soothed when reunited with parents. | Inconsistent parenting in which parents are often disengaged except during times of infant exploration, at which time parents become overly intrusive. |
| Disorganized (D) | Infants do not actively explore environment in parents' presence. Infants are distressed at parents' separations, but of maltreating parents often demonstrate confused and contradictory behaviors upon reunions. The majority of infants express their disorientation with dazed facial expressions. | Parenting that is frightening to the infant. |

*Note:* Descriptions in groups A, B, and C taken from Berk (1997). Descriptions in Group D based on Solomon & George (1999).

# Attachment and Ethnicity/Culture

One of the core tenets of attachment theory is that the attachment relationship is evolutionarily adaptive and is a universal phenomenon. Cross-cultural research does suggest that all infants form secure or insecure attachments. Furthermore, there is extant evidence that the number of children who form a secure pattern of attachment is proportionately comparable across cultures. In America, Africa, China, Israel, Japan, and Western Europe approximately two-thirds of children form secure attachments to their caregivers (van Ijzendoorn & Sagi 1999).

Results from international studies, however, suggest that specific types of insecure attachments vary across cultures. Studies conducted in Japan and Germany form the basis for international comparisons of attachment patterns and discussions of potential influences of culture on attachment behaviors. In Japan, a higher proportion of children are classified as ambivalent and a lower proportion classified as avoidant than in American and Western European cultures. In Germany, on the other hand, a higher proportion of children are classified as avoidant and a lower proportion as ambivalent than in American and Japanese cultures (Levine 2001). These differences in attachment distributions in Germany and Japan are theorized to relate to differences in parenting styles in the two cultures. German parents tend to leave their children for extended periods of time and encourage self-reliance at an early age, whereas Japanese parents foster skin-to-skin contact in infancy and encourage interdependence.

# Determinants of Attachment Styles

Children's initial attachment relationships reflect the interactive patterns and styles of parents and children. Both parents and children play roles in the development of attachments. However, parental caretaking behaviors are the most significant determinants of children's attachment styles. The majority of studies conducted on attachment and parenting focus on mother–child interactions.

Certain mother–child interactions in early infancy promote attachment through biological processes. In particular, nipple grasp, sucking, orogustatory stimulation by milk, and ventral-to-ventral (stomach/chest to stomach/chest) body contact are factors in the formation of attachment (Polan & Hofer 1999). Close ventral-to-ventral

contact between a mother and child releases the neurochemical oxytocin in both the mother and child. Oxytocin, in turn, induces feelings of comfort and closeness in mother and child that contributes to the formation of attachment between the two (Nelson & Panksepp 1998). The importance of early mother–infant physical contact for attachment formation is vividly demonstrated in an experimental study by Anisfeld, Casper, Nozyce and Cunningham (1990) with low-income inner-city mothers of newborn infants. In this study, an experimental group was given soft baby carriers, and a control group was given rigid carriers. The soft carriers increased physical contact between mothers and infants. At 13 months, 83% of the babies in the experimental group were securely attached to their mothers compared with only 39% of the control group babies.

After the early infancy period, maternal behaviors continue to influence the quality of the mother–child attachment relationship (see Table 6.3). Children whose mothers respond sensitively and appropriately to their needs form secure attachments because they are confidant that they will be protected and that their needs will be met. On the other hand, children whose mothers ignore

*Table 6.3*    Disorders of Attachment

| Title | Source | Description |
|---|---|---|
| Reactive attachment disorder | DSM-IV (2001) | This disorder involves failure to initiate social interactions or indiscriminate friendliness with strangers that begins at age 5 or younger. It is characterized by 1) pathogenic treatment by the caregiver before age 5; 2) lack of an attachment relationship before age 5; and 3) persistent turmoil in all relationships (Greenberg 1999). |
| Nonattachment | DSM-IV (2001) Lieberman & Zenah (1999) | This disorder describes children who do not show a preferred attachment figure and who have cognitive abilities at or above the level of 10 to 12 months. |
| Disordered attachments | Lieberman & Zenah (1999) | These disorders are characterized by deviations in secure-base behavior. |
| Disrupted attachments | Lieberman & Zenah (1999) | This refers to extreme grief reactions after the loss of an attachment figure prior to age 3. |

their dependency pleas develop avoidant attachments because they are not confident that their mothers will respond to their needs. To avoid being rejected and distressed when their needs are unfilled, these children learn to suppress the expression of affect (Cassidy & Kobak 1988). Children whose mothers respond inconsistently to their needs develop ambivalent attachments because they are anxious about their mothers' availabilities and afraid that their mothers will be unresponsive or unsuccessful in meeting their needs (Weinfield et al. 1999). These children become dependent, angry, and clingy in attempts to maintain close proximities to their mothers who are not consistently available.

Children tend to form disorganized attachments when their mothers have experienced personal loss and difficult life circumstances (Lyons-Ruth, Bronfman, & Parson 1999). This association is rooted in the fact that mothers who are unresolved to trauma or loss are more likely to partake in frightening caregiving behaviors (Jacobvitz & Hazen 1999). Fearful maternal behaviors place children in an unresolvable paradox because fear activates children's attachment behavioral systems; however, their primary attachment figure is the source of fear (Lyons-Ruth et al. 1999). These infants are thus unable to form coherent behavioral strategies to deal with the fear (Main & Hesse 1990).

# Stability in Attachment Styles

After 18 months, children's attachment styles tend to be relatively stable. Due to assimilation, a process by which novel experiences and situations are integrated into already present schemas, children's models of relationships are resistant to change (Bretherton & Munholland 1999). As children mature, modest changes in their environments may adjust but not completely alter their models of specific relationships (Bowlby 1988).

Waters (1978) conducted one of the first studies of attachment stability. Observing infants with their mothers in the Strange Situation at 12 and 18 months, Waters found differences over time in discrete attachment behaviors, such as frequency of looking, but 96% concordance in security status. Similarly, Main and Cassidy (1988) found high concordance (82%) in attachment ratings between 12 months and 6 years.

As children mature, their attachment classifications continue to reflect the quality of their relationships with primary caregivers. However, the manifestations of attachment styles change over time. By the early school years, children with each of the attachment styles evidence distinct behaviors. Securely attached children are comfortable communicating their feelings and needs to their caregivers and are able to seek comfort from them (Main & Cassidy 1988). Avoidantly attached children are minimally communicative about personal concerns and reluctant to express dependency needs with caregivers. Children with avoidant attachments also tend to demonstrate more anger, negative affect, and aggression than children with other attachment styles (Weinfield et al. 1999). Ambivalently attached children often exhibit exaggerated dependency needs but are not easily soothed by attachment figures and do not feel comfortable with closeness to attachment figures. Ambivalent children also tend to be less forceful and confident, more hesitant in the face of novelty, and generally evidence more anxiety than children with other attachment styles (Weinfield et al. 1999). Disorganized children develop coherent methods to have their attachment needs met by 6 years of age. Most behave in a controlling manner toward their caregivers. These controlling strategies may either be punitive or caregiving. Children with controlling punitive strategies direct their caregivers usually either in a rejecting or humiliating manner. On the other hand, children with controlling caregiving strategies behave in an extremely cheerful or solicitous manner (Jacobvitz

& Hazen 1999). These behaviors bring children into contact with their caregivers to ensure that caregivers will attend to their needs.

## Maternal Stress and Depression

Various maternal experiences and traits impact children's attachment styles through their effect on maternal caregiving behaviors. In particular, mothers' past attachment relationships, stress levels, and depressive symptoms are related to their parenting behaviors associated with children's attachment styles. Children's attachment patterns with their mothers tend to be similar to those of their mothers with their own mothers (e.g., Ainsworth & Eichberg 1991, Benoit & Parker 1994, van Ijzendoorn 1995). Mothers incorporate caregiving experiences with their children into their preexisting models of attachment, developed through their interactions with their own mothers. This association is referred to as the *intergenerational transmission of attachment* (George & Solomon 1999).

Parental stress also has a profound effect on the quality of children's attachments due to its negative impact on maternal sensitivity and responsivity. Maternal stress is related to hostility, anger, irritability, and mistrust of and alienation from one's children (Conger 1984). Data from studies of mother–child dyads among mothers with high and low levels of reported stress indicate that children from high-stress dyads tend to form insecure attachments, whereas those from low-stress dyads tend to develop secure attachments (DeMulder et al. 2000; Teti et al. 1991). Children whose mothers evidence high levels of stress are particularly likely to develop ambivalent attachments due to inconsistent maternal care (Moss et al. 1996).

Parental depression is also associated with less positive parent–child interactions. Depressed mothers are less sensitive and engaged in their interactions with their children than are nondepressed mothers (DeMulder & Radke-Yarrow 1991). Results from a large-scale study, the NICHD Study of Early Care and Youth Development, showed that both women who were sometimes depressed as well as those who were chronically depressed were less sensitive in their interactions with their children than were mothers who were never depressed (NICHD ECCRN 1999). In several studies, children whose mothers were depressed evidenced higher rates of attachment insecurity, in particular disorganized attachment, than children whose mothers were not depressed (DeMulder & Radke-Yarrow 1991, Radke-Yarrow et al. 1985).

## Parental Separations and Attachment

Handling physical separations is a challenge for parents and young children. Children's separation anxiety peaks at 15 months when they begin to develop attachments. At this point, children demonstrate separation protests in the form of crying when their primary caretakers leave and resist even short periods of separation, such as at bed time. Children may continue to protest physical separations from primary caretakers throughout the second year. However, brief periods of physical separation between children and parents are beneficial for children's development of psychological separatism and are not detrimental to the attachment relationship.

One of the first prolonged periods of separation for most children in the United States is entry into child care (NICHD 1999). A debate used to exist in the literature regarding whether prolonged periods of separation between mother and child may be detrimental for the child's development of a secure attachment. Critics suggest that frequent separations from their mother will undermine children's trust in their mothers' responsiveness. Numerous studies have been conducted to research the potential association between nonmaternal child care and child attachment. Several studies conducted in the 1980s demonstrated associations between early and extensive child care and increased rates of insecure attachment between 12 and 18 months (Belsky & Rovine 1988, Clarke-Stewart 1989, Lamb & Sternberg 1990). However, results from studies conducted in the 1990s failed to demonstrate an association between nonmaternal care and attachment insecurity (Roggman et al. 1994, Symons 1998). Furthermore, results from the largest, most comprehensive study of child care to date demonstrated no main effects of child care on infant–mother attachment security, measured at 15 and 36 months. However, in this study, child care was important in its interaction with several family factors. In particular, infants were less likely to be securely attached to their mothers at 15 months when low maternal sensitivity and/or responsivity was combined with poor-quality child care, more than one child-care arrangement, or more than minimal hours in care (more than 10 hours per week) (NICHD Early Child Care Research Network 1997). Similarly, when maternal sensitivity was low, more hours per week in care modestly increased the risk of ambivalent attachment at 36 months (NICHD Early Child Care Research Network 1998).

Children's experiences of transition into child care, however, may impact the effect of child care on children's attachment security. Rauh, Ziegenhain, Muller, and Wijnroks (2000) examined the effect of experiences of transitions into child care on change in attachment classifications. They found that a change from a secure to insecure pattern was associated with abrupt transitions into child care but not with gradual transitions. Abrupt transitions were defined by long attendance hours with little or no maternal company in the child care center during the initial period in care. Gradual transitions were defined by short attendance hours with long periods accompanied by the mother during the initial period in care.

## Marital Conflict, Divorce, and Single Parenthood

Extensive evidence exists that supportive spousal relationships when children are young are associated with caring and sensitive parenting styles that correlate with attachment security (Erel & Burman 1995). Children from families whose parents have satisfying marriages are more likely to develop secure attachments than those from families whose parents have less satisfying marriages. This association appears to hold across cultures and economic groups (Belsky 1999).

Longitudinal studies of marital satisfaction and quality of parent–child attachments indicate powerful long-term effects. For example, data from one study demonstrated that at 1 to 3 years of age, children whose mothers reported higher levels of marital satisfaction and lower levels of marital conflict prenatally were more likely to be securely attached than children whose mothers reported lower levels of prenatal marital satisfaction (Howes & Markman 1989). Results from another study showed that high levels of marital conflict prenatally, and at 3 months postpartum, were associated with disorganization in mother–child attachment relationships at 1 year (Owen & Cox 1997). Marital quality also appears to be associated with the quality of young children's attachments to mothers after the birth of a sibling. In particular, results from one study showed that high levels of marital accord subsequent to the birth of a second child were associated with first-born attachment security (Teti et al. 1996). Due to the long-term implications of marital satisfaction for children's attachments, parental divorce may be associated with children's insecure attachments.

Several studies have been conducted to examine the effects of parental divorce on children's attachment relationships. In general, parental divorce is associated with insecure attachments between children and their mothers and fathers

(Solomon & George 1999). Divorce may impact children's attachments through parental conflict. For example, in one study, high levels of conflict and low levels of communication between divorcing parents were associated with infant attachment insecurity, disorganized attachment in particular (Solomon & George 1999). Furthermore, results from other studies demonstrate no impact of divorce itself on children's attachment relationships when controlling for amount of marital conflict. In particular, results from one study indicated similar attachment styles among children whose parents were divorced and whose parents were married yet reported high levels of conflict in their marriage (Emery 1982). Therefore, marital discord, rather than divorce, may be detrimental for children's developments of secure attachments.

Few studies have been conducted to examine the potential effects of single parenthood on the quality of infant–mother attachments; however, results from one study indicated a higher prevalence of insecure attachments among children of single versus married mothers. Specifically, 67% of children with married mothers developed secure attachments compared to 25% with single mothers (Gaffney et al. 2000). Associations between single parenthood and attachment insecurity may reflect high levels of stress experienced by single parents, who may lack child care and financial assistance, and probably varies as a function of the timing of single parent status.

## Attachment and Parental Death

The death of a parent has a profound impact on a young child's attachment behavioral system. Young children, like adults, go through three stages after the loss of a parent: protest, despair, and detachment (see Table 6.4). Young children who fail to reach the detachment stage and cannot resolve their grief over the loss of an attachment figure may develop an attachment disorder. These children demonstrate disrupted attachments, show prolonged periods of grief reactions, and are unable to form or sustain attachments with other caregivers.

Children's reactions to a parent's death also reflect the history and dynamics of their relationships. Children with disorganized attachments to their parents before their deaths tend to experience intense fright after the death. In particular, disorganized children often conceive of their parents in frightening terms such as visiting ghosts who may scare them (Normand et al. 1996). On the other hand, children with secure attachments before the parent's death appear better able to reflect and organize their feelings and to view their

*Table 6.4*   Stages of Grieving After Parental Death

| Stage | Description |
| --- | --- |
| Stage 1: Protest | Children demonstrate prolonged periods of anxiety, anger, and denial and continuously search for the parent. When these reactions lessen, the child enters the second stage of grieving. |
| Stage 2: Despair | Children demonstrate extreme sadness and withdrawal. These reactions are the consequences of the failure of protest to bring about the return of the lost attachment figure. |
| Stage 3: Detachment | Children regain an interest in other activities and relationships. This is the defensive inhibition of attachment responses that have not brought back the lost attachment parent. |

deceased parents as positive forces that remain in their lives (Silverman & Nickman 1996).

# Consequences of Attachment to Primary Caregivers

The quality of children's attachment relationships has implications for their development. In particular, children's early attachment relationships influence their developing self-representations and self-confidence and guide their relational choices, expectations, and behaviors toward others. Children's early attachment relationships may also influence their physical development.

A majority of research concerns the role of attachment on children's social competence. In multiple studies, researchers have demonstrated that children with secure attachments look for and expect caring and encouraging interactions with others. Secure children thus act in manners that invite such support from others and evidence high levels of social competence. Children with insecure attachments, on the other hand, expect little from others and behave in ways to discourage support (Thompson 1998). For example, children with insecure attachments often behave more aggressively toward teachers in early elementary school than children with secure attachments (Sroufe et al. 1983). Furthermore, insecurely attached children are more likely to engage in negative peer interactions than securely attached children (Pastor 1981).

Several investigators have observed the role of specific attachment styles in children's social and relational development. Results from the majority of these studies demonstrate that disorganized attachment is an extremely powerful risk factor for the development of behavior problems. Young children with disorganized attachments tend to be more incompetent in play and conflict resolution than securely, avoidantly, and ambivalently attached peers (Lyons-Ruth et al. 1993). Furthermore, children with disorganized attachments

tend to lack coherent strategies for initiating play with peers (Jacobvitz & Hazen 1999).

Children's early attachment relationships predict later school-age behavior problems. Generally, children with secure attachments are less likely to demonstrate behavior problems in elementary school than those with insecure attachments (Sroufe 1983). Insecurity poses a stronger risk for boys. For example, insecurely attached males are more likely than insecurely attached females to behave aggressively with peers (Cohn 1990). Researchers who have examined the implications of specific attachment styles report that disorganized attachment is the strongest predictor of behavior problems (Carlson 1998, Moss et al. 1996).

Children's early attachment relationships also have serious implications for their physical and psychological development. In particular, attachment styles are associated with infants' abilities to cope with stress. Securely attached children tend to handle stress better than insecurely attached children. Associations between attachment security and stress reactivity have been theorized to reflect children's IWMs of relationships. In particular, securely attached children may more easily self-soothe during times of stress through recollections of previous sensitive caregiver–child interactions.

Differences in stress responses among children with varying attachment styles are reflected in their cortisol levels. Cortisol is a hormone secreted by the actions of the hypothalamic-pituitary-adrenocorticol (HPA) axis, released in response to stressors (Gunnar & Nelson 1994). Securely attached children tend to have lower cortisol levels than insecurely attached children after a stressful experience, indicating these children's lower levels of stress reactivity compared to insecurely attached children. For example, in one study, insecurely attached children demonstrated elevated levels of cortisol after the Strange Situation procedure when compared with securely attached children (Spangler & Grossman 1993). Furthermore, results from several studies indicate that children with disorganized attachments have significantly elevated cortisol levels, compared to securely attached children, after short periods of separation (Herstgaard et al. 1995, Spangler & Grossman 1993). Results from these studies suggest that infants with disorganized attachments are most vulnerable to stressful situations. Differences in children's stress responses have implications for their physical development because increased levels of cortisol can lead to damage of the hippocampus (DeBellis et al. 1999).

# Attachment and Multiple Caregivers

The significance of the primary attachment figure in the formation of attachment relationships is at the core of attachment theory. Children do, however, develop attachments to other caregivers in their lives. Initially researchers and theorists focused on mother–child and father–child attachment relationships. Bowlby (1980) and Ainsworth (1967) stated that children first develop an attachment to their mother, typically the primary caregiver, and then to their father. Children may use both their mothers and fathers as secure bases from which to explore the environment; however, children tend to demonstrate a preference for their mothers in times of stress (Lamb 1977). This preference probably reflects more extended periods of time that children tend to spend with their mothers, as compared with their fathers.

Data from studies of mother–infant and father–infant attachment patterns demonstrate low to modest concordance between attachment patterns children have with their parents (Belsky et al. 1984, Grossman et al. 1981, Lamb et al. 1982, Fox et al. 1991). Similar to mother–child attachments, paternal sensitivity is a significant predictor of attachment security. However, associations between paternal sensitivity and security of attachment tend to be lower than those between maternal sensitivity and security of attachment (van Ijzendoorn & DeWolff 1997). This weaker association between paternal sensitivity and security of attachment may demonstrate varying parenting roles in which mothers and fathers engage. In particular, fathers often engage in more socializing and less caretaking activities with their children than do mothers.

Although infants' most important attachment relationships are usually with their parents, various other individuals may become attachment figures for children. Bowlby (1980) stated three main propositions related to multiple attachments in childhood: 1) most children form several attachment relationships; 2) the number of potential attachment figures is limited; 3) an attachment hierarchy exists among young children's attachment relationships such that primary attachment figures are those individuals who most frequently attend to children's needs. Additionally, according to Bowlby, attachment relationships with primary attachment figures are most highly correlated with individuals' later functioning.

Child care providers and early elementary school teachers are often alternative attachment figures for children (Howes & Hamilton 1992, Howes et al. 1998, Pianta et al. 1995). The development of attachment relationships in child care seems to be an analogous process to that of mother–infant attachment development. At the beginning of child care, children direct their attachment behaviors toward the caregiver; however, their behaviors tend to be sporadic. With extended time in settings, their behaviors become more organized (Howes 1999). Children tend to form more secure relationships with child care providers the more time they spend with them (Raikes 1993). Although concordance between styles of mother–child and child care provider–child attachment exists, the association is not strong. In fact, studies suggest that children with prior maladaptive maternal relationships may form secure attachment relationships with alternative caregivers (Howes & Segal 1993).

No studies have been conducted to examine the process of attachment relationship formation between early elementary school teachers and children. However, data from multiple studies demonstrate that young children do form attachments to teachers (Anderson et al. 1981, Howes & Hamilton 1992, Lynch & Cicchetti 1992, Pianta 1994, Pianta & Nimetz 1991). Again, weak associations between mother–child attachment styles and teacher–child attachment styles are reported (Pianta 1999).

## Adoption and Foster Care

Attachment theory has predominately been used to explain relationships between mothers and their biological children. Hundreds of thousands of infants in the United States though are adopted and placed in foster care each year. Infants adopted before or during the optimal period for attachment development, 6 to 9 months, engage in the same processes of attachment formation with their caregivers as infants do with their biological mothers (Howes 1999). Furthermore, infants adopted in the first few months of life show the same distributions of attachment security as infants care for by their biological parents (Singer et al. 1985). Children, adopted before 6 months of life by sensitive caregivers also tend to form secure attachments regardless of the number of former foster care placements (Singer et al. 1985; Howe 2001).

There are very few studies with children who have been adopted after infancy. The majority of studies that have been conducted, however, indicate that children adopted after 2 years of age also develop attachments with caregivers. However, these children usually do not progress through all the stages of attachment formation. Specifically, these children's relationships with alternative caregivers begin as goal-corrected partnerships

(reciprocal relationships) (Greenberg 1999). Furthermore, the quality of attachments that earlier- and later-adopted children form may be different. Research demonstrates that prior to age 6 is a critical period for children's attachment development. A child that has not developed an attachment to a stable adult during this age will likely suffer from significant emotional difficulties and have difficulties forming secure attachments throughout life. No study has been conducted to examine the security of children's attachments adopted after a specific age. However, results from studies of adopted individuals indicate that age at placement is associated with security of attachment such that individuals adopted after 2 years of age are more likely to be insecurely attached to their adopted caregivers (Howe 2001).

Some adopted children, and most foster care children, experience not only changes in caregivers but also have been victims of abuse. Infants and young children with prior insecure or disordered attachments who are removed from abusive surroundings tend to develop more optimal attachments to alternative caregivers. These attachments are likely to be secure when caregivers are sensitive and responsive to their needs. For example, in one study, researchers found that 47% of toddlers taken from maternal custody, due to abuse or neglect, and moved to a high-quality shelter with high adult–child ratios formed secure attachments with alternative caregivers within 2 months of placement (Howes & Segal 1993).

## Disorders of Attachment

Although the majority of children develop either secure or insecure attachments to primary caregivers, some children demonstrate clinical attachment disorders (see Table 6.3). Groups of researchers have identified different classifications of attachment disorders. Attachment disorders may result from the lack of an important attachment relationship, significant changes in the quality of care by a primary attachment figure, or traumatic distortions or losses of attachment figures in childhood.

Two types of attachment disorders are outlined in the *Diagnostic and Statistical Manual of Mental Disorders IV* (DSM-IV) (American Psychiatric Association 1994): *reactive attachment disorder of infancy or early childhood* (*RAD*) and *nonattachment*. RAD, as outlined in the DSM-IV, involves the avoidance of social interactions or the demonstration of contradictory social responses. The age of onset for this disorder is 5 years or younger. Two types of RAD have been identified: *inhibited* and *disinhibited*. Inhibited RAD is characterized by hypervigilance and fear that is demonstrated by extreme withdrawal. Disinhibited RAD, on the other hand, is characterized by indiscriminate friendliness and lack of attachment to a caregiver who is sought out to provide feelings of safety and security (Greenberg 1999). RAD is typically associated with long-term hospitalization without the presence of strong protective factors (i.e., almost daily visits by parents, the daily involvement of a specific nurse or aide). Children can also evidence this disorder when their parents are depressed or have substance abuse problems. The disorder of nonattachment involves children who do not demonstrate an attachment to any one person. Reasons for children's nonattachments are unclear; however, possible reasons are previous negative and/or unresponsive interactions with attachment figures.

Based on attachment theory and research, Lieberman and Zeanah (1999) developed an additional taxonomy of attachment disorders. This taxonomy was created to capture more varying types of attachment disorders than those presented in the DSM-IV (Greenberg 1999). Lieberman and Zeanah (1999) outlined three different types of attachment disorders: *nonattachment*, *disordered attachment*, and *disrupted attachment*. The characteristics of nonattachment, described by Lieberman and Zenah, are the same as those defined in the DSM-IV; however, they include the stipulation that children have the cognitive abilities of a 10- to 12-month-old child. This requirement is included to differentiate attachment disorders from cognitive and developmental disorders (Greenberg, 1999).

Lieberman and Zenah also outlined two additional types of attachment disorders: disordered attachment and disruption of attachment. Three subtypes of disordered attachments were identified. These include *inhibition*, demonstrated by clinging to an attachment figure and minimal exploration; *reckless self-endangerment*, demonstrated in failure to use an attachment figure as a secure base in times of risk; and *role reversal*, demonstrated in children's extreme anxiety related to their attachment figures' well-beings (Greenberg 1999). Lastly, disrupted attachment disorder is based on the premise that loss of a primary attachment figure in infancy is pathogenic. However, specific descriptions of how normal grief reactions differ from pathological ones have not been provided (Greenberg 1999).

# Intervention Programs and the Application of Attachment Theory

Attachment theory and research has influenced clinical practice, in that family interventions often focus on the development of security. An example of an intervention program based on attachment theory is the Infant–Parent Program (IPP) at the Child Development Project at the University of Michigan. Families participating in this program often face poverty, joblessness, homelessness, substance abuse, and violence. Approximately 30% of the families are referred to the program from child protective services and 15% from juvenile or family court. Children often suffer from separation anxiety and uncontrolled anger. A subset of the children suffers from RAD. The IPP is a demonstration program designed to develop and evaluate infant–parent psychotherapy as a treatment for relational disorder of infancy. Participation in this program involves a parent and child engaging in therapy sessions. Sessions are largely unstructured, with themes allowed to unfold through interactions with the parent and child. Joint play, questions, developmental guidance, and expressions of support are used by clinicians to assist parents in altering inflexible, contracted, and distorted notions of their children and to develop more developmentally suitable and emotionally supportive interactions with their children. The goal of these interventions is to assist the children in becoming more securely dependent on their parents. A randomized treatment outcome study with a subsample of participants demonstrated significant differences between treatment and control groups in children's avoidance, resistance, and anger directed at their mothers (Lieberman & Zeanah 1999).

A second intervention program based on attachment theory is The Child Trauma Research Project (CTRP). This program utilizes age-modified infant–parent psychotherapy to evaluate and help children, ages 5 years and younger, who have witnessed domestic violence. The program includes the mother and child. The clinical objectives are to assist the mother in entering into and understanding the child's thoughts, to assist the child and mother in forming a narrative of their experience together, and to provide the mother and child with a protected space to enact their conflicts and discover more constructive ways to resolve them. An evaluation of the program is currently being conducted (Lieberman & Zeanah 1999).

Additional programs have been designed based on attachment theory to encourage positive and sensitive parent–child interactions. Very little assessment data are available on these programs. Preliminary data, however, suggest that these programs assist mothers in engaging in sensitive and responsive interactions with their children (Lieberman & Zeanah 1999).

# References

Ainsworth, M. D. S. (1967). *Infancy in Uganda: Infant care and the growth of attachment.* Baltimore: Johns Hopkins University Press.

Ainsworth, M. D. S., Blehar, M., Waters, E., & Wall, S. (1978). *Patterns of attachment: A psychological study of the strange situation.* Hillsdale, NJ: Erlbaum.

Ainsworth, M. D. S., & Eichberg, C. G. (1991). Effects on infant-mother attachment of mothers' unresolved loss of an attachment figure or other traumatic experience. In C. M. Parkes, J. Stevenson-Hinde, & P. Marris (Eds.), *Attachment across the life cycle* (pp. 161–183). London: Routledge.

Anderson, C. W., Nagel, P., Roberts, M., & Smith, K. (1981). Attachment in substitute caregivers as a function of center quality and caregiver involvement. *Child Development* 52, 53–61.

Anisfeld, E., Casper, V. Nozyce, M., & Cunningham, N. (1990). Does infant carrying promote attachment? An experimental study of the effects of increased physical contact on the development of attachment. *Child Development* 61, 1617–1627.

Belsky, J. (1999). Infant-parent attachment. In J. Cassidy & P. Shaver (Eds.), *Handbook of attachment: Theory, research and clinical applications* (pp. 141–162). New York: The Guilford Press.

Belsky, J., & Cassidy, J. (1994). Attachment: Theory and evidence. In M. Rutter & D. Hay (Eds.), *Development through life: A handbook for clinicians* (pp. 373–402). Oxford: Blackwell.

Belsky, J., Garduque, L., & Hrncir, E. (1984). Assessing performance, competence, and executive capacity in infant play: Relations to home environment and security of attachment. *Developmental Psychology* 20, 406–417.

Belsky, J., & Rovine, M. J. (1988). Nonmaternal care in the first year of life and the security of infant-parent attachment. *Child Development* 59, 157–167.

Benoit, D., & Parker, K. (1994). Stability and transmission of attachment across three generations. *Child Development* 65(5), 1444–1456.

Berk, L. E. (1997). *Child Development* (4th ed.). Boston: Allyn and Bacon.

Bowlby, J. (1969/1980). *Attachment and loss: Volume 1, Attachment.* New York: Basic Books.

Bowlby, J. (1988). *A secure base: Clinical applications of attachment theory.* London: Routledge.

Bretherton, I. & Munholland, K. (1999). Internal working models in attachment relationships: A construct revisited. In *Handbook of attachment: Theory, research and clinical applications* (pp. 89–115). New York: The Guilford Press.

Carlson, E. A. (1998). A prospective longitudinal study of disorganized/disoriented attachment relationships in maltreated infants. *Developmental Psychology 25*, 525–531.

Carlson, V., Cicchetti, D., Barnett, D., & Braunwald, K. (1989). Disorganized/disoriented attachment relationships in maltreated infants. *Developmental Psychology 25*, 525–531.

Cassidy, J., & Kobak, R. (1988). Avoidance and its relation to other defensive processes. In J. Belsky & T. Nezworski (Eds.), *Clinical implications of attachment* (pp. 300–336). Hillsdale, NJ: Erlbaum.

Chisholm, K., Carter, M. C., Ames, E. W., & Morison, S. J. (1995). Attachment security and indiscriminately friendly behavior in children adopted from Romanian orphanages. *Development and Psychopathology 7*, 283–297.

Clarke-Stewart, K. A. (1989). Infant day-care: Maligned or malignant? *American Psychologist 44*, 266–273.

Cohn, D. A. (1990). Child-mother attachment of six-year-olds and social competence at school. *Child Development 61*, 152–162.

Conger, R. (1984). Perception of child, child-rearing values, and emotional distress as mediating links between environmental stressors and observed maternal behavior. *Child Development 55*, 2234–2247.

DeBellis, M. D., Keshavan, M. S., Clark, D. B., Casey, B. J., Giedd, J. N., Boring, A. M., et al. (1999). Developmental traumatology part II: Brain development. *Biological Psychiatry 45*, 1271–1284.

DeMulder, E. K., Denham, S., Schmidt, M., & Mitchell, J. (2000). Q-sort assessment of attachment security during the preschool years: Links from home to school. *Developmental Psychology 36*, 274–282.

DeMulder, E. K., & Radke-Yarrow, M. (1991). Attachment with affectively ill and well mothers: Concurrent behavior correlates. *Development and Psychopathology 3*, 227–242.

Diagnostic and Statistical Manual of Mental Disorders (4th ed.). (2000). Washington, DC: American Psychiatric Association.

Emery, R. E. (1982). Interparental conflict and the children of discord and divorce. *Psychological Bulletin 92*, 310–330.

Erel, O., & Burman, B. (1995). Interrelatedness of marital relations and parent-child relations. *Psychological Bulletin 118*, 108–132.

Fox, N. A., Kimmerly, N. L., & Shafer, W. D. (1991). Attachment to mother/attachment to father: A meta-analysis. *Child Development 52*, 210–225.

Gaffney, M., Greene, S., Wieczorek-Deering, D., & Nugent, K. (2000). The concordance between mother-infant attachment at 18 months and attachment 10 years later among married and single mothers. *Irish Journal of Psychology 21*(3–4), 154–170.

George, C., & Solomon, J. (1999). Attachment and caregiving. The caregiving behavioral system. In *Handbook of attachment: Theory, research and clinical applications* (pp. 649–671). New York: The Guilford Press.

Greenberg, M. (1999). Attachment and psychopathology in childhood. In *Handbook of attachment: Theory, research and clinical applications* (pp. 469–497). New York: The Guilford Press.

Grossman, K. E., Grossman, K., Huber, F., & Wartner, U. (1981). German children's behavior towards their mothers at 12 months and their fathers at 18 months in Ainsworth's Strange Situations. *International Journal of Behavioral Development 4*, 157–181.

Gunnar, M., & Nelson, C. (1994). Event-related potentials in year-old infants. *Child Development 65*(1), 80–94.

Hertsgaard, L., Gunnar, M., Erickson, M. F., & Nachimas, M. (1995). Adrencorticol responses to the Strange Situation in infants with disorganized/disoriented attachment relationships. *Child Development 66*, 1100–1106.

Howes, C. (1999). Attachment relationships in the context of multiple caregivers. In *Handbook of attachment: Theory, research and clinical applications* (pp. 671–688). New York: The Guilford Press.

Howes, C., & Hamilton, C. E. (1992). Children's relationships with caregivers: Mothers and child care teachers. *Child Development 53*, 859–878.

Howes, C., Hamilton, C. E., & Phillipsen, L. C. (1998). Stability and continuity of child-caregiver relationships. *Child Development 69*, 418–426.

Howes, C., & Markman, H. J. (1989). Marital quality and child functioning: A longitudinal investigation. *Child Development 60*, 1044–1051.

Howes, C., & Segal, J. (1993). Children's relationships with alternative caregivers: The special case of maltreated children removed from their homes. *Journal of Applied Developmental Psychology 17*, 71–81.

Howe, D. (2001). Age at placement, adoption experience and adult adopted people's contact with their adoptive and birth mothers: An attachment perspective. *Attachment & Human Development 3*, 222–237.

Jacobvitz, D., & Hazan, N. (1999). Developmental pathways from infant disorganization to childhood peer relationships. In J. Solomon & C. George (Eds.), *Attachment disorganization*. New York: Guilford Press.

Lamb, M. E. (1977). Father-infant and mother-infant interaction in the first year of life. *Child Development 78*, 157–181.

Lamb, M. E., Hwang, C. P., Frodi, A., & Frodi, M. (1982). Security of mother- and father-infant attachments and its relation to sociability with strangers in traditional and non-traditional Swedish families. *Infant Behavior and Development 5*, 355–367.

Lamb, M., & Sternberg, L. (1990). Do we really know how day-care affects children? *Journal of Applied Developmental Psychology 11*, 351–379.

Lamb, M., Thompson, R., Gardner, W., & Charnov, L. (1985). *Infant-mother attachment: The origins and developmental significance of individual differences in Strange Situation behavior.* Hillsdale, NJ: Lawrence Erlbaum Associates.

LeVine, R. A. (2001). Culture and personality studies, 1918–1960: Myth and history. *Journal of Personality* 69, 803–818.

Lewis, M., Feiring, C., McGuffog, C., & Jaskir, J. (1984). Predicting psychopathology in six-year-olds from early social relations. *Child Development* 55, 123–136.

Lieberman, A. F., & Zeanah, C. H. (1999). Contributions of attachment theory to infant-parent psychotherapy and other interventions with infants and young children. In *Handbook of attachment: Theory, research and clinical applications* (pp. 555–575). New York: The Guilford Press.

Lynch, M., & Cicchetti, D. (1992). Maltreated children's reports of relatedness to their teachers. In R. C. Pianta (Ed.), *Relationships between children and nonparental adults: New directions in child development* (pp. 81–108). San Francisco: Jossey-Bass.

Lyons-Ruth, K., Alpern, L., & Repacholi, B. (1993). Disorganized infant attachment classification and maternal psychosocial problems as predictors of hostile-aggressive behavior in the preschool classroom. *Child Development* 64, 572–585.

Lyons-Ruth, K., Bronfman, E., & Parsons, E. (1999). Maternal frightened, frightening, or atypical behavior and disorganized infant attachment patterns. *Monographs of the Society for Research in Child Development 64(3),* 67–96.

Main, M., & Cassidy, J. (1988). Categories of response to reunion with the parent at age 6: Predicted from infant attachment classifications and stable over a one-month period. *Development Psychology* 21, 407–412.

Main, M., & Hesse, E. (1990). Parents' unresolved traumatic experiences are related to infant disorganized attachment status: Is frightened and/or frightening parental behavior the linking mechanism? In M. T. Greenberg, D. Cicchetti, & E. M. Cummings (Eds.), *Attachment in the preschool years: Theory, research, and intervention* (pp. 161–182). Chicago: University of Chicago Press.

Main, M., & Solomon, J. (1986). Discovery of a new, insecure-disorganized/disoriented during the Ainsworth Strange Situation. In M. T. Greenberg, D. Cicchetti, & E. M. Cummings (Eds.), *Attachment in the preschool years: Theory, research, and intervention* (pp. 121–160). Chicago: University of Chicago Press.

Marcus, R. F. (1991). The attachments of children in foster care. *Genetic, Social, and General Psychology Monographs* 117, 355–397.

Marvin, R. S. (1977). An ethological-cognitive model for the attenuation of mother-child attachment behaviors. In T. M. Alloway, L. Krames, & P. Pliner (Eds.), *Advances in the study of communication and affect (Vol. 3). The development of social attachment.* New York: Plenum Press.

Marvin, R., & Britner, P. (1999). Normative development: The onotogeny of attachment. In *Handbook of attachment: Theory, research and clinical applications* (pp. 44–68). New York: The Guilford Press.

McCartney, K., & Dearing, E. (2002). Attachment. In N. J. Salkind & L. H. Margolis (Eds.), *Child Development* (pp. 32–37). Farmington Hills, MI: Macmillan.

Moss, E., Parent, S., Gosselin, C., Rousseau, D., & St-Laurent, D. (1996). Attachment and teacher-reported behavior problems during the pre-school and early school-age period. *Development and Psychopathology* 8, 511–525.

National Institutes of Child Health and Human Development (NICHD) Early Child Care Research. (1998). The effects of infant child care on infant-mother attachment security: Results of the NICHD study of early child care. *Child Development* 69, 1145–1170.

National Institutes of Child Health and Human Development (NICHD) Early Child Care Research. (1997). The effects of infant child care on infant-mother attachment security: Results of the NICHD study of early child care. *Child Development* 68, 860–879.

Nelson, E., & Panksepp, J. (1998). Brain substrates of infant-mother attachment: Contributions of opioids, oxytocin and norepinephrine. *Neuroscience and Biobehavioral Reviews* 22, 437–452.

Normand, C. L., Silverman, P. R., & Nickman, S. L. (1996). Bereaved children's changing relationships with the deceased. In D. Klass, P. R. Silverman, & S. L. Nickman (Eds.), *Continuing bonds: New understandings of grief* (pp. 87–111). Washington, DC: Taylor & Francis.

Owen, M. T., & Cox, M. J. (1997). Marital conflict and the development of infant-parent attachment relationships. *Journal of Family Psychology 11(2),* 152–164.

Pastor, D. L. (1981). The quality of mother-infant attachment and its relationship to toddlers' initial sociability with peers. *Developmental Psychology* 17, 326–335.

Pianta, R. C. (1999). *Enhancing relationships: Between children and teachers.* Washington, DC: American Psychological Association.

Pianta, R. C. (1994). Patterns of relationship between children and kindergarten teachers. *Journal of School Psychology* 32, 15–32.

Pianta, R., & Nimetz, S. (1991). Relationships between children and teachers: Associations with classroom and home behavior. *Journal of Applied Developmental Psychology* 12, 379–393.

Pianta, R. C., Steinberg, M., & Rollins, K. B. (1995). The first two years of school: Teacher-child relationships and deflections in children's classroom adjustment. *Development and Psychopathology* 7, 295–312.

Polan, J., & Hofer, M. (1999). Psychobiological origins of infant attachment and separation responses. In J. Cassidy and P. Shaver (Eds.), *Handbook of Attachment*. New York: Guilford.

Radke-Yarrow, M., Cummings, E. M., Kuczynski, L., & Chapman, M. (1985). Patterns of attachment in two- and three-year-olds in normal families and families with parental depression. *Child Development* 56, 884–893.

Raikes, H. (1993). Relationship duration in infant care. *Early Childhood Research Quarterly* 8(3), 309–325.

Rauh, H., Ziegenhain, U., Muller, B., & Wijnroks, L. (2000). Stability and change in infant-mother attachment in the second year of life: Relations to parenting quality and varying degrees of day care experience (pp. 251–276). In P. M. Crittenden & A. H. Claussen (Eds.), *The organization of attachment relationships: Maturation, culture, and context*. New York: Cambridge University Press.

Roggman, L., Langlois, J., Hubbs-Tait, L., & Rieser-Danner, L. (1994). Infant day-care, attachment and the "file drawer problem." *Child Development* 65, 1429–1443.

Rutter, M., & O'Connor, T. (1999). Implications of attachment theory for child care. In *Handbook of attachment: Theory, research and clinical applications* (pp. 823–845). New York: The Guilford Press.

Silverman, P. R., & Nickman, S. L. (1996). Introduction: What's the problem? In D. Klass, P. R. Silverman, & S. L. Nickman (Eds.), *Continuing bonds: New understandings of grief* (pp. 3–25). Washington, DC: Taylor & Francis.

Singer, L. M., Brodsinsky, D. M., Ramsay, D., Steir, M., & Waters, E. (1985). Infant-mother attachment in adoptive families. *Child Development* 55, 1573–1551.

Solomon, J., & George, C. (1999). The caregiving system in mothers. *Attachment and Human Development* 1(2), 171–190.

Solomon, J., George, C., & de Jong, A. (1995). Children classified as controlling at age six: Evidence of disorganized representational strategies and aggression at home and at school. *Development and Psychopathology* 7, 447–463.

Spangler, G., & Grossmann, K. E. (1993). Biobehavioral organization in securely and insecurely attached infants. *Child Development* 64, 1439–1450.

Sroufe, L. A. (1997). Psychopathology as outcome of development. *Development and Psychopathology* 9, 251–268.

Sroufe, L. A. (1996). *Emotional development*. Cambridge, England: Cambridge University Press.

Sroufe, L. A. (1983). Individual patterns of adaptation from infancy to preschool. In M. Perlmutter (Ed.), *Development and policy concerning children with special needs: Minnesota symposium on child psychology* (Vol. 16). Hillsdale, NJ: Lawrence Erlbaum Associates.

Sroufe, L., Fox, N., & Pancake, V. (1983). Attachment and dependency in developmental perspective. *Child Development* 54, 1615–1627.

Stern, D. (1977). *The first relationship*. Cambridge, MA: Harvard University Press.

Symons, D. K. (1998). Post-partum employment patterns, family-based care arrangements, and the mother-infant relationship at age two. *Canadian Journal of Behavioral Science* 30, 121–131.

Teti, D., Sakin, J., Kucera, E., Corns, K., & Das Eiden, R. (1996). And baby makes four. *Child Development* 67, 579–596.

Teti, D. M., Nakagawa, M., Das, R., & Wirth, O. (1991). Security of attachment between preschoolers and their mothers: Relations among social interaction, parenting stress, and mothers' sorts. *Developmental Psychology* 27, 440–447.

Thompson, R. A. (1998). Early sociopersonality development. In W. Damon (Series Ed.) & N. Eisenberg (Vol. Ed.), *Handbook of child psychology: Vol. 3. Social, emotional and personality development* (5th ed., pp. 25–104), New York: Wiley.

Turner, P. J. (1991). Relations between attachment, gender and behavior with peers in preschool. *Child Development* 62, 1475–1488.

Wartner, U.G., Grossmann, K., Fremmer-Bombik, E., & Suess, G. (1994). Attachment patterns at age six in South Germany: Predictability from infancy and implications for preschool behavior. *Child Development* 65, 1014–1027.

van Ijzendoorn, M. H. (1995). Of the way we are: On temperament, attachment, and the transmission gap: A rejoinder to Fox. *Psychological Bulletin* 117, 411–415.

van Ijzendoorn, M. H., & de Wolff, M. S. (1997). In search of the absent father: Meta-analysis of infant-father attachment. A rejoinder to our discussants. *Child Development* 68, 604–609.

Van Ijzendoorn, M. H., & Sagi, A. (1999). Cross-cultural patterns of attachment. In *Handbook of attachment: Theory, research and clinical applications* (pp. 713–734). New York: The Guilford Press.

Waters, E. (1978). The reliability and stability of individual differences in infant-mother attachment. *Child Development* 49, 483–494.

Weinfield, N. S., Sroufe, A., Egeland, B., & Carlson, E. (1999). The nature of individual differences in infant-caregiver attachment. In *Handbook of attachment: Theory, research and clinical applications* (pp. 68–89). New York: The Guilford Press.

# Chapter 7

# Cognitive Development

John Travers

Mark Twain once said, "Always do right. This will gratify some people, and astonish the rest." Twain, in his delightful tales, frequently offered insightful views of human nature, cleverly interweaving mental and moral guideposts with story themes. His examples of the mental abilities of children are superb. Do you recall the memorable scene where Tom Sawyer was desperately trying to avoid whitewashing Aunt Polly's fence?

*One of Tom's friends, Ben Rogers, passed by, imitating the "Big Missouri" riverboat. When Ben sympathized with him for having to work, Tom looked at him and said, "What do you call work?"*

*His friend asked, "Why ain't that work?" Tom neatly dodged the question and asked, "Does a boy get a chance to whitewash a fence every day?" By that time Ben was jumping up and down in his eagerness to paint. When that happened, Tom gave up the brush with reluctance in his face but alacrity in his heart.*

*And while that late steamer, Big Missouri (his friend), worked and sweated in the sun, the retired artist sat on a barrel in the shade close by, dangled his legs, munched his apple, and planned the slaughter of more innocents.*

What else can we do but acknowledge a sophisticated and subtle mind at work? The question that intrigues us, however, is how children and adults acquire this remarkable ability to think, reason, and solve problems. From the early phases of a mother's pregnancy when a child's brain is forming neurons at a rate so amazingly rapid that it defies imagination to the days of later adulthood when that same brain is fighting deterioration, human beings are experiencing quantitatively and qualitatively different types of cognitive development.

The themes of cognitive psychology have become so widely accepted and so carefully studied that an enormous body of literature—both theoretical and experimental—has resulted. Flavell (1999, pp. 22–23) has identified three waves of research:

1. The first surge of interest evolved from the seminal work of Piaget. As we mentioned in Chapter 1, his belief that it was possible to explain the development of children's thinking presented new, challenging horizons for researchers to explore.

2. The second major movement began in the 1970s and arose from studies of

metacognition, which refers to that time when children begin to realize how their minds work. In other words, children begin to think about their thinking.

3. The third and current phase that began in the 1980s is research into theory-of-mind development. Examining the rationale for theory of mind, cognitive psychologist David Bjorklund (2000) has stated that a theory of mind implies more than a collection of concepts. What is inherent in these ideas is a framework that enables children to recognize different activities of their minds: dreams, memories, imagination, beliefs, and having some means of accounting for the actions of other people. In this way, children learn to "read the minds of others" and understand the tremendous power residing in the ability to think. It is a process that continues throughout the life span (Bjorklund 2000, p. 214).

Thus our task is clearly defined for us: How can we identify these cognitive changes, and how do individuals proceed through the various stages of cognitive development—that is, what are the psychological mechanisms involved in cognitive development? To guide us in our answers to these questions, we trace the path of cognition by

- exploring several of the outstanding theories intended to explain cognitive progress;

- weaving the biological basis of cognition throughout the various developmental epochs;

- examining the outstanding characteristics of cognitive development; and

- analyzing the relationship between language and cognition.

As we do, we'll also be concerned with how the path of cognitive development impacts the manner in which your clients react to programs, treatments, and suggestions. Their ability to pay *attention* to what you say, to *recall* the advice you

give them, and to *understand* what they are supposed to do are examples of how cognitive development affects the outcome of diagnosis and treatment.

The search for the course of cognitive development begins by examining the developmental aspects of the theories we discussed in Chapter 1.

# Cognitive Development— The Theories

The theories that we discuss in this section are among the most influential in the field of cognitive development. Although the basic ideas of Piaget and Vygotsky were presented in Chapter 1, in this chapter we look more closely at their thoughts on development itself. We also consider the work of neo-Piagetian thinker Kurt Fischer and conclude with an analysis of information processing theory. First, however, let's return to the world of Jean Piaget.

## Piaget and Cognitive Development

As was mentioned in Chapter 1, Piaget believed that cognitive development means passage through four stages of development, the first of which is the *sensorimotor* period, which occurs in infancy. The remarkable cognitive changes of the first two years of life occur within a sequence of six stages when the child is struggling with *egocentrism,* that tendency to see the world only from their point of view. Very young children lack social orientation. They speak at and not to each other, and two children in conversation may be discussing utterly unrelated topics. (Likewise, egocentric adults know that other viewpoints exist, but they disregard them.) The egocentric child simply is unaware of any other viewpoint.

Infants "know" in the sense of recognizing or anticipating familiar, recurring objects and happenings; and they "think" in the sense of behaving toward these objects and events with mouth, hand, eye, and other sensory-motor instruments in predictable, organized, and often adaptive ways. A good example can be seen in the way babies follow the mother with their eyes and how often they smile at the mother's face, expecting pleasant consequences.

## FEATURES OF THE SENSORIMOTOR PERIOD

Several characteristics of the *sensorimotor* period help to explain the beginnings of how infants think according to Piaget. Infants initially don't have a sense of object permanence. An object or person removed from their field of vision ceases to exist. Imagine an infant playing with a teddy bear. If you move it behind a chair and out of sight, the infant simply stops searching for it. This explains babies' pleasure when someone plays hide-and-seek with them. When hidden, the face no longer exists because the baby has not acquired object permanence.

Gradually, as they move about their environment, crawling and walking, they realize that there's a distance between the objects they're using to steady themselves. In this way, they develop concepts of space and time. For example, how many times have you seen infants pull themselves up by a chair, drop to the floor, crawl some distance, and then pull themselves up by using a table? By moving from object to object, they learn about space and the time it takes to move from object to object.

As children use their growing sensorimotor intelligence, they begin to find order in their universe. They distinguish their own actions as causes, and they begin to discover events that have their causes elsewhere, either in other objects or in various relationships between objects. This helps them to develop the concept of causality. For example, infants will push a toy truck and watch it roll, gradually realizing that their own actions caused the truck to roll. As they cognitively move through the six subdivisions of the sensorimotor period, they progress from reliance on reflex actions (such as grasping and sucking) to a basic understanding of the world around them and manifesting the first signs of representing their world through language. Table 7.1 summarizes the six subdivisions of the sensorimotor period.

Consequently, progress through the sensorimotor period leads to four major accomplishments:

- *Object permanence:* Children realize that permanent objects exist around them; something out of sight is not gone forever.
- *A sense of space:* Children realize environmental objects have a spatial relationship.
- *Causality:* Children realize a relationship exists between actions and their consequences.
- *Time sequences:* Children realize that one thing comes after another.

By the end of the sensorimotor period, children move from purely sensory and motor functioning (hence the name *sensorimotor*) to a more symbolic kind of activity.

## PIAGET AND THE CHILDHOOD YEARS

Piaget believed that during these years children pass through the *preoperational* and *concrete operational* periods. For Piaget, the great accomplishment of the preoperational period (2 to 6 years) is a growing ability to represent, which is how we record or express information. For example, the word "car" is a *representation* because it represents a certain idea. Pointing an index finger at a playmate and saying "Stick 'em up" is also an example of representation. Other activities typical of preoperational children reflect their use of internal representation and include the following (Piaget & Inhelder 1969):

- *Deferred imitation:* Preoperational children can imitate some object or activity that they have previously witnessed.
- *Symbolic play.* Children enjoy pretending that they are asleep or that they are someone or something else. (Piaget argued eloquently for recognizing the importance of play in a youngster's life.)

*Table 7.1*   Characteristics of the Sensorimotor Period

**The Six Subdivisions of This Period**

| | |
|---|---|
| Stage 1 | During the first month the child exercises the native reflexes, for example, the sucking reflex. Here is the origin of mental development, for states of awareness accompany the reflex mechanisms. |
| Stage 2 | Piaget referred to stage 2 (from 1 to 4 months) as the stage of primary circular reactions. Infants repeat some act involving the body, for example, finger sucking. (Primary means first, circular reaction means repeating the act.) |
| Stage 3 | From 4 to 8 months, secondary circular reactions appear; that is, the children repeat acts involving objects outside themselves. For example, infants continue to shake or kick the crib. |
| Stage 4 | From 8 to 12 months, the child "coordinates secondary schemes." Recall the meaning of schema—behavior plus mental structure. During stage 4, infants combine several related schemata to achieve some objective. For example, they will remove an obstacle that blocks some desired object. |
| Stage 5 | From 12 to 18 months, tertiary circular reactions appear. Now children repeat acts, but not only for repetition's sake; now they search for novelty. For example, children of this age continually drop things. Piaget interpreted such behavior as expressing their uncertainty about what will happen to the object when they release it. |
| Stage 6 | At about 18 months or 2 years, a primitive type of representation appears. For example, one of Piaget's daughters wished to open a door but had grass in her hands. She put the grass on the floor and then moved it back from the door's movement so that it would not blow away. |

- *Drawing:* Piaget thought children of this age project their mental representations into their drawings. Highly symbolic, their artwork reflects the level of their thinking and what they are thinking.

- *Mental images:* Mental images appear late in this period because of their dependence on internalized imitation. Children of this age form images that reproduce objects and events, but they cannot anticipate any changes. This reflects the nature of their cognitive structures and level of cognitive functioning.

- *Language:* For preoperational children, language becomes a vehicle for thought. Children of this age need ample opportu-

nities to talk with adults and with each other. (See the language section of this chapter.)

In the *concrete operational period* (7 to 11 years), children overcome the limitations of the preoperational period and display operational thinking; that is, they can reverse their thinking. Among children's cognitive achievements of these years are the following:

- *Conservation* appears. Recalling Piaget's famous water jar problem, children in the concrete operational stage can mentally pour the water back. By reversing their thinking in this manner, they *conserve* the basic idea: the amount of water remains the same regardless of the shape of the container.

- *Seriation* means that concrete operational children can arrange objects by increasing or decreasing size.
- *Classification* enables children to group objects with some similarities within a larger category. Brown wooden beads and white wooden beads are all beads.
- *Reversibility* enables children to retrace their thoughts.
- *Numeration* means that children understand the concept of numbers; for example, children understand oneness—that one boy, one girl, one apple, and one orange are all one of something.

## PIAGET AND THE STAGE OF FORMAL OPERATIONS

From a theoretical perspective, Piaget's stage of formal operations is a fruitful beginning for any analysis of adolescent thought. According to Piaget, the *formal operational* period, during which the beginnings of logical, abstract thinking appear, commences at about 11 or 12 years of age. During adolescence and the appearance of formal operations, youngsters demonstrate an ability to reason realistically about the future and to consider possibilities that they actually doubt. Teenagers look for relationships among events, they separate the real from the possible, they test their mental solutions to problems, and they feel comfortable with verbal statements. For example, when younger children are asked to assume that coal is white, they reply that coal has to be black, whereas adolescents accept the unreal assumption and reason from it. Thus the period's great achievement is a release from the restrictions of the tangible and the concrete (Elkind 1994).

In one experiment, children were given a cue stick, a cue ball, and a billiard-type table with several targets on it. The children were asked to hit the target with the cue ball by bouncing it off the side (banking their shots). When asked about what had happened, concrete operational children explain in very tangible terms: "If I hit it this way" (demonstrates), "it goes that way" (again demonstrates). Formal operational children, on the other hand, search for explanatory principles: "The rebound depends on the angle at which I held the cue stick" (Piaget and Inhelder 1969).

Some adolescents, however, may still be concrete operational, or only into the initial stages of formal operations. They have just consolidated their concrete operational thinking and continue to use it consistently. Unless they find themselves in situations that demand formal operational thinking (such as science and math classes), they continue to be concrete operational thinkers. As Elkind noted (1984, p. 221), learning how to use formal operations takes time and practice with a blend of concrete and abstract materials.

## FEATURES OF THE FORMAL OPERATIONAL PERIOD

There are several essential features of formal operational thinking.

1. *The ability to separate the real from the possible* distinguishes the formal operational child from the concrete operational. Adolescents try to discern all possible relations in any situation or problem and then, by mental experimentation and logical analysis, attempt to discover which are true. Flavell (1963) noted that there is nothing trivial in the adolescent's accomplishment; it is a basic and essential reorganization of thought processes that permits the adolescent to exist in the world of the possible.

2. *Adolescent thinking is propositional,* which means that adolescents use not only concrete data, but also statements or propositions that contain the concrete data. Dealing with abstract concepts no longer frustrates them. For example, a teacher could ask a class of adolescents a question such as *You've been appointed to a*

*committee that oversees a drug prevention program in your school. What are some new, but realistic, ideas you would suggest?* and expect that the students will be able to respond. Also, their increasing ability to deal with "if this–then that" statements may cause them to argue more vigorously about any controversial matter such as drug use, school programs on sexual conduct, or political matters.

3. *Adolescents attack a problem by gathering as much information as possible and then making all the possible combinations of the variables that they can.* They proceed as follows. *First,* they organize data by concrete operational techniques (classification, seriation). *Second,* they use the results of concrete operational techniques to form statements or propositions. *Third,* they combine as many of these propositions as possible. (These are hypotheses, and Piaget often refers to this process as hypothetico-deductive thinking.) *Fourth,* they then test to determine which combinations are true.

To illustrate these abilities, Piaget devised a series of famous experiments, one of which is the pendulum problem. Subjects are shown a pendulum hanging from a string. They're provided with strings of varying lengths and different weights. They're told that they can change the length of the string, the weight of the pendulum, the height from which it's released, and the amount of force used to push the pendulum. Then they are asked to discover what determines how fast the pendulum swings.

Young children (preoperational) attack the problem randomly, usually deciding that speed depends on how hard they push it. Middle childhood children (concrete operational) find that the length of the string is critical, but they can't divorce other factors, such as their push, from their reasoning. Adolescents (formal operations), however, vary one factor at a time, finally learning that the length of the string determines the speed of the pendulum.

### CRITICISMS OF PIAGET

Although Piaget has left a monumental legacy, his ideas have not gone unchallenged. Piaget was a believer in the stage theory of development; that is, development is seen as a sequence of distinct stages, each of which entails important changes in the way a child thinks, feels, and behaves. (See Chapter 1 for a discussion of stage theory.) However, the acquisition of cognitive structures may be gradual rather than abrupt and is not a matter of all or nothing; for example, a child is not completely in the sensorimotor or preoperational stage. Also, because stage theory equates the psychological structures of any stage with stability, it offers no explanation for the psychological mechanisms that account for variability and change in cognitive development (Fischer & Bidell 1998, p. 490). Human beings frequently depart from the consistency predicted by stage theory.

Developmental psychologists have grown increasingly skeptical of stage theory because of questions concerning the nature of the stages, the meaning of structure, combination of structures, and so on. Also, evidence has accumulated that children reach levels of cognitive competence earlier than Piaget realized. Specifically, it is difficult, if not impossible, to prove the existence of cognitive structures by simply analyzing behavior. Too often the behavior contradicts the theoretical structures. Also, explanations of how individuals pass from one stage to another remain weak. Nevertheless, Piaget's monumental contributions forever changed the way in which we look at children.

## Fischer and Skill Theory

Beginning with the assumption that the complexity of human behavior creates special problems for social scientists and leads to oversimplifications of explanations, Fischer and Bidell (1998) proposed a theory that focuses on the *dynamic structures of human behavior.* Defining psychological structure as the organizational property of dynamic systems of activity, Fischer and Bidell (1998, p. 471), as we have seen, disagree sharply with the static nature of stage theory.

These researchers believe that the concept of dynamic skill captures the characteristics of psychological structures in a more familiar manner and helps to explain specific patterns of developmental variability. Defining skill as the capacity to act in an organized way in a specific context, these authors believe that such variability emerges from the principles of constructive dynamics (Fischer & Bidell 1998). For example,

1. Skills in any context make up a hierarchy, with earlier acquired skills incorporated into a new, inclusive whole.

2. Skills are intended for use in specific contexts.

3. Skills are at multiple levels, depending on level of development.

Fischer, a cognitive psychologist at the Harvard Graduate School of Education, has spent many years studying the relationship between the appearance of new mental abilities and changes in the rate of brain growth. As a result of his research, Fischer believes he has found evidence for at least 12 brain growth spurts between birth and 21 years of age. He reached his conclusions based on studies of the growth of head size and brain activity (using EEG readings and increases in the density of synaptic junctions). The 12 brain growth spurts are as follows (Fischer & Rose 1998).

During *infancy,* Fischer has identified the ages at which seven of the brain growth spurts occur: 3 to 4 weeks, 7 to 8 weeks, 10 to 11 weeks, 15 to 18 weeks, 8 months, 12 months, and 20 months. Infancy is a time of extraordinary growth. Children are born with all their senses ready to go and immediately begin to absorb stimulation coming from this exciting new world: objects to watch and follow; a loving, caring person who will do anything to keep them happy; pleasant sounds to listen to; anytime they're hungry, food magically appears; they're rocked, hugged, and carried around; when they're tired, they simply tune out everybody and everything and go to sleep. But best of all, they're learning. Their brain cells are forming at an incredible rate and making connections with all kinds of neighboring cells.

At about 7 or 8 months, they suddenly find that they can crawl and creep, giving them whole new worlds to explore. At 12 months—wonder of wonders—they can pull themselves up, view their universe from a whole new perspective, and start to take steps that lead to new horizons. They begin to command their dominion with words and to interact verbally with those loving objects around them. Finally, as they approach 2 years, they begin to embark on the world of ideas—they start to think about all these wonderful things in their world.

During the *childhood years,* two brain growth spurts appear: at 4 years and 7 years. At 4 years of age, children understand much more about the world around them and they organize this information in a different manner. They're probably experiencing some type of preschool world and beginning to decide which of their playmates they like and which of they don't. They can run, jump, chase others, and PLAY! With their steadily growing cognitive abilities, they imagine all kinds of playmates and engage in fantastic activities. They have now experienced the 5 to 7 shift, that is, children's thinking after age 7 seems to be different from their thinking before age 5 (Sameroff & Haith 1996, p. 3). They are now more engaged in the symbolic world. Finally, in *the later years,* Fischer believes that brain growth spurts occur at 11 years, 15 years, and 20 years.

Perhaps the most significant feature of this chronology is to note how the brain is doing its part in all of these exciting phases of development. Whether a child is learning to walk, talk, or form relationships, the brain is ready to supply all of the neural firepower needed to be successful. If our brains are to function as they must to survive, doesn't it seem reasonable that to meet the challenges of a complex world new neural connections are constantly needed? That's where the environment comes in. Children especially must experience those stimuli that positively affect their ability to form the vital connections that facilitate emotional security, learning and remembering, solving problems, and adjusting to the challenges that lead to fulfillment. Understanding the mechanisms of cognitive development helps you, as a health care provider, to care for children in a manner that integrates how they make sense of the world.

## Vygotsky and Development— The Cultural Perspective

We presented several of the basic themes in Vygotsky's theory in Chapter 1, and if you understand his fundamental ideas, you'll be able to grasp how his theory works. He identified dual paths of cognitive development: *elementary processes* that are basically biological and *psychological processes* that are essentially sociocultural. Children's behaviors emerge from the intertwining of these two paths. For example, brain development provides the physiological basis for the appearance of external or egocentric speech, which gradually becomes the inner speech children use to guide their behavior.

### Basic Themes in Vygotsky's Theory

Three fundamental assumptions run through Vygotsky's work: the unique manner in which he identified and used the concept of development, the social origin of mind, and the role of speech in cognitive development.

**The Concept of Development**    Vygotsky's *concept of development* is at the heart of his theory. He thought that elementary biological processes are qualitatively transformed into higher psychological functioning by developmental processes. In other words, such behaviors as speech, thought, and learning are all explained by development. Speech serves as an example.

The "noises" that babies make in their speech development—crying, cooing, babbling—are accompanied by physical movement. Children gradually begin to point at objects and adults tell them the name—ball, cup, milk. First words come, then children start to string words together, talk aloud, and finally use speech much the way adults do. Instead of seeing a series of independent accomplishments, Vygotsky viewed these changes as *a series of transformations brought about by developmental processes.* Consequently, a developmental analysis of speech helps to provide clues as to how speech and thought are interrelated.

**The Social Origin of Mind**    To understand cognitive development, we must examine *the social and cultural processes* shaping children (Wertsch & Tulviste 1992). But how do these processes affect cognitive development? Vygotsky argued (1978) that any function in a child's cultural development appears twice, on two planes: first, in an interpsychological category (social exchanges with others), and, second, within the child as an intrapsychological category (using inner speech to guide behavior).

What happens to transform external activity to internal activity? For Vygotsky, the answer is to be found in the process of *internalization.* As he stated, the transformation of an interpersonal process (egocentric speech) into an intrapersonal process (inner speech) is the result of a long series of developmental events (Vygotsky 1978, p. 57). He termed this internalization process "the distinguishing feature of human psychology," the barest outline of which is known.

**The Role of Speech in Cognitive Development**    Although Vygotsky lacked hard data to explain this belief, he believed that *speech* is one of the most powerful tools humans use to progress developmentally.

*. . . .the most significant moment in the course of intellectual development, which gives birth to the purely human forms of practical and abstract intelligence, occurs when speech and practical activity, two previously completely independent lines of development, converge (Vygotsky 1978, p. 24).*

## VYGOTSKY AND LANGUAGE DEVELOPMENT

Vygotsky's ideas concerning language development offer a clear insight into his interpretation of development. In his important contribution, *Thought and Language* (1962), he clearly presented his views about the sequence of language development, which he believed encompassed four stages: *preintellectual speech, naive psychology, egocentric speech,* and *inner speech.*

1. *Preintellectual speech:* Preintellectual speech refers to the elementary processes (crying, cooing, babbling, bodily movements), the biological sources that gradually develop into more sophisticated forms of speech and behavior. As human beings we have an inborn ability to develop language, which must then interact with the environment if language development is to fulfill its potential. Michael Cole (1996) employs a garden metaphor to help explain these issues. Think of a seed planted in damp earth in a jar and then placed in a shed for 2 weeks. The seed sprouts, a stem emerges, and leaves appear. But for further development the plant must now interact with sunlight.

2. *Naïve psychology:* Vygotsky referred to the second stage of language development as naïve psychology, in which children explore the concrete objects in their world. At this stage, children begin to label objects around them and acquire the syntax of their speech. They only gradually acquire an understanding of the verbal forms they have been using; that is, they realize that language influences their thinking and shapes their relationships with others.

3. *Egocentric speech:* Around the time that children turn 3 years old, egocentric speech emerges. This is a form of speech in which children carry on lively conversations, whether or not anyone is present or listening to them. As Vygotsky noted (1962, p. 46), egocentric speech is speech on its way inward but still mostly outward.

4. *Inner speech:* Finally, speech turns inward (inner speech) and serves an important function in guiding and planning behavior. For example, think of a 5-year-old girl asked to get a book from a library shelf. The book is just out of her reach, and as she tried to reach it, she murmurs to herself, "Need a chair." After dragging a chair over, she climbs up.

   You can see how speech accompanies her physical movements, guiding her behavior. In 2 or 3 years, the same girl, asked to do the same thing, will probably act the same way, with one major exception: She won't be talking aloud. Vygotsky believed she would be talking to herself, using inner speech to guide her behavior, and for difficult tasks she undoubtedly would use inner speech to *plan her behavior.* In many cases, children who aren't permitted these vocalizations *can't accomplish the task!* In fact, the more complex the task, the greater the amount of egocentric speech.

What does this mean for work with your clients? As people, particularly children, acquire new knowledge and skills, they move to higher levels of understanding and achieve greater control over their mental activities. By being aware of their growing consciousness and the self-regulation of their thought processes, you help to produce desirable changes in their behavior that contribute to improved health practices. In other words, the interaction between an active child and an active social environment leads to healthy developmental change.

We turn our attention now to information-processing theorists and how they interpret the journey through the challenges and accomplishments of cognitive development.

## The Information Processing Model

What is happening in the human head to produce human cognition? This question posed by well-known cognitivist John Anderson (1993) appears in the first chapter of his book on human cognition and is the fundamental guide to the rest of his work. It is also the basic question in cognitive development: What are the structures and content of human knowledge, and what are the developmental mechanisms that propel humans through progressive knowledge states (Klahr & Macwhinney 1998)? The following quotation by cognitive psychologist Robert Sternberg is a good starting point to answer this question.

*Information processing theorists seek to understand cognitive development in terms of how people of different ages process information (i.e., decode, encode, transfer, combine, store, retrieve it), particularly when solving challenging mental problems (Sternberg 2002, p. 462).*

There is a major difference between the work of the information-processing theorists and Piaget, Fischer, and Vygotsky. Information-processing theorists do not attempt to provide a comprehensive explanation of cognitive development as did the other theorists we discussed. The information-processing theorists focus on cognitive processes such as attention, memory, and language that change over time and help to explain cognitive development.

Piaget, as we have seen, argued forcefully that cognitive development proceeds by progression through discrete stages. Information-processing theorists, however, argue just as strongly that cognitive development occurs as individuals improve such cognitive processes as attention and memory.

Consequently, any mental activity that involves noticing, taking in, mentally manipulating, storing, combining, retrieving, and acting on information describes information processing. Changes in these processes explain cognitive development and reflect changes either in the hardware (memory, speed of processing, etc.) or software (the ability to use strategies). Thus the foundation on which information processing is built consists of assumptions about the manner in which humans acquire, store, and retrieve information (Bjorklund 2000, p. 118).

In your work with your clients, the ideas of information-processing theorists offer several helpful suggestions.

- If you are giving instructions to clients, both children and adults, be sure you have their undivided attention. Be aware that medications and anxiety can affect attentiveness.

- From your interactions with individual clients, you should have acquired a good grasp not only of what they remember, but also how they go about memorizing. Try to capitalize on this knowledge.

- Encourage your clients to use strategies that are both effective and compatible with their age and needs.

In working with clients of any age, it's important to assess a person's readiness to not only take in information and advice that you are providing, but to use that information and advice at home. It is also important to remember that sometimes the client and the family members may receive the same information you provide but in a different form, leading to disagreements about the health care regimen later at home. Some suggestions for teaching and talking with clients and family members include the following:

- Be sure you have a client's and/or family member's undivided attention. Remember that medications, anxiety, and distractions in a hospital or clinic can limit attentiveness.

- As you talk with clients and families, assess what they know and understand about what you have told them. Ask them to repeat it back in their own words. Ask them how they best remember things and capitalize on their own strategies. For example, some people need everything written down.

- Become familiar with developmentally appropriate strategies for remembering that apply to clients in the age group with which you usually work. How an 8-year-old remembers and uses information differs from a 50-year-old—although both may benefit from similar strategies! For example, visual clues to take medications can include putting a note on the bathroom mirror or leaving the toothbrush next to the medicine bottle.

As we complete this section, remember that information-processing theorists believe that *all* thinking is information processing. The task, then, is to determine what cognitive processes are involved in the selection of successful solutions and how they change over time. Our goal in the remainder of the chapter is to discuss—as much as space permits—the cognitive processes that lead to the successful solution of problems.

# Cognitive Development— The Processes

In the 21st century it's almost a cliché to state that we cannot understand the workings and development of the human mind unless we take into consideration its underlying neurophysiological foundation. The tremendous surge in neuroscientific interest and research has provided data that offer current—and potential—insights into the secrets of human cognition. Consequently, it seems relevant, if not crucial, to review the beginnings of our neurological substrate.

## The Biological Beginnings

*At a recent soccer game, I asked Lindsey, a nine-year-old player, to describe for me what she thought as she was racing down the field. I'm not sure I understood everything she said. (Lindsey is very polite and is quite patient with the curious questions of adults.) After looking at me quizzically, she said that first she would have to decide whether to pass or shoot. "I'd pass if I had to go through the defense, Lauren would pass back and I'd score. Or she would shoot and I'd be there for the rebound if she missed. But if there were no defense, I'd take the shot. If our goalie made a good save and a good drop kick out to me, I'd do a scissors to get by the defense and shoot. But if someone got behind the defense, I'd pass." GOALLLL!!!*

What does this have to do with cognitive development and the brain? Everything. Imagine the thoughts—the cognitive processes—of these two players as they had to make a split-second decision on what to do for their team. They certainly had to give intense attention to what they were doing. Memory had to enter into their decision—what had happened in previous similar situations? This means that the hippocampus area of the brain, which is crucial for memory, becomes active. Clearly, problem solving was necessary, which demands involvement by the frontal area of the cerebral cortex. Were the young girls excited? Of course, that goes without saying. Consequently, the brain part known as the amygdala swings into action.

Everything we think, do, and feel has its basis in the brain. Unfortunately, this is also true when things go wrong. One of the most famous cases in the history of psychology concerns a 9-year-old boy known as HM. Knocked down by a bicycle, he suffered head injuries that eventually led to repeated epileptic attacks. His condition worsened to the point where he was having 10 blackouts and a major seizure every week. At 27 years of age, HM was almost completely incapacitated. The decision was made to remove the inner part of the temporal lobe on both sides of the brain, a region that included the hippocampus. It turned out to be one of those cases where we say that the operation was a success but the patient suffered irreversible damage. The epileptic seizures became less in number and intensity, but HM suffered a devastating loss of memory from which he never recovered. Since that time, studies have clearly linked the hippocampus to memory (Gazzaniga et al. 1998).

For better or worse, the brain is tightly bound to all aspects of our lives. The neuroscientist Lise Eliot (2000) nicely summarizes this reality when she notes that every decision parents make relates to their child's brain development: whether to have a glass of wine during pregnancy, whether to smoke during pregnancy, when to return to work, what kind of school their child should attend, how much television they should watch. These thoughts about the powerful role that the brain plays in cognitive development are important reminders of the interactive nature of development. Remember, however, the genes may pass on the genetic program that forms the nervous system, the brain may direct a child's behavior, but experience ultimately determines the quality and extent of brain development.

## The Brain and Cognition, Cognition and The Brain

When you think of the complexity of the brain, it's stunning to realize how quickly neural development occurs. The neuroscientist Marian Diamond (1998) summarizes the rapid growth in this way: If fertilization occurred on Monday, by Thursday the embryo would consist of 30 cells clustered together. By Saturday, this cluster of cells (a blastocyst) would have started digging into the woman's uterine wall. By Tuesday of the following week the endoderm, mesoderm, and ectoderm would be emerging. This happens before the woman misses her first period. Unknowingly she may have consumed alcohol, continued smok-

ing, and used some type of drug, all of which can damage the developing embryo. Summarizing, then, the stages in this initial phase of nervous system development are as follows.

- The process begins with the induction of the neural plate, which can only occur during a limited time, usually about the beginning of the third prenatal week.

- The neural tube forms and its top expands into the brain as we know it, while the rest of the tube will become the spinal cord.

- Nerve cells begin to form in the neural tube (a process called *cell proliferation*). For a baby to be born with 100 *billion* neurons, nerve cells must be produced during pregnancy at an average rate of 250,000 per minute!

- The nerve cells at this stage are called neurons, and they begin to leave the neural tube and travel to their destination in the developing brain. This process is called *cell migration,* which typically commences during the seventh prenatal week. Some of the neurons travel tremendous distances in the brain, for example, equal to the distance from Boston to San Francisco.

- The neurons now embark on their task of forming 1000 trillion connections in a child's brain.

- A pruning process quickly sets in and million of neurons and connections perish, which is nature's way of insuring survival of the fittest neurons.

- An infant's brain is about 25% of its adult weight at birth, which means that 75% of its continued growth and development will be in direct contact with the environment.

- Brain enrichment is an idea whose time has come. A child is born with about 1000 trillion brain connections, but by age 10 that number is down to 500 trillion, which under normal circumstances remains fairly constant for most of the remaining years. The original number was mainly due to nature's generous oversupply to insure that a child would be able to make all the connections it needed.

Think of the figures we've so casually mentioned.

- 200 billion brain cells in the fetal brain by the fifth month.
- 100 billion brain cells in a newborn baby's brain.
- One trillion glia cells in a baby's brain. (These are support cells.)
- 1,000 trillion connections in a baby's brain.

As you can see, at about the fifth prenatal month, estimates are that a fetus has developed 200 billion brain cells. What happened to cause the fetus to lose 100 billion brain cells in the space of the four remaining months of pregnancy? The answer lies in the number of brain cells or neurons that nature originally produces in all our brains.

Nature has manufactured billions of brain cells more than will be needed to guarantee that the brain will be able to form enough connections for all the needed abilities and skills that demand new connections and to meet the challenges at birth. The neurons that don't make connections simply die. This exercise in survival (some connections die, some connections survive) continues throughout our lives, giving new and critical meaning to the expression "Use it or lose it." Recall Darwin's famous belief in the survival of the fittest—the fittest of our neurons are those that make connections and survive. The lesson for all of us is: Keep busy, seek challenges, stay alert.

Now, however, let's examine several of those processes that play a key role in cognitive development.

## The Role of Attention

Early on a beautiful September morning, I met my child psychology class in front of the university library. I had asked the research staff of the library to introduce the first-year students to the mysteries of the computer facilities. Because I had previously assigned them a term paper, they were properly motivated for the session.

After a humorous but pertinent overview, the librarians broke the class into three sections so that everyone would have some hands-on time with the computers and the various programs. As I moved from group to group, I was struck by the individual differences in attention. A few class members were obviously tired by this ghastly early morning intrusion into their lives and their attention soon faded. Some were easily distracted by the movement in the library as other students entered and commenced their work at nearby tables and computers. I would say about one-half the group was intensely focused on the computers and the instructions they were receiving.

I'm sure you can guess the purpose of this introduction: You can help your clients attend to what's really important by becoming familiar with how they attend. For example, vision, hearing, and touch are probably the three most important sensor systems, *but* patients undoubtedly differ on which of these systems they prefer. Their preferences influence what they attend to and help to identify their learning style. You have your own preferences; for example, you may prefer a certain temperature, intensity of lighting, or time of day to work. You may need everything systematically arranged, whereas someone else requires much less structure. These differences suggest that unless you have circumstances that match your individual preferences, you may miss the significant clues in your environment. *Your clients react in exactly the same manner.* Remember: *What people attend to determines what they do.*

## What Is This Attention We Should Be Attending To?

To give you some idea of how long scientists have been struggling to untie the attentional knot, consider the fairly recent past. About 100 years ago, America's premier psychologist, William James, when asked about attention, replied:

*Everyone knows what attention is. It is the taking possession by the mind, in clear and vivid form, of one out of what seems several simultaneously possible objects or trains of thought.*

James' statement is interesting on two accounts: First, it tells us that psychologists have been wrestling with this topic for centuries; second, James really doesn't tell us in his response anything we didn't know.

For example, the famous "cocktail party" effect. Imagine you're standing in a crowded room, people are sipping their drinks, and you're talking to one person. The noise level is high and you have to concentrate on your partner to understand what she's saying. By means of your concentration (called selective attention), you're able to carry on a conversation. This is what James was talking about, but it doesn't help to explain why or how you paid attention. Why did you concentrate on that one person? Was it something about her appearance, the subject she was discussing, your own interests, a desire to be polite, or all of the above?

To answer these and similar questions, Ross Thompson (1998), a neuroscientist at the University of Nebraska, after studying the way in which temperament or personality interacts with the environment, concludes the following:

- Temperament (a unique and stable style of behaving) influences how a person selects and responds to different aspects of the environment (individuals, settings, activities,

etc.), in other words, what she attends to. This in turn will affect how she will respond.

- A person's temperament may mesh well or poorly with the demands of the social setting. The goodness-of-fit between temperament and environment has a major impact on personality and adjustment. As the environment changes dramatically through the years, changes have powerful effects on what individuals attend to.

- Temperament colors how individuals perceive and think about the environment and what attracts their attention.

- Temperament may interact with environmental influences in a way we simply don't understand.

With these ideas in mind, let's turn to the various types of attention that psychologists have identified.

## Types of Attention

Psychiatrist Nancy Andreasen (2001) refers to attention as the "spotlight" of the brain. That is, attention enables people to decide what is important, what is needed, and what is dangerous, *but* it also helps them to ignore everything else. Andreasen goes on to point out that attention is central to the cognitive processes your clients constantly use. But we also know that none of us can sustain a burning attention in all of our activities. Consequently, she suggests that there are different types of attention, with different characteristics, which can alert you to a person's current state of alertness.

- *Sustained attention* refers to concentration for lengthy periods of time. A good example of this would be a client's continued concentration on a physical problem or a scheduled operation several weeks away.

- *Directed attention* refers to concentrating on a particular feature in the environment under the influence of some external force. For example, you try to stress the importance of maintaining a schedule of daily corrective exercises.

- *Selective attention* refers to the ability to consciously concentrate on something that is personally important. The cocktail party is a good example. Amid all the hubbub of ongoing conversations, I hear my name spoken and I select that stimulus to concentrate on. Remember that selective attention focuses on people, objects, and activities that people find highly important.

- *Divided attention* refers to the attempt to concentrate on several things at the same time. There are both good and bad features of divided attention. If you've ever watched a football game, you probably recall seeing one team kicking the ball to the other. Occasionally the player who is supposed to catch the ball drops it. Divided attention at work! The player looks at the ball while simultaneously trying to see if any opposing player is close enough to tackle him.

- *Focused attention* refers to the need to zero in on some task that simply has to be done. For example, maintaining a schedule of prescribed medication requires focused attention. How often have you suddenly thought, "Did I take my blood pressure pill this morning?"

When you think about attention in this manner it explains a great deal about behavior. For example, if a client can't concentrate on the instructions you've given, improvement is sure to suffer. If he can't, or refuses to, listen to your advice, troublesome behavior could result. Thinking about these issues helps to explain the importance and the complexity of attention. The more you know about it, the better you can shape a client's environment so that developmentally appropriate materials and techniques are used that match their interests, abilities, and developmental level. This is the only path to ensuring the focused attention that patients need to move successfully through a challenging environment, one composed of diverse, distracting, and often disturbing stimuli.

## Memories Are Made of This

*Most of us probably will never forget where we were on September 11, 2001. That tragic event is burned into the minds and hearts of Americans in a way that we'll never forget. I had an early class that morning and when I returned to my office several students were waiting to discuss their term papers. It was a pleasant, light-hearted meeting; none of us had a hint of the tragedy that was unfolding while we talked. I turned on my computer to check my e-mails and was immediately overwhelmed by a number of messages detailing the horror of what had happened in New York.*

How important is memory in our lives? Would you agree with Eric Kandel (Squire & Kandel 2000) when he states that without memory we're really nothing—no sense of self, no sense of a personal history, no sense of certainty? Just a vague sense of bewildered frustration. In some of my recent work, I was talking with a stroke victim who summarized his predicament in words hard to forget. "John, you don't know what's it's like to wake up in the morning and not know who you are, or what happened yesterday. No matter how exciting yesterday might have been, I can't remember it. It's as if nothing happened; there's no yesterday."

As we begin a brief excursion into the world of memory, here are four guiding principles that have emerged from recent research (Eliot 2000).

1. *The brain as a whole is involved in memory;* memories don't reside in one particular location.

2. Memories are reproduced in the same manner as they were formed (psychologists refer to this as *retrieval*).

3. Memories are stored in the brain's *synapses,* which are the connections between neurons.

4. These synaptic connections can be strengthened through use, and new synaptic processes can be formed by learning.

## How Does Memory "Work"?

In the innocent days of past years, we naively believed that memories were simply stored in one location and each memory was conveniently assigned to a brain cell(s). Today, however, unraveling the secrets of memory hidden in brain systems and synaptic connections is seen as a daunting but achievable task. Here is where we currently stand with regard to the relationship between brain and memory.

What we usually think of as a memory—recall of information, figures, people—which is often called *explicit memory,* requires the action of several brain parts: the hippocampus, the thalamus, the temporal lobes, and the frontal lobes of the cortex. In other words, explicit memory is memory for facts. Explicit memory (also called *declarative memory*) works on stored information that can be retrieved by concentrated recollection and the use of various cues and strategies. Richard Restak (2001), a neuroscientist who comments frequently on the latest brain research, points out the hippocampus and the medial temporal lobe are critical brain areas for the formation and storage of explicit memories.

Daniel Schacter (1996), chairperson of the Psychology Department at Harvard and a noted memory researcher, believes that it is only toward the end of the first year that infants give evidence of explicit memory. For example, you're in a restaurant enjoying a leisurely dinner when a young couple is seated next to you and the hostess is carrying an infant seat. You're intrigued by the behavior of your 1-year-old neighbor. Suddenly she knocks the toy from her tray. But she pauses *and looks down to the floor for the toy.* The moment

of truth: This infant is displaying a capacity for explicit memory, no matter how limited.

Another type of memory, much more obscure and difficult to analyze—think of how you learned to ride a bike—is often called *implicit memory* and involves the cerebellum, the amygdala, and the motor cortex. Implicit memory is almost automatic; we really don't think about it. When we require the information needed to perform this kind of task, such as riding a bike, we're not aware of consciously searching for specific steps that will help us to remember. It may have taken us a long time to acquire the skill, but, once mastered, doesn't demand any effort to be retrieved. (This sort of memory is called *implicit, nondeclarative, memory without record,* or *knowing how.*) We don't recall where, when, and how we learned it.

Implicit memory may also have a powerful emotional accompaniment, which explains the involvement of the amygdala. We previously mentioned how the storage of memories can be colored by the emotions and circumstances surrounding the original experience. A good example of this emotional involvement is the anxiety or panic attack. Individuals who have had vivid and disturbing events in their lives (war, accident) may have frightening flashbacks called *posttraumatic stress disorders.* For no plausible reason, they suddenly have feelings that range from intense physical reactions (pounding heart, drenched in sweat) to a sense of impending death. In these cases the amygdala is involved, explaining the emotional feelings that accompany the flashback.

Explicit and implicit memory storage use different brain systems and strategies for storing memories. Researchers now realize that the entire nervous system is engaged in the formation of memories. The neuroscientist Lise Eliot (2000) summarizes this newly recognized dilemma when she states that the entire nervous system must be involved because information storage is a fundamental property of all neurons. All memories are stored as synaptic changes somewhere in the brain.

The challenge in research is to trace the neural systems involved and identify the underlying changes that occur. Researchers are probing the neural systems that support both implicit and explicit memory. As they do, they're discovering how changes take place during learning and how these changes are maintained in memory. Here's what we think your clients do to remember (*encode*), to retain (*storage*), and to remove that information from storage (*retrieval*) (Squire & Kandel 2000).

## ENCODING INFORMATION

To be able to recall effectively, individuals must have first placed the information in their memory system. This process, called encoding, is accomplished just as its name implies. People pay attention to something and, if desired, they turn that something into a biological code that we're still trying to unravel. The more attentive they are, the more they concentrate, the more time they spend on analyzing details, the deeper and more long-lasting will be the memory.

The cognitive neuroscientist Michael Gazzaniga and his colleagues (1998) believe that encoding seems to require two separate stages—*acquisition* and *consolidation.* Acquisition is our immediate reaction to the sights, sounds, and other stimulation that we register. But to transfer these sensations to long-term memory requires watching, listening, rehearsing—that is, consolidation.

Thus there is clear evidence that the more individuals process information—watching, listening, rehearsing, acting on it—the more deeply the memory will be embedded. The neuroscientists Squire and Kandel (2000) conclude that memory is better the more we have a reason to study, the more we like what we are studying, and the more we bring the full force of our attention to the learning. If you can accustom your clients to attack learning tasks in this manner, they'll almost automatically build in retrieval cues that will prove to be of enormous help in the future.

## STORAGE

You can help your clients to store their memories as accurately as possible and to retrieve them as fully as possible. When they try to remember something, here's a quick overview of what happens in their brains. After they encode information, they must retain it—somehow, somewhere—if it is to be useful to them. *The individual connection between two neurons is the elementary unit of storage* (Squire and Kandel 2000). Consequently, how you can help your clients strengthen synaptic connections becomes one of your key goals in working with them to improve their memorization techniques.

Remember that there is no one, special place where memories are permanently stored. Memory is stored in the neural systems that initially recorded it. That is, the brain regions that first responded to stimulation are the same brain regions that process it for storage. It's important to remember, however, that the brain areas that originally contributed to the memory may not have been strengthened to the same degree. If you think about this in relation to your client's memories, you can understand what it implies for their ability to recall: why some elements of a memory are lost, why some are distorted, and what they must do to make their memories permanent.

**Types of Memory Used in Storage.** The various names given to memory storage depend on the time each holds information in storage. Psychologists typically use three memory stores for their analysis: sensory memory, short-term memory, and long-term memory.

- *Sensory memory:* Sensory memory holds information for only a fraction of a second. Two things then happen: either the information is lost or you rehearse it sufficiently to transfer it either to short-term or long-term memory (Santrock 2004). A particularly interesting and useful aspect of sensory memory is the distinction it makes between visual and auditory information. Sensory memory will hold visual information for only a second or two without rehearsal, but may retain auditory information for up to 30 seconds.

- *Short-term memory.* Short-term memory refers to the process by which information is retained for a brief period of time or is transferred to long-term memory. Recent studies suggest that short-term memory consists of two components: *immediate memory* and *working memory.*

*Immediate memory* refers to that information that we pay attention to now (what we see, hear, feel at this moment) and then hold in memory. In other words, the incoming information registers on our brains. Immediate memory retains this data for about thir 30 seconds and can hold about seven items. George Miller, a well-known Harvard psychologist, wrote a famous article entitled, *The Magic Number Seven, Plus or Minus Two.* Since then psychologists have believed that the extent of our immediate memory is from five to nine items. (Remember, however, that seven numbers are not the same as seven general categories.)

*Working memory* becomes active as an individual "works on" the information and begins the transfer to short-term memory. Working memory can stretch the retention of information by repetition, or rehearsal, and help it to survive for several moments. Thanks to recent animal research we now think that the frontal lobes of the brain are involved. Some psychologists argue that working memory and short-term memory are essentially identical. But Yale University neuroscientist Patricia Goldman Rakic (1995) believes that the holding action of the frontal lobes is actually what we mean by working memory.

- *Long-term memory:* Long-term memory refers to information that is retained for a significant time. That's the easy part. Much more difficult is to explain how information moves from short-term to long-term memory. Let's imagine you take your 7-year-old to a major league baseball game for the first time. (Boy or girl, it makes no difference.) As I type this, I visualize Fenway Park in Boston, soon to be abandoned for a more dazzling, modern field. You never forget your first visit to this beautiful green diamond. (Incidentally, this a good example of explicit memory: famous left field wall, scoreboard, bullpens, etc.)

Note that I said, "You'll never forget your first visit to Fenway Park." Why? Your visual pathways activated areas of the cortex in the frontal lobe and also in the temporal lobe. The temporal lobe now begins the process of transforming the information about the ball park with the help of the cortical areas. How does this occur?

Neuroscientists have learned that short-term memory becomes long-term memory only if a "consolidation switch" is thrown. This consolidation switch stimulates specific genes to form new proteins. If you think about your own memory for a moment, you'll recall how easy it is to forget something if you didn't take the time to rehearse it. It's during this interval that the necessary genes are turned on and new proteins manufactured.

Here is another way to think about this process. How often have you heard that an athlete was "dinged," a term that is frequently applied to football and hockey players and usually implies a mild concussion. Imagine that a football player is hit very hard. If you ask that player what happened immediately after being hit, he can usually tell you about the play. If you ask him about the same play 30 or 40 minutes after being hit, he frequently can't tell you. In other words, the details of the play made it into short-term memory, but could not last long enough to transfer to long-term memory.

## RETRIEVAL

From what we've said about encoding and storage, you may well conclude that retrieving information is a simple matter of recalling data from the various locations where it was originally stored. Unfortunately, it's not that simple. *The cues that you use for retrieval may only recall some parts of the stored information.* The cues may be so weak that the original memory may now return in a distorted form. (e.g., I remember that I was wearing a gray sport jacket when it happened. Sorry. It was a brown jacket.)

The significance of cues for retrieval goes far in explaining why scientists believe that, as Squire and Kandel (2000) note, retrieval is essentially a creative and reconstructive process. Also, your mood and emotions at the time you originally stored information has a strong impact on retrieval. If you were happy when you stored that memory, you probably remember the positive aspects of whatever it was. For retrieval to be truly effective, the cues used should be as faithful as possible to the original memory. In other words, the encoding and retrieval cues should be as similar as possible.

**How Does Retrieval Work?**    To fully understand retrieval, two procedures require discussion: recall and recognition. Recall is a process in which we must reach into memory, with no given cues, to retrieve information. Recognition, however, demands that we identify previously learned material by differentiating among retrieval cues. Multiple choice tests are a good example of a recognition task. Remembering (!) the distinction between these two processes will help you and your clients in forming strategies.

As a result of decades of research, speculation, and common sense reasoning, we can make certain generalizations that should help your clients with retrieval. Among them are the following:

- *Similarity of material can cause interference.* For example, many medications have similar names. When working with clients, help them to devise a strategy to differentiate among various pills. For example, color coding bottle caps can help distinguish between two medications that are similar in name or appearance.

- *Meaningful material aids recall.* Make instructions, schedules, and the like as meaningful as possible in the context of their lives. Once you know a client, you can then use people and circumstances to bring meaning to their efforts. For example, ask about daily routines or events that would help a person to remember that it's time to take a medication or to check blood sugar levels.

- *Time on task helps your clients to remember.* There's no avoiding the implications of time; your clients must spend focused time on your instructions, suggestions, and programs. Watch them; make sure conditions are as positive as possible; if they need it, help them to concentrate. There is no substitute for focused time on instructions, suggestions, questions, and responses.

- *Rehearsal (going over something repeatedly) is an important memory strategy.* We have discussed this repeatedly, but it bears repetition: If the synaptic connections where memory is stored are to function effectively in retrieval, then your clients must rehearse. Again, try to make it as pleasant and meaningful as possible by using memory aids that have personal meaning for your client.

- *Memory strategies can help people remember.* Try to devise as many helpful hints and suggestions as possible for devising strategies that will improve your client's memories. For example, placing pills in pill organizers that are sorted by the day and hour, posting written notes, or placing the toothbrush next to the medication bottle all are meaningful memory strategies.

## FORGETTING

Forgetting, unfortunately, is a normal process and different from an abnormal loss of memory occasioned by shock or brain injury. Under normal daily conditions, what causes individuals to forget previously acquired material? Neuroscientists are still searching for clues that will help us to untangle this memory knot. Studies are attempting to determine what changes in brain cells and synaptic connection when forgetting occurs. Current theories and research point to these likely explanations.

- *Forgetting as an actual loss of information:* Some of the synaptic changes and brain cell modifications are lost. New information reshapes existing connections and these changes cause loss due to the passage of time, which probably accounts for the loss of information or at least the modification of the original learning. As previously mentioned, these changes are slowed depending on the strength of the initial connection.

- *Forgetting as cue-dependent:* Retrieval failure is caused by a lack of pertinent and usable cues. For example, when your clients encode and store facts about a proposed exercise schedule, they have a better chance of remembering them if they have linked meaningful cues to the facts. "You used to read when you came home from work. Why not put a book on a treadmill and do both?"

- *Forgetting because of interference.* Psychologists agree that most forgetting happens because new learning interferes with past learning. Interference can be either retroactive (the interference is produced by learning that occurs after the memory event) or proactive (it is produced by learning that occurred before the memory event).

## FALSE MEMORY

Elizabeth Loftus, a psychologist at the University of Washington (Seattle), then 44 years old, had been falsely told by a relative that when her mother drowned in their swimming pool, she was the one who had discovered the body. She hadn't remembered, but now, she relates, she had vivid memories of her mother floating face down in the pool, police cars, and flashing lights. But her brother called her a few days later and told her it was all a mistake; her aunt had found the body.

Loftus was stunned. If she, as a highly trained psychologist, could be so easily fooled, what did that mean for the average person? She addressed this question in a fascinating series of experiments. Initially, she asked older parents to identify several events in the early years of their children's lives. She then presented these incidents to their now adult children, but she also included an episode that was false. She told them they had been lost in a shopping mall until found by another adult and returned to their parents. They were crying, frightened, and bewildered when found. About 25% of the subjects agreed that this had happened, and some of them even added more graphic details.

These studies caused instant and heated controversy. Those who as adults claimed that they had been abused as children felt they were being branded as liars. Loftus was subjected to extended criticism both from some of her academic colleagues and those involved in these unfortunate circumstances. How fragile is memory? Are these cases always false? Obviously not. Are they always true? Obviously not. Each case requires intensive scrutiny, but they illustrate once again not only the importance of memory in our lives but also the need for continued research that addresses these issues.

If you are able to help your clients by improving their thinking about attention and memory, can you apply these insights to the problems they face?

# Improving Problem-Solving Behavior

I recently was asked to give a talk to a group—nurses, social workers, teachers—on thinking skills and problem-solving strategies. To begin, I presented the following problem:

*Two motorcyclists are 100 miles apart. At exactly the same moment they begin to drive toward each other for a meeting. Just as they leave, a bird flies from the front of the first cyclist to the front of the second cyclist. When it reaches the second cyclist, it turns around and flies back to the first. The bird continues flying in this manner until the cyclists meet. The cyclists both travel at the rate of 50 miles per hour, while the bird maintains a constant speed of 75 miles per hour. How many miles will the bird have flown when the cyclists meet?*

Examining this problem, you may immediately begin to calculate distance, miles per hour, and constancy of speed. Actually, this is not a mathematical problem; it's a word problem. Carefully look at it again. Both riders will travel for one hour before they meet; the bird flies at 75 miles per hour; therefore, the bird will have flown 75 miles. No formula or calculations are needed, just a close examination of what is given.

The talk was in the evening. They were tired, and not too attentive. Then they became downright mad at themselves for not getting the correct answer. Now I had their attention, and they were determined not to be tricked again. I next asked them to think of something that had frustrated them recently—in other words, a problem—and how they had felt if they couldn't reach a solution.

## WHAT KINDS OF MISTAKES DO INDIVIDUALS MAKE?

Most errors are made not because children and adults lack information about the problems but mainly because they don't attend to the problem or fully employ their reasoning processes. For example, try this problem.

*In a different language, liro cas means red tomato, dum cas dan means big red barn, and xer dan means big horse. What is the word for barn in this language? (a) dum (b) liro (c) cas (d) dan (e) xer*

Here we have a fairly simple problem, but one demanding a systematic comparison of phrases and a careful matching of words. Poor problem solvers often jump at the first clue, with the result that they choose b, c, d, or e.

Among the most common sources of error are the following:

- *Failure to observe and use all the relevant facts of a problem.* Did you account for each word in the language problem?

- *Failure to adopt systematic, step-by-step procedures.* The problem solver may skip steps, ignore vital information, and leap to a faulty conclusion. Did you make a check, or some other mark, against each word?

- *Failure to perceive vital relationships* in the problem. Did you discover the pattern that led to *dum* as the correct answer?

- *Frequent use of sloppy techniques in acquiring and applying vital information.* Did you guess at the meanings of any of the words? Did you try to eliminate the irrelevant words?

## CHARACTERISTICS OF GOOD PROBLEM SOLVERS

Solving a problem occurs when a person has a particular goal in mind that can't be attained immediately because obstacles are present. Thus there are four criteria needed for problem solving to occur: goals, obstacles, strategies for overcoming the obstacles, and an evaluation of the results (Bjorklund 2000). We know a great deal about problem-solving strategies today, and this knowledge can be of great value to your clients who obviously are faced with physical and psychological problems. How they react to these situations goes a long way toward their recovery.

But we also know that some children and adults don't do well with problems because they're afraid of them. "I'm just not smart enough"; "I never could do these." Here is a good example. Group the following numbers in such a way that when you add them, the total is 1,000.

8 8 8 8 8 8 8 8

Unintimidated elementary school children get the answer almost immediately. Some of you won't even bother trying; others will make a halfhearted effort; still others will attack it enthusiastically. What is important is how you think about a problem. In the eights problem, think of the only number of groups that would give you 0 in the units column when you add them—five groups. Try working with five groups and you will eventually discover that

888 + 88 + 8 + 8 + 8 gives you 1,000.

Many of the daily problems children face are vague and ill defined, and if they lack problem-solving strategies, their task is next to impossible. Recent research indicates that most children devise a wide variety of strategies to solve their problems and, depending on the nature of the task, they'll select what they think is the most appropriate strategy. This has led to *the adaptive strategy choice model* of Robert Siegler (1998). Those strategies that produce successful solutions increase in frequency, while those that do not decrease in frequency. Children have multiple strategies available at all ages, but a child's age dictates which strategies are most frequently used.

Many developmental features come into play during the life span to enhance the cognitive skills of human beings. Attention dramatically improves as your clients learn to shut out distractions and concentrate on the immediate task. Short-term memory span increases as they acquire and use various memory strategies. They are becoming more capable of transferring ever increasing amounts of information to long-term memory by strengthening synaptic connections (Squire & Kandel 2000). With these ideas in mind, let's now turn to several suggestions for improving the problem-solving skills of your clients.

**Improving Problem-Solving Skills.** Many models have been proposed to help people solve a wide variety of problems. Often these models employ acronyms to assist people in problem solving (e.g., SAC—Strategic Air Command; NATO—North Atlantic Treaty Organization; HOMES—The names of the Great Lakes: Huron, Ontario, Michigan, Erie, Superior). For our purposes we'll use an acronym that you'll remember easily and transfer to any problems or teach to others. The acronym is *DUPE* and its intent is to convey the message: *Don't let yourself be deceived.* The meaning of each letter is as follows:

*D—Determine* just exactly what is the nature of the problem. Too often meaningless elements in the problem deceive us; it is here that attention to detail is so important. How would you go about solving this problem?

*There is a super psychic who can predict the score of any game before it is played. Explain how this is possible.*

This problem, taken from Bransford and Stein (1993), poses a challenge to most of us because, as the authors noted, a reasonable explanation is difficult to generate. If you are having difficulty, it is probably because you have made a faulty assumption about the nature of the problem. You were not asked about the final score; the score of any game before it is played is 0 to 0. We deliberately presented a tricky problem to stress that you must attend to details.

*U—Understand* the nature of the problem. Realizing that a particular problem exists is not enough; you must also comprehend the essence of the problem if your plan for solution is to be accurate. For example, we frequently hear that a pupil's classroom difficulties are due to hyperactivity. Thus the problem is determined; but understanding the cause of the hyperactivity—physical, social, psychological—requires additional information. Here is an example of the need to understand the nature of a problem.

*Tom either walks to work and rides his bicycle home or rides his bicycle to work and walks home. The round trip takes one hour. If he were to ride both ways, it would take 30 minutes. If Tom walked both ways, how long would a round trip take?*

This problem illustrates a basic problem-solving strategy of dividing a problem's information into subgoals to help understand what's required. Think for a moment: What are the givens? How long would it take to ride one way? (15 minutes) How long is a round trip? (1 hour) How long does it take to walk one way? (45 minutes) How long is the round trip if Tom walked both ways? (45 + 45 = 90 minutes)

*P—Plan your solution.* Now that you know that a problem exists and you understand its nature, you must select strategies that are appropriate for the problem. It is here that memory plays such an important role (Siegler, 1998).

*E—Evaluate your plan,* which usually entails two phases. First you should examine the plan itself in an attempt to determine its suitability. Then you must decide how successful your solution was.

We come now to the final topic: the careful use of language in communicating with people of all ages.

## Language and Cognitive Development

We begin with a word of caution: We're probably safe in saying that our genes propel us into a language world, and our brains assume direction of the process, but—and it's a major warning—it's experience that shapes the final outcome. If you recall our work in Chapter 1, we stressed that children exposed to a stimulating environment will develop a richer network of connections in the brain than children whose experiences are more limited. Exactly the same pattern applies to their language: Humans are programmed to receive verbal stimulation, which then enhances their language ability.

*Learning to talk is probably the greatest intellectual leap of an individual's life: It opens up a new universe of questions, reasoning, social communication, and opinions for (better or worse!) that punch all other types of learning into warp speed and make a child finally seem like a full-fledged person. While language is in many ways a distinct module of the human mind and brain, it is also the critical foundation for much of what we consider to be intelligent behavior. The more we understand how the language organ of the brain develops, the better we can foster this most important basis of a person's intellectual development (Eliot 2000, p. 354)*

The relationship between language and cognition is one that has long challenged investigators because of the issues they share: the kinds of categories formed, the attentional mechanisms acquired, and the possibility of dependent interactions between cognitive and language achievements, among others.

### The Language Areas

Understanding the brain's role in language seems to be a simple matter, probably because we're still learning about it! Beginning in 1864, we confidently identified certain parts of the brain as performing specific language functions. It was then that the French neurologist Paul Broca, working with stroke victims whose speech had been impaired and who suffered from paralysis of the right side of the body, determined that "we speak with the left hemisphere." Broca's area (in the left frontal lobe), as it came to be known, is thought to be responsible for the production of speech.

In 1876, the German psychiatrist Karl Wernicke described a section of the brain that receives incoming speech sounds. Called Wernicke's area (in the temporal lobe), it is responsible for interpreting and translating the speech sounds just heard and putting together the words for a reply. This composition is then passed on to Broca's area through a bundle of nerve fibers.

But that isn't the end of it. The motor area of the brain now becomes involved and causes movements of the face, tongue, jaw, and throat. And, of course, our speech is often quite emotional. Think of it this way: Someone begins to talk to you and these speech sounds immediately are transferred to Wernicke's area. You understand what was said and think about a reply. When you decide to respond, your message is transferred to Broca's area along a pathway of nerve fibers where a plan for vocalizing your ideas is formed. Parts of the motor cortex are now alerted and the appropriate muscles of the mouth, lips, tongue, and the larynx swing into action and you make your answer.

Language seems to be a function of the left cerebral hemisphere. John Ratey (2001), a clinical professor of psychiatry at Harvard Medical School, believes that language mainly resides in the left hemisphere for about 90% of the population. About 5% have their main language in the right hemisphere, and another 5% split their language functions between both hemispheres. Remember, however, that both hemispheres are connected by the corpus callosum and both hemispheres are involved in language production. For example, the right hemisphere, mainly responsible for our emotional state, determines the emotional reactions of the speaker.

This so-called classical model of the brain–language relationship, however, has been challenged by recent research, so today no one is quite sure what Broca's or Wernicke's area specifically does. Although we still accept the general idea that certain brain areas are responsible for certain behaviors, current studies have made us uncomfortable with the neat answer that "Broca's area does this" or "Wernicke's area does that." Thanks to data supplied by EEG studies, PET scans, CAT scans, and MRIs, a different picture is emerging. We now think that language functions are spread throughout the brain much more than we originally thought. Possible solutions to the problem of how these brain areas work together in our language world remain elusive. Questions of how the brain organizes movement and emotions as we listen, read, speak, and write still remain unanswered.

The part of the brain identified as Wernicke's area (associated with interpretation and comprehension) seems to develop more rapidly than Broca's area. The neural pathway connecting Wernicke's area to Broca's area develops even more slowly. Children simply can't put their ideas into words because their brain won't let them. This makes practical sense if you think about that old saying: "He knows more than he's saying." Parents, psychologists, and linguists have long believed that children's speech doesn't accurately reflect what they know. Children know many more words and meanings than they can actually say.

Regardless of age, clarity of communication should be your goal. Both adults and children demonstrate noticeable individual differences in the expression and comprehension of language. Consequently, in your instruction and explanations you should formulate your message in terms designed to match the linguistic and cognitive levels of your clients. Once children have acquired the basics of their language, at about 5 years of age, you begin to encounter a bewildering range of language skills that result from differences in ability, environment, education, role, and physical condition, among others. The effort you make to match your language to the receptive level of your clients, and to interpret the language of others, may well spell success or failure of treatment.

# Conclusion

As we conclude this brief excursion into the mysteries of cognitive development, we should note that although horror stories abound about the decline of cognitive abilities during the later years, fortunately recent studies, such as the Seattle Longitudinal Study (Schaie 1994), paint a more promising picture. They clearly show that those individuals who maintain their levels of cognitive functioning continue to engage in mental activities, whether it's careful reading of newspapers, doing crossword puzzles, or facing new challenges (such as learning to use a computer). Mental stimulation reaches across all ages and all aspects of development, supporting and furthering the quality of the later years.

*At a special session of the British House of Lords, Winston Churchill was honored on his ninetieth birthday. As he descended the stairs of the amphitheater, one of the lords turned to another and said, "They say he's really getting senile." Churchill stopped, turned to them and said in a stage whisper loud enough for many to hear, "They also say he's deaf."*

Research suggests that as people enter these years, their physical stamina, memory, and cognitive processing don't decline as much as previously thought. (For an example of this research, see Schaie 1994). Although some aspects of cognitive functioning lose a degree of efficiency (speed of processing for example), such losses in a healthy 60-, 70-, or 80-year-old are more than offset by gains in knowledge and skill due to experience, a positive ending to our exploration of the cognitive world.

# References

Anderson, J. (1993). *Rules of the mind.* Hillsdale, NJ: Erlbaum.

Andreasen, N. (2001). *Brave new brain.* New York: Oxford.

Baillargeon, R. (1987). Object permanence in 3-1/2 and 4-1/2 month old infants. *Developmental Psychology 23,* 655–664.

Bjorklund, D. (2000). *Children's thinking.* Belmont, CA: Wadsworth.

Bransford, J., & Stein, B. (1993). *The IDEAL problem solver.* New York: Freeman.

Chugani, H. (1996). Neuroimaging of developmental nonlinearity and developmental pathologies. In R. Thatcher, G. Lyon, J. Rumsey, & N. Krasnegor (Eds.), *Developmental neuroimaging: Mapping the development of brain and behavior.* San Diego, CA: Academic Press.

Cole, M. (1996). *Cultural psychology.* Cambridge, MA: Harvard University Press.

Diamond, M. (1998). *Magic trees of the mind.* New York: Harper.

Eliot, L. (2000). *What's going on in there? How the brain and mind develop in the first five years of life.* New York: Bantam.

Elkind, D. (1994). *Understanding your child.* Boston: Allyn and Bacon.

Elkind, D. (1984). All dressed up and no place to go. Reading, MA: Addison-Wesley.

Fischer, K., & Rose, S. (1998). Dynamic development of coordination of components in brain and behavior: A framework for theory and research. In K. Fischer & G. Dawson (Eds.), *Human behavior and the developing brain.* New York: Guilford.

Fischer, K., & Bidell, T. (1998). Dynamic development of psychological structures in action and thought. In R. M. Lerner (Ed.), *Handbook of child psychology: Volume 1. Theoretical models of human development.* New York: John Wiley.

Flavell, J. (1963). *The developmental psychology of Jean Piaget.* New York: Van Nostrand.

Flavell, J. (1999). Cognitive development: Children's knowledge about the mind. In J. Spence, J. Darley, & D. Foss (Eds.), *Annual review of psychology.* Palo Alto, CA: Annual Reviews.

Gazzaniga, M., Ivry, R., & Mangun, G. (1998). *Cognitive neuroscience: The biology of the mind.* New York: Norton.

Klahr, D., & Macwhinney, B. (1998). Information processing. In W. Damon (Series Ed.), D. Kuhn, & R. Siegler (Volume Eds.), *Handbook of child psychology: Volume 2. Cognition, perception, and language.* New York: John Wiley.

Piaget, J., and Inhelder, B. (1969). *The psychology of the child.* New York: Basic Books.

Rakic, P. (1995). Corticogenesis in human and nonhuman primates. In M. Gazzaniga (Ed.), *The cognitive neurosciences.* Cambridge, MA: MIT Press.

Ratey, J. (2001). *A user's guide to the brain.* New York: Pantheon.

Restak, R. (2001). *The secret life of the brain.* Washington, DC: Joseph Henry Press.

Sameroff, A., & Haith, M. (1996). *The five to seven year shift.* Chicago: University of Chicago Press.

Santrock, J. (2004). *Life-span development.* New York: McGraw-Hill.

Schacter, D. (1996). *Searching for memory.* New York: Basic Books.

Schaie, K. (1994). The course of adult intellectual development. *American Psychologist* 49, 304–313.

Santrock, J. (2000). *Children.* New York: McGraw-Hill.

Siegler, R. (1998). *Children's thinking.* Upper Saddle River, NJ: Prentice Hall.

Squire, L., & Kandel, E. (2000). *Memory: From mind to molecules.* New York: Scientific American Prress.

Sternberg, R. (2002). *Cognitive psychology.* Belmont, CA: Wadsworth.

Thies, K., & Walsh, M. (1999). A developmental analysis of cognitive appraisal of stress in children and adolescents with chronic illness. *Child Health Care* 28, 15–32.

Thompson, R. (1998). Early sociopersonality development. In W. Damon (Series Ed.) & N. Eisenberg (Volume Ed.), *Handbook of child psychology: Volume 3. Social, emotional, and personality development.* New York: John Wiley.

Vygotsky, L. (1962). *Thought and language.* New York: Wiley.

Vygotsky, L. (1978). *Mind In Society.* Cambridge, MA: Harvard University Press.

Wertsch, J. & Tulviste, P. (1992). L. S. Vygotsky and contemporary developmental psychology. *Developmental Psychology* 28(4), 548–557.

# Chapter 8

# Nutrition and the Behavior of Children: Food for Thought

Elizabeth Metallinos-Katsaras

Dr. Kathleen Gorman

Understanding a child's behavior is a complex process. Any elementary text of child development recognizes not only the unique individual characteristics of the child (e.g., biological, cognitive, social, and self-processes) but also the wealth of influences beyond the child (e.g., parents, siblings, extended family members, schools, and neighborhoods) that contribute to the developmental process. In this chapter we summarize what is known about one such factor, nutrition, and its effect on behavior. This chapter primarily focuses on nutritional deficits and their effects on behavior, although some other special nutrition topics relevant both to children and this audience will also be addressed.

In today's culture, nutrition is commonly believed to have direct effects on behavior. Hence, it is not uncommon to hear (or to have actually made) such statements as "breakfast is the most important meal of the day" or "Jamie gets hyped whenever he eats sugar" or "children can't learn on an empty stomach." Popular beliefs about the effects of nutrition on children's behavior often bear little resemblance to the body of research that has sought to examine this relationship. Given the implications of such beliefs for clinical practice and the fact that many social programs have

grown out of the theory that nutrition is a critical factor in children's development, it is important to scrutinize the evidence.

Understanding the limits of our knowledge in this area is important for clinical practitioners because they are in the position to provide accurate health information to patients. Their expertise in health care and their frequent contact with patients provide an important venue for disseminating information and modifying parental and children's behavior when necessary. At the same time, practitioners can be valuable teachers to assist in modifying erroneous perceptions regarding nutrition's effect on children's behavior.

Malnutrition refers to a condition that results from an "excess, imbalance, or deficit of nutrient availability in relation to tissue needs" (Dietz & Trowbridge, 1990). More recently the terms *undernutrition* (the deficit of nutrient availability) and *overnutrition* (the excess) have been used; however, these terms have not always been used consistently. For example, protein energy malnutrition refers to a deficiency in protein and energy, not excess.

The basis for research on the relationship between nutrition and behavior has generally been the idea that there is an optimal amount of nutrients that is required for healthy development and that a diet deficient (or in excess) in nutrients is likely harmful. In this chapter we focus primarily on nutrient deficiencies for a number of reasons. First, until recently, the prevalence of children suffering worldwide from undernutrition far exceeded those experiencing overnutrition. Further, the available research on the relationship between nutrition and behavior has focused on the effects of nutritional deficiencies rather than nutritional excess. Finally, although overnutrition has gained attention in recent years, the research on overnutrition has concentrated primarily on identifying the causes of overeating and on the consequent health outcomes rather than on any potential cognitive and behavioral effects.

In the section addressing potential effects of nutritional deficits, we begin by providing background definitions, information on prevalence, and the theoretical rationale for the research on the effects on behavior. The section deals with four main topics: protein energy malnutrition (PEM), micronutrient (i.e., vitamin and mineral) deficiencies, breast milk, and hunger/food insecurity.

1. PEM generally refers to conditions of widespread undernutrition and is usually diagnosed by poor growth (weight and height). PEM is often studied at the population level; individuals with PEM may, but do not necessarily, suffer from specific nutrient deficiencies as well.

2. Micronutrient deficiencies (MND), on the other hand, refer to a specific nutrient deficiency, sometimes diagnosed through a combination of biochemical and clinical indicators. The section on MND covers iron deficiency anemia and iodine as well as other less well-studied nutrients.

3. The next section considers the research on breast milk and its effects on cognitive development in infants. Although bottlefed infants are not typically considered under-

nourished, the research on the effects of breast milk are based on the hypothesis that breast milk provides an optimal source of nutrition and anything other than breast milk may in fact be nutritionally deficient.

4. Finally, we cover the topic of hunger and food insecurity. Increasing levels of childhood poverty throughout the United States have resulted in a recent surge of research on the effects of poverty on children's development, with specific attention to issues of hunger and food insecurity.

In the latter part of the chapter we discuss special topics in nutrition and behavior, so called because they cannot be classified into one general topic but rather represent several areas of current interest and controversy. They are included because health care providers are often queried about them and can dispel prevailing misconceptions. This portion of the chapter is divided into three sections: multivitamin and mineral supplements, sucrose, and food additives. It highlights the relevant research exploring their relation to behavior.

One final clarification is required. This chapter uses the term *behavior* to refer to a diverse array of outcomes that have been studied in association with nutrition, including cognition, achievement, activity, and attention. Depending on the nutritional issue being examined, the behavioral outcome varies. For example, low energy intake during gestation and infancy is often believed to affect children's overall cognitive function, whereas short-term hunger and intake of specific nutrients (e.g., sugar) are more often thought to affect attention and activity levels. Admittedly, one of the challenges of the malnutrition and behavior research is to begin to specify more clearly the specific behavioral outcomes associated with specific nutrient deficiencies (Gorman, 1995). Nonetheless, the current state of the research is fairly nonspecific and in most cases does not allow for such distinctions. In almost all of the research, the use of a variety of assessments has been solely for the purpose of establishing whether there are differences between those with a nutritional deficiency and those without a nutritional deficiency, and not for purposes of diagnosis or intervention. In other words, be it assessment techniques such as the Bayleys, the Griffiths, the McCarthy, or the Vineland, the aim of the research is to identify a direct causal association to an outcome, without a specific hypothesis about the area of behavior affected.

# Nutritional Deficits

In this chapter we use the term *nutritional deficits* to include both undernutrition (i.e., nutrient deficiencies) as well as dietary deficits with potential to lead to a deficiency. The nutrients referred to herein include both macronutrients (i.e., energy-yielding nutrients such as protein, fat, carbohydrates) and micronutrients (i.e., vitamins and minerals).

In general, undernutrition is believed to be causally related to behavioral outcomes. Furthermore, the hypothesized causal link is generally supported by basic bench science demonstrating physical or neurochemical changes caused by the nutritional deficiencies. Nutrient deficiencies affect biochemical processes and growth and, when severe, have clinical manifestations. Thus, sometimes they are diagnosed by laboratory tests, other times by growth faltering, and still others by specific clinical signs.

Establishing the existence and the nature of the causal link between nutritional deficits and behavior is complicated by the fact that said deficits rarely occur in isolation. Children who are undernourished are likely to come from families or homes characterized by factors well known to pose risks to optimal development of children (e.g., low levels of education and income). Although the role of the environment has long been recognized as an explanatory factor in the association between undernutrition and development, only recently has the research attempted to build environmental variation into the designs and explore the interactions between nutrition and environmental variables. The significance of this statement will become more evident, for example, in the section on breast milk, where differences between those who choose to breastfeed and those who do not may in fact account for the observed cognitive benefits often noted in breastfed infants.

The literature on undernutrition comes primarily from low-income countries and provides evidence for the effects of nutrient restrictions on infant and child development. It is important to note that any discussion of the effects of nutrition requires attention to issues of both quality and quantity. The term *malnutrition* often conjures up the image of children from war-torn, impoverished countries, who demonstrate severe degrees of nutritional deprivation: dispigmentation of the skin, emaciation, bloated stomachs, and so on. Although certainly critical, these children represent relatively few of the majority of undernourished children in the world and rarely (except for circumstances of severe neglect) are observed within the United States. Nonetheless, undernutrition (of the mild-to-moderate form) that results in stunting and low weight for age, is more common worldwide, including in the United States.

Recent estimates (2000) suggest that 150 million children (28%) under the age of five suffer from malnutrition in the developing world (UNICEF, 2002). In the United States, data from the Pediatric Nutrition Surveillance System 1997 (U.S. Department of Health and Human Services, 1997) on low-income children and families show the prevalence of low height for age among children under 2 years of age to be twice as high as that expected within the general population, and an overall prevalence of iron deficiency anemia of between 15% and 25% for this population. Although the high prevalence of anemia and growth stunting within this sample may reflect, in part, the successful targeting efforts of at-risk populations (e.g., data are collected among participants in the Supplemental Nutrition Program for Women, Infants and Children [WIC], which gives preferential enrollment to high nutritional risk families), the evidence indicates that a large number of children in the United States are at elevated levels of health and nutritional risk.

## Protein-Energy Malnutrition

PEM is a deficiency of protein, energy, or both and is caused by either recent severe food restriction (acute PEM) or by long-term food deprivation (chronic PEM). Indicators of PEM include low height for age (i.e., stunting) and/or low weight for height (i.e., wasting) (Whitney & Rolfes, 2002).

There remains little doubt that severe levels of protein-energy malnutrition adversely affect the psychomotor and cognitive development in children as well as long-term school learning and achievement (Grantham-McGregor, 1995; Levitsky & Strupp, 1995). What is less clear, and of greater relevance to this chapter, is whether less severe forms of undernutrition can also affect behavior. Several large field studies were conducted in low-income countries during the 1960s and 1970s to test the hypothesis that improved nutrition at different developmental periods was associated with improved cognitive performance (Gorman, 1995). In each study, children at nutritional risk were supplemented and compared with children who remained unsupplemented. Overall, a summary of the results suggests small, yet statistically significant, effects on a variety of developmental outcomes (e.g., mental and motor development, preschool cognitive function) (Gorman, 1995).

During the 1980s, better-designed studies and the use of improved statistical analyses strengthened the conclusions that nutrition has an independent effect on behavior (Gorman, 1995; Husaini et al., 1991; Pollitt & Oh, 1994; Pollitt, Watkins, & Husaini, 1997). For example, one study in Jamaica looked at the effects of improved

diet, as well as psychosocial stimulation on young children's behavior, over a period of 2 years. After 2 years, children who received both nutritional supplementation and psychosocial stimulation scored significantly better than the other groups and most similarly to a matched group of children without a history of malnutrition. The use of children with different nutritional histories and multiple treatment conditions in a randomized study highlights the significance of individual differences and potential interactive effects of interventions. However, a follow-up of these children at 4 and 8 years later showed few enduring effects of the nutritional intervention and seemed to indicate more enduring effects of the psychosocial stimulation. That is, children whose mothers had higher vocabulary scores showed increased effects of nutritional supplementation on cognitive performance (Grantham-McGregor, Walker, Chang, & Powell, 1997). By the time the children were about 12, only the effects of psychosocial stimulation remained (Walker et al., 2000).

Data from a study in Guatemala provides additional support for the interactions between nutrition and behavior. In this study, children who had been given a high-calorie/high-protein supplement throughout the first several years of life had significantly better performance in adolescence on various psychoeducational tests (e.g., reading, numeracy, vocabulary, and general knowledge) as compared to children who had received a low-calorie supplement (Pollitt et al., 1993). More important, the effects of the supplementation varied by levels of socioeconomic status (SES) and by schooling history. That is, children from the poorest families seemed to benefit the most from the supplementation and performed similarly to those from higher SES homes. In addition, children with more exposure to school (beyond 3 years) showed greater benefits of the supplementation than those with fewer years of schooling.

Taken together, the results of these studies provide evidence for the effects of nutritional supplementation on cognitive development. Further, the results illustrate the potential for long-term effects of nutrition and the role that the environment (i.e., characteristics of families, home, school) plays in mediating such a relationship. In other words, the effects of improved nutrition will be determined in part by the environment (e.g., parenting, socioeconomic status, quality of schooling) in which the intervention takes place. In thinking about the applications of such research, one might argue that attention to nutritional deficiencies alone may be insufficient, and that efforts to intervene on behalf of undernourished children will require multi-focal interventions targeted at parental behavior and school quality as well as the individual's health, nutrition, and cognitive status.

One of the most promising areas of research attempting to explain the pathway between malnutrition and behavior has focused on assessing the role of activity and motor development as a mediator in this relationship (Gorman, 1995). The basic hypothesis is that poorly nourished children interact less with their environment due to reduced energy and activity levels. The idea is that children who engage less, who less frequently explore, play, and interact with the people and things in their environment, will be less stimulated in their development and, hence, perform less well on developmental assessments. Limited research on this question has provided some support for these ideas (Jamaica, Indonesia), but studies are relatively new and future research is needed.

## Iron Deficiency Anemia and Other Micronutrient Deficiencies

Iron has historically been the most extensively studied micronutrient deficiency in relation to behavior in children. This is not surprising given the fact that it is still one of the most common micronutrient deficiencies in the world (Centers for Disease Control and Prevention, 2002) and continues to be a problem among certain popula-

tions in developed countries such as the United States. Data from the National Health and Nutrition Examination Survey (NHANES) 1999–2000 indicated that 7% of toddlers ages 1 to 2 years and 9% to 16% of adolescent girls and women of childbearing age were iron deficient based on laboratory tests of iron status (Centers for Disease Control and Prevention, 2002; Looker, Dallman, Carroll, Gunter, & Johnson, 1997). The elevated risk among toddlers during a time considered sensitive for cognitive development (i.e., the first 2 years of life) has provided the impetus for the infancy period being the most common target for research of the behavioral effects of iron deficiency anemia, or IDA. Much less has been done on preschool and school-aged children.

### IRON DEFICIENCY ANEMIA

Consistently it has been shown that IDA infants score lower on the Bayley Scales of mental and motor development in comparison to nonanemic infants (Grantham-McGregor & Ani, 2001). It has also been found that children's achievement, among both preschool and school-aged subjects, is poorer for formerly anemic children than nonanemic children (Grantham-McGregor & Ani, 2001; Hurtado, Claussen, & Scott, 1999; Lozoff, Jimenez, Hagen, Mollen, & Wolf, 2000). What has been difficult to establish, however, is whether iron deficiency anemia per se is the cause of these differences because children who are IDA are more likely to also have been exposed to a range of social, health, and environmental risk factors. Much like infants with general undernutrition, infants and children with IDA are more likely to be poor, exposed to lead, and live in a less stimulating environment. In addition, they are less likely to have access to high-quality educational opportunities (e.g., day care, schools) (Grantham-McGregor & Ani, 2001). All of these can independently and adversely affect development (Grantham-McGregor & Ani, 2001; Duncan & Brooks-Gunn, 1997; Huston, Garcia Coll, & McLoyd, 1994).

The best evidence for establishing an effect of IDA on development comes from studies using randomized controlled trials in infants and children. The results, however, have not always been consistent. In some, IDA infants treated with iron show significant gains in developmental scores as compared to IDA infants receiving placebo (Idjradinata & Pollitt, 1993). In others, no effects of the iron were found. Two studies are illustrative. The first was a clinical trial of iron supplementation in Indonesian infants (12–18 months) (Idjradinata & Pollitt, 1993). At baseline, IDA infants scored significantly lower on both Bayley's Mental Development Index (MDI) and the Psychomotor Development Index (PDI) than either iron-replete or iron-deficient nonanemic infants. After being supplemented with iron the IDA infants' iron status improved, as did developmental indicators. In fact, after supplementation the IDA infants' scores on the MDI and PDI improved so much that there were no longer significant differences between the three groups. Conversely, the IDA-placebo-treated infants continued to score significantly lower than all other groups on both the MDI and PDI. This study also included infants with iron deficiency but not anemia. Iron supplementation did not have any effect on the developmental scores of this group.

The second study, conducted in Costa Rica, again showed that IDA infants scored significantly lower on the MDI and PDI than iron-replete infants at baseline. However, unlike the Indonesian study, these differences persisted even after 3 months of iron therapy (Lozoff et al., 1987). Closer examination of the data revealed that despite iron therapy, not all children responded similarly, and whereas some infants' IDA was reversed with iron supplementation, others still showed biochemical signs of iron deficiency (Lozoff, 1989). The infants whose IDA was completely reversed ($n = 9$) scored similarly to the iron-sufficient infants on the MDI and PDI, whereas infants whose deficiency was not completely corrected continued to score significantly

lower than the iron-sufficient infants. The implication is that the reason for the lack of improvement on cognitive test scores after treatment was because IDA had not been corrected. Although fewer in number, some studies on children beyond infancy (e.g., preschool and school-aged) also show a relationship between IDA and measures of intelligence and other cognitive processes (e.g., discrimination learning tasks, visual recall) (Bruner, Joffe, Duggan, Casella, & Brandt, 1996; Lucas, Morley, & Isaacs, 2001; Pollitt, Leibel, & Greenfield, 1983; Pollitt, Saco-Pollitt, Leibel, & Viteri, 1986; Seshadri & Gopaldas, 1989; Soewondo, Husaini, & Pollitt, 1989). Generally the studies on preschool and school-age children provide support for the contention that IDA in later childhood can affect children's behavior.

In summary, taken together all the evidence from numerous studies supports the contention that iron deficiency anemia has an adverse effect on cognitive development. The effects of iron supplementation have been observed on a wide range of outcomes from performance on global tests of intelligence to specific cognitive processes and central nervous system development. Still, the research has not consistently found that developmental outcomes improve with iron supplementation, and frequently children with a history of IDA continue to perform more poorly than their nonanemic peers. Imperative then for clinical practice is the need to prevent IDA via early detection and treatment in order to minimize the possibility of functional consequences of this nutritional deficiency.

## IODINE, ZINC, AND OTHER MICRONUTRIENT DEFICIENCIES

The summary of the research on iron and iron deficiency anemia indicates it is one of the most thoroughly studied micronutrient deficiencies and the best understood with regard to its effects on behavior in humans. Other nutrients also have detrimental effects on behavior, while still others have the potential to affect behavior, but most haven't been sufficiently or adequately studied. For example, on the one hand it is well established that severe levels of maternal iodine deficiency results in cretinism, deafness, and poor motor and cognitive outcomes for the fetus (Bleichrodt et al., 1987; Boyages et al., 1989; Cao et al., 1994; Fierro-Benitez, 1986; Pharoah, Connolly, Ekins, & Harding, 1984). Among populations where iodine deficiency is endemic, iodine supplementation before pregnancy or during the first trimester results in improved developmental outcomes (Cao et al., 1994). For this reason, in most industrialized countries, as well as many lower-income countries, efforts to promote iodination of salt have received priority as a public health effort and been extremely successful. On the other hand, much less is known about the potential effects of mild-to-moderate levels of iodine deficiency.

Similarly, it is not yet clear whether zinc deficiency affects cognitive development despite a number of parallels to malnutrition. For example, zinc deficiency is associated with delays in growth as well as lethargy, apathy, and slow movement. In laboratory animals (e.g., rhesus monkeys), zinc-deprived animals had lower activity levels, longer response times, and impaired success at learning tasks as compared to controls (Golub et al., 1985; Golub et al., 1996). One major barrier to conducting research on zinc in humans is the fact that there is not a definitive marker of zinc deficiency (Institute of Medicine, 2001). Thus, much of the research in this area has been conducted on laboratory animals (i.e., rats and monkeys) in whom zinc deficiency is induced by providing a zinc-deficient diet; less research has been conducted in infants and children.

Several zinc intervention studies (primarily randomized controlled trials) conducted on infants or toddlers at nutritional risk (i.e., those born low birth weight (<2500 grams) or with evidence of past or current nutritional deprivation) have noted effects on motor development scores (Black, 1998), time spent in high-movement activities (Sazawal et al., 1996), and activity

(Benton, Griffiths, & Haller, 1997). Among school-aged nutritionally at-risk children, one intervention study (Penland et al., 1997) reported a significant improvement in scores on several neuropsychological tests (i.e., Continuous Performance Task, oddity learning, tapping, tracking), while another (Penland, 2000) found a significant effect of zinc on reasoning (i.e., fewer trials were needed to learn simple concepts). In contrast, another study of stunted school-age boys found no effect of zinc supplementation either on attention or academic performance (Gibson, et al., 1989). Because of the difficulty of identifying zinc deficiency in many cases, children being supplemented may not be deficient. There is no reason to expect effects of zinc supplementation on cognition if zinc status is adequate. This also makes it difficult for clinicians to identify children who have zinc deficiency; at best, children who have other evidence of malnutrition (inadequate dietary intake, poor growth) are probably at risk for zinc deficiency.

Despite our brief attention to other micronutrients, our knowledge of the roles of specific nutrients throughout the life span is constantly being revised. For example, during the past 10 years there has been attention given to the preventative effects of folate on the development of neural tube defects. As a result, the Food and Drug Administration mandated fortification of folate in grain products. Such changes in policy are expected to result in a decline in neural tube defect incidence. This illustrates that there continues to be incalculable potential for expansion of our knowledge in this area

## Breast Milk

Many of the studies on malnutrition have focused on food intakes during early childhood. Many of these early childhood studies have attempted to understand nutritional effects on cognitive development during infancy by focusing on breastfeeding and the properties of breast milk; underlying beliefs that breast milk is the optimal food source for infants form the basis for these studies. Implicit in these beliefs is the idea that formula may be deficient in some nutrients important for development, even though this has not been explicitly shown. Again, popular literature has tended to frequently tout the widespread benefits of breast milk for the young infant. Although the benefits of breast milk on immune function, morbidity, growth, and infection are well established (Lucas et al., 1997; Rider, Samuels, Wilson, & Homer, 1996), the evidence for its effects on mental development, particularly among healthy infants, is less convincing (Jacobson, 1999; Jacobson, Chiodo, & Jacobson, 1999; Rogan & Gladen, 1993).

The research on the effects of breast milk on cognitive function is complicated by two main factors. First, it is impossible to conduct an experimental study on breastfeeding using a rigorous design because one cannot randomly assign mothers to treatment groups (Rogan & Gladen, 1993; Greene et al., 1995; Horwood & Fergusson, 1998; Mortensen, Michaelsen, Sanders, & Reinisch, 2002). Complicating this design weakness further is the fact that mothers who choose to breastfeed are different from mothers who choose not to breastfeed on a number of factors. For example, mothers who choose to breastfeed and mothers who bottle feed differ in age, socioeconomic status, education, and ego development (Greene et al., 1995; Horwood & Fergusson, 1998; Mortensen et al., 2002; Morrow-Tlucak, Haude, & Ernhart, 1988), all factors also known to affect infant developmental outcomes. As a result, research controlling for these variables has resulted in a reduction in the magnitude of associations between breastfeeding and mental development (Greene et al., 1995; Mortensen et al., 2002; Morrow-Tlucak et al., 1988; Taylor & Wadsworth, 1984). The evidence suggests that, in fact, it is likely that the parents who choose to breastfeed convey additional benefits to their children (through genetic endowment, behavior, or provision of opportunities) and that the observed bene-fits have little or nothing to do with the properties of breast milk. Furthermore, the association between breastfeeding and cognition is no longer significant when maternal IQ and parenting skills are also taken into consideration (Rogan & Gladen, 1993). In other words, studies that seem to establish a relationship between breastfeeding and cognition without considering these other factors are likely making assumptions about the effects of breast milk that are unwarranted.

However, one series of studies has attempted to control for many of these confounding variables (Lucas et al., 1990; Lucas et al., 1992; Lucas, Morley, & Cole, 1998). Lucas and his colleagues conducted a series of studies using preterm, low-birth-weight infants (<1850 grams) in Great Britain. In these studies, infants of nonbreastfeeding mothers were randomly assigned to either a standard full-term or a special preterm formula (designed to more closely mimic the properties of breast milk than standard formula), while infants whose mothers chose to provide breast milk were also randomly assigned to one of two supplemental formula groups for a period of 4 weeks. In this way, differences between breast milk and formula could be compared as well as differences in standard versus preterm formula. In an assessment of the infants at 18 months, comparisons between formula types demonstrated significant benefits of preterm as compared to full-term formula on the Psychomotor Development Index (PDI) of Bayley (Lucas et al., 1990). Similarly, among infants receiving supplementary feeding in addition to breast milk, those who had received preterm formula scored higher on the social quotient from the Vineland than those receiving full-term formula. When subjects were combined, comparisons between full-term and preterm formula indicated advantages of preterm formula on the PDI and the Vineland social maturity scale.

In a follow-up assessment at age 7, comparisons were made between infants of mothers who chose to provide breast milk and those who did not on the Wechsler Intelligence Scale for

Children (revised for UK) (Lucas et al., 1992; Lucas et al., 1998). According to the authors, similar percentages of infants in each group had received the different types of formulas. Initial findings show a 10-point advantage on each of the IQ scales (verbal, performance, and overall IQ) for those in the breast milk group. In a subsequent analysis between formula groups (Lucas et al., 1998), the authors report that males showed a benefit of the preterm formula as compared to full-term formula on language development. There was an apparent dose-response to the preterm formula, suggesting that the more formula ingested, the greater the developmental gains.

The authors conclude that the combined results of this study, showing both benefits of breast milk over formula and benefits of preterm formula over standard formula, provide strong evidence that these benefits are attributable to specific properties of breast milk (Lucas et al., 2001). These conclusions are further strengthened by the fact that all infants were fed by nasogastric tube, hence controlling for any potential behavioral differences associated with the act of breast-feeding. Additionally, the results of these studies have advanced a number of theories regarding specific properties of breast milk, most specifically long chain polyunsaturated fatty acids, and their association with brain development (Crawford, 1993; Lucas, 1990; Kretchmer, Beard, & Carlson, 1996).

Research on specific mechanisms and nutrient properties is ongoing. In the meantime, practitioners can derive several recommendations from this work. First, it is important to keep in mind that there are numerous health reasons to promote breastfeeding among new mothers if at all possible. Further, it is likely that the nutritional needs of at-risk infants, particularly those who are born premature and with very low birth weights, are of critical concern to their healthy development. At the same time, there is little current evidence that the effects of breast milk on cognitive development observed in these studies composed entirely of preterm, very-low-birth-weight infants would generalize to otherwise healthy full-term infants.

## Hunger and Food Insecurity

On October 30, 2002, the World Health Organization identified hunger as the number one health risk facing the world, affecting 170 million children and resulting in 3.4 million deaths in the year 2000 alone. In the U.S., estimates suggest that 20 million adults and 13 million children (10.5% of all U.S. households) are food insecure due to lack of resources (USDA Food Security in the United States, 2003). Members of these households report experiencing uncertain availability or access to food on a regular basis. Additionally, of these 11 million food-insecure households, approximately 3.3 million suffered from food insecurity that was so severe as to be classified as "hungry." In these households, the 5.6 million adults and 2.7 million children often miss meals or reduce the size of their meals due to lack of resources.

*Hunger* is typically defined as the "uneasy or painful sensation caused by a recurrent or involuntary lack of food. . ." (USDA, 2002) due to lack of resources. *Food insecurity* refers to the inability to acquire adequate and safe foods in socially acceptable ways. All people who experience hunger (i.e., people who skip meals or reduce their food intake due to lack of necessary resources) are considered food-insecure; not all those who are food-insecure experience hunger. Hunger and food insecurity are caused primarily by poverty. With approximately 1 out of every 6 children in the U.S. living in poverty, it is clear that hunger poses a serious problem for large numbers of children (Children's Defense Fund, 2002).

In general, there is increasing evidence that hunger affects children's psychosocial and academic functioning (Kleinman et al., 1998; Murphy et al., 1998; Murphy et al., 1998). Although the mechanisms for such associations are still unclear, it has been hypothesized that reduced food intake resulting in hunger may have an immediate metabolic or hormonal effect on cognitive function (e.g., memory or attentional processes) as well as potential long-term effects of cumulative dietary deficiencies (Pollitt, 1995). Methodologically, the association is difficult to establish because children who are at risk for hunger are frequently exposed to a wide variety of other risk factors (e.g., poverty) that are also associated with poor cognitive function and school performance. Two types of designs have been used to assess the effects of hunger on cognition, and each will be reviewed separately. In both types of studies reviewed, breakfast is the treatment variable. Breakfast has been shown to be a key component of a good diet by providing an important portion of the days' calories and nutrients (Hunter, 1994; Nicklas, Bao, Webber, & Berenson, 1993). Its absence is considered to have potential effects on learning and school performance. Various surveys of children's eating habits suggest that anywhere from 5% to 26% of school-aged children frequently skip breakfast (McIntyre, 1993; Sampson, Sujata, Meyers, & Houser, 1995).

## Experimental Studies

The first type of study assesses whether the condition of hunger affects cognitive function, and these studies focus on measuring children's response to fasting (e.g., eating or not eating breakfast) conditions. These studies vary on a number of factors, including children's ages and nutritional histories. Furthermore, such studies have been conducted among both low-income (developing) populations, where exposure to malnutrition is common, as well as well-nourished populations, such as those found in the U.S. In general, the studies attempt to control for the children's diet by testing them under fasting conditions and then again after eating on similar measures.

For example, a number of studies have focused specifically on glucose and cognition. It has been argued that because the brain has a high requirement for glucose relative to other organs (Benton, 2001), the provision or availability of glucose before cognitive tasks may be particularly critical. The results of these studies are mixed, and weakness in study design further complicates their interpretation. In two studies it was unclear whether subjects had eaten breakfast (Benton, Owens, & Parker, 1994; Owens & Benton, 1994), and in another, the nutritional content of the breakfast was not controlled (Donohoe & Benton, 1999). Interestingly, research using animal models finds a U-shaped relationship between blood glucose and memory; at both high and low doses of glucose, the ability to retain learned information is impaired (White & Wolraich, 1995). Although this type of relationship could account for the mixed findings, it is unclear whether this relationship would be replicated in children. Finally, other studies have reported a positive relationship between glucose tolerance and cognitive performance (Donohoe & Benton, 2000). Given what is known about individual differences in diet and glycemic effect, research on glucose studies of fasting and cognition must include consideration of previous diet.

Other studies have looked at time lag between fasting and performance, whereas still others have tried to separate out the effects of current and prior nutrition. In one such study in Jamaica, McGregor and colleagues (Simeon & Grantham-McGregor, 1989) tested the effects of missing breakfast on cognitive function among children of different nutritional histories: previously severely malnourished (based on prior hospitalization), stunted (suggesting previous chronic undernutrition of a moderate magnitude), and nonstunted controls. All children were tested under both a breakfast condition and a tea-only condition. Results showed that both stunted and previously malnourished groups of children performed similarly, and that missing breakfast resulted in lower test performance on verbal fluency and coding in these subjects. In contrast, the nonstunted controls' math performance and MFFT efficiency scores improved as a function of missing breakfast. In a separate study, using a cross-over design, poorly nourished Jamaican children performed significantly better on tests of verbal fluency (but not visual search, digit span, or speed of processing) after eating breakfast, as compared to well-nourished children (Chandler, Walker, Connolly, & Grantham-McGregor, 1995).

In summary, the results of well-controlled studies appear to indicate that fasting has effects on short-term memory that do not necessarily generalize to other domains of cognitive function. In addition, these effects likely vary as a function of previous nutritional risk (Simeon & Grantham-McGregor, 1989; Chandler et al., 1995, Pollitt, Cueto, & Jacoby, 1998). Notably, it is unclear whether the reported effects are of meaningful magnitude, whether they can be sustained over time, or whether they are uniformly adverse. At least four studies have reported some small improvement in performance on certain tasks among healthy children under fasting conditions. Finally, although the results of several studies indicate that children at higher nutritional risk may be more susceptible to the effects of hunger (Simeon & Grantham-McGregor, 1989), this finding has not been consistent (Lopez et al., 1993).

## SCHOOL-BASED PROGRAM EVALUATIONS

The second type of studies reviewed here assess whether provision of food to children at nutritional risk can affect school performance. These studies have primarily been conducted using the food assistance and feeding programs in schools that target low-income children in an attempt to reduce hunger and thereby improve school performance. One of the underlying assumptions of the school-based programs is the idea that children who come to school hungry will have a more difficult time paying attention in school (Pollitt, 1995). With the introduction of federally funded nutrition assistance programs in the schools and, in particular, the School Breakfast Program, in-

vestigators have been able to use these interventions as an alternative model to assess the effects of breakfast on school performance as well as to evaluate the effectiveness of the investment.

Data from evaluations of school breakfast programs have provided support for their benefits (Meyers et al., 1989). In one study, data on achievement, absenteeism, and tardiness collected before the initiation of school breakfast programs were compared with similar data after the school breakfast program. As compared to nonparticipants, children participating regularly in the school breakfast program showed significantly higher performance on the Comprehensive Test of Basic Skills (CTBS) and lower rates of absenteeism and tardiness. Most notably, even after controlling for a large number of potentially confounding variables (e.g., sex, ethnicity, family size, income, pretest CTBS scores), the school breakfast program continued to show independent effects on the outcomes. One limitation of this study is that participation was voluntary, and this introduced a potential self-selection bias that could not be taken into account in the analyses.

In a two-state, three-school evaluation of the breakfast program, researchers found initial differences in academic performance between students with high participation in the school breakfast program (i.e., those who typically ate school breakfast) as compared to those with lower participation rates (Murphy et al., 1998) on a wide range of assessments including test scores, indicators of depression and anxiety, hyperactivity, and attendance. After introducing Universal School Breakfast (making the program free for all students in the school), program participation rates increased 100%. The authors report that after 4 months of this breakfast program, students who frequently ate school breakfast showed improved rates of attendance and punctuality, decreased rates of psychosocial symptoms, and improved academic functioning (math grades) as compared to those who ate breakfast infrequently. Although suggestive, multiple methodological problems (nonrandom design, small sample sizes, loss of subjects, and no control for usual breakfast consumption) prohibit the ability to establish any causal relationship between breakfast and student behavior. It is likely that children who chose to eat breakfast are significantly different in a number of ways from those who do not eat breakfast.

Several studies from low-income countries suggest that children's performance (Richter, Rose, & Griesel, 1997; Vera Noriega et al., 2000) and attendance (Pollitt et al., 1996) improve with the introduction of a breakfast program, although based on the designs these effects are likely the result of increased motivation rather than any specific nutritional effect. A comprehensive review of 15 school feeding programs in developing countries (Levinger, 1984; Levinger, 1994) examined the association of school feeding with school attendance, participation, and achievement with inconclusive results. Results of this review highlight the difficulties associated with the implementation and evaluation of school feeding programs. Shortcomings likely to account for low program impact include inadequate targeting, food substitution rather than supplementation, inadequate supplementation (not meeting nutritional needs), poor administration and inefficient program implementation, and lack of nutrition education.

In sum, despite the absence of strong support for a direct impact of school feeding programs on school performance, consideration of the issues noted above in both programming and evaluation is likely to lead to more robust findings (Levinger, 1994). It should not be surprising that program evaluations of school feeding programs have not yielded strong effects on learning given the limitations of study designs available in school-based research. Furthermore, although one would expect that children at highest risk might benefit the most from such programs, this hypothesis has not been adequately tested. In other words, school-based studies frequently combine all children—those who eat breakfast at home with those who

eat at school and those who do not eat breakfast—without any ability to control for the amount or quality of the breakfast consumed or the previous days' intake. Finally, the expectations for the effects of such programs should be more realistic. Many studies have demonstrated rather consistent effects of school breakfast on attendance, absenteeism, and school participation. Attendance and absenteeism are critical factors for evaluation and should be studied as both important outcomes as well as potential mediating factors in the long-term effects on school achievement.

# Special Topics in Nutrition and Behavior

In addition to research on nutrient deficiencies and their effects on behavior, there is some research and numerous anecdotal accounts of the effects of sugar, nonnutrient additives, and indiscriminate supplementation of vitamins and minerals on children's behavior. Because these grew more out of popular opinion and specific case reports than scientific research, some of the reported studies and their proponents do not have their contentions grounded in sound scientific research. Although there are numerous potential foods and nonnutrients that have been espoused as affecting behavior, such as multivitamin (MV)/mineral supplementation, we have chosen to discuss sugar and additives in this chapter because they have been the most widely discussed and, we believe, misunderstood.

## Multivitamin Mineral Supplementation

Over the past 20 years, a number of researchers have proposed that giving a multivitamin/mineral supplement indiscriminately to otherwise seemingly healthy children improves their performance on intelligence tests. The hypothesis driving much of this research is that a subset of the population has compromised cognitive functioning because they are deficient in one or more micronutrients even though, based on the normal clinical screenings such as growth monitoring, biochemical tests, or clinical examination, the children appear healthy.

The design of these studies runs counter to traditional practice in designing a well-controlled experiment, which is to

1. have some theory as to why a specific nutrient would affect cognitive performance, and why delays might exist despite any other indication of deficiency;

2. identify which children are deficient in that nutrient; and

3. conduct a randomized controlled intervention trial.

Although some studies have provided some support for improved cognitive performance with MV/mineral supplementation (Benton et al., 1997; Benton et al., 1995; Nelson, 1992; Schoenthaler et al., 1990; Schoenthaler et al., 2000), others have not (Nelson, 1992; Schoenthaler et al., 1990; Nelson et al., 1990). Given the implications that such an association would have for clinical practice or public health policy, and the fact that it runs counter to nutrition recommendations for children (ADA, 2003), it is important to closely scrutinize the evidence.

The evidence for the positive effects of MV/mineral supplementation come from several studies in which healthy children have been mass supplemented for differing lengths of times (6 weeks to 12 months) and with a varying combination of nutrients and levels (i.e., 10%–200% of the recommended daily allowance [RDA] depending on the study). Although several early studies concluded that MV/mineral supplementation significantly improved nonverbal intelligence of preschoolers and school-aged children (Nelson, 1992; Schoenthaler et al., 1990; Peritz, 1994), a critical examination of the research reveals methodologic shortcomings that call the va-

lidity of these conclusions into question. For example, studies failed to document convincing evidence of a nutritional deficiency (Benton et al., 1997; Benton et al., 1995; Nelson, 1992; Schoenthaler et al., 1990; Peritz, 1994), to control for confounding factors or bias that may have influenced the results (Benton et al., 1995; Schoenthaler et al., 1990; Peritz, 1994), and to provide a rationale for the nutrient composition of the supplementation (Benton et al., 1997; Benton et al., 1995; Nelson, 1992; Schoenthaler et al., 1990). Further, in some cases, the "effects" are the result of a lack of normal improvement one would see over time and with practice among the placebo group rather than improved performance resulting from supplementation (Nelson, 1992; Schoenthaler et al., 1990).

Three studies were conducted that attempted to address some of the limitations of previous studies by matching on baseline cognitive measures, and/or on anthropometric indicators of nutritional status, and/or assessing blindness to treatment (i.e., whether the subjects and parents were aware of the treatment they were getting) (Nelson, 1992; Schoenthaler et al., 2000; Nelson et al., 1990). Two showed no effect of MV/mineral supplementation on nonverbal intelligence (Nelson, 1992; Nelson et al., 1990), whereas one demonstrated a significant effect (Schoenthaler et al., 2000). When one examines the data in the latter study carefully, it becomes evident that there are some areas of potential bias that may account for the results seen; many of these are illustrative of the research supporting a positive effect of MV/mineral supplementation.

For example, in one randomized, double-blind placebo-controlled trial, 388 school-aged children (6–12 year olds) were mass supplemented for 3 months with a MV/mineral tablet, including between 50% and 67% of the RDA. However, a potentially biased group of only 63% of the original sample was included in the final analyses due to an *a priori* decision to exclude data from six testers who did not meet specific criteria (Schoenthaler et al., 2000). At the post-test, both groups of children on average showed an improvement in IQ scores. However, there was a statistically significant between-group difference ($p < 0.038$) of 2.47 favoring the group receiving the MV/mineral supplement. Subsequent analysis revealed that this difference was primarily due to a subset of the children whose increase in IQ score was greater than 15 points. Over a third of those randomized to MV/mineral (35%) exhibited such an increase as compared to 21% of those given placebo. The proportions were significantly different ($p < 0.01$) between groups, and the authors contended that the significant increase among the MV group was likely due to improved nutrition among a subset of poorly nourished children despite a lack of any nutritional assessment evidence (i.e., biochemical evidence) to support this claim. The fact that 21% of the placebo group showed similarly large IQ improvements (>15 points) raises questions about underlying reasons or problems with study design or implementation that could account for this large improvement in performance among those who didn't receive the supplementation.

In conclusion, careful scrutiny of the research reveals too many potential biases to conclude that supplementation with MV/minerals improves intelligence test scores of the general pediatric population. Nonetheless, one common finding was that in several different studies, a particular subset of those supplemented exhibited a large change in test scores. It may well be that a subset of children are deficient in a specific nutrient or nutrients and hence respond favorably to treatment. However, although the data supporting this hypothesis are intriguing, they are by no means conclusive, and further research with better-controlled designs are necessary. In addition, the multivitamin research is limited by the fact that it does not allow us to identify a specific nutrient. Indiscriminate supplementation of most essential vitamins and minerals is neither a feasible nor an acceptable clinical or public health practice. Hence, at this point in time, based on this body of research one would not provide a MV/mineral supplement to children unless there is dietary, biochemical, or anthropometric evidence of a risk for a deficiency and then for the purposes of improving overall nutritional status and health rather than for making children "smarter."

## Sucrose

If a group of children happens to be particularly rambunctious, one frequently hears parents or teachers ask "How much sugar did you have today?" Interestingly, the evidence for the strongly held belief by parents and teachers that sugar causes behavioral changes in children, particularly hyperactivity, is weak. The best test of the effects of sugar on behavior come from double-blind challenge trials, in which children are given sugar or a nonsugar substance (placebo) and are tested and/or observed by parents or teachers. Although anecdotal reports are rampant with claims that sugar causes hyperactivity in children, very few studies using this type of design have shown any adverse effects of sugar in the expected direction (ADA, 2003).

Several have reported no effect of sucrose on behavior (ADA, 2003; Wolraich et al., 1995) while still others have reported effects in the opposite direction as those hypothesized, that is, a decrease in activity and an increase in drowsiness in children after sugar ingestion (Wolraich, Wilson, & White, 1995; Wolraich et al., 1994; Rapoport, 1986). Several potential explanations have been offered for this lack of uniformity in the research findings, including differences in subjects (i.e., various ages, some normally active and some diagnosed with ADD or ADHD), state characteristics (fasting, non-fasting), study design issues (dosage of sucrose, differences in research settings, amount of time elapsed between challenge and testing, the placebo used), and the behavioral measures utilized. In addition, some (Saravis et al., 1990) but not all (Wolraich et al., 1995; Rapoport, 1986) researchers have reported that aspartate, the most commonly used placebo, may also cause behavioral changes.

One of the underlying assumptions of such research is that children with specific behavior problems such as attention deficit disorder (ADD) and hyperactivity may be particularly sensitive to the effects of sugar. Despite this assumption, many studies have examined samples composed primarily of normally active (without ADD or hyperactivity) children, whereas fewer have focused specifically on samples of children diagnosed with ADD, with or without hyperactivity.

In six double-blind sucrose-challenge studies in normal children, two found no effects of sucrose on behavior (ADA, 2003; Saravis et al., 1990), two showed what might be considered positive effects (Wolraich et al., 1995; Rapoport, 1986), and two others showed negative effects (ADA, 2003; Kruesi et al., 1987). Among the studies reporting adverse effects of sugar consumption, weaknesses in design may account for such findings. For example, in one study, the differences found were between the high-sucrose and low-sucrose condition. After the high-sucrose challenge, girls (but not boys) made a greater number of errors on the Paired Associates task than when on the low-sucrose challenge; there were no differences between high sucrose and aspartate (i.e., placebo) (Kruesi et al., 1987). In addition, teachers perceived significantly greater activity in the high-sucrose versus low-sucrose challenge. There were no effects of the high-sucrose challenge on other cognitive measures, fidgeting, or the Abbreviated Conner's Teacher's Rating Scale (used to diagnose hyperactivity). One of the weaknesses of this study is that children are likely aware of the differences because they can taste the sweetness; this awareness has the potential for affecting the children's behavior. Hence, it is not clear whether it was the sucrose per se or their awareness that affected the results observed.

Studies that have examined the effects of sucrose on children diagnosed with ADD with or without hyperactivity have shown very little support (ADA, 2003; Rosen et al., 1988; Girardi et al., 1995) that sugar causes hyperactivity in this group of children. In a study of 7- to 10-year-old hyperactive boys, there was no effect of a sucrose challenge on performance on a sustained attention test (CPT), paired associate learning, matching familiar figures, fine or gross motor movements, or the draw-a-line slowly or draw-a-line fast tests (ADA, 2003). Another study using hyperactive boys attending a day treatment program for hyperactive children (ADA, 2003) reported no differences in behaviors during recreational periods, academic performance, or teacher ratings based on sucrose challenge. In still another study that also used tests of attention among children with ADD, an oral 5-hour glucose tolerance test found no effect of glucose on the CPT, although, interestingly, the catecholamine response to the glucose was significantly lower in those with ADD than in the control group (Rosen et al., 1988). Finally, the results of a recent meta-analysis of studies using designs that met set criteria that defined scientific rigor concluded that the available evidence does not support a relationship between sugar consumption and behavior or cognitive performance of children (ADA, 2003).

Despite all the research to the contrary, there has been an obvious resistance of parents and teachers to fully accept such a conclusion. In some ways this is understandable because high sugar consumption often accompanies events that elicit high activity levels among children. Often, then, what should be attributed to the event (i.e., birthday party) is attributed instead to the cake. Illustrative is the results of a study of 5- to 7-year-old boys who were reported to be sugar sensitive. Although all children got a placebo (aspartame), half the mothers were told that their children were given a large dose of sugar and the other half were told that their children were given placebo. Mothers who were told that their sons received sugar rated their children as significantly more hyperactive than those who were told that their children were given a placebo. Videotapes failed to corroborate their perceptions (Wender & Solanto, 1991).

Thus, the research often does not support parental perception regarding effects of sucrose. This is true whether we are talking about children diagnosed with ADD and/or hyperactivity or normally active children. Reported positive effects of elimination diets in treating ADD children may be due to the concurrent elimination of other substances such as caffeine or allergens and not the elimination of sucrose (Hoover & Milich, 1994). Although there may be a highly specific subgroup of children that is sensitive to sucrose, the bulk of the available research has not yet identified this group.

## Food Additives

In addition to sugar, food additives have frequently been implicated as causes of children's behavioral problems and, specifically, hyperactivity. Although data from correlational studies and open trials, where normal diets are replaced with additive-free diets (the Feingold diet), have provided support for such an association, the evidence that the food additives per se are the cause of the reported improvements in behavior are limited by the generally weaker study designs used in this area (Kanerak, 1994). For example, one cannot exclude the possibility that either parental or children's perceptions, or changes in the amount of attention a child gets, or some other factors that are changing throughout the treatment may be the actual causes of the improvements. Knowledge of the treatment in and of itself can greatly influence expectations and perceptions and, ultimately, the reports that comprise the data used in these studies. Furthermore, many other factors may also change with dietary manipulations, making it impossible to directly link the food additives per se to behavioral change. For example, it's been reported that when children are put on elimination diets they suddenly receive much more attention from caregivers and this may improve behavior (Schnoll, Burshteyn, & Cea-Aravena, 2003).

Two other types of studies offer a better test of the association between food additives and behavior: dietary studies and challenge studies. Dietary studies include two randomly assigned diets (similar in taste), one with additives and one without; in challenge studies, the subject is provided either a food with additives or an additive capsule after being on a non-additive diet for a specified period of time. Of 11 studies using these two techniques to test for the effect of a single or a class of substances (i.e., artificial colors) in children diagnosed with hyperactivity, only three found an effect of the challenge on the child's behavior (Levitsky & Strupp, 1985). In those studies, two showed effects on teachers' ratings of child behavior (Levitsky & Strupp, 1985).

More recently, studies have employed a standardized technique of "double-blind placebo-controlled food challenge" (DBPCFC) to diagnose adverse food reactions (Boris & Mandel, 1993). This procedure includes an elimination diet and a subsequent reintroduction of the suspected food (or additive) and may also include allergy skin testing. Although a well-controlled design, this technique does not always enable the investigator to identify any one item or specific substance, but rather to identify a food or a class of foods to which the individual may be sensitive. Three studies using this technique provide limited support for either specific food sensitivities of *some* children with ADD (Bock et al., 1988; Carter et al., 1993) and/or sensitivity to food additives, although effects were often seen in only a subgroup of children.

In summary, the available evidence does not support the contention that food additives adversely affect the behavior of hyperactive children. What does seem to be true, however, is that a small subset of hyperactive children may be particularly sensitive to some foods and/or food additives, and these children may benefit from a modified diet.

# Conclusions and Applications

So what does all this mean to health care professionals whose goal is to improve the health and well-being of patients? First, what is clear is that the relationship between nutrition and children's behavior is complex. The degree to which nutrition will have an effect on behavior seems to be moderated by other environmental factors, many of which vary from one group of children to the next. The end result of this complexity is that the results of different studies frequently seem to contradict each other despite their apparent similarities in study design. As our understanding of the factors influencing development grows, our ability to design studies that can isolate the effect of nutrition on behavior and development will improve.

Nonetheless, the current research provides fairly strong evidence that there is an association between nutrition and behavior. More specifically general malnutrition, iron deficiency anemia, and iodine deficiency can adversely affect children's development and behavior. At the same time, the evidence for the effects of zinc deficiency or hunger on behavior among at-risk children is suggestive but not conclusive.

First of all, it is important to keep in mind that parents who are concerned about their children's behavior need reassurance. Many times parents are looking for that one answer that is the cause of their child's problem—whether it is sugar, vitamins, or too much food. Rarely will the answer be so simple.

For example, parents of a child who has already been identified with a nutritional deficiency such as IDA should be encouraged to treat it adequately. Parents who understand that the consequences for lack of treatment may include not only anemia and its behavioral consequences (e.g., lethargy) but also cognitive consequences may be more highly motivated to comply with the some-

times difficult regimen of daily dosages, particularly with young children.

At the same time, parents who complain about more general behavioral problems and raise a potential nutritional possibility as a cause for the behavioral problem require different responses. For example, a parent who worries that the child eats too much or too little may have a legitimate concern. It may not, however, be related to the child's behavior (i.e., there is little evidence that hyperactivity is the result of too much sugar). However, parents of children with particular food allergies and sensitivities may want to consider the effects that certain foods may have in relation to their children's behavior. In cases where all else fails, dietary changes may in fact result in behavior change, but even in these instances it may be the result of a shift in attention and family dynamics rather than a direct nutrient effect.

Alternatively, a child who rarely eats breakfast but who is generally healthy and shows no other behavior problem is likely at little risk. While breakfast consumption should be promoted because it provides a significant portion of the child's daily nutrient needs, more than likely this child meets her dietary needs in other ways (e.g., through late morning snacks, an early and adequate lunch). However, a child who rarely eats breakfast and also shows learning and/or attention problems, low motivation or interest, or lethargy may benefit from eating breakfast and having an improved diet. Many children are undernourished as a result of limited economic resources, lack of adequate choices in the home, lack of supervision at mealtimes, and low participation (or access) to school meals programs. Children from such families may benefit from more regular dietary intakes, either through school meals programs or more organized meals in the home, or additional resources to help parents acquire the necessary means to provide for their family.

This advice should not be interpreted as minimizing the importance of good nutrition to overall health. Nor should the possibility that a child is deficient in nutrients be overlooked. Good nutrition is important both to prevent health problems as well as to minimize the possibility that nutritional deficiencies might impair optimum cognitive development. It is also important to identify children at risk so that nutrition interventions can occur before the development of deficiencies or before deficiencies become chronic and severe. What we learn from the literature, however, is that nutrition is one interconnecting piece of the complex biological and environmental puzzle that interacts to determine a child's development.

# References

ADA. (n.d.). Retrieved July 2003 from http://www.eatright.org/Public/NutritionInformation/92_13216.cfm.

Al-Dahhan, J., Jannoun, L., & Haycock, G. B. (2002). Effect of salt supplementation of newborn premature infants on neurodevelopmental outcome at 10–13 years of age. *Archives of Disease in Childhood, 86*, 2, pF120(4).

Benton, D., Owens, D. S., & Parker, P. Y. (1994). Blood glucose influences memory and attention in young adults. *Neuropsychologia, 32*, 595–607.

Benton, D., Fordy, J., & Haller, J. (1995). The impact of long-term vitamin supplementation on cognitive functioning. *Psychopharmacology, 117*, 298–305.

Benton, D., Griffiths, R., & Haller, J. (1997). Thiamine supplementation mood and cognitive functioning. *Psychopharmacology, 129*, 66–71.

Benton, D. (2001). The impact of the supply of glucose to the brain on mood and memory. *Nutrition Reviews, 59*, S20–S21.

Black, M. M. (1998). Zinc deficiency and child development. *Am J Clin Nutr, 68*, 464S–9S.

Bleichrodt, N., Garcia, I., & Rubio, C., et al. (1987). Developmental disorders associated with severe iodine deficiency. In Hetzel, B. S., Dunn, J. T., & Stanbury, J. B. (eds). The prevention and control of iodine deficiency disorders (pp. 65–84). Amsterdam: Elsevier Science Publishers.

Bock, S. A., Sampson, H. A., & Atkins, F. M., et al. (1988) Double-blind, placebo-controlled food challenge (DFPCFC) as an office procedure: a manual. *J Allergy Clin Immunol, 82*, 986–997.

Boris, M., & Mandel, F. S. (1993). Foods and additives are common causes of the attention deficit hyperactive disorder in children. *Ann Allergy, 72*, 462–468.

Boyages, S. C., Collins, J. K., & Maberly, G. F., et al. (1989). Iodine deficiency impairs intellectual and neuromotor development in apparently normal persons: a study of rural inhabitants of north-central China. *Med J Australia, 150*, 676–682.

Bruner, A. B., Joffe, A., Duggan, A. K., Casella, J. F., & Brandt, J. (1996). Randomized study of cognitive effects of iron supplementation in non-anemic iron-deficient adolescent girls. *Lancet, 348*, 992–996.

Carter, C. M., Urbanowicz, M., & Hemsley, R., et al. (1993). Effects of a few food diets in attention deficit disorder. *Arch Dis Child, 69*, 564–568

Cao, X. Y., Jiang, X. M., & Dou, Z. H., et al. (1994). Timing of vulnerability of the brain to iodine deficiency in endemic cretinism. *N Engl J Med, 331*,1793–44.

Centers for Disease Control and Prevention. (2002). Iron Deficiency—United States, 1999–2000. *MMWR, 51*, 897–899.

Chandler, A. K., Walker, S. P., Connolly, K., & Grantham-McGregor, S. (1995). School breakfast improves verbal fluency in undernourished Jamaican children. *J Nutr, 125*, 894–900.

Children's Defense Fund. (2002). Every child deserves a fair start. http://www.childrensdefense.org/fairstart-povstat1.htm (accessed May 22, 2002).

Crawford, M. A. (1993). The role of essential fatty acids in neural development: implications for perinatal nutrition. *J Clin Nutr, 57*(suppl), 703S–710S.

Dietz, W. H., & Trowbridge, F. L. (1990). Symposium on the identification and prevalence of undernutrition in the United States: introduction, Bethesda (MD). *American Institute of Nutrition* (pp 917–8).

Donohoe, R. T., & Benton, D. (1999). Cognitive functioning is susceptible to the level of blood glucose. *Psychopharmacology, 145*, 378–385.

Donohoe, R. T., & Benton, D. (2000). Glucose tolerance predicts performance on test of memory and cognition. *Physiology & Behavior, 71*, 394–401.

Duncan, G. J., & Brooks-Gunn, J. (1997). *Consequences of Growth Up Poor.* NY: Russell Sage Foundation.

Fierro-Benitez. (1986) Long-term effects of correction of iodine deficiency on psychomotor and intellectual development. In Dunn, J. T., Pretell, E. A., Daza, C. H., & Viteri, F. E. (eds), *Towards the Eradication of Endemic Goiter, Cretinism, and Iodine Deficiency* (pp. 182–200). Washington, DC: PAHO Publication No. 502.

Gibson, R. S., Smit Vanderkooy, P. D., & MacDonald, A. C., et al. (1989). A growth-limiting, mild zinc-deficiency syndrome in some southern Ontario boys with low height percentiles. *Am J Clin Nutr, 49*, 1266–1273.

Girardi, N. L., Shaywitz, S. E., Shaywitz, B. A., Marchione, K., Fleischman, S. J., Jones, T. W., et al. (1995).

Blunted catecholamine responses after glucose ingestion in children with attention deficit disorder. *Pediatric Res, 38*(4), 539–542.

Golub, M. S., Gershwin, M. E., & Hurley, L. S., et al. (1985). Studies of marginal zinc deprivation in rhesus monkeys: infant behavior. *Am J Clin Nutr, 42,* 1229–1239.

Golub, M. S., Takeuchi, P. T., Keen, C. L., Hendrickx, A. G., & Gershwin, M. E. (1996). Activity and attention in zinc-deprived adolescent monkeys. *Am J Clin Nutr, 64,* 908–15.

Gorman, K. S. (1995). Malnutrition and cognitive development: evidence from experimental/quasi-experimental studies among the mild-to-moderately malnourished. *J Nutr, 125*(8S), 2239S–2244S.

Grantham-McGregor, S. (1995). A review of existing studies of the effect of severe malnutrition on mental development. *Nutr, 125*(8S), 2223S–2228S.

Grantham-McGregor, S. M., Walker, S. P., Chang, S. M., & Powell, C. A. (1997). Effects of early childhood supplementation with and without stimulation on later development in stunted Jamaican children. *Am J Clin Nutr, 66,* 247–253.

Grantham-McGregor, S., & Ani, C. (2001). A review of studies on the effect of iron deficiency on cognitive development in children. *J Nutr, 131,* 649S–668S.

Greene, L. C., Lucas, A., & Barbara, E., et al. (1995). Relationship between early diet and subsequent cognitive performance during adolescence. *Biochem Soc Trans, 23,* 376S.

Hoover, D. W., Milich, R. (1994). Effects of sugar ingestion expectancies on mother-child interactions. *J Abn Child Psyc, 22*(4), 501–515.

Horwood, J., & Fergusson, D. M. (1998). Breastfeeding and later cognitive and academic outcomes. *Pediatrics, 101,* 9–20.

Hunter, B. T. (1994). The importance of breakfast. *Cons Resear Maga, 77,* 8–10.

Hurtado, E. K., Claussen, A. H., & Scott, K.G. (1999). Early childhood anemia and mild or moderate mental retardation. *Am J Clin Nutr, 69,* 115–119.

Husaini, M. A., Karyadi, L., & Husaini, Y. K., et al. (1991). Developmental effects of short-term supplementary feeding in nutritionally-at-risk Indonesian infants. *Am J Clin Nutr, 54,* 799–804.

Huston, A. C., Garcia Coll, C. T., & McLoyd, V. C. (1994). Children and Poverty, *Child Development* (special issue), 65 (2)

Idjradinata, P., & Pollitt, E. (1993). Reversal of developmental delays in iron-deficient anaemic infants treated with iron. *Lancet, 341,* 1–4.

Institute of Medicine (2001), Shaping the future for health, dietary reference intakes for Vitamin A, Vitamin K, arsenic, boron, chromium, copper, iodine, iron, manganese, molybdenum, nickel, silicon, vanadium and zinc. National Academy Press.

Jacobson, S. W. (1999). Assessment of long-chain polyunsaturated fatty acid nutritional supplementation on infant neurobehavioral development and visual acuity. *Lipids, 34,* 151–160.

Jacobson, S. W., Chiodo, L. M., & Jacobson, J. L. (1999). Breastfeeding effects on intelligence quotient in 4- and 11-year-old children. *Pediatrics, 103,* 71–82.

Kanerak, R. (1994). Does sucrose or aspartame cause hyperactivity in children? *Nutr Rev, 52,* 173–175.

Kleinman, R. E., Murphy, M. J., Little, M., & Pagano, M. E., et al. (1998). Hunger in children in the United States: potential behavioral and emotional correlates. *Pediatrics, 101,* 97–105.

Kretchmer, N., Beard, J. L., & Carlson, S. (1996). The role of nutrition in the development of normal cognition. *Am J Clin Nutr, 63,* 997S–1001S.

Kruesi, M. J. P., Rapoport, J. L., & Cummings, E. M., et al. (1987). Effects of sugar and aspartame on aggression and activity in children. *Am J Psychiatry, 144,* 1487–1490.

Levinger, B. (1984). *School Feeding Programs: Myth, Reality and Potential.* Unpublished document. March 10, 1984.

Levinger, B. (1984) *School Feeding Programs: A Look at Nutritional Impact.* Unpublished document. April 24, 1984.

Levinger, B. (1994). *Nutrition, Health and Education for All.* United Nations Development Programme.

Levitsky, D., & Strupp, B. (1985). *Nutrition and the behavior of children.* In Walker W.A., Watkins J.B. (eds). Nutrition in pediatrics: Basic science and clinical applications, 1st ed. (pp 357–372). Boston: Little, Brown.

Levitsky, D., & Strupp, B. (1995). Malnutrition and the brain: Changing concepts, changing concerns. *Nutr, 125*(8S), 2212S–2221S.

Looker, A. C., Dallman, P. R., Carroll, M. D., Gunter, E. W., & Johnson, C. L. (1997). Prevalence of iron deficiency in the United States. *JAMA, 277*(12), 973–977.

Lopez, I., de Andraca, I., & Perales, C. G., et al. (1993). Breakfast omission and cognitive performance of normal, wasted and stunted schoolchildren. *Eur J Clin Nutr, 47,* 533–542.

Lozoff, B., Brittenham, G. M., & Wolf, A. W., et al. (1987). Iron deficiency anemia and iron therapy effects on infant developmental test performance. *Pediatrics, 79,* 981–995.

Lozoff, B. (1989). Methodologic issues in studying behavioral effects of infant iron-deficiency anemia. *Am J Clin Nutr, 50,* 641–654.

Lozoff, B., Jimenez, E., Hagen, J., Mollen, E., & Wolf, A. W. (2000) Poorer behavioral and developmental outcome more than 10 years after treatment for iron deficiency in infancy. *J Pediatrics, 105*(4), 1–11.

Lucas, A. (1990). Does early diet program future outcome? *Acta Paediatr Scand, 365* (suppl), 58–67.

Lucas, A., Morley, R., & Cole, T. J., et al. (1990). Early diet in preterm babies and developmental status at 18 months. *Lancet, 335,* 1477–1481.

Lucas, A., Morley, R., & Cole, T. J., et al. (1992). Breast milk and subsequent intelligence quotient in children born preterm. *Lancet, 339,* 261–264.

Lucas, A., Fewtrell, M. S., & Davies, P. S. W., et al. (1997). Breastfeeding and catch-up growth in infants born small for gestational age. *Acta Paediatr, 86,* 564–569.

Lucas, A., Morley, R., & Cole, T. J. (1998). Randomized trial of early diet in preterm babies and later intelligence quotient. *BMJ, 317,* 1481–1487.

Lucas, A., Morley, R., & Isaacs, E. (2001). Nutrition and mental development. *Nutrition Review, 59,* S24–S33.

McIntyre, L. (1993). A survey of breakfast-skipping and inadequate breakfast-eating among young school-children in Nova Scotia. *Can J Public Health, 84,* 410–414.

Meyers, A. F., Sampson, A. E., Weitzman, M., et al. (1989). School breakfast program and school performance. *Am J Dis Child, 143,* 1234–1239.

Morrow-Tlucak, M., Haude, R. H., & Ernhart, C. B. (1988). Breastfeeding and cognitive development in the first 2 years of life. *Soc Sci Med* (Great Britain; Pergamon Press), *26,* 635–63.

Mortensen, E. L., Michaelsen, K. F., Sanders, S. A., & Reinisch, J. M. (2002). The association between duration of breastfeeding and adult intelligence. *JAMA, 287,* 2365–2371.

Murphy, M. J., Pagano, M. E., & Nachmani, J., et al. (1998). The relationship of school breakfast to psychosocial and academic functioning. *Arch Pediatr Adolesc Med, 152,* 899–907.

Murphy, M. J., Wehler, C. A., Pagano, M. E., & Little, M., et al. (1998). Relationship between hunger and psychosocial functioning in low-income American children. *J Am Acad Child Adolesc Psychiatry, 37,* 163–170.

Nelson, M., Naismith, D., & Burley, V., et al. (1990). Nutrient intakes, vitamin and mineral supplementation in British schoolchildren. *Br J Nutr, 64,* 13–22.

Nelson, M. (1992). Vitamin and mineral supplementation and academic performance in schoolchildren. *Proc Nutr Soc, 51,* 303–313.

Nicklas, T. A., Bao, W., Webber, L. S., & Berenson G. S. (1993). Breakfast consumption affects adequacy of total daily intake in children. *J Am Diet Assoc, 93,* 886–891.

Owens, D. S., & Benton, D. (1994). The Impact of Raising Blood Glucose on Reaction Times. *Neuropsychobiology, 30,* 106–113.

Penland, J. G., Sandstead, H. H., Alcock, N. W., Dayal, H. H., Chen, X. C., Li, J. S., et al. (1997). A preliminary report: Effects of zinc and micronutrient repletion on growth and neuropsychological function of urban Chinese children. *J Amer Coll Nutr, 16*(3), 268–272.

Penland, J. G. (2000). Behavioral Data and Methodology Issues in Studies of Zinc Nutrition in Humans. *J. Nutr, 130,* 361S–364S.

Peritz, E. (1994). The Turlock vitamin-mineral supplementation trial: a statistical re-analysis. *J Biosoc Sci, 26,* 155–164.

Pharoah, P., Connolly, K., Ekins, R. P., & Harding, A. G. (1984). Maternal thyroid hormone levels in pregnancy and the subsequent cognitive and motor performance of children. *Clin Endocrinol, 21,* 265–270.

Pollitt, E., Leibel, R. L., & Greenfield, D. B. (1983). Iron deficiency and cognitive test performance in preschool children. *Nutr Behav, 1,* 137–146.

Pollitt, E., Saco-Pollitt, C., Leibel, R. L., & Viteri, F. E. (1986). Iron deficiency and behavioral development in infants and preschool children. *Am J Clin Nutr, 43,* 555–565.

Pollitt, E., Gorman, K. S., & Engle, P. L., et al. (1993). Early Supplementary Feeding and Cognition. *Monogr Soc Res Child Devel, 58,* 1–118.

Pollitt, E., & Oh, S. Y. (1994). Early supplementary feeding, child development and health policy. *Food Nutr Bull, 15,* 208–214.

Pollitt, E. (1995). Does breakfast make a difference in school? *J Am Diet Assoc, 95,* 1134–1139.

Pollitt, E., with Mari Golub, Kathleen Gorman, Sally Grantham-McGregor, David Levitsky, Beat Schurch, et al. (1996). A reconceptualization of the effects of undernutrition on children's biological, psychosocial, and behavioral development. *Social Policy Report, X,* 1–21.

Pollitt, E., Jacoby, E. R., & Cueto, S. (1996). School breakfast and cognition among nutritionally at-risk children in the Peruvian Andes. *Nutr Reviews, 54,* S22–S26.

Pollitt, E., Watkins, W. E., & Husaini, M. A. (1997). Three-month nutritional supplementation in Indonesian infants and toddlers benefits memory function 8 years later. *Am J Clin Nutr, 66,* 1357–1363.

Pollitt, E., Cueto, S., & Jacoby, E. R. (1998). Fasting and cognition in well-nourished and undernourished schoolchildren: a review of three experimental studies. *Am J Clin Nutr, 67*(suppl), 779S–784S.

Rapoport, J. L. (1986). Diet and hyperactivity. *Nutr Rev, 44*(suppl), 158–162.

Richter, L. M., Rose, C., & Griesel, R. D. (1997). Cognitive and behavioral effects of a school breakfast. *S Afr Med J, 87,* 93–100.

Rider, E., Samuels, R., Wilson, K., & Homer, C. (1996). Physical growth, infant nutrition, breastfeeding, and general nutrition. *Curr Opin Pediatr, 8,* 293–297.

Roa, R., & Georgieff, M. K. (2000). *Early nutrition and brain development.* In Nelson Ca (ed). The effects of early adversity on neurobehavioral development: The Minnesota symposia on child psychology; Vol 31 (pp 1–30). Lawrence Erlbaum Associates.

Rogan, W. J., & Gladen, B. C. (1993). Breast-feeding and cognitive development. *Early Hum Dev, 31,* 181–193.

Rosen, L. A., Bender, M. E., & Sorrel, S., et al. (1988). Effects of sugar (sucrose) on children's behavior. *J Consult Clin Psychol, 56,* 583–589.

Sampson, A. E., Sujata, D., Meyers, A. F., & Houser, R. (1995). The nutritional impact of breakfast consumption on the diets of inner-city African-American elementary school children. *J Natl Med Assoc, 87,* 195–202.

Saravis, S., Schachar, R., & Zlotkin, S., et al. (1990). Aspartame: effects of learning, behavior, and mood. *Pediatrics, 86,* 75–83.

Sazawal, S., Bentley, M., Black, R. E., Dhingra, P., George, S., & Bhan, M. K. (1996). Effect of zinc supplementation on observed activity in low socioeconomic Indian preschool children. *J Pediatrics, 98,* 1132–1137.

Schnoll, R., Burshteyn, D., & Cea-Aravena, J. (2003). Nutrition in the treatment of attention-deficit hyperactivity disorder: A neglected but important aspect. In: *Applied Psychology and Biofeedback, 28*(1), 63–75

Schoenthaler, S. J., Amos, S. P., & Eysenck, H. J., et al. (1990). Controlled trial of vitamin-mineral supplementation: effects on intelligence and performance. *Person Indiv Diff, 12,* 351–352.

Schoenthaler, S. J., Bier, I. D., Young, K., Nichols, D., & Jansenns, S. (2000). The effect of vitamin-mineral supplementation on the intelligence of American schoolchildren: A randomized, double-blind placebo-controlled trial. *The Journal of Alternative and Complementary Medicine, 6*(1), 19–29.

Seshadri, S., & Gopaldas, T. (1989). Impact of iron supplementation on cognitive functions in preschool and school-aged children: the Indian experience. *Am J Clin Nutr, 50*(suppl), 675–681.

Simeon, D. T., & Grantham-McGregor, S. (1989). Effects of missing breakfast on the cognitive functions of school children of differing nutritional status. *Am J Clin Nutr, 49,* 646–653.

Soewondo, W., Husaini, M., & Pollitt, E. (1989). Effects of iron deficiency on attention and learning processes in preschool children: Bangdung Indonesia. *Am J Clin Nutr, 50*(suppl), 667–673.

Strupp, B., & Levitsky, D. (1995). Developmental psychobiology: theoretical premises that help in the understanding of the effect of malnutrition on development. *Nutr, 125*(8S), 2221S–2232S.

Taylor, B., & Wadsworth, J. (1984). Breast feeding and child development at five years. *Dev Med Child Neurol, 26,* 73–80.

Uauy, R., & de Andraca, I. Human milk and breast feeding for optimal mental development. Unpublished manuscript. INTA University of Chile.

UNICEF: World summit for children, 2002, Retrieved May 22, 2002 from http://www.childinfo.org/eddb/malnutrition/index.htm.

USDA: Food security measurements: Concepts and definitions. Economic Food Security Briefing Room. Retrieved May 22, 2002 from http://www.ers.usda.gov/briefing/FoodSecurity.

USDA Food Security in the United States: Conditions and trends. Retrieved 2003 from http://www.ers.usda.gov/Briefing/FoodSecurity/trends.

U.S. Department of Health and Human Services. Pediatric nutrition. 1997 Executive Summary: 1–6.

Vera Noriega, J. A., Ibanez, S. E. D., & Ramos, M. O. P., et al. (2000). Evaluacion de los efectos de una programa de desayunos escolares en atencion y memoria. *Arch Lat Am Nut, 50,* 35–41.

Wachs, T. D. (1993) Effects of mild to moderate malnutrition on human development: correlation studies. Paper prepared for the IDECG task force meeting on the effects of protein-energy malnutrition on cognitive development, December 6–10, Davis, CA.

Walker, S. P., McGregor, S. M., & Powell, C. A., et al. (2000). Effects of growth restriction in early childhood on growth, IQ, and cognition at age 11 to 12 years and the benefits of nutritional supplementation and psychosocial stimulation. *J Pediatr, 137,* 36–41.

Wender, E. H., & Solanto, M. V. (1991). Effects of sugar on aggressive and inattentive behavior in children with attention deficit disorder with hyperactivity and normal children. *Pediatrics, 88,* 960–966.

White, J. W., & Wolraich, M. (1995). Effect of sugar on behavior and mental performance. *Am J Clin Nutr, 62*(suppl), 242S–9S.

Whitney, E. N., & Rolfes, S. R. (2002). Understanding Nutrition 9th edition. *422, 432–434, 441*

Wolraich, M. L., Lindgren, S. D., & Stumbo, P. J., et al. (1994). Effects of diets high in sucrose or aspartame on the behavior and cognitive performance of children. *N Engl J Med, 330,* 301–307.

Wolraich, M. L., Wilson, D. B., & White, J. W.. (1995). The effect of sugar on behavior or cognition in children. *JAMA, 274*(20), 1617–1621.

# Chapter 9

# Motor Development

Jean Eckrich
Scott Strohmeyer

Understanding the processes involved in the achievement of motor skills has developed from a multidisciplinary approach. Developmental psychologists along with biologists, and now kinesiologists, have sought to understand movement behavior across the life span. Historically, the field has looked at these movement changes from a product perspective, or the outcome of the movement behavior. Recently, however, focus has shifted to the process aspects of motor development and the underlying mechanisms allowing or causing changes. Additionally, it is now accepted that changes in motor behavior must be explained by additional factors rather than by changes in the central nervous system alone. This multifaceted philosophy for understanding the developing individual has been identified as *dynamical systems theory*. The underlying premise of this theory is to understand all elements that may influence development.

Clark (1994) has identified factors that help explain changes in motor behavior as constraints and further separated them into three categories: (1) *organism*, (2) *environmental*, and (3) *task constraints*. Organism constraints are described as those constraints related to the structure and function of the body. Certainly, the body's size and shape affect movement as do the anatomical features of the skeletal system. Balance is affected in early childhood because of body proportions and resulting location of the center of mass. Additionally, various physiological measures influence the acquisition of motor skills as well as changes in movement across the life span. For instance, muscular strength is one physiological measure that may affect the development of walking. On the other end of the continuum, decreases in muscular strength may affect the ability to rise from a chair. All systems (i.e., muscular, respiratory, cardiovascular, perceptual, nervous, etc.) affecting a movement response must have developed to a critical level for the individual to be able to accomplish a skill or remain at that critical level for the maintenance of the skill. Additionally, these systems must be able to self-organize to accomplish a given task. Although the development of the organism is essential for the acquisition of motor skills, the interaction with the environment and the demands of the task also impact skill development.

Environmental constraints include those constraints in the physical and sociocultural environments of the mover. These include such factors as the lighting or temperature of the environment as well as the influences of gravity. However, environmental constraints also can include a wide array of circumstances that are influenced by other individuals. For instance, opportunities for practice as well as the quality of instruction received are affected by peers, family members, coaches, and teachers. Opportunities to practice, quality of instruction received, and affiliations also influence the type of reinforcement given (Clark, 1994; Gallahue & Ozmun, 2002).

The interactive role of the demands of the movement task with the organism and the environment must also be considered when examining motor skill acquisition and completion (Gallahue & Ozmun, 2002). The goals of a particular movement such as speed or accuracy influence the mover and his/her response. Certainly, the purpose of the movement response also impacts the response. For instance, some movement responses must meet guidelines of a particular sport, such as the arm and leg action for a soccer throw-in. While the goals and purpose are important, implements such as bats, rackets, and/or balls affect the mover. The size, shape, and weight of an implement all factor into the success an individual may have and/or alter the movement response (Clark, 1994).

It is no longer appropriate to examine one particular system or mechanism to explain motor behavior. It is best understood as a dynamic process with improvements and decrements in movement abilities related to the change in constraints (Clark, 1994). The complex relationship of the organism, environment, and task must be explored to gain a full understanding of the abilities and limitations of the mover.

# Factors Affecting Motor Development

Various factors influence the development of motor skills throughout the life span. Some of these factors have the ability to impact the process of

how the movement occurs as well as the underlying changes, such as improved balance or increased nerve conduction velocity, affecting the movement response. Others have the ability to impact the product or the movement outcome. The movement outcome or product is often the focus because many individuals are only concerned with how fast, how high, or how far. It is essential to understand motor development from both perspectives because each is critical in exploring the changes in movement, whether it is an infant struggling to achieve locomotion or an elite athlete functioning effortlessly or an elderly person striving to maintain independence. Therefore, sociocultural factors, physiological functioning, and perceptual motor abilities and their role in changes in the movement process and/or movement product are highlighted. However, other factors such as normal growth can alter the movement response and enhance or be detrimental to the product. Disuse and disability often associated with older adults also alters movement responses.

## Sociocultural Influences

Sociocultural influences affect the development of the motor domain by shaping attitudes, beliefs, and opportunities. These influences include significant others, personal attributes, and socialization situations (Greendorfer, 2002). Significant others include important individuals and or groups such as family members, peers, teachers, and coaches. They have the ability to encourage or discourage certain motor behaviors (Haywood & Getchell, 2001).

In early childhood, the family is the primary socializing agent. Parents have a strong capacity to shape children's interests and attitudes (Welk, Wood, & Morss, 2003). Although the research has not been conclusive regarding the specific roles of mothers and fathers, children's behaviors are often reflective of their parents' interests. Certainly, an interesting trend to follow will be the role of mothers because many of them will have had greater opportunities to participate in physical activity than in previous generations, and there are fewer barriers associated with female participation in physical activity.

Although the family serves as the first socializing agent, peers also play a role throughout childhood. If the peer group is involved in physical activities, the individual often is as well (Haywood & Getchell, 2001). Teachers and coaches also have the potential to contribute to the socialization process. Youth who have had a negative experience in physical education or youth sport programs generally choose not to participate in physical activity as adults.

Greendorfer (2002) identified personal attributes as key factors in sport socialization. Throughout childhood, attributes such as self-efficacy and perceptions of competence are greatly influenced by significant others (Haywood & Getchell, 2001). There is a greater likelihood that children will persist in physical activities if they have greater levels of self-esteem and perceptions of competence. Because children rely so heavily on the adults in their lives for information, it is essential that these adults give appropriate and constructive feedback and make appropriate attributions related to the movement performance.

Children's socialization is also affected by their social situations. The environment can be conducive to an active or passive lifestyle. Exploring and playing outside provide opportunities to practice and develop gross motor skills. Cold weather areas are favorable for the development of certain motor skills, whereas warm weather areas are beneficial for the development of other motor skills. Urban environments will also be conducive to the development of yet other motor skills (Haywood & Getchell, 2001). The availability and types of various toys as well as the play environment affect the choices of children's activities. The prominence of computer games has been hypothesized to contribute to the sedentary lifestyle

of children and subsequent health problems. Sex role stereotypes can and are often introduced through the types of games and toys in the play environment.

Peer groups play a prominent role in the socialization process throughout older childhood and adolescence while the role of family, teachers, and coaches diminishes slightly (Greendorfer, 2002). Throughout this developmental stage, adolescents are becoming more independent and group affiliation often is a factor. Therefore, activity selection as well as sport dropout can be more a factor of belonging than interest (Gallahue & Ozmun, 2002). Peer groups continue to play a significant role throughout adulthood in decisions about movement opportunities. As young adults transition to new jobs, new locations, and new households, the peer group and spouses can influence activity patterns. However, other factors are important as concerns about health become more prevalent through middle and older adulthood (Gabbard, 2000). Personal attributes also continue to influence participation patterns. Experiences in childhood and adolescence greatly influence levels of self-efficacy and perceptions of competence related to physical activity and often affect adult activity patterns.

## Physiological Functioning

Motor development is often assessed through an analysis of a movement process as well as the movement product. Various physiological factors affect a movement response by impacting the movement process and/or movement product. For instance, a lack of shoulder flexibility can affect the range of motion of the arms in an overarm throw, which would result in an immature throwing pattern and likely affect the distance of the throw. An individual can have a very mature movement pattern for jumping but the actual distance of the jump may be poor for a variety of reasons, including a lack of muscle strength.

Therefore, it is essential to understand various physiological changes that occur across the life span. The physiological components of fitness are discussed later in this chapter.

## *Perceptual Changes*

Motor behavior is enhanced by improvements in the perceptual system. These changes occur throughout childhood. The stimuli received through the various senses allows for the processing of information and the subsequent motor response. For example, infants and young children develop the capability to process information from various sensory receptors that allow for an awareness of body position. This ability assists in the development of balance and subsequently in the development of walking, hopping, and so on. Similarly, motor behavior can be negatively affected by deficiencies in the perceptual system that occur through illness, disability, and/or aging. For example, declines in visual ability affect the ability to move in settings with reduced light, as well as the ability to track moving objects.

Although the anatomical features of the visual system are adult-like early in life, particular characteristics such as depth perception, spatial orientation, and perception of movement all develop throughout childhood. Visual input is essential to the tracking of an object for a catch as well as object deflection skills like hitting a baseball.

### KINESTHESIS AND PERCEPTUAL INTEGRATION

An awareness of movement and body position is referred to as kinesthesis and is the ultimate outcome of a functioning kinesthetic system. However, the kinesthetic system is not well understood because it is not a single sensory system (Gabbard, 2000). Various sensory receptors such as golgi tendon organs, joint receptors, muscle spindles, and vestibular apparatus contribute to the kinesthetic system. Improvements in body awareness (knowledge of body parts as well as their capabilities, limitations, and relationship to each other), spatial awareness (knowledge of the body's location in space), temporal awareness (development of a temporal pattern within movements), directional awareness (recognition of two separate sides of the body, an awareness of external space, and the ability to project the body to intended areas of space), and vestibular awareness (ability to achieve and sustain equilibrium) affect movement responses (Gabbard, 2000). These abilities are critical for the development of motor skills. Examples include the skills that are executed throughout the life span such as walking, which requires balance; jumping, which requires the projection of the body into space; and running, which requires a temporal pattern.

Auditory perception is not as closely linked to motor development as visual and kinesthetic perception (Gabbard, 2000). However, skillful movers often use auditory information. For instance, auditory location is one characteristic of auditory perception and may help a soccer player become aware of an approaching defender or allow a tennis player to sense the pace of the return by the sound of the ball on the racket.

Equally important as the development of each individual system is perceptual integration. Although partially functional at birth, perceptual integration develops throughout childhood and adolescence (Gabbard, 2000). A key indicator of perceptual integration is the ability to receive stimuli in more than one form and process all sources of information to shape a movement response. For instance, the utilization of kinesthetic and visual information enhances the ability to return a tennis or volleyball serve.

### CHANGES ACROSS LIFE SPAN

Changes in the perceptual system begin approximately in middle adulthood with some changes in the visual system and greater changes occurring with more advanced age. Gabbard (2000) summarized the following changes in perception with aging: 1) visual perception decreases in acuity, sensitivity to light, visual information processing, and perception of movement; 2) auditory perception decreases in sensitivity to high and low frequencies; and 3) kinesthetic perception decreases in touch sensitivity, weight discrimination, and balance.

Movement is affected by the changes in the perceptual system as well as by perceptions of competence associated with these changes. For example, older adults generally exhibit greater toe out positions, shorter stride lengths, and velocity decreases while walking. Certainly, some of these changes may be necessary due to decreases in balance. However, they can also occur because of a fear of falling, which may also limit other activity choices. Another example of the impact of decrements in the perceptual system is with the ability to intercept a moving object. Cluttered visual backgrounds make it more difficult to identify the targeted object, such as in tennis, which negatively impacts performance. An understanding of perceptual changes is critical to help the elderly individual develop and/or maintain an active lifestyle or for a community or organization to design a movement environment that minimizes the impact of these changes.

# Components of Health-Related Fitness

The focus of this section is on components of health-related fitness, which include cardiorespiratory endurance, muscular strength, muscular endurance, flexibility, and body composition. Changes in body systems throughout childhood, such as increased muscular strength, have the potential to enhance movement performances by the application of greater forces. Similarly, changes in body systems throughout adulthood also affect health-related fitness in these individuals. For the adult, the effects of the aging process on physiological function tend to lead to declines in motor performances that were maximized in early adulthood.

## Cardiorespiratory Endurance

Cardiorespiratory endurance is the ability of the cardiovascular and respiratory systems to take in, deliver, and utilize oxygen for sustained physical work (Payne & Isaacs, 2002). It has a prominent role in physical health because cardiovascular disease is a significant health care issue. At the same time, it is an essential component of many aerobic activities such as running, biking, and swimming. Despite limitations, cardiorespiratory endurance is often assessed by measures to estimate or determine maximum oxygen consumption or uptake, which is the "largest amount of oxygen that a human can consume at the tissue level" (Payne & Isaacs, 2002, p. 178). It is often expressed in absolute values (L/min) or in relation to body weight (ml/kg/min). Normal developmental changes affect cardiorespiratory endurance, as do physical activity levels.

Absolute maximum oxygen uptake improves throughout childhood. When maximum oxygen consumption is expressed in relation to body weight, these absolute changes throughout childhood are minimal in boys and may actually decrease in girls (Rowland, 1996). Increases in heart volume, lung size, and blood volume all factor into the changes in maximal aerobic power. As a result, there are improvements in performance of endurance activities such as running throughout childhood (Rowland, 1996).

Peak absolute maximum oxygen uptake occurs in late adolescence for males and late childhood to early adolescence in females (Wilmore & Costill, 1994). When maximum oxygen consumption is expressed relative to body weight, it plateaus in males between 6 and 26 years of age and declines in females at approximately 13 years old (Wilmore & Costill, 1994). Increases in heart size, blood volume, working capacity, vital capacity, and metabolic rates are documented in both genders during adolescence. However, males will exhibit greater increases in all parameters (Wilmore & Costill, 1994). As a result, improvements in performance of endurance activities such as running, swimming, and soccer will be observed throughout adolescence.

Physiological decreases related to cardiovascular endurance can be seen in early adulthood. Maximum oxygen consumption will decrease at a rate of approximately 10% per decade beginning after the age of 25 (Wilmore & Costill, 1994). Physically active adults who maintain body composition, however, maintain a higher maximum uptake than sedentary adults and can reduce the rate of decline to about 5% per decade (Wilmore & Costill, 1994). Reductions in maximal heart rate during strenuous exercise as one ages may partially explain decreases in maximum oxygen uptake (Spirduso, 1995). Other possible causes for decreases in maximum oxygen uptake could be due to age-related changes: loss of muscle mass, inability of the body to redirect blood from organs to working muscles, and deficiencies of the muscle to use oxygen (Spirduso, 1995). Exercise has been shown to prevent, delay, or even reverse a substantial amount of physiological aging (Rowe & Kahn, 1987). In sedentary adults who have begun to exercise, aerobic capacity can be restored to acceptable levels (Posner, Gorman, Klein, & Woldow, 1986).

## Muscular Strength and Endurance

Muscular strength and endurance are important components of many movements. For example, a baseline of strength is needed to achieve various motor milestones such as lifting the head or walking. Severe decrements in strength may eliminate the ability to stand from a sitting position or climb stairs and affect independent living for the elderly. A lack of strength can also increase the risk of falls in the elderly. In addition to motor tasks related to general function (i.e., lifting, walking, standing, rising from a seated position, falls), the product or movement outcome of many other motor skills can be also be affected by strength levels. Jump heights, throwing distances, and running velocities can all be enhanced by greater levels of strength.

Various factors can affect muscular strength throughout childhood, including muscle size and neural adaptations. Children's absolute muscle size increases, and subsequent improvements in muscular strength are observed (Rowland, 1996). Previous controversy over the appropriateness of strength training for children has been eliminated. The American Academy of Pediatrics (2001) has supported properly designed and supervised resistance training programs for children. Improvements in strength are seen in children as a result of training, and these changes are generally associated with neurological changes rather than muscle hypertrophy before adolescence (Rowland, 1996). Muscular endurance is associated with muscular strength, and improvements are also seen in this area throughout childhood (Gabbard, 2000).

Muscle strength improves throughout adolescence. Muscle size increases with growth, and parallel increases in strength are also observed. However, gender differences manifest themselves shortly after the onset of puberty. The onset of puberty exposes males to the effects of sex hormones that will influence muscular structure and size. Muscle weight is approximately 27% of body weight in male children. In the adolescent male, muscle weight increases to about 40% of total body weight (Vrijens, 1978). Strength differences between the sexes continue throughout the life span.

During early and middle adulthood, muscle strength and endurance remain fairly constant. However, after the age of 45, significant declines in strength and endurance occur. Over the next 20 years, approximately 20% of grip strength will be lost (Shepard, 1981). Maintenance of muscle strength is achieved best in muscles that are used for daily activity, isometric contractions, eccentric contractions, slow velocity contractions, repeated low-level contractions, and strength maneuvers using small joint angles. Declines are more readily observed in muscles used infrequently (movements that are very specialized), dynamic strength moves (activities requiring maximum force production), concentric contractions (muscle-shortening activities), rapid velocity contractions (speed movements), power production (production of large amounts of force when time is a factor), and strength maneuvers using large joint angles (force production activities when the muscle is significantly longer than resting length) (Spirduso, 1995). Men also seem to lose strength more slowly than women. Strength training can enhance muscle strength at any age. Exercise has been shown to slow the effects of muscle loss. Resistance training can improve muscle strength at any age.

## Flexibility

Flexibility factors into the range of motion of joints and can enhance or restrict mobility, which will affect movement processes and products. For example, mature throwing patterns will not be achieved if there is a lack of flexibility of the shoulder. The evidence regarding developmental changes throughout childhood is not consistent. The most significant discrepancy is a determination of the age at which declines in flexibility begin. A key limitation to the research has been a result of examining the flexibility of different body joints. The evidence is quite conclusive that flexibility is joint specific. It also appears that physical activity patterns may have a greater impact on flexibility changes throughout childhood than age itself (Gabbard, 2000).

Peak flexibility of the hamstrings is attained in the late teens or early 20s (Payne & Isaacs, 2002). Throughout adolescence, increased flexibility has been observed with females performing better than males in sit-and-reach flexibility (Ross & Gilbert, 1985; Ross & Pate, 1987). The mechanism for gender inequities is unknown but could

be related to the types of activities in which a person might participate. Flexibility, however, can be improved at any age through proper exercise routines.

Flexibility during the adult years (~20–60 years) shows a tendency to decrease. Declines in flexibility occur primarily as a result of not moving joints through the full range of motion for everyday living (Haywood & Getchell, 2001). Three factors that appear to influence flexibility most are physical activity, inherent effects of aging, and degenerative joint diseases such as osteoarthritis (Gabbard, 2000; Haywood & Getchell, 2001). However, a number of investigations have found that flexibility can be enhanced at any age with targeted stretching protocols (Brown & Holloszy, 1991; Germain & Blair, 1983; Munns, 1981; Raab, Agre, McAdam, & Smith, 1988).

## Body Composition

There has been increased interest in the body composition of children in recent years. Health concerns have been expressed as data support claims that a greater percentage of children are obese than in the past (Boreham & Riddoch, 2001; Haywood & Getchell, 2001). Recognizing these concerns, it is important to note that motor development and performance are also affected. Developmental delays of motor skills were observed in babies that were identified as fat using the Svenger's index of body weight (Jaffe & Kosakov, 1982). Higher percentages of body fat have been associated with poorer performances in cardiovascular endurance activities as well as muscular endurance activities (Haywood & Getchell, 2001). In addition, excess fat can limit range of motion and subsequently affect the quality of a movement performance.

Boys and girls display similar increases in fat free mass throughout childhood while body fat percentage declines in early childhood (Rowland,

1996). During later childhood, girls show a rise in body fat that continues throughout adolescence, whereas boys show a slight increase followed by a decline (Rowland, 1996).

Adolescence is a period of rapid change in body composition, and significant differences between the sexes will manifest themselves at this stage of development. Body composition changes in adolescence lead to differences in performance characteristics between males and females. Brooks and Fahey (1985) identified various differences between the sexes that arise during adolescence. Males will tend to 1) have a lower percentage of body fat; 2) possess greater muscle mass; 3) exhibit greater weight; 4) be taller; 5) have wider shoulders, longer arms and legs; and 6) have narrower hips. Body fat percentage will continue to increase for females throughout adolescence, while males will peak and then show a slight decline (Rowland, 1996). Unfortunately, ". . .body fat adds to the mass of the body without contributing to force-producing capacity" (Gabbard, 2000, p. 303). Therefore, due to apparent mechanical advantages, males may be more inclined to perform better at sprinting, jumping, and throwing where longer levers and stronger musculature produce relatively greater rotational torque for proficient exhibition of these motor skills. Females, on the other hand, are more proficient at motor skills requiring a greater degree of balance (Gabbard, 2000).

"For the average person, gains in body weight and fat begin gradually in the late 20s and continue to increase until approximately the age of 55 or 60, when they show signs of decreasing" (Gabbard, 2000, p. 340). Typically, the average person will increase in body weight and fat by 15% from 20 to 60 years of age. This value is the same for men and women. The effects of weight gain and increased body fat are nebulous. Increases in body fat are often associated with impaired cardiac functioning. Increasing body fat is inversely related to moving total body weight. Because fat is not involved in force production, it

simply becomes excess weight that must be moved during locomotion activities (Gabbard, 2000). Regular exercise and a proper diet assist individuals in maintaining lean body mass (Haywood & Getchell, 2001). Body composition is continually changing throughout life. Unfortunately, for the aging adult, lean body mass is being lost and body fat increases. Training programs can slow the loss of lean body mass, but not reverse losses entirely.

# Early Motor Behavior

Gabbard (2000) and Haywood and Getchell (2001) have characterized movements during infancy as spontaneous and reflexive in nature. These movements are followed by the development of postural control, rudimentary locomotion, and manual control.

## Spontaneous Movements

Spontaneous movements are those that occur without any apparent purpose or stimulus (Piek & Carman, 1994). These movements are generally repetitive in nature and are often referred to as rhythmical stereotypies (Thelen, 1979). Stereotypies have been divided into the major segments of the body including: 1) legs and feet; 2) arms, hands, and fingers; 3) torso; and 4) head and face (Thelen, 1979). Although the movements appear quite random, there is a temporal component. The onset, peak movements, and decline of the different stereotypies appear to be related "with transitions between no voluntary control over the limb or body segment and adaptive and intentional control" (Thelen, 1996, p. 141). Thelen (1979) identified 47 distinct stereotypical movement patterns. Two of the most frequently observed stereotypies are kicking and waving type movements (Piek & Carman, 1994; Thelen, 1979).

Thelen (1979) found that infants in prone or supine positions often would make rhythmical movements with their legs and feet. The most common movement was that of rhythmical kicking, and various forms occur such as simultaneous leg kicking, alternate leg kicking, and single leg kicks. These movements were generally the earliest developed and were observable as early as 4 weeks of age, peaked between 24 to 32 weeks, and decreased in frequency during the last 8 to 10 weeks of the first year.

Hand and arm movements were the next most frequently observed movement (Thelen, 1979). Different forms of movement occurred such as arm waving, banging against a surface, hand and finger flexion, and so on. Thelen determined that arm movements generally developed before hand movements. Arm and hand movements peaked around 34 to 42 weeks. Additional frequently observed movements involved the torso (i.e., rocking) and hand and face movements (i.e., nodding and head shaking).

Much uncertainty exists about the specific role of stereotypies in the development of voluntary movement. It is apparent that the spontaneous movements of infancy regress before goal-directed and purposeful movements. However, a key finding is that these rhythmical movements involve neuromuscular coordination and that many of the patterns of stereotypies are similar to those seen in adult movements (Haywood & Getchell, 2001).

## Reflexes

Reflexes are involuntary movements that are a response to particular stimuli (Haywood & Getchell, 2001). They can be elicited in the fetus and are observable in infants. They are primarily controlled subcortically. Payne and Isaacs (2002) have identified key reasons to study and understand reflexes, including their role in nourishment and protection as well as their determination of neurological development. Whereas some reflexes last a lifetime, such as blinking, others are strictly categorized as infant behavior. These reflexes are generally identified as primitive, postural, or lo-

comotor. The most common reflexes with responses to stimuli, functioning times, and warning signs are identified in Table 9.1. Use of a timetable can serve as an important marker for determining the integrity of the central nervous system (Gallahue & Ozmun, 2002).

Gallahue and Ozmum (2002) have identified four different criteria that would create concern about normal neurological functioning and maturation. These include:

1. Preservation of a reflex beyond the age at which it should have been inhibited by cortical control

2. Complete absence of a reflex

3. Unequal bilateral reflex responses

4. Responses that are too strong or too weak (p. 122)

## Motor Milestones

As the central nervous system develops, voluntary movement gradually appears. Throughout the first year of life, there are periods when the voluntary movements overlap with reflexes and stereotypies (Gabbard, 2000). However, reflexive movements related to infancy are almost nonexistent after the first year of life. The development of voluntary movements is one indication that higher brain centers are functioning (Gallahue & Ozmun, 2002).

Motor milestones are achieved in a cephalocaudal and proximodistal pattern. Head and trunk control occurs before standing, and arm movements occur before thumb opposition. These skills develop in an orderly fashion, although their onset is quite variable. Using dynamical systems as a model to explain the acquisition and onset of rudimentary behaviors, organism, task, and environmental constraints must be explored. Organism constraints are critical and appear to have the most influence in the first year (Clark, 1994). The development of various systems including the muscular system, central nervous

*Table 9.1* INFANTILE REFLEXES

Infantile Reflexes

| Reflex/ Reaction | Starting Position (if important) | Stimulus | Response | Time | Warning Signs |
|---|---|---|---|---|---|
| **Primitive Reflexes** | | | | | |
| Asymmetrical tonic neck reflex | Supine | Turn head to one side | Same-side arm and leg extended | Prenatal to 4 months | Persistence after 6 months |
| Symmetrical tonic neck reflex | Supported sitting | Extend head and neck; Flex head and neck | Arms extend, legs flex Arms flex, legs extend | 6 to 7 months | |
| Doll-eye | | Flex head | Eyes look up | Prenatal to 2 weeks | Persistence after first days of life |
| Palmar grasping | | Touch palm with finger or object | Hand closes tightly around object | Prenatal to 4 months | Persistence after 1 year; asymmetrical reflex |
| Moro | Supine | Shake head, as by tapping pillow | Arms and legs extend, fingers spread; then arms and legs flex | Prenatal to 3 months | Presence after 6 months; asymmetrical reflex |
| Sucking | | Touch face above or below lips | Sucking motion begins | Birth to 3 months | |
| Babinski | | Stroke sole of foot from heel to toes | Toes extend | Birth to 4 months | Persistence after 6 months |
| Searching or rooting | | Touch cheek with smooth object | Head turns to side stimulated | Birth to 1 year | Absence of reflex; persistence after 1 year |
| Palmar-mandibular (Babkin) | | Apply pressure to both palms | Mouth opens; eyes close; head flexes | 1 to 3 months | |
| Plantar grasping | | Stroke ball of foot | Toes contract around object stroking foot | Birth to 12 months | |
| Startle | Supine | Tap abdomen or startle infant | Arms and legs flex | 7 to 12 months | |

## Table 9.1 CONTINUED

### Infantile Reflexes

| Reflex/Reaction | Starting Position (if important) | Stimulus | Response | Time | Warning Signs |
|---|---|---|---|---|---|
| **Postural Reactions** | | | | | |
| Derotative righting | Supine | Turn legs and pelvis to other side | Trunk and head follow rotation | From 4 months | |
| Labyrinthine righting reflex | Supine | Turn head sideways | Body follows head in rotation | From 4 months | |
| | Supported upright | Tilt infant | Head moves to stay upright | 2 to 12 months | |
| Pull-up | Sitting upright, held by 1 or 2 hands | Tip infant backward or forward | Arms flex | 3 to 12 months | |
| Parachute | Held upright | Lower infant toward ground rapidly | Legs extend | From 4 months | |
| | Held upright | Tilt forward | Arms extend | From 7 months | |
| | Held upright | Tilt sideways | Arms extend | From 6 months | |
| | Held upright | Tilt backwards | Arms extend | From 9 months | |
| **Locomotor Reflexes** | | | | | |
| Crawling | Prone | Apply pressure to sole of one foot or both feet alternately | Crawling pattern in arms and legs | Birth to 4 months | |
| Walking | Held upright | Place infant on flat surface | Walking pattern in legs | Birth to 5 months | |
| Swimming | Prone | Place infant in or over water | Swimming movement of arms and legs | 11 days to 5 months | |

*Reprinted by permission, from K. M. Haywood & N. Getchell (2001). Life span motor development (3rd ed). Champaign, IL: Human Kinetics, p. 90.*

system, and perceptual system is essential. However, environmental and task constraints are also relevant. Opportunities must exist for skills to develop, and the task must be appropriate to the organism (i.e., small ball versus a big ball).

An understanding of the milestones is important in the clinical setting. Whereas the acquisition of the motor milestones is quite variable, a delay in several motor areas may be an indication of developmental problems with particular concern in the maturation of the nervous system (Haywood & Getchell, 2001). However, development is truly dependent on the ability of the various systems to self-organize. The mover must be able to do so in the context of the environment and required task. Delays in motor milestone achievement could be an indication of other de-velopmental concerns, including the coordination of the systems or a deficiency in any one system. A disability could also alter the general timetable for motor milestone achievement.

## STABILITY

Lifting the head, sitting alone, and progressing through other milestones until one achieves the ability to stand upright unassisted are critical skills. Stability is essential for the development of movement and other motor skills. The ability to walk will not occur without postural control. Additionally, stability aids skills such as reaching and grasping. This allows the body to be put in position to free the arms and hands for reaching and grasping (Payne & Isaacs, 2002). The various rudimentary tasks related to stability and approximate age of onset for each are in Table 9.2.

### *Table* 9.2    RUDIMENTARY STABILITY ABILITIES

#### Developmental Sequence and Approximate Age of Onset of Rudimentary Stability Abilities

| Stability Tasks | Selected Abilities | Approximate Age of Onset |
|---|---|---|
| Control of head and neck | Turns to one side | Birth |
| | Turns to both sides | 1 week |
| | Held with support | 1st month |
| | Chin off contact surface | 2nd month |
| | Good prone control | 3rd month |
| | Good supine control | 5th month |
| Control of trunk | Lifts head and chest | 2nd month |
| | Attempts supine-to-prone position | 3rd month |
| | Success in supine-to-prone roll | 6th month |
| | Prone-to-supine roll | 8th month |
| Sitting | Sits with support | 3rd month |
| | Sits with self-support | 6th month |
| | Sits alone | 8th month |
| | Stands with support | 6th month |
| Standing | Supports with handholds | 10th month |
| | Pulls to supported stand | 11th month |
| | Stands alone | 12th month |

*Reprinted by permission, from D. L. Gallahue & J. E. Ozmun (2002).* Understanding motor development: Infants, children, adolescents, adults *(5th ed). Boston: McGraw Hill, p. 139.*

*Figure 9.1*   Developmental Sequences for Walking

**INITIAL**

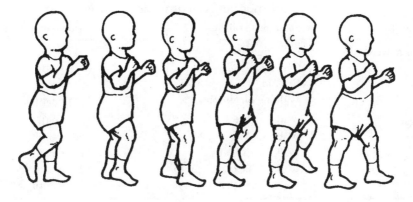

**ELEMENTARY**

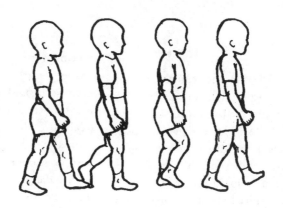

**MATURE**

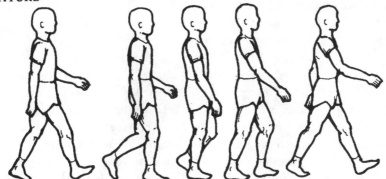

*Reprinted by permission, from D. L. Gallahue & J. E. Ozmun (2002).* Understanding motor development: Infants, children, adolescents, adults *(5th ed). Boston: McGraw Hill, p. 231.*

*Table 9.3*    RUDIMENTARY LOCOMOTOR ABILITIES

### Developmental Sequence and Approximate Age of Onset of Rudimentary Locomotor Abilities

| Locomotor Tasks | Selected Abilities | Approximate Age of Onset |
|---|---|---|
| Horizontal movements | Scooting | 3rd month |
| | Crawling | 6th month |
| | Creeping | 9th month |
| | Walking on all fours | 11th month |
| Upright gait | Walks with support | 6th month |
| | Walks with handholds | 10th month |
| | Walks with lead | 11th month |
| | Walks alone (hands high) | 12th month |
| | Walks alone (hands low) | 13th month |

*Reprinted by permission, from D. L. Gallahue & J. E. Ozmun (2002).* Understanding motor development: Infants, children, adolescents, adults *(5th ed). Boston: McGraw Hill, p. 141.*

## LOCOMOTION

Infancy is also marked by the acquisition of basic skills related to locomotion such as creeping, crawling, and upright walking. Initial movements are very unskilled. However, they provide an important means of exploring one's surroundings. Developing the ability to walk is a key example of progression from immature to mature movement patterns. Initial efforts are marked by many falls. Key descriptors of early walking include 1) a wide base of support with toe out positions; 2) arms in a high guard position; 3) limited range of motion in the trunk, legs, and hips; and 4) short steps (Gabbard, 2000). A wide base of support and out-toeing provides a more stable and larger base of support for the inexperienced walker. Holding the arms high without much arm swing reduces the changes in body position that can disrupt balance. Limited ranges of motion and short steps assist in limiting the time of one leg support (see Figure 9.1, Initial).

As the individual becomes more experienced with walking, control of stability becomes less of a conscious concern. As a result, the base of support will narrow, out-toeing decreases; range of

motion in the trunk, legs, and hips increases; and stride length also increases (see Figure 9.1, Elementary). Mature walking patterns are not evident until approximately 4 to 5 years of age (Gabbard, 2000). This stage of development is exhibited when the individual walks with a narrow base of support, reflexive arm swing, elongated gait, and a pronounced heel–toe contact with each footstrike (see Figure 9.1, Mature). Approximate onset of appearance for walking and other basic locomotor skills are identified in Table 9.3.

## MANIPULATION

Reaching, grasping, and releasing are three general skills related to manual control. These skills are essential in the accomplishment of many skills of daily living but also important as they provide another method to explore the environment (Payne & Isaacs, 2002). Initial arm and hand movements are categorized as stereotypies and reflexes. However, goal-directed movements begin at approximately 4 months of age with significant progress made in the next 2 months (Gabbard, 2000). The ability to grasp progresses from a very crude movement response involving

*Table 9.4*    Rudimentary Manipulative Abilities

### Developmental Sequence and Approximate Age of Onset of Rudimentary Manipulative Abilities

| Manipulative Tasks | Selected Abilities | Approximate Age of Onset |
|---|---|---|
| Reaching | Globular ineffective reach | 1st to 3rd month |
| | Definite corralling reach | 4th month |
| | Controlled reach | 6th month |
| Grasping | Reflexive grasp | Birth |
| | Voluntary grasp | 3rd month |
| | Two-hand palmar grasp | 3rd month |
| | One-hand palmar grasp | 5th month |
| | Pincer grasp | 9th month |
| | Controlled grasp | 14th month |
| | Eats without assistance | 18th month |
| Releasing | Basic release | 12th to 14th month |
| | Controlled release | 18th month |

*Reprinted by permission, from D. L. Gallahue & J. E. Ozmun (2002). Understanding motor development: Infants, children, adolescents, adults (5th ed). Boston: McGraw Hill, p. 144.*

both arms and hands to a skillful response requiring thumb opposition (Gabbard, 2000). Initial movements of releasing involve the dropping of an object. This is evident in the very early stages of grasping an object. Controlled releasing of an object occurs much later and would be defined as skillful at approximately 18 months of age. The progression of manual control is outlined in Table 9.4.

# Childhood

Early, middle, and later childhood is marked by further refinement of the basic rudimentary skills of stability, locomotion, and manipulation; improvements in perceptual abilities; and changes in physiological functioning. This further development provides more effective ways for children to explore the environment, understand their surroundings, create a greater movement repertoire such as combining fundamental skills, and move toward greater independence.

## Fundamental Motor Skills

As fundamental motor skills such as throwing, catching, and striking develop, various descriptors are used to identify individuals at an initial, elementary, or mature stage of development. The differences in the performance of basic motor skills are quite apparent when working with children in this stage of development. Gallahue and Ozmun (2002) have identified three separate categories of differences. These include between-child differences, which reinforces the basic developmental principle of individuality. A second category includes between-pattern differences for an individual child. The child may be at an initial stage for jumping and a mature stage for throwing. Differences such as these are often related to opportunities and other environmental influences. Finally, within-pattern differences also manifest themselves, which sometimes creates greater challenges for understanding.

An example would be when a child uses an elementary stage upper body action and a mature lower body action for the performance of a kick. Possible explanations for within-pattern differences are: "(a) incomplete modeling of the movement of others, (b) initial success with the inappropriate action, (c) failure to require an all-out effort, (d) inappropriate or restricted learning opportunities, or (e) incomplete sensorimotor integration" (Gallahue & Ozmun, 2002, p. 187).

## STABILITY

After the basic skill of standing upright is achieved, childhood is marked by greater improvements in stability. This includes the ability to change body position, adapt to changes in body position, and maintain balance with a smaller base of support. These abilities can be categorized as either axial or postural.

*Axial movements, or non-locomotor, movements are orientation movements of the trunk or limbs while in a static position. Twisting, turning, bending, stretching, and swinging are axial movements. Postures are other body positions that place a premium on the maintenance of equilibrium while in a position of static or dynamic balance. Standing, sitting, inverted supports, rolling, stopping, dodging, and landing as well as beam walking, stick balancing, and one-foot balances are dynamic or static balance postures (Gallahue & Ozmun, 2002, p. 188).*

Balance develops throughout childhood. This is evidenced by observing the significant postural sway of toddlers while walking and contrasting this postural sway with the more refined movement response achieved by elementary school children. Another example of stability development is in beam walking. Giacalone and Rarick (1985) studied dynamic balance in preschool children. Children were asked to walk on a balance beam at different heights, with different widths, and with different slopes. Improvements with age were seen when averaging performances across all conditions.

However, stability is task specific. Some of the challenges in assessing stability are related to proper measurement. Certainly, there can be changes in process that are much more difficult to assess than the changes in product. For instance, kinesthetic information becomes more important and visual information less important in balance activities as children grow (Haywood & Getchell, 2001). Children's vestibular awareness and body awareness are two ways that children receive kinesthetic information to allow for static and dynamic balance without visual information. These abilities are critical because the development of stability above basic rudimentary levels is essential for the accomplishment of fundamental motor skills such as skipping, hopping, kicking, and throwing.

## LOCOMOTION

Walking, running, jumping, skipping, hopping, galloping, and sliding encompass the repertoire of locomotor skills attained and refined throughout childhood. They are used for basic needs such as transporting the body from one location to another, but they are also used for exploration, discovery, and play. They later serve as a foundation for more complex motor skills associated with specific sport and movement tasks such as throwing, kicking, and so on. The development of each of the locomotor skills is dependent upon the interaction of the task, organism, and environment. For example, balance may be a rate limiter for hopping, and sociocultural influences can affect the development of skipping in boys.

After a rudimentary level of walking is achieved, further refinement begins in the second year of life. A pattern that includes rigid arms in a high-guard position and steps that create a wide base of support is replaced with a more efficient pattern that lowers the arms and narrows the base of support. Descriptions of mature walking include changes in process and product (see Figure 9.1). Haywood and Getchell (2001, pp. 122–123) have identified the following characteristics for proficient walking:

- Absolute stride length increases, reflecting greater application of force and greater leg extension at push-off. Also, as children grow, increased leg length contributes to a longer stride.

- Planting the foot flatly on the ground changes to a heel-then-forefoot pattern.

- The individual reduces out-toeing and narrows the base of support laterally to keep the forces exerted in a forward–backward plane.

- The skilled walker adopts the double knee-lock pattern to assist the full range of leg motion.

- The pelvis rotates to allow the full range of leg motion and oppositional movement of the upper and lower body segments.

- Balance improves and forward trunk inclination is reduced.

- The skilled walker coordinates oppositional arm swing (with the arms extending at the sides) with the movement of the legs.

Shumway-Cook and Woollacott (2001, p. 367) have identified three requirements for successful locomotion, which include "(a) the ability to generate a rhythmic stepping pattern to move the body forward (progression), (b) postural control (stability), and (c) the ability to adapt gait to changing task and environmental requirements (adaptation)." The emergence of mature gait has been identified by some as early as 5 years of age (Gabbard, 2000) to 7 years of age (Shumway-Cook & Woollacott, 2001).

In recent years there has been increased concern about the external loads that children are carrying while walking. Children commonly carry books, school supplies, and athletic equipment in backpacks. Negrini, Carabalona, and Sibilia (1999) found that the average load carried by children in Italy with an average age of 11.6 years was 22% of their body weight. These findings are of concern because of the increase in back pain in children and adolescents. In a study in the United States, Pascoe and colleagues (1997) found that 65.5% of 11- to 13-year-old children identified the weight that they carry as heavy and 29.5% consider the

weight as medium. Over 60% of these children self-reported muscle soreness and 50.8% reported back pain. Hong and Brueggemann (2000) found changes in trunk lean and a prolonged recovery time for blood pressure with loads of 15% and 20% of body weight in 10-year-old-boys and recommended that loads of no more than 10% of body weight be carried by this population.

Running requires the development of sufficient strength to propel the body off the ground and to accept body weight on landing. Additionally, the development of the nervous system is necessary to help coordinate the rapidly moving body parts (Payne & Isaacs, 2002). Balance is also critical to receive the body weight on a limited base of support and to transfer the weight in order to facilitate a flight phase (Haywood & Getchell, 2001). Early running attempts are characterized by limited leg swing, stiff uneven strides, absence of a flight phase, incomplete support leg extension, arms raised, out-toeing, and a wide base of support (Gallahue and Ozmun, 2002) (see Figure 9.2, Initial).

Although mature walking patterns must not be present for an individual to begin running, developmental changes in the running pattern are relatively congruous with developmental changes in the walking pattern. Mature running patterns are characterized by an increase in stride length, a decrease in the lateral base of support, a predominance of sagittal plane movements, and greater range of motion (Haywood & Getchell, 2001). These changes are similar in purpose to the changes that occur in development of the mature walking pattern (see Figure 9.2). Additional improvements throughout childhood include a decrease in vertical movements, an increase in duration of the nonsupport phase, an improvement in the placement of the contact foot in relation to the center of mass, and better use of the arms (Gabbard, 2000).

There are many variations of the skill of jumping. The first observable form is that of a leap, which involves a one-foot takeoff and a landing on the opposite foot and is observable at about

*Figure 9.2*   Developmental Sequences for Running

**INITIAL**

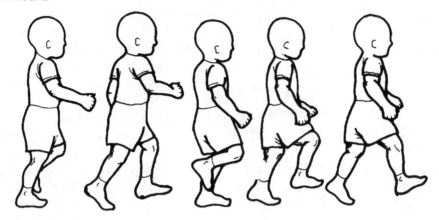

**ELEMENTARY**

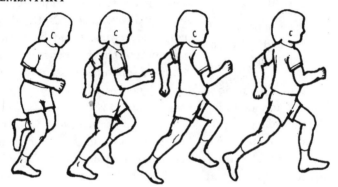

**MATURE**

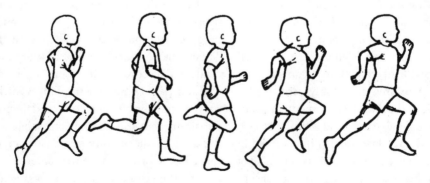

*Reprinted by permission, from D. L. Gallahue & J. E. Ozmun (2002). Understanding motor development: Infants, children, adolescents, adults (5th ed). Boston: McGraw Hill, p. 233.*

2 years of age (Gabbard, 2000). Children also perform vertical jumps and long jumps for distance. Both of these forms in a mature stage require the ability to direct force in a manner that will give the intended flight, coordinate arm and leg action, and receive force at landing by flexion of the ankles, knees, and hips (Haywood & Getchell, 2001). Hopping has been identified by Gabbard (2000) as a form of jump. It is the most difficult of all jumps because it requires takeoff and landing on one foot. Force to propel the body must be generated by one leg, and balance must be maintained on a minimal base of support (Haywood & Getchell, 2001).

Galloping, sliding, and skipping are the remaining locomotor skills developed throughout childhood. Each requires some combination of walking, running, hopping, and leaping (Gabbard, 2000). Galloping is the first one to emerge, followed by sliding, and skipping generally develops last. Galloping and sliding have some similarities but the obvious difference is in the direction of movement. Haywood and Getchell (2001) have identified these as asymmetric gaits because the mover spends more time on one leg than on the other; that is, each phase is not 50%. Sliding is considered more difficult because the mover is facing in one direction and moving in another (Payne & Isaacs, 2002). Another difficulty in the development of these skills is the ability to exert different amounts of force from each leg (Haywood & Getchell, 2001). The ability to lead with the nondominant leg takes longer to develop in comparison to skills in which one leads with the dominant leg.

Skipping is generally the last observable locomotor skill. It requires a step and hop on one foot followed by the same movement on the other foot (Haywood & Getchell, 2001). A rate limiter for skipping may be the neuromuscular system because the skill does not develop until the body "can coordinate the two limbs as they alternately perform asymmetric tasks" (Haywood & Getchell, 2001, p. 142).

## MANIPULATION

Throughout early, middle, and later childhood, the ability to manipulate various objects develops and becomes more refined. The terms used to define gross motor skills such as throwing, catching, and striking vary; Haywood and Getchell (2001) identify these as *ballistic skills,* whereas Payne and Isaacs (2002) define these as *fundamental object-control skills,* and Gallahue and Ozmun (2002) as well as Gabbard (2000) refer to these as *manipulative skills.*

These fundamental motor skills are used for play, games, and sport. Clark (1994) has classified these into *object projection skills* and *interception skills.* Throwing is an object projection skill that can take many different forms, such as underhand, sidearm, and overarm. The goal of the throw can be for speed, accuracy, and/or both speed and accuracy. Clark (1994) further classified object interception skills into *object deflection* and *object reception* skills. The main objective of object deflection skills is to intercept an object and direct the object away such as in kicking and striking. The goal of object reception skills such as catching and trapping is "intercepting an object for the purpose of collecting the object" (Clark, 1994, p. 252).

All individuals do not achieve a mature movement pattern for these skills. However, throughout childhood, it is very possible for children to develop in all these areas. Environmental constraints including opportunities for practice, types of reinforcement, and quality of instruction all factor into the mastery of these skills. The application and reception of force also put demands on the neuromuscular system as strength and balance are required (Clark, 1994). Physical size factors into skills such as throwing and receiving an object. Figure-ground perception as well as depth perception and other perceptual skills are necessary for interception skills (Clark, 1994). Children learn to catch with one hand or two as well as to catch larger and smaller balls. They learn to throw a ball at different trajectories with different speeds. They develop the ability to kick a stationary ball and a moving ball. Some of these skills in more advanced forms also require the child to be able to achieve these goals while moving.

Children are simultaneously refining their fine motor skills. This includes the ability to complete tasks such as handwriting, eating, and dressing. These skills require the development of the coordination of the shoulder, elbow, and wrist (Clark, 1994). The palmar grasp utilized for holding writing implements is replaced by the dynamic tripod (i.e., holding the implement with three fingers), which allows for specialized finger movement and occurs at around the age of seven (Payne & Isaacs, 2002). They have noted developmental trends in handwriting including "an increase in upright posture, more stable trunk and hand, and an increase in the likelihood of holding the hand below the line of writing and in line with the forearm" (p. 293). Improvements in printing, writing, and proper spacing of letters as well as drawing are enhanced by the ability to gain control of the small muscles of the hand and wrist. Activities requiring bimanual control or the use of both hands first develop for symmetric functions (e.g., rolling a ball, catching) followed by asymmetrical functions (e.g., throwing) and are associated with the development of hand preference (Gabbard, 2000).

# Adolescence

Adolescence is a time of rapid physical change in the development of the individual. It is at this point in the life cycle when the individual may experience growth spurts that lead to adolescent awkwardness (Payne & Isaacs, 2002). Balance can be disrupted for up to 6 months (Tanner, 1990), and performance in motor tasks can also decline during these maximum growth stages (Beunan, et. al., 1988; Ostyn, Simons, Beunen, Renson, & Gerven, 1980). Episodes of chaotic behavior (i.e., loss of balance, declines in coordination, etc.) are most likely due to rapid growth in the musculo-

skeletal system and the inability of the neurological systems to adapt quickly to the rapidly changing constraints of the developing musculoskeletal system. Although adolescent awkwardness has been shown to exist, it is more frequently associated with males but is not a universal phenomenon (Beunan & Malina, 1988). Beunan and Malina (1988), in follow-up testing of young adults, found that movement response declines were temporary. As a result, individuals responsible for motor assessment of adolescents should exercise caution when interpreting motor performance during this rapid growth period.

## Fundamental Motor Skills

Gabbard (2000) stated that, "The period from later childhood through adolescence is characterized by several growth and development milestones, many of which are manifested in significant improvements in motor skill performance" (p. 300). At this stage of development, the adolescent begins to build upon the fundamental movement abilities acquired in childhood. The adolescent's movement evolves to produce greater product (sport skill) performance. Fundamental motor skill patterns are generally considered mature in exhibition, but refinements may still be developing in late-maturing individuals. Differences in motor patterns are believed to be dependent upon maturation of the individual (Gabbard, 2000; Haywood & Getchell, 2001; Payne & Isaacs, 2002). Differences may also be a result of experience in performing the fundamental patterns.

Sex-related differences are also observed during the adolescent years. Differences in product performance generally favor males (Gabbard, 2000; Haywood & Getchell, 2001; Payne & Isaacs, 2002). Motor performance of males tends to improve throughout adolescence on a wide variety of skills. Females, on the other hand, mature earlier, and motor performance peaks at adult levels around 14 years of age (Haubenstricker, Wisner, Seefeldt, & Branta, 1997). Evidence exists that the female will plateau if not decline slightly in motor performance after peak performance is exhibited (Malina & Bouchard, 1991; Thomas, Nelson, & Church, 1991).

Differences in performance between genders as the adolescent enters adulthood can be attributed to a variety of biological, structural, cultural, and sociological factors. Biologically, males are larger, possess less body fat and more muscle, and transport oxygen more efficiently than females (Gabbard, 2000). This would put females at a disadvantage for activities involving horizontal (e.g., running, galloping) or vertical (e.g., jumping, leaping) movements of the body (Smoll & Schutz, 1990; Thomas et al., 1991). Body fat adds weight to the body but does not provide force production. This limits the relative amount of force-producing muscle available to the mover. Structurally, the longer legs and arms of the male allow him to produce greater leverage and rotational torque for throwing and striking tasks. The females' lower center of mass is beneficial for greater stability (Gabbard, 2000).

## STABILITY

Stability generally improves during adolescence. However, it is context specific.

As one proceeds through adolescence, there is a tendency to rely less on visual information and rely more on kinesthetic feedback, such as spatial and temporal awareness, to regulate stability (Haywood & Getchell, 2001). The ability to statically balance oneself tends to increase with age to approximately 18 years of age (Williams, 1983). Stability is developed through participation in specialized movement skills, which will then be integrated into the execution of specific and complex movements (i.e., sports and worksite contexts).

## LOCOMOTION

The adolescent years are characterized by applying fundamental locomotion patterns in more specialized activities. Walking, running, jumping, hopping, and sliding have been refined to the point that they are now used in a wider variety of environments. Specifically, many of these fundamental locomotor skills are now applied to the sport setting. Again, the development of each of the locomotor skills is dependent upon the interaction of the task, organism, and environment. Balance and skeletal and/or muscular maturation may serve as rate limiters in sport-specific proficiency.

Walking at this stage of development is proficient in its execution (see Figure 9.1, Mature). Some product-related aspects of the walk may improve, such as walking velocity, because of changes in size, but the overall movement pattern remains relatively the same. Individual variations in walking patterns are more a function of social or cultural factors than physical differences between individuals.

Running speed continues to develop during adolescence until a plateau is reached. Exactly when the running pattern is exhibited in its most mature pattern depends upon the experience level of the individual.

## MANIPULATION

Adolescence is a time of further refinement of manipulative abilities. Fundamental motor skills used in play, games, and sport will take on specialized qualities based upon environmental constraints of experience in specialized skills, types of reinforcement, and quality of instruction. It is at this age when the individual may become extremely proficient in a particular sport or movement pattern, due to interest and or experiences. However, anthropomorphic characteristics of the individual may determine one's abilities in throwing, catching, kicking, and/or other projection or reception tasks. The adolescent continues to improve with respect to balance, strength, depth perception, tracking, and anticipation. All are important factors in the development of specialized movement patterns (Clark, 1994).

Fine motor patterns have been fairly well established before adolescence. Again, experience with particular motor patterns (i.e., writing, spacing, etc.) will show the greatest refinements. Accuracy in reaching and grasping has become perceptually based in middle childhood (McDonnell, 1979) and will continue to remain as such unless constraints such as strength, balance, visual acuity, and so on become a concern (Haywood & Getchell, 2001).

# Early to Middle Adulthood

Early adulthood is when most individuals reach their peak in physical performance and health. It is during this stage of the life cycle that "peak motor performance" is attained (Gabbard, 2000). Most physical best performances are attained during the early stages of this life cycle, and declines occur in relative weight lifted, running velocity, and the like due to decreases in physiological functioning. Unlike the motor development of young individuals, movement patterns usually remain consistent through early old age (~60 yrs.) (Haywood & Getchell, 2001; Gabbard, 2000). Very few changes in movement process occur throughout early and middle adulthood. "Extrinsic factors continue to play a larger role as individuals proceed through adulthood, leading to greater variability among individuals in older adulthood" (Haywood & Getchell, 2001, p. 61). Generally, lifestyle, injury, and/or changes in body weight may result in changes in motor patterns (Haywood & Getchell, 2001). There is a significant lack of research concerning motor development in this age category. A possible explanation for limited research might be that because stability in motor behaviors for healthy individuals varies so little, rewards of research may be minimal. Whereas motor development of children, adolescents, and the aged may lead to lifetime quality, the apparent need for information on adults is not so imminent.

## Fundamental Motor Skills

Fundamental motor skills in early and middle adulthood develop on an individual basis.

Generalizations about developmental trends cannot be made about this age category mainly because there is a lack of research with this cohort (Haywood & Getchell, 2001). Changes in gait, jumping, throwing, and catching may result from opportunities to use particular skills, exercise, injury, and changes in body weight. Some individuals may never reach mature levels of performance. This is due in part to the lack of opportunity to participate in developmental activities as a child or adolescent. Maintaining and/or developing these skills at this stage of the life cycle also will depend on motivation to participate in physical activity and opportunity to practice. Gender differences may still exist, but again, motivation and opportunities to use skills can narrow the gap in performance differences between the sexes.

### STABILITY

Until approximately 60 years of age, static control of posture improves (Payne & Isaacs, 2002). Body sway when standing, on the other hand, is often used to determine an individual's ability to maintain balance. Stability during this stage of the life cycle is very well maintained with minimal adjustments taking place during perturbations. Both visual and kinesthetic feedbacks are used to maintain balance. During rhythmic or expected movement, the adult will use visual information to stabilize the head and upper body and muscles around the ankle to adjust stability at the base of support (Buchanan & Horak, 1999). During slow or minimal perturbations in balance, the young or middle-aged adult will use muscles about the ankle to maintain balance, but muscles at the hip will be employed if perturbations are large or quick (Horak, Nashner, & Diener, 1990; Kuo & Zajac, 1993).

### LOCOMOTION

Normal walking patterns will remain fairly constant across the life span barring any physical impairments. Chronological age is not a good predictor of change in gait patterns. Rather, changes in gait can be predicted readily more by health status (Engle, 1986), physical inactivity (Larish, Martin, & Mungiole, 1988), and pathological conditions. Adults, however, tend to walk more slowly than children. It is believed that this is more an economy of effort change in gait pattern than further motor development (Craik, 1989; Winter, 1983). That is, the adult walkers slow their velocity by allowing the momentum caused by pendular action of the lower limb to create the walking motion instead of pulling the leg forward. Thus, less energy is needed to walk.

Khattab (1980) also examined walking differences between children and adults. She found that adults had considerably fewer balance problems than children, possibly due to a relatively lower center of mass height for adults. Adults also were found to be more efficient although less energetic walkers. Adults took longer strides because of their longer leg length, used less hip flexion and extension during the stride, and required less rearward force to slow the forward momentum after a heel strike. These factors support the conclusion that adult walkers are more economical than children.

Mature running patterns can be maintained throughout early and middle adulthood. However, in those individuals approaching old age, older runners will not flex the knee or hip as much, will develop shorter stride lengths, take fewer strides, and generally slow down (Nelson, 1981) (see Figure 9.2). Rate limiters in running are the same as they are for walking. Running also requires greater generation of force and a greater requirement to maintain dynamic balance. Thus smaller changes in the rate limiters of strength and balance may lead to the disappearance of this skill in later parts of this developmental stage (Haywood & Getchell, 2001).

### MANIPULATION

Reaching and grasping will remain important motor skills throughout the life of an individual. One's career and other daily tasks may involve the ability to manipulate objects. Kaurenen and Vanharanta (1996) investigated reaching in adults aged 21 to 71 years. They found that reaction time, movement speed, and tapping speed (repetitive finger movement to a designated target) all decreased as one got older. They also noted declines in coordination of the hands and feet. Grip strength also declined with age. Significant declines, however, did not occur until after the age of 50 years. Grasping objects, on the other hand, remains consistent throughout the life cycle. Strength and joint impairment can act as rate limiters in one's ability to reach and grasp.

## The Aging Adult

Old age is a time of significant declines in the motor abilities of the individual. Lean body mass decreases; fast twitch muscle fibers that are recruited for speed, power, and strength activities decrease; nerve conduction speed slows; vision changes; kinesthetic receptors change; and musculoskeletal problems such as arthritis become limiting factors in motor performance. There seems to be a general consensus that significant declines in motor performance begin around 50 to 60 years of age, although some individuals will show significant declines before this age. Generally, disease, strength, injury, or lifestyle are determinants in motor behavior changes.

*The differences in physical function of old adults is striking. Capacities range from the frail older adult living in a long-term care facility, who experiences severe difficulty walking, bathing, and dressing, to an 80-year-old living independently, who can run a 26.2 mile marathon race in a masters' track meet. The concept of "average" ability for a specific age group becomes less and less appropriate for individual performance with increasing age (Spirduso, 1995, pp. 28–29).*

Physically active individuals can slow the decline in motor performance but cannot stop these declines. Care, therefore, must be exercised when assessing older adult motor development. Factors such as ethnicity, gender, and health status will confound interpretations. It has been shown that the aging adult will respond favorably to intervention and practice. However, for long-term benefits to be experienced, changes in behavior must become lifestyle practices (Spirduso, 1995).

## Fundamental Motor Skills

Movement patterns in the young adult and the middle-aged adult are relatively stable for an individual and quite varied or unpredictable as far as trends can be discerned for that age group as a whole. Motor development of the aging adult becomes somewhat more predictable. Although physically active older adults can slow the decline in motor performance, many physiological factors make it more and more difficult to maintain high levels of performance. Sedentary individuals will show the greatest declines in the absence of other mitigating factors (Gabbard, 2000; Haywood & Getchell, 2001; Gallahue & Ozmun, 2002).

When throwing, older adults will decrease in range of motion and velocities. In an investigation conducted by Williams, Haywood, and VanSant (1990, 1991), older adults were found to be only moderately advanced with respect to the developmental stages of throwing (see Figure 9.3). Velocities were comparable with velocities that 8- to 9-year-old children could generate on similar throwing tasks. Men were more advanced with respect to the developmental sequences and ball velocities were higher. It is commonly held that skill performance for older adults is in a state of consistent decline. In another study conducted by Williams, Haywood, and VanSant (1998), a group of older adults was observed over a period of 7 years. They found that throwing performance in older adulthood is relatively stable with small changes in performance being more typical than large declines.

With respect to striking skills (i.e., tennis serve), Haywood and Williams (1995) found in two groups of older adults (62–68 years and 69–81 years) that there were no significant differences between the groups in motor development and ball velocities. Further, no differences due to gender were found. Again, evidence of significant decline with age was not observed in skills that are used repeatedly. Flexibility also was determined and no differences were found between groups. Findings from these studies would suggest that well-practiced skill performance can be maintained for older adults.

Can the older adult improve performance in new skills? Evidence exists that new skills can be learned by older adults, but practice sessions must be structured and more numerous (Cerella, 1990; Spirduso, 1995). Obviously, motivation to perform becomes a factor, as well as physical and physiological abilities. To see long-term benefits, the older adult must make the new skill performance a lifestyle decision because skill can be quickly lost without practice (Spirduso, 1995).

### STABILITY

Adults over the age of 60 experience a decline in their ability to maintain balance. Older adults sway more than young adults when standing upright and when leaning (Hasselkus & Shambes, 1975; Perrin, Jeandel, Perrin, & Bene, 1997), time of response increases after perturbation or body position changes, and sequence of muscular response varies as one ages (Perrin et al., 1997). The older adult will tend to correct the upper body before the lower body when balance is perturbed. This response is opposite that of younger adults (Perrin et al., 1997). Possible factors influencing a decline in the ability to balance include changes in various body systems, particularly in vision, nerve conduction speed, and muscle strength.

As a result of the inability to efficiently maintain balance, older adults are more prone to falls than any other age cohort. In adults over the age of 65, one-third to one-half will fall at least once a year (Nickens, 1985; Perry, 1982). Falls are

*Figure 9.3*    Developmental Sequences for Throwing

**INITIAL**

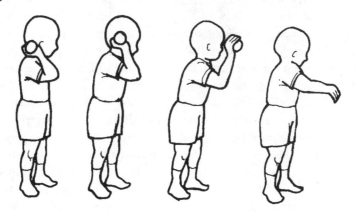

**ELEMENTARY**

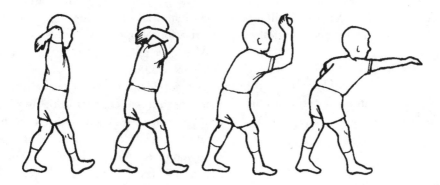

**MATURE**

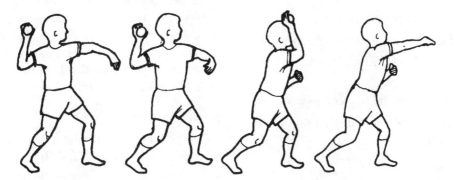

responsible for over 80% of fractures in the elderly and are the leading cause of accidental death over the age of 75 years (Spirduso, 1995). Characteristics that define individuals who are prone to falling include women; individuals who take more steps to turn 360 degrees; individuals who must push off when rising from a chair; individuals using antidepressants (Lipsitz, Jonsson, Kelley, & Koestner, 1991); and individuals who have unusually weak muscles particularly in the hip adductors, knee extensors, knee flexors, and ankle dorsiflexors (MacRae, Lacourse, & Moldavon, 1992). Medication usage can also predispose one to falls (Spirduso, 1995).

Physical exercise can contribute to the prevention of falling in the aging adult. Spirduso (1995) outlined the basic components of a physical exercise program that will help prevent falling in older adults. She stated that a proper physical exercise program will

- Strengthen leg and back muscles;
- Enhance reflex and motor synergy postural reactions;
- Improve gait;
- Increase flexibility;
- Maintain body weight;
- Improve mobility to avoid unexpected perturbations in balance;
- Decrease cardiovascular disease risks;
- Reduce the risk of postural hypotension;
- Lower the probability of needing medication;
- Enhance sleep and reduces insomnia; and
- Raise self-confidence in physical abilities (p. 179).

## LOCOMOTION

In a series of studies examining walking patterns over the age of 60 years, Murray, Drought, and Kory (1964); Murray, Kory, Clarkson, and Sepic (1966); and Murray, Kory, and Sepic (1970) found that older men walked with a gait pattern similar to that of younger men with some exceptions. Step lengths for older men were approximately 3 cm shorter; they toed out approximately 3 degrees more; and there was less ankle extension and less pelvic rotation. Older women indicated the same differences when compared to younger women. Schwanda (1978) confirmed these findings and also presented data that most other factors of proficient walking (i.e., stride rate, time for recovering-leg swing, support time, and vertical deviations) remain consistent as one ages. It would seem then that individual differences are the result of disease, disuse, or injury. Balance and fear of falling may also work to limit the opportunities an older adult takes to walk (Haywood & Getchell, 2001). Additionally, desires to enhance balance may also factor into the increased muscle coactivation of opposing muscle groups observed in the gait of the elderly (Shumway-Cook & Woollacott, 2001).

For individuals who continue to run in old age, there are minimal changes in the movement pattern. Nelson (1981) found that the older adult would not flex at the ankle, knee, or hip as much as a younger runner. The older adult exhibits shorter and fewer strides and overall tends to be slower than their younger counterparts. Rate limiters for running are the same for all developmental stages and include the need for greater force generation and dynamic balance. For these reasons, the skill of running may disappear altogether for the older performer. There are examples, however, of individuals performing into their 90s in running events. These are rare cases.

## MANIPULATION

The ability to reach and grasp for the older adult is often important for daily activity and independence. After the age of 50, reaction time, movement speed, and tapping speed decrease and the aging adult will also experience declines in coordination of the hands and feet. Roy, Winchester, Weir, and Black (1993) also found that the older adult slows down more at the end of a reach than young adults. They speculated that this may allow for more corrections by the older adult. The ability to grasp objects remains consistent throughout the life cycle; however, declines in grip strength that occur with aging (Kauranen & Vanharanta, 1996) and/or joint impairment can act as rate limiters in one's ability to reach and grasp.

Fine motor manipulations in such skills as handwriting (Contreras-Vidal, Teulings, & Stelmach, 1998) and crafts such as crocheting will see little decline in ability with age. Coordination of the fingers and wrist may decline slightly with age, but these skills do not require a great deal of speed or accuracy to be executed successfully. Limiting factors in fine motor skills will predominantly include disuse and disease.

In skills that involve rapid aiming (e.g., monitoring and manipulating complex displays), older adults will increase the time of deceleration or the movement time to a target, especially if accuracy is important. Time of acceleration or the initial phase of the movement response is less and not as forceful. This leads to more adjustments being made in the final manipulation. Young adults, on the other hand, accelerate and decelerate equally and use much more force in the acceleration phase (Vecruyssen, 1997). Practice is critical for the older adult. Compensation can be made for slowing by knowing locations of buttons and levers extremely well (Haywood & Getchell, 2001).

## Concluding Remarks

Motor development has been described in recent years from a life span approach. The continuum includes various stages of development such as the reflexive behaviors of infants, the movement refinements in childhood and adolescence, and the declines in movement responses in the elderly. Although there are similarities in movement sequences such as the development of motor milestones, there also is great individuality in movement responses. Some individuals develop to

the point of general functioning for activities of daily living, whereas others become elite athletes.

A key element in understanding movement responses across the life span is the recognition of the role of organism, environment, and task constraints, which are continually changing. These constraints combine to affect the acquisition of new skills and the skillfulness of the movement response as well as the inability to perform a previously acquired skill. This dynamical systems theory provides a strong model for understanding the underlying processes related to motor development. Technological advances in kinetic and kinematic analyses allow for greater opportunities to study movement. In addition, factors such as an aging society, an increased emphasis on health promotion, and societal changes such as reductions in gender biases necessitate additional study, which should provide greater insights into motor development.

## References

American Academy of Pediatrics. (2001). Strength training by children and adolescents. *Pediatrics, 107,* 1470–1472.

Beunen, G., & Malina, R. M. (1988). Growth and physical performance relative to the timing of adolescent spurt. In K. B. Pandolf (Ed.), *Exercise and sport sciences reviews.* New York: Macmillan.

Beunen, G., Malina, R. M., Van't Hof, M. A., Simons, J., Ostyn, M., Renson, R., et al. (1988). *Adolescent growth and motor performance: A longitudinal study of Belgian boys.* Champaign, IL: Human Kinetics.

Boreham, C., & Riddoch, C. (2001). The physical activity, fitness and health of children. *Journal of Sport Sciences, 19,* 915–929.

Brooks, G. A., & Fahey, T. D. (1985). *Exercise physiology: Human bioenergetics and its applications.* New York: Macmillan.

Brown, M., & Holloszy, J. O. (1991). Effects of a low-intensity exercise program on selected physical performance characteristics of 60- to 71-year-olds. *Aging, 1,* 129–139.

Buchanan, J. J., & Horak, F. B. (1999). Emergency of postural patterns as a function of vision and translation frequency. *Journal of Neurophysiology, 81,* 2325–2339.

Cerella, J. (1990). Aging and information-processing rate. In J. E. Birren & K. W. Schaie (Eds.), *Handbook of the psychology of aging* (3rd ed., pp. 201–221). New York: Academic Press.

Clark, J. E. (1994). Motor development. In V. S. Ramachandran (Ed.), *Encyclopedia of human behavior* (Volume 3, pp. 245–255). New York: Academic Press.

Contreras-Vidal, J. L., Teulings, H. L., & Stelmach, G. E. (1998). Elderly subjects are impaired in spatial coordination in fine motor control. *Acta Psychologica, 100,* 25–35.

Craik, R. (1989). Changes in locomotion in the aging adult. In M. H. Woollacott & A. Shumway-Cook (Eds.), *Development of posture and gait across the life span* (pp. 176–201). Columbia, SC: University of South Carolina Press.

Engle, V. F. (1986). The relationship of movement and time to older adults' functional health. *Research in Nursing and Health, 9,* 123–129.

Gabbard, C. P. (2000). *Lifelong motor development* (3rd ed.). Boston: Allyn and Bacon.

Gallahue, D. L., & Ozmun, J. C. (2002). *Understanding motor development: Infants, children, adolescents, adults* (5th ed.). Boston: McGraw Hill.

Germain, N. W., & Blair, S. N. (1983). Variability of shoulder flexion with age, activity, and sex. *American Corrective Therapy Journal, 37,* 156–160.

Giacalone, W. R., & Rarick, G. L. (1985). Dynamic balance of preschool children as reflected by performance on beam-walking tasks. *Journal of Genetic Psychology, 146,* 307–318.

Greendorfer, S. L. (2002). Socialization processes and sport behavior. In T. S. Horn (Ed), *Advances in sport psychology* (2nd ed, pp. 371–401). Champaign, IL: Human Kinetics.

Hasselkus, B. R., & Shambes, G. M. (1975). Aging and postural sway in women. *Journal of Gerontology, 30,* 661–667.

Haubenstricker, J. L., Wisner, D., Seefeldt, V., & Branta, C. (1997). Gender differences and mixed-longitudinal norms on selected motor skills for children and youth. *Journal of Sport & Exercise Psychology: 1997 NASPSPA Abstracts, 19,* S63.

Haywood, K., & Getchell, N. (2001). *Life span motor development* (3rd ed.). Champaign, IL: Human Kinetics.

Haywood, K., & Williams, K. (1995). Age, gender, and flexibility differences in tennis serving among experienced older adults. *Journal of Aging and Physical Activity, 3,* 54–66.

Hong, Y., & Brueggemann, G. P. (2000). Changes in gait patterns in 10-year-old boys with increasing loads when walking on a treadmill. *Gait and Posture, 11,* 254–259.

Horak, F. B., Nashner, L. M., & Diener, H. C. (1990). Postural strategies associated with somatosensory and vestibular loss. *Experimental Brain Research, 82,* 167–177.

Jaffe, M., & Kosakov, C. (1982). The motor development of fat babies. *Clinical Pediatrics, 21,* 619–621.

Kauranen, K., & Vanharanta, H. (1996). Influences of aging, gender, and handedness on motor performance of upper and lower extremities. *Perceptual and Motor Skills, 82,* 515–525.

Khattab, E. (1980). The effect of aging on selected kinematic and kinetic parameters of gait. In J. M. Cooper & B. Haven (Eds.), *Proceedings of the biomechanics symposium* (p. 348–349) Indianapolis: Indiana University.

Kuo, A. D., & Zajac, F. E. (1993). Human standing posture: Multi-joint movement strategies based on biomechanical constraints. *Progress in Brain Research, 97,* 349–358.

Larish, D. D., Martin, P. E., & Mungiole, M. (1988). Characteristic patterns of gait in the healthy old. In J. A. Joseph (Ed.), Central determinants of age related declines in motor function. *Annals of the New York Academy of Sciences, 515,* 18–31.

Lipsitz, L. A., Jonsson, P. V., Kelley, M. M., & Koestner, J. S. (1991). Causes and correlates of recurrent falls in ambulatory frail elderly. *Journal of Gerontology: Medical Sciences, 46,* M114–M122.

MacRae, P. G., Lacourse, M., & Moldavon, R. (1992). Physical performance measures that predict faller status in community-dwelling older adults. *Journal of Occupational and Sports Physical Therapy, 16,* 123–128.

Malina, R. M., & Bouchard, C. (1991). *Growth maturation and physical activity.* Champaign, IL: Human Kinetics.

McDonnell, P. M. (1979). Patterns of eye-hand coordination in the first year of life. *Canadian Journal of Psychology, 33,* 253–267.

Munns, K. (1981). Effects of exercise on the range of joint motion in elderly subjects. In E. L. Smith & R. C. Serfass (Eds.), *Exercise and aging: The scientific basis.* Hillside, NJ: Enslow.

Murray, M. P., Drought, A. B., & Kory, R. C. (1964). Walking patterns of normal men. *Journal of Bone and Joint Surgery, 46-A,* 335–360.

Murray, M. P., Kory, R. C., Clarkson, B. H., & Sepic, S. B. (1966). Comparison of free and fast speed walking patterns of normal men. *American Journal of Physical Medicine, 45,* 8–24.

Murray, M. P., Kory, R. C., & Sepic, S. B. (1970). Walking patterns of normal women. *Archives of Physical Medicine and Rehabilitation, 51,* 637–650.

Negrini, S., Carabalona, R., & Sibilia, P. (1999). Backpack as a daily load for schoolchildren. *The Lancet, 354,* 1974.

Nelson, C. J. (1981). *Locomotor patterns of women over 57.* Unpublished master's theses, Washington State University, Pullman.

Nickens, H. (1985). Intrinsic factors in falling among the elderly. *Archives of Internal Medicine, 145,* 1089–1093.

Ostyn, M., Simons, J., Beunen, G., Renson, R., & Van Gerven, D. (Eds.) (1980). *Motor development of Belgian secondary schoolboys.* Leuven: Leuven University Press.

Pascoe, D. D., Pascoe, D. E., Wang, Y. T., Shim, D., & Kim, C. K. (1997). Influence of carrying book bags on gait cycle and posture of youths. *Ergonomics, 40,* 631–641.

Payne, V. G., & Isaacs, L. D. (2002). *Human motor development* (5th ed.). Boston: McGraw Hill.

Perrin, P. P., Jeandel, C., Perrin, C. A., & Bene, M. C. (1997). Influence of visual control, conduction, and central integration on static and dynamic balance in healthy older adults. *Gerontology, 43,* 223–231.

Perry, B. C. (1982). Falls among the elderly: A review of the methods and conclusions of epidemiologic studies. *Journal of the American Geriatrics Society, 30,* 367–371.

Piek, J. P., & Carman, R. (1994). Developmental profiles of spontaneous movements in infants. *Early Human Development, 39,* 109–126.

Posner, J. D., Gorman, K. M., Klein, H. S., & Woldow, A. (1986). Exercise capacity in the elderly. *American Journal of Cardiology, 57,* 52C–58C.

Raab, D. M., Agre, J. C., McAdam, M., & Smith, E. L. (1988). Light resistance and stretching exercise in elderly women: Effect upon flexibility. *Archives of Physical Medicine and Rehabilitation, 69,* 268–272.

Ross, J. G., & Gilbert, G. G. (1985). The national children and youth fitness study: A summary of findings. *Journal of Physical Education, Recreation and Dance, 56,* 45–50.

Ross, J. G., & Pate, R. R. (1987). The national children and youth fitness study II: A summary of findings. *Journal of Physical Education, Recreation and Dance, 58(9),* 51–56.

Rowe, J. W., & Kahn, R. L. (1987). Human aging: Usual and successful. *Science, 237,* 143–149.

Rowland, T. W. (1996). *Developmental exercise physiology.* Champaign, IL: Human Kinetics.

Roy, E. A., Winchester, T., Weir, P., & Black, S. (1993). Age differences in the control of visually aimed movements. *Journal of Human Movement Studies, 24,* 71–81.

Schwanda, N. A. (1978). *A biomechanical study of the walking gait of active and inactive middle-age and elderly men.* Unpublished doctoral dissertation. Springfield College, Springfield, MA.

Shepard, R. J. (1981). Cardiovascular limitations in the aged. In E. L. Smith & R. C. Serfass (Eds.), *Exercise and aging: The scientific basis* (pp. 19–29). Hillsdale, NJ: Enslow.

Shumway-Cook, A., & Woollacott, M. H. (2001). *Motor control: Theory and practical applications* (2nd ed.). Philadelphia: Lippincott Williams & Wilkins.

Smoll, F. L., & Schutz, R. W. (1990). Quantifying gender differences in physical performance: A developmental sequence. *Developmental Psychology, 26,* 360–369.

Spirduso, W. W. (1995). *Physical dimensions of aging.* Champaign, IL: Human Kinetics.

Tanner, J. M. (1990). *Fetus into man.* Cambridge, MA: Harvard University Press.

Thelen, E. (1979). Rhythmical sterotypies in normal human infants. *Animal Behavior, 27,* 699–715.

Thomas, R. J., Nelson, J. K., & Church, G. (1991). A developmental analysis of gender differences in health-related physical fitness. *Pediatric Exercise Science, 3,* 28–42.

Vecruyssen, M. (1997). Movement control and speed of behavior. In A. D. Fisk & W. A. Rogers (Eds.), *Handbook of human factors and the older adult* (pp. 55–86). San Diego: Academic Press.

Vrijens, J. (1978). Muscle strength development in pre- and postpubescent age. In J. Borms & M. Gebbelinck (Eds.), *Pediatric Work Physiology.* New York: Karger.

Welk, G. J., Wood, K., & Morss, G. (2003). Parental influences on physical activity in children: An exploration of potential mechanisms. *Pediatric Exercise Science, 15,* 19–33.

Williams, H. G. (1983). *Perceptual and motor development.* Englewood Cliffs: Prentice-Hall.

Williams, K., Haywood, K., & VanSant, A. (1990). Movement characteristics of older adult throwers. In J. E. Clark & J. H. Humphrey (Eds.), *Advances in motor development research* (Volume 3, pp. 29–44). New York: AMS Press.

Williams, K., Haywood, K., & VanSant, A. (1991). Throwing patterns of older adults: A follow-up investigation. *International Journal of Aging and Human Development, 33,* 279–294.

Williams, K., Haywood, K., & VanSant, A. (1998). Changes in throwing of older adults: II. *Journal of Aging and Physical Activity, 4(2),* 194–202.

Wilmore, J. H., & Costill, D. L. (1994). *Physiology of sport and exercise.* Champaign, IL: Human Kinetics.

Winter, D. A. (1983). Biomechanical motor patterns in normal walking. *Journal of Motor Behavior, 15,* 302–330.

# Chapter 10

# Psychosocial Development: Adolescence and Sexuality

John Dacey

Deborah Margolis

Adolescence is a period of biological, psychological, cognitive, and social change. Adolescents are members of families; ethnic, racial and religious groups; school communities; peer groups; and broader society. Therefore, to fully understand adolescent development we must acknowledge the many contexts within which adolescents live and grow. Adolescence is an exciting period of growth and change; it can also be a challenging developmental period both for the adolescents and for those with whom they come in contact. The convergence of biological, psychological, social, and cultural factors during adolescence can pose a major challenge for health care providers charged with meeting the needs of adolescent patients.

It is impossible to talk about adolescent development without considering changes in physical and cognitive development. Puberty is probably the most visible change associated with adolescence. Puberty presents challenges as adolescents grapple with changes to their bodies. Health care providers can help adolescents manage changes associated with puberty by providing adequate information about these changes. Beyond the obvious physical changes of adolescence, some of the most profound changes take place in how adolescents think about themselves and their world. Their increasing capacity to think abstractly impacts the way that they consider, explore, and interact with the world around them.

This chapter provides an overview of adolescent psychosocial development. The interaction of physical and cognitive development with other developmental issues of adolescence is explored throughout the chapter. Key issues in adolescent development are addressed, including sense of self, relationships with families and peers, and sexuality, with special attention to problems encountered by adolescents that will likely bring them into contact with health providers.

## Identity and Self-Concept

To better understand adolescent development, it is crucial to explore the constructs of self and identity. The self has been of major interest to psychologists for many decades. William James (1890/1950) presented a model of the self that remains useful in understanding the links between the development of self-concept and personal identity. Self-concept can be defined as the thoughts and beliefs about one's physical, social,

191

and psychological qualities. Self-concept is one of the basic components of identity development. Therefore, a clear, realistic, and integrated self-concept provides the groundwork for healthy identity development. This would suggest the need to help parents and other caregivers appropriately support adolescents so that feelings of self-adequacy can develop.

## Impact of Cognitive Changes on Self-Concept

The adolescent's self-concept changes in many ways throughout the adolescent years. That is, how an individual describes "who I am" at age 12 will be very different from the self-description at age 19. The changes that take place in self-concept during those years are due in large part to the cognitive changes that are also taking place. Growth in abstract and hypothetical thinking affects the way in which adolescents describe themselves. Advances in social-cognitive processes, including social comparison, perspective taking, and self-awareness, also contribute to the changing self-concept. Cognitive abilities to compare oneself with others emerge in middle childhood and increase in adolescence as the teen encounters more complex and varied groups of individuals with whom to compare the self. According to Selman (1980), abstract thinking contributes to developments in perspective taking (or the ability to understand a situation from another person's point of view). Perspective taking enhances self-understanding because the adolescent can step outside an immediate situation and look at herself or himself as others would.

Harter (1990, 1993, 1999) believes that the more advanced reasoning skills of the adolescent influence self-concept in both positive and negative ways. Advances in social comparison, for example, lead to the realization that one is not as good as one's peers in many activities. With social cognitive advances that permit critical self-evaluation according to the standards of others,

the adolescent may suffer from an awareness that others hold negative views of him or her. Advanced social reasoning skills can also help adolescents behave in more socially acceptable ways. For some adolescents, changes in the way they think about themselves contribute to occasional emotional problems such as depression and anxiety.

Social-learning theorists such as Albert Bandura view the self as developing in a different way. Social-learning theorists suggest that the self is based mainly on the expectations people believe that others have for them and whether those expectations are reasonable. Our attitude toward self is learned and can be greatly influenced by whether we think we can succeed and whether we think other people think we can succeed. *Self-efficacy* is the name Bandura gives to self-expectations, or beliefs about what can be accomplished as a result of our efforts.

These beliefs influence how we behave and thus have implications for health care practice. For example, if weight loss is recommended, those patients who believe they will be successful will try harder. This effort helps them to succeed. In turn they are more self-confident. They are then perceived by others as successful and will be expected to continue to succeed. Because self-efficacy influences what a person will attempt and how well a person will actually perform, developing a strong and positive sense of self-efficacy is very important. Bandura calls this process through which beliefs, behavior, and environment affect one another *reciprocal determinism.*

## Erikson's Concept of Self

According to Erik Erikson, the main task of the adolescent is to achieve a *state of identity.* Erikson (1958, 1959, 1963, 1968, 1969; Erikson & Coles, 2000) refers to identity as a state toward which one strives. In a state of identity, the various aspects of self-concept are in agreement with each other. According to Erikson, *repudiation* of choices is another essential aspect of reaching personal identity. In any choice of identity, the selection we make means that we have repudiated (given up) all the other possibilities, at least for the present. All of us know people who seem unable to do this. They cannot keep a job, they are not loyal to their friends, they are unable to be faithful to a spouse. For them, "the grass is always greener on the other side of the fence." Interestingly, Erikson suggests that identity confusion is far more likely in a democratic society because there are so many choices, which would suggest that identity development is socially constructed.

Erikson sees late adolescence as a period of moratorium—a "time-out" period during which the adolescent experiments with a variety of identities, without having to assume responsibility for the consequences of any particular one. Erikson stated that indecision is an essential part of the moratorium. Tolerance of it leads to a positive identity. Some youths, however, cannot stand the ambiguity of indecision. This leads to premature foreclosure. The adolescent who makes choices too early or internalizes the choices of others may come to regret them and is especially vulnerable to identity confusion in later life.

## Cultural Identity

Cultural identity is that part of self-concept that comes from the knowledge and feelings about belonging to a particular cultural group. Cultural identity includes self-identification (whether I describe myself as Latino) and a sense of belonging (how close do I feel toward other people in my cultural group). It also involves an attitude toward and involvement with one's cultural group (Phinney, 1990). Adolescents growing up in a society in which the dominant culture differs from their culture of origin face additional challenges in creating and integrating a positive ethnic identity with a strong and positive self-identity. Such adolescents ask themselves not only, "Who am I?" but also such questions as "Who am I as an African American?" or "as a Latino?"

Experts believe that a positive sense of cultural identity can help adolescents feel good about themselves in the face of discrimination and threats from the larger society. Some findings suggest that higher levels of cultural identity are related to better psychological adjustment and higher self-esteem (Parham & Helms, 1985; Phinney, 1989, 1990; Phinney & Alipuria, 1990; Phinney & Chivira, 1995; Roberts et al., 1999). Ohye and Henderson Daniels (1999) believe that there is still much work needed to understand the complex issues of race, ethnicity, and class. These researchers suggest that studies of adolescent females have been largely restricted to white females (Ohye & Henderson Daniels, 1999).

## Gender Identity

Gender identity is a person's self-identification as male or female and results largely from those physical characteristics that are part of our biological inheritance—the traits that make us males or females. Genitals and facial hair are examples of characteristics that affect gender identity. Gender role, on the other hand, develops largely from the specific gendered traits that are considered mainstream at any given time in a given culture. For example, in our culture, expression of emotion differs by gender, although there is no known physical cause for this difference. Gender-role behavior is the extent to which a person's behaviors, occupations, and interests are considered masculine or feminine according to cultural norms. Sexual orientation refers to a person's choice of sexual partner of the same sex (homosexual), of the opposite sex (heterosexual), or both sexes (bisexual).

It is possible for people to accept or reject their gender identity and/or their gender role. Some people are perfectly happy with their gender identity, but do not like their culturally constructed gender role. Research indicates that while gender roles may be modified by differing cultural expectations, gender identity is fixed within the first 4 to 5 years of a child's development (Money &

Ehrhardt, 1972). Once a child's gender identity has been established, it is unlikely to change, even when biological problems occur. Even in extreme cases of chromosome failure, gender identity is not affected. In almost all cases, adolescents desperately want medical treatment so they can keep their gender identities. Although gender identity becomes fixed early in life, gender roles usually undergo changes as the individual matures. The relationships between the roles of our two genders also change and have altered considerably in the past few decades.

Pressures to behave in gender-appropriate ways often increase in adolescence. Carol Gilligan and colleagues (Brown & Gilligan, 1992; Gilligan, Lyons, & Hanmer, 1990) believe that this creates a dilemma for adolescent girls. Adolescent girls feel an increased need to conform to female gender-role expectations in order to be accepted by peers. They become aware that feminine interpersonal qualities are not as highly valued by society as masculine characteristics. Nolen-Hoeksema, Girgus, & Seligman (1991) suggest that adolescent girls who feel that they must hide their competence to win the acceptance of adolescent boys and adults also have feelings of hopelessness, helplessness, and depression. Pipher (1994) also suggests that there are risks to mental health when the true selves of adolescent girls become lost when young women are faced with the choice to be true to themselves or be accepted by others.

Recent literature and research looking at the development of boys (e.g., Pollack, 1998) suggests that societal expectations of gendered behavior limits boys as well as girls. Pollack (1998) describes what he calls the "boy code" as "the outdated and constricting assumptions, models, and rules about boys that our society has used since the nineteenth century" (p. 6). Pollack believes that the "boy code" places boys in what he calls a "gender straitjacket" (p. 6) and limits boys' ability to be as connected to others as they would like and need to be. Pollack also describes a "mask"

(p. 5) behind which boys hide their true feelings. He believes that boys become so good at wearing the "mask" that they are not necessarily even aware of their true feelings.

## Social Cognition, Egocentrism, and Self

Social cognition involves the thinking that we do about how we relate to others. Some theorists suggest that adolescents have a particularly idiosyncratic way of viewing the way they relate to others, which has been referred to as *adolescent egocentrism*, a term coined by Elkind (1978). For Elkind, the term adolescent egocentrism suggests that adolescents have a tendency to exaggerate the importance, uniqueness, and severity of social and emotional experiences. It also suggests that adolescents become very interested in and focused on themselves. This trait, which begins in early adolescence and becomes more prominent during the middle teen years (Elkind & Bowen, 1979), is composed, according to Elkind, of two specific factors: *imaginary audience* (Montgomery & others, 1996; Rycek, Stuhr, McDermott, Benker, & Schwartz, 1998; Vartanian, 1997) and *personal fable* (Vartanian, 1997). Adolescent egocentrism is an important construct for health care providers to understand because it may help to understand much of adolescent behavior, especially with regard to risk-taking behavior and compliance (or lack of compliance) with safety and health-related measures.

### THE IMAGINARY AUDIENCE

With increased interest in the self and a growing ability to imagine what others might think, which are both characteristics of adolescent cognitive development, adolescents often feel like they are "on stage." Performing for an imaginary audience, the adolescent's imagination often goes to extremes. Adolescents often begin to assume or imagine that everyone around is noticing and scrutinizing every aspect of behavior and appearance (Montgomery & others, 1996; Rycek, et al., 1998; Vartanian, 1997). It is not unusual for adolescents to believe with certainty that everyone around them notices each of their physical "imperfections" (e.g., a bad haircut, pimples, braces, glasses). It is also not unusual for adolescents to believe that others are staring at them. When watching adolescents in public places you may notice that they appear to behave as if they are on stage (singing or laughing loudly). Thus, the imaginary audience does not necessarily refer to negative attention but rather to the adolescent belief that they are always being watched and noticed. Adolescents may believe that notice brings acclaim and popularity in some situations and negative judgments causing them to be ostracized in others. When thinking about some aspects of health care we should consider the imaginary audience. If adolescents believe that others are always watching, they may not be likely to comply with health care regimens that they think will attract scrutiny or other negative attention. For example, diabetic adolescents (especially young adolescents) are loathe to test blood glucose (or have their diabetes mentioned) in any situation that includes their peers for fear of being viewed as freaks (Thies, 1996). By later adolescence, teens seem to be a bit more comfortable and are more willing to test blood glucose at least among friends or discreetly at the back of a classroom (Thies, 1996; Thies & Walsh, 1999).

## THE PERSONAL FABLE

In addition to the imaginary audience, there is a second component of adolescent egocentrism known as the personal fable. Many adolescents seem to make up stories about themselves, which become their own personal fables (Vartanian, 1997). These fables tend to involve the adolescents' belief that they are unique and therefore extremely different from people around them. As a result, they cannot believe that anyone else could possibly understand how they are feeling or relate to their experience. Thus, the feelings of uniqueness involved in the personal fable may contribute to a sense of being special and invincible but can also create a sense of isolation. These feelings become important to consider from a health care perspective.

For example, an adolescent struggling with a difficult family situation may feel very isolated, believing that nobody could possibly understand or relate to the experience. Similarly, a teen who is experiencing health problems may well believe that she or he is the only one in such a situation. Support groups for teens experiencing health issues may help to address these issues. On the other hand, the personal fable can pose a health care challenge because it may cause adolescents to believe that their uniqueness leads to invincibility. It can be difficult to convey the importance of safety precautions to adolescents because they seem often to believe that "it won't happen to me." This attitude potentially impacts adolescent behavior and may increase risk-taking behavior as teens may recognize risks to others but fail to acknowledge risks to themselves. Examples would include risky sexual behavior, drinking and driving, and drug experimentation.

An additional issue to explore when considering the personal fable as it relates to health care is the tendency to make heroes out of sick children and adolescents. Given the adolescent tendency to feel special and different, we might consider the wisdom of playing into this tendency especially if it becomes a setup for later disappointment. Although there are no simple, easy answers or solutions, it certainly seems worthy of consideration.

## PERSPECTIVE TAKING

Teenagers may have problems working with others because of their egocentric thinking. Robert Selman (1976, 1980) has added a great deal to Elkind's theory of adolescent egocentrism with his concept of perspective taking, which suggests the ability to look at a situation from another person's point of view. Perspective-taking is an important part of social cognition and seems to increase with cognitive development in adolescence. In some ways, perspective taking is the antithesis of egocentric thinking and may perhaps provide the antidote to some of the pitfalls of adolescent egocentrism. Understanding adolescent ability to engage in perspective taking can provide health care providers an opportunity to maximize communication with adolescents.

# Self-Esteem and Competence in Adolescence

Whereas self-concept answers the question "Who am I?", self-esteem answers the question "How do I feel about who I am?" Persons with high self-esteem like and accept themselves. According to Campbell and Lavallee (1993), well-defined self-concept leads to high self-esteem, which in turn often leads to successful behavior (Rosenberg, 1985). It is important to understand that identity development in general and the development of self-concept and self-esteem in particular occurs within the larger social and cultural context, where cultural and/or ethnic identity, sexual identity, and the impact of gender roles are also central to the adolescent's self-definition and self-evaluation.

Harter (1990; 1993; 1999; Harter, Whitesell, & Junkin 1998) suggests that, in general, high self-esteem results when teens are doing well in areas where success is important to them. For example, if appearance and athletics are important, adolescents must do well in those areas to feel good about themselves. Conversely, if success in a particular area is not considered important, doing poorly will not cause bad feelings. Harter's research suggests that physical appearance, being liked by others of the same age, and doing well in sports are most important to adolescent self-esteem. In recent work by Harter and colleagues (1998), teens with higher self-worth were more able to discount their weaknesses than were adolescents with lower feelings of self worth.

Positive self-esteem develops when parents, teachers, friends, and other people who are considered important believe in adolescents and expect them to succeed. Research also suggests that social support is an important variable in the development of self-esteem (DuBois, et al., 2002). During early adolescence, although the opinion of parents remains important, the importance of opinions of classmates and peers increases. Whereas for early adolescents, self-esteem depends heavily on the attitudes of others, older adolescents develop a firmer sense of their own beliefs and attitudes, so they are less dependent on the attitudes of others. Persons with low self-esteem seem to be most susceptible to the opinions of others in determining how they feel about themselves at a particular point in time (Campbell & Lavallee, 1993).

Harter's research (1993) suggests that the domains of competence rated least important by adolescents—doing well in school and behaving well—are those rated as most important by parents. This difference in priorities creates an obvious conflict and may pose a threat to self-esteem. Because perceived support and approval from both classmates and parents are central to adolescent self-esteem, balancing the priorities of each group can be a challenge. When adolescents forfeit competence or fail to meet expectations in areas deemed important by significant others, such as parents and peers, the adolescent may perceive an accompanying loss of support. Thus, the adolescent who disappoints parental expectations for school success may feel a loss of parental support and approval. Similarly, the adolescent who does not meet the expectations and social norms of peers may also experience a loss of support from peers. Interestingly, Markstrom (1999) has found that religious involvement is related to positive self-esteem. Perhaps religious involvement provides some adolescents with a sense of connection and belonging, which heightens feelings of support and approval and thus impacts self-esteem.

Self-esteem changes during adolescence. Petersen and associates (1991) and Brooks-Gunn (1991) suggest that many early adolescents experience "simultaneous challenges" that can negatively affect self-esteem. These challenges include social events such as changing schools, changes in parent–adolescent relationships, and biological changes associated with puberty. Physical maturation in early adolescence may also negatively affect self-esteem, especially in girls. Early adolescent girls may not be ready to deal with the new expectations people have of a person who has reached puberty (for example, an increased interest in the opposite sex). Eccles, Barber, Jozefowicz, Malenchuck, & Vida (1999) found that both boys and girls experience a decrease in self-esteem that coincides with the transition to middle or junior high school. Alerting parents, teachers, and other important adults to the developmental challenges often triggered by school transitions could enable the influential adults in the lives of adolescents to better support adolescents during these transitions.

## Gender and Self-Esteem

Many researchers have suggested that the level of self-satisfaction and self-esteem reported by adolescents is generally lower than that of elementary school children. However, the decline in self-satisfaction and self-esteem is greater for adolescent girls (Gilligan et al., 1990). Eccles and colleagues (1999) noted that adolescence presents risks and opportunities for both boys and girls. These researchers found that girls' self-esteem dropped more than boys'; however, they found that both boys and girls suffer from decreases in self-esteem. Interestingly, these researchers further suggest that girls seem to be more negatively affected by failures and concern about failures than boys. This finding would suggest that girls might be less likely than boys to try new things or take risks, which in turn could limit their future academic and career possibilities.

From a health care perspective it would be important to think about the implications for engaging in risk-taking behavior. Kling, Hyde, Showers, & Buswell (1999) reviewed a large number of studies on gender differences in self-esteem and found that male scores were higher on standard measures of global self-esteem but that the gender differences were relatively small. This finding would suggest that there has been more attention paid to the relatively small gender differences than to the relatively large gender similarities.

A number of explanations have been given for adolescent gender differences in self-esteem. Eccles and colleagues (1999) believe that puberty places young women at increased risk because of the narrow standards of beauty in American society. In addition, they found that many adolescent girls still believe that high achievement conflicts with what is considered femininity. Brooks-Gunn (1991) suggests that girls who experience high levels of conflict in the parent–daughter relationship and are early maturers appear to be at greatest risk for greatest loss in self-esteem and psychological distress during adolescence. Early maturation means that these girls are experiencing weight gain earlier than their peers, thereby increasing dissatisfaction with physical appearance. Petersen and associates (1991) point out that girls often mature earlier than boys and are more likely to experience puberty prior to the transition to middle school. Girls, therefore, are more at risk because they experience both puberty and school change at the same time.

Sadker and Sadker (1991) suggest that many educational practices and teacher behaviors negatively affect the self-esteem and academic achievement of girls. Boys, for example, are often given more attention and instruction by teachers and parents. Girls often receive praise for the neatness and appearance of their work, whereas boys receive more praise for the quality of their ideas. Girls seem to be rewarded for silence and passivity. Boys conclude that adults hold males in higher regard. Girls, on the other hand, learn that adults assume females cannot achieve at the same level as males.

*Gender Gaps,* a 1999 report published by the American Association of University Women (AAUW) as a follow-up to the 1992 AAUW report *How Schools Shortchange Girls,* suggests that although there has been some improvement in terms of gender equity in schools, gaps remain. Consequently, young women remain at high risk for decreased self-esteem. The above findings certainly suggest that gender role socialization and societal expectations play a crucial role in the development of self-esteem. This is a potentially an important finding from the perspective of intervention because roles and expectations, though entrenched, can be changed, and parents and other meaningful adults in the lives of adolescents can be instructed about the importance of such change.

Carol Gilligan and colleagues (1990) believe that adolescent girls often conceal their true feelings, which results in loss of self-esteem. The researchers found that at age 11, the girls expressed their opinions with much self-confidence. By age 15 and 16, the girls were much less certain and answered many questions by saying, "I don't know." Gilligan and colleagues believe that adolescent girls hold back their real feelings, especially anger or resentment, in order to obtain approval, popularity, and attention at home and at school. In her best-selling book *Reviving Ophelia,* Mary Pipher (1994) also suggests that the true selves of adolescent girls may become lost when young women are faced with the choice to be true to themselves or be accepted by others. This concealment of real feelings can have important implications for health care. If girls learn that they must always be quiet, calm, kind, and offer socially acceptable answers to questions, they may be unwilling and eventually unable to share their true feelings. This could prevent accurate assessment of both physical and mental health situations.

## Race and Self-Esteem

Research on the self-esteem of racial minorities has focused on African American youths. Early research assumed that poverty, low status, and perceived discrimination would result in low self-esteem. In an early study, Clark and Clark (1947) found African American children more interested in playing with white dolls than with dolls of their own color. This was interpreted as evidence of low self-esteem. Those results have since been interpreted as a reflection more of the racial prejudice of society and less of the children's feelings about themselves. Most recent studies suggest that there are no self-esteem differences among racial and ethnic groups (Phinney & Rosenthal, 1992). Phinney and Rosenthal (1992) further suggest that the self-esteem of ethnic and racial minorities is influenced by a number of factors including the achievement of a committed ethnic identity, the presence of a strong and positive ethnic community with which to become involved, and gender-role expectations.

Recent research indicates that African American girls showed no evidence of decline in self-esteem at early adolescence (Eccles et al., 1999). In fact, these researchers found that African American girls have higher self-esteem than European American girls and African American boys. African American girls scored higher on measures of confidence in their femininity, masculinity, popularity, and physical attractiveness, whereas their European American counterparts scored higher on measures of worry about weight and social self-consciousness (Eccles et al., 1999). These differences suggest that the drop in self-esteem often linked with early adolescence is not inevitable but rather is socially constructed. Again, this speaks to the importance of intervention and education. Parents, caregivers, educators, and health care providers need to acknowledge the power of societal messages. Media, for example, is pervasive and powerful, replete with messages about what young people should look like and how they should behave.

## Self-Concept and Social Competence

Although social competence has been defined in a variety of ways, the simplest definition is the ability to interact effectively with others. Socially competent people are able to make and keep friends and to accomplish their goals when relating to others. For adolescents, social competence is an important part of self-concept. Among the eight dimensions of adolescent self-concept identified by Harter (1990), social acceptance by peers together with physical appearance were most related to feelings of positive self-esteem. Adolescents who feel accepted by their peer group and their parents are likely to feel good about themselves.

Adolescents with low self-esteem are more likely to be disliked and rejected by peers. They are more likely to be shy and are less likely to be selected as leaders in clubs and social activities. Difficulties in social competence are not likely to disappear after adolescence. Growing research evidence suggests that adolescents who have poor peer relationships are more likely to have adjustment difficulties in adulthood.

Identity involves exploration (a loosening of parental control) and commitment (self-defined and integrated). Independence need not be the only end product; interdependence and connection have an important part in maturity for both men and women. Many psychologists view the self as the foundation of mental health. According to Carl Rogers (1971), for example, people feel good about themselves when their view of themselves fits well with the feedback they get from those around them. Psychological difficulties develop when parents, teachers, siblings, and friends are unwilling to accept a person the way he or she is. Rogers went so far as to argue that "unconditional positive regard," which means total acceptance of the child as a person, is necessary to the development of a psychologically healthy self.

The teen who confronts the multiple changes of adolescence with a healthy sense of self is better prepared to meet the challenges that accompany this period of rapid physical and psychological change. We need to consider the many changes that take place during adolescence.

# Families and Peers

As adolescents spend less time with the family and more time interacting with the larger world, they encounter a broader range of values and ideas. In conjunction with the cognitive changes occurring during adolescence, the exposure to different ideas often contributes to an examination of parental values and teachings. As a result, adolescents begin to question and challenge parental views and develop ideas of their own. No longer are parents viewed as all-knowing authorities. Optimally, over time, adolescents develop more mature and realistic views of their parents as persons with particular skills, talents, and knowledge, who deserve their respect but who can also make mistakes.

## Autonomy and Support Within Families

Reaching a state of psychological autonomy is an important developmental task for adolescents. Disagreement exists, however, about the type of family environment that is most conducive to the development of autonomy. Traditional psychoanalytic theorists (Blos, 1979; Freud, 1958) have long argued that the development of healthy autonomy is achieved through a loosening of family ties. More recently, theorists and researchers (Grotevant & Cooper, 1986; Larose & Boivin, 1998; Sim, 2000; Youniss, 1989) have argued that healthy autonomy is promoted by positive and supportive parental relationships. Thus, it is connection to and support from parents that allows for the expression of both positive and negative feelings, which foster social competence and personal responsibility.

## CONFLICT

Adolescence is often stereotypically described as a period of storm and stress, rebellion, and conflict with parents and other adults. This belief is based mainly on early theories, popularized by G. S. Hall and Sigmund and Anna Freud. Anna Freud (1969a) who studied troubled adolescents, noted that conflict with parents was common and concluded that was a normal and necessary part of adolescence. She believed that the biological changes of puberty set off this conflict, which was needed so that adolescents could become independent from their families. Adolescents who got along well with their parents were thought to be immature. A different view has been suggested by research with normal adolescents (Arnett, 1999). Such research has suggested that the majority of adolescents admire their parents, turn to them for advice, and feel loved by them. Families reporting significant difficulties with adolescents often also had problems before their children reached adolescence. Ary, Duncan, Duncan, & Hops (1999) found that families experiencing high levels of conflict were more likely to have low levels of parent–child involvement.

Conflict, especially when dealt with appropriately and productively within the context of meaningful connection, is not necessarily problematic. Laursen (1995) suggests that some conflict is part of all significant interpersonal relationships in which mutual needs must be negotiated. Sagrestano, McCormick, Paikoff, & Holmbeck (1999) found that parents reported more conflict than their children did, which suggests that adults and teens may assess conflict differently. Laursen, Coy, & Collins (1999) also suggest that there are multiple dimensions to conflict: *conflict rate, conflict affect* (or intensity), and *total conflict.* These researchers found that amount of conflict decreases from early to late adolescence but that the intensity of the remaining conflict increases from early to middle adolescence.

Minor conflicts and disagreements with parents may actually help adolescents to establish in-

dependence (Smetana, Yau, Restrepo, & Braeges, 1991). Conflict may help adolescents to develop interpersonal negotiation skills and independent thinking, as long as the argument takes place within a supportive and accepting family environment (Allen, Hauser, Bell, & O'Connor, 1994; Hauser & Bowlds, 1990). When parents are hostile, the adolescent is likely to feel rejected and avoid further discussion and interaction with parents. From this perspective, the critical issue is not that minor conflicts take place, but how adolescents and their parents interact to resolve these conflicts. Source of conflict, type of conflict, and ability to resolve conflict along with degree of family connectedness and support are important considerations for health care providers who may be asked to assess adolescent–parent situations.

Although the research suggests that most parents and adolescents do not fight excessively, there is evidence that conflict increases somewhat in early adolescence for a brief period of time. In many families, early adolescence is a period of bickering and squabbling (Steinberg, 1981, 1987, 1988). In general, early adolescents express less affection toward their parents, spend less time with them, and bicker more when they are together. Arguments between adolescents and parents generally decline toward the end of puberty. Although these arguments seem to support the psychoanalytic belief that the changes of puberty trigger conflict, such conflicts tends to be minor and are not like the storm and stress described by G. S. Hall and Sigmund and Anna Freud. It is important to note that bickering often takes place while adolescents are still quite close to their parents. Some theorists believe that this helps adolescents to make new close friendships outside the family without breaking family ties (Steinberg, 1990).

Petersen (1985), however, believes that it is overlapping factors rather than puberty itself that cause parent–child conflicts in early adolescence. Life changes, such as a change of school, are taking place in the adolescent's life. Middle school poses new challenges, and adolescents face many new expectations socially and academically. Meeting these new expectations combined with the stresses of puberty can also create risks for depression and other mental health concerns (Ge, Conger, & Elder; 2001). Dekoric, Noom, & Gordon (1997) found that parents and adolescents had consistently different expectations of developmental tasks and that level of conflict was associated with these differences in developmental expectations. Adolescents often feel ready to make decisions for themselves, whereas parents and caregivers appropriately feel that adolescents are still in need of structure and guidance. For example, an adolescent may feel that a curfew of 11:00 p.m. is overly restrictive, whereas a caregiver believes that such a curfew is reasonable and wise. Again, the differing expectations of adolescents and adults as a natural source of conflict is important to note for health care providers.

## ATTACHMENT TO PARENTS

It seems clear that some degree of discord between parents and adolescents is likely to occur occasionally. Feelings of support and connection to parents as well as ability to resolve conflict appear to help adolescents develop a healthy sense of psychological autonomy (DuBois et al., 2002). Allen and colleagues (1994) maintain that parent–adolescent relationships that are characterized by both autonomy and support are most healthy for adolescent development. Larose and Boivin (1998) found that teens with perceived security to parents at the end of high school maintained this feeling of security even after leaving home for college. In addition, these feelings of security were positively associated with emotional adjustment outside the family. Therefore, helping parents and teens to forge supportive relationships would seem a worthwhile goal.

These findings are consistent with attachment theory (Ainsworth, Blehar, Walters, & Wall, 1978; Bowlby, 1969). Attachment theory (see Chapter 6) has been popular in helping psychologists, educators, and other scientists understand parent–child relationships during early childhood. According to this view, a trusting relationship with one's parent or caretaker gives the child feelings of security and self-confidence. Parents who are sensitive, warm, and responsive to their young children and who support their independence help them develop secure attachments. In this model, independence results from closeness and secure attachment.

Attachment theory has also been applied to parent–adolescent relationships. Research has suggested that when teens develop more friends outside the family, they do not cut themselves off from their families. Furthermore, their ties to parents do not make them dependent. Rather, when adolescents feel that their parents believe in them and will help them out if they need it, they may be more self-confident and more willing to try new activities. Research indicates that adolescents with secure parental attachment have higher self-esteem and are more socially competent than those with insecure attachments (Armsden & Greenberg, 1987; Kenny, 1987; Kenny & Donaldson, 1991; Kobak & Sceery, 1988). In addition, secure parental attachments may contribute to positive views of self and lower levels of depressive symptoms among adolescent boys and girls (Kenny, Moilanen, Lomax, & Brabeck, 1993).

## Friends, Peers, and Risk-Taking Behavior

In adolescence, the young person is more likely to confide feelings and problems to close friends than to parents. Appropriate parental monitoring and guidance around peer issues can help to protect teens from some of the risks of increased peer influence (Bogenschneider, Wu, Raffaelli, & Tsay, 1998; Flannery, Williams, & Vazsonyi, 1999). Lack of parental or adult supervision and monitoring in the after-school hours can have negative effects on adolescent behavior and peer relationships. Young teens who lack adult supervision are more likely to engage in risk-taking behaviors and get into trouble (Bogenschneider et al., 1998; Flannery et al., 1999). In addition, young adolescents can be astute about whether their parents agree with each other around issues of child rearing (Johnson, Shulman, & Collins, 1991; Scaramella, Conger, & Simons, 1999; Steinberg, 1987). Thus, parents must develop the skills necessary to cooperate around child-rearing issues. When parents are able to make these adjustments, they are better able to manage the conflicts that occur in this area (Jacobson & Crockett, 2000; Paikoff & Brooks-Gunn, 1991; Steinberg, 1987).

Older views of adolescence, especially Erikson's, Anna Freud's, and Blos' theories, stress that emotional separation from parents should be the goal of adolescence. From these perspectives, identity is formed through detaching emotionally from the family and shifting affection to peers. Within the framework of these principles, an adolescent who is respectful of parents and emotionally attached to them is considered to lack maturity (Baumrind, 1991a). Several sociologists and psychologists have criticized this view because it emphasizes the value of separation from others and downplays the need in humans at all stages of life for connectedness and a sense of community (Bellah, Madsen, Sullivan, Swidler, & Tipton, 1985; Gilligan, 1982; Gilligan et al., 1990; Kenny, 1987; Kenny & Donaldson, 1991; Lasch, 1979, Pollack, 1998; Pipher, 1994).

### IDENTIFYING WITH PEERS

Peer pressure and group conformity can produce both positive and negative influences on adolescent friendships. Involvement in antisocial or delinquent behavior, beginning to smoke and use alcohol or other drugs, becoming prematurely sexually active, or limiting one's efforts in school to prevent being ostracized are all risk factors of adolescent peer pressure. Involvement in community service and other idealistic causes, avoidance of drugs and alcohol, as well as interest in school achievement can also be related to (positive) peer pressure. Recent research suggests that parent involvement and supervision is a key variable when considering the impact of peer pressure (Bogenschneider & others, 1998; Flannery & others, 1999).

Pombeni and others (1990) confirmed that adolescents usually choose to associate and identify with those who are like themselves, and who have similar problems, values, and hopes for the future. It appears that teens who suffer the insecurity of scant or absent emotional support from parents are willing to pay a higher price for acceptance by peers. Given the importance of friendships during adolescence, Brendgen and colleagues (2000) compared teens with deviant friends, teens without deviant friends, and teens with no friends. These researchers found that adolescents with deviant friends tended to be delinquent more often than teens without deviant friends. They also found that teens with deviant friends were as likely as teens with no friends to be depressed. The crowd that an adolescent associates with allows her or him to try out a particular identity (Brendgen et al., 2000; Kinney, 1999).

Peers can give young adolescents a clearer idea of how they appear to others at a time when they are very sensitive to the imagined judgments of others (Pugh & Hart, 1999; Talwar, Nitz, & Leruer, 1990). Peers may also give much appreciated support and encouragement in times of difficulty, especially those times when parents are not made aware of the problem. The quality of relationships established in the teenage years has been shown to continue to have an effect much later in life (Pugh & Hart, 1999). Thus, issues of peers and peer pressure have long-term implications.

## Dating Behaviors

In earlier childhood, cross-gender friendships to the exclusion of same-gender friendships can be a source of social difficulty, but by adolescence this difficulty is no longer apparent (Kuttler, La Greca, & Prinstein, 1999). Before graduating from high school, most adolescents have entered into dating relationships (Savin-Williams & Berndt, 1990). Dating can refer to group activities or single-couple experiences. Montgomery and Sorell (1998) found that amount of dating experienced varied by age. Adolescents reported being "in love" about half of the times they reported being in an ongoing relationship. Interestingly, the researchers also found that boys reported falling in love earlier and more often than girls.

Perceptions of dating and romance seem to be age and gender related. Young adolescents may confuse cross-gender friendships and romantic relationships, but this distinction is clarified by late adolescence (Shulman & Scharf, 2000). Younger adolescents, especially girls, often develop crushes on an older adolescent or adult. Crushes seem to provide a means of expressing affection to someone outside the immediate family. They are generally intensely felt, but do not last long because other crushes take their place. During early adolescence, the object of affection (a crush or sweetheart) often is not even aware of this admiration. By mid-adolescence, both partners are generally aware of the other's affection. There is an increased openness and communication of affection between partners. Steady dating is most common among late adolescents.

# Adolescents and Sexuality

Adolescence is accompanied by increases in sexual arousal, interest, and behavior. Increased interest in sexuality results from both biological and social factors. Hormonal changes, for example, stimulate sexual interest and motivation. They also contribute to changes in physical appearance and attractiveness to members of the opposite sex. Changes in physical appearance and attractiveness indirectly affect sexual behavior as young adolescents suddenly find themselves becoming the objects of sexual attention. Social factors, including expectations and controls that limit opportunities for sexual behavior, also have an influence on the ways in which sexual interest is expressed.

The timing and incidence of sexual expression is largely determined by sociocultural norms. Considerations, therefore, of what is normal sexual behavior and desirable types and levels of sexual expression at different ages are related to sociocultural norms and moral and ethical belief systems (Miller & Dyk, 1993). Cultural changes of the last 40 years, commonly referred to as the sexual revolution, have changed some cultural norms regarding sexual expression and behavior. Although sexuality is a normal part of adolescent development, sexual behavior is accompanied by significant risks.

## Heterosexual Behavior

*Heterosexuality* is the preference for intimate interpersonal relationships and sexual interaction with members of the opposite sex. Adolescent heterosexual behavior most often begins with less intimate behaviors and progresses to higher levels of intimacy. Findings from studies (McCabe & Collins, 1984; Smith & Udry, 1985) reveal that noncoital behaviors, such as hugging and kissing, then fondling and petting, typically precede sexual intercourse. In general, boys report greater desire for sexual intimacy on a first date than do girls. As girls' commitment to a relationship increases, however, their desire for sexual intimacy generally increases, becoming similar to the desires reported by boys. However, some researchers (Tolman, 1999) believe that insufficient attention has been paid to desire in adolescent girls because the assumption is often made that adolescent boys are interested in sex and adolescent girls are interested in love.

Looking at adolescent attitudes toward timetables for sexual activity, Feldman, Turner, & Araujo (1999) found that most participants believed that sexual activity should happen with serious rather than casual partners. Paradoxically, most participants also reported that their own sexual activity had often been with casual partners. This finding raises important questions about the possible discrepancy between attitudes toward sexual activity and actual behavior. By the middle to late teens, most adolescents have engaged in a fairly predictable sequence of sexual experiences, often including sexual intercourse.

Although sexuality develops throughout life, first intercourse is viewed by most as the key moment in sexual development. When this moment occurs is influenced by numerous factors. For example, the more the adolescent engages in risk behaviors such as drug and alcohol abuse and delinquency, the earlier first intercourse is likely to take place (Santelli, Brener, Lowry, Bhatt, & Zabin, 1998; Savin-Williams, 1994). The statistics about age at first intercourse vary, but all research confirms that this experience occurs at a younger age than it did for previous generations (Besharov & Gardiner, 1997; Carnegie Corporation, 1995). One difficulty with such research is that it relies on self-report, which is often not reliable. In a recent study of honesty in self-reporting, Siegel D. (1998) found that some middle school students admitted that they had not been honest when completing a sexual behavior questionnaire. The researchers found that 78% of middle school boys and 94% of girls reported honesty; 14% of the boys who admitted dishonesty overstated their sexual behavior and 8% of the girls admitting dishonesty understated their behavior.

## FACTORS THAT CONTRIBUTE TO HETEROSEXUAL ACTIVITY

There are numerous opinions about why youngsters are engaging in sexual behavior at earlier ages. Some theorists point to changes in social context and suggest that adolescents today learn about sexuality much earlier and from more sources than in the past. Sexually explicit magazines, rock music videos, advertisements displaying sexual situations, movies depicting sexually graphic material, and the Internet are all part of the everyday culture. The women's movement and its focus on double standards about acceptable sexual behavior for women versus men also con-

tributed to the social context of teens today. However, when adolescents are asked to explain how they decided to first have sex, they do not say "the social context." Instead they talk about relationships and their own sense of their developing self. Tolman (1999) believes that we need to pay closer attention to the relational aspects of sexuality in order to better understand teen sexual behavior.

Many studies have found that family as well as other environmental factors influence adolescent sexual activity (Lammers, Ireland, Resnick, & Blum, 2000). Lammers and colleagues (2000) found that dual-parent families, higher socioeconomic status, academic achievement, religiosity, feeling cared for by parents and other adults, and high parental expectations were all associated with later onset of sexual activity. It is important to remember that these are not causal factors but rather variables that have been found to be associated with sexual activity.

A number of studies have looked at the relationship between sexual communications among family members and sexual behavior (Dittus, Jaccard, & Gordon, 1999; Feldman & Rosenthal, 2000; Raffaelli, Bogenschneider, & Flood, 1998; Whitaker & Miller, 2000). All have found that parents can have a powerful effect on their children's behavior, including those who are in their late teens, when the parent–child interaction is good and talk about sexuality is direct. This is an important finding with implications for parenting and health care situations. The meaningful adults in the lives of adolescents must be willing to speak with adolescents about sexuality and sexual behavior, but parents and other caregivers often feel uncomfortable in such situations. Health care providers can model appropriate communication skills around sensitive topics and open lines of communication.

## Homosexual Behavior

Although most research on adolescent sexuality and sexual behavior focuses on heterosexual teens, not all adolescent sexual activity is between males and females. Same-gender sexual activity often occurs as part of the adolescent process of sexual exploration. For most children from the age of 7 to about 13, best friends, the ones with whom they dare to be intimate, are people of the same sex. Feelings become especially intense between ages 10 and 12 when young people enter puberty and feel a growing need to confide in others. It is only natural that they are more trusting with members of their own sex who share their experiences. Occasionally these close feelings result in overt sexual behavior. One study found this to be true more than one-third of the time (Janus & Janus, 1993). In most cases, this behavior results from curiosity rather than from a homosexual orientation.

Sexual behavior thus differs from sexual orientation or identity. A *homosexual* is a person who prefers sexual interaction and intimate, interpersonal relationships with members of the same sex. The majority of persons who come to identify themselves as homosexual have engaged in heterosexual sex, usually during adolescence (Savin-Williams, 1998). Some youths become aware of their homosexual orientation before engaging in homosexual sex or even in any sexual activity at all (Savin-Williams & Rodriguez, 1993). By late adolescence and young adulthood, sexual orientation determines the gender of a sexual partner on a much more consistent basis. Research suggests that one's sexual orientation as either heterosexual, homosexual, or bisexual develops gradually from childhood through adulthood, with approximately 8 to 10 percent of young people in the United States identifying themselves as homosexual or bisexual at some point in their lives (D'Augelli, 1988). Unfortunately, gays, lesbians, and bisexuals live in a society full of stereotypes about homosexuality. These stereotypes create increased risk for gay and lesbian adolescents.

## SELF-AWARENESS OF HOMOSEXUALITY

Historically, psychologists believed that homosexuality did not emerge until adulthood. Studies of male homosexuals reviewed in the *Journal of the American Medical Association* (Remafedi, 1988),

however, indicate that this belief was the result of interviews with teens, most of whom were ashamed or otherwise unwilling to tell about their feelings on the subject. Beaty (1999) found that gay teens with close relationships to parents came out sooner than those teens who did not feel close to their parents. This finding would reinforce the idea that lack of disclosure or later disclosure is not necessarily a reflection of later emergence of homosexuality. Boxer, Cook, & Herdt (1999) studied self-identification of 202 gay and lesbian adolescents ages 14 to 20. These researchers found a mean age of 16.7 for males and 16.0 for females for self-identification. This finding suggests that many young people may self-identify as gay or lesbian long before they disclose their homosexuality to others.

Current studies are in remarkable agreement that at least one-third of all males have had "a homosexual experience that resulted in an orgasm" at least once during their adolescent years. About 10% "are exclusively homosexual for at least three years between the ages of 16 and 55" (p. 222). Janus and Janus (1993) found that 22% of men and 17% of women have had at least one homosexual experience. On the other hand, other studies have found that only 1% are exclusively homosexual throughout life (Muir, 1993).

Savin-Williams and Rodriguez (1993) believe that the age at which youths become aware of their homosexuality is dropping because of the increased visibility of gays and lesbians in our culture. Although most gays and lesbians are aware of their sexual feelings and orientations during adolescence, most do not disclose this to others until the college years or later. According to one study of gay college men, fewer than half had disclosed that they were gay to family members (D'Augelli, 1993). Parents are often not the first people to whom a gay or lesbian adolescent discloses, nor are siblings (Savin-Williams, 1998). Mothers are often told before fathers, and mothers report knowing about their children's sexual orientation (whether or not they have been told) more often than fathers (Savin-Williams, 1998).

Savin-Williams (1998) believes that disclosure to family members is one of the most critical events in the life of a gay or lesbian teen.

People who achieve an early and positive acceptance of their gay or lesbian identity evidence high self-esteem (Beaty, 1999; Boxer et al., 1999). It is not clear whether coming to terms with one's sexual identity enhances feelings of self-esteem or whether those with high self-esteem are better able to accept their homosexual identity (Savin-Williams & Rodriguez, 1993). It is clear, however, that developing a healthy sexual identity and maintaining positive self-esteem are often more complicated for the gay or lesbian adolescent, who must struggle with problems of stigma and stereotypes. Communication of one's sexual orientation to significant others is important to the development of a positive gay or lesbian identity. The psychological distress that accompanies the process of achieving a gay or lesbian identity is less when the environment is accepting of homosexuality (Boxer, Cohler, Herdt, & Irvin, 1993). Adolescents who have difficulty accepting their own homosexuality or fear the consequences of revealing their homosexuality to others may lie or conceal their sexual orientation. This occurs at great cost to feelings of self-esteem and well-being.

### REVEALING HOMOSEXUAL ORIENTATION

Revealing a homosexual orientation is accompanied with significant risks, however. Loss of friendships, threats to physical safety, loss of parental emotional and financial support, and restriction of career choices are some of the possible consequences. Because of the risks of self-disclosure and the importance of support, it may not be wise to pressure adolescents to acknowledge and reveal their homosexual orientation before they are ready (Savin-Williams, 1998; Savin-Williams & Rodriguez, 1993). There is some evidence that younger gay or bisexual male adolescents (those less than 18 years old) whose parents have knowledge of their child's sexuality may suffer more negative psychosocial consequences—such as having higher rates of substance abuse, dropping out of school, or requiring psychiatric hospitalization—compared to their older (18 years and older) gay peers (Remafedi, 1988). Among older adolescents and young adults, self-disclosure of one's sexual orientation to parents and feelings of psychological well-being are associated with secure parental attachments (Beaty, 1999; Holtzen, Kenny, & Mahalik, 1995).

Homosexuality poses special problems and risk factors for teens. In response to societal stereotypes and prejudices, gay males and lesbians frequently express feelings of isolation from family, peers, and social/educational institutions (Boxer et al., 1999; D'Augelli & Rose, 1990; Martin & Hetrick, 1988). Social isolation and a lack of identity with other people have been associated with suicide, for which gay and lesbian adolescents appear to be at risk (Savin-Williams, 1994). Trotter (1999) suggests that gay and lesbian youth are two to six times more likely to attempt suicide and that 30% of gay and bisexual men have attempted suicide. Lock and Steiner (1999) found that gay, lesbian, and bisexual adolescents were at increased risk for problems of both mental and physical health. It is important to remember that those psychological difficulties experienced by some gay and lesbian teens are because of societal prejudices and stressors, not because homosexuality is a mental illness. There is little institutional support for homosexual youths. Schools often do not recognize the existence of homosexual adolescents (Boxer et al., 1999). Clearly, health care providers must explore their own assumptions about homosexuality so that they can develop supportive attitudes and behaviors toward gay and lesbian adolescents.

## Sex Education

The term "sex education" usually suggests courses taught at schools, and although these courses might be one means of educating children and adolescents about sex, it should not be the only means. Health care providers could play an important role in helping children and adolescents develop healthy attitudes, accurate information, and good decision-making strategies. Peers are usually reported to be the most common source of sex information for adolescents. This is a definite problem because peers are often an inaccurate source of information (Treboux & Busch-Rossnagel, 1990). Additionally, teens are likely to act according to how they believe their friends are acting, and yet their perceptions of their friends actions may be inaccurate (Brooks-Gunn & Paikoff, 1993).

For example, the notion that "everybody is doing it" may cause teens to engage in sexual behavior to "be like everybody else" when, in fact, everybody is not doing it. Young teens also learn about sex and sexuality through media exposure. Today's teens have access to a tremendous amount of sexually explicit material and information (Carpenter, 1998). Unfortunately, the media's portrayal of sex and sexuality is often incomplete, with little focus on relationships, responsibility, and consequences.

Many parents of adolescents today may be responding to pressures and concerns about teenage sexuality. Such parents strive to model openness in talking about sex. However, even parents who want to be able to discuss sex with their children may not always communicate openly. Feldman and Rosenthal (2000) found that parents and adolescents evaluated parent communication about sex differently. They found that parents evaluated their communication more positively than their teens. Parents may believe that they are effectively communicating with their adolescents, but adolescents may not feel that the communication is effective. This gap in communication may be due in part to a lack of practice in and comfort with talking about sex. Here too, health care providers can be helpful in providing guidance for parents about how to approach sensitive topics and conversations.

# Teen Pregnancy and Parenthood

Teen pregnancy is one of the obvious risks of adolescent sexual behavior. Although pregnancy is not the only risk and not all sexually active adolescents become pregnant, approximately half of all first pregnancies happen within 6 months after sexual activity begins. Many teens continue not to use birth control after their first sexual experience (Roye, 1998). It seems that many of the factors that influence whether teens use birth control are the same as those that influence sexual activity. Teens who do not get along with their parents, who are not doing well in school, and whose friends are teenage parents are less likely to use birth control methods. Teenagers who are able to talk with their parents about sexuality and family planning are more likely to use birth control consistently and effectively (Jorgensen, 1993). Unclear understanding about how and when pregnancy occurs also results in poor use of birth control. Feelings of guilt and fear and concerns about the negative effects of contraceptives lead some adolescents away from their use. Because sexual desire among girls is generally not acknowledged, some adolescent girls have few strategies for handling it (Brooks-Gunn & Paikoff, 1993).

Girls are frequently portrayed as the victims of male sexual desires. They are responsible for protecting themselves from the sexual advances of their male companions. Interestingly, while traditional social controls, such as adult supervision and chaperoning may no longer exist, feelings about obtaining birth control remain ambivalent. As a result, many adolescent girls and boys continue to engage in unprotected sexual activity.

Most of what we know about teenagers' attitudes about birth control has been learned from teenage girls; we know very little about boys' attitudes. Boys may know little about reproduction, the menstrual cycle, and contraceptive methods (Blau & Gullotta, 1993). Given that a single male teenager has the potential to impregnate multiple teenage girls, and that both males and females are involved in sexual activity that leads to pregnancy, we cannot afford to place the entire burden on girls and ignore adolescent boys in our research and contraceptive education. Health care providers can be wonderful sources of information and education for both male and female adolescents.

## Teen Parenthood

Teen parenthood is a major health care concern in our society. Although teenage parenthood was not uncommon in the past, the number of unmarried teenage parents remains high and creates risks for the parent(s) who are still teens, as well as for their children. Interestingly, we often make the assumption that when teenagers become pregnant the pregnancy is accidental. However, it is important to recognize intentional teen pregnancy as a growing area of social concern that needs to be addressed. Many young teenage mothers view having a child as a way to meet their needs for love and affection (Corcoran, Frankline, & Bell, 1997). Pregnancy may also be seen as a way to maintain a relationship. Sadly, adolescents alienated from their families and desperately in need of support and connection may see having a child as a way to create a loving relationship that is otherwise absent in their lives (Williams & Vines, 1999).

The solution to the problem of teenage pregnancy and parenthood is not a simple one. To solve the problem we must address issues of access and power. In addition, we have to solve problems of education and poverty regardless of race and socioeconomic status. However, from a more immediate standpoint, we must also address the many adolescent myths at play around sexual behavior. Health care providers can be important agents for addressing these myths.

For example, many teens believe that they cannot get pregnant having sex for the first time. It is important to remember, as mentioned above, that approximately half of all first pregnancies happen within 6 months after sexual activity begins and that many teens continue not to use birth control after their first sexual experience (Roye, 1998). Others believe that using contraception may diminish sexual pleasure. Many others have not developed skills or had practice talking about sexual relationships and are therefore uncomfortable talking to partners about using contraception.

Beyond pregnancy prevention, we must also consider ways to help teenage mothers provide their babies with the needed emotional, intellectual, and physical care while also enabling the mothers to continue their education. These factors often make a difference in the future of the mothers and their children. Increased attention must also be paid to the often forgotten adolescent fathers who may or may not be involved in the lives of the children they were instrumental in helping to create.

### TEENAGE FATHERS

Whether a teenage father remains involved with his child may also depend on support from his own family and the family of the teenage mother (Furstenberg, 1994). Family members typically give opinions as to whether the pregnancy should be terminated and whether they believe the relationship between the teenage parents will survive. The mother's family, believing the father will not be reliable, may be quick to point out his failings. They may be protective of their daughter and grandchild. The father's family may warn the father of the difficulties of parenting and suggest that he may not actually even be the father. When both families offer support, because they approve of the father or believe it is in the newborn child's best interest, fathers are more likely to remain involved.

## Adolescent Victimization

Unfortunately, the victimization of adolescents is common (Elders & Albert, 1998). Adolescents are at risk for victimization, including rape and sexual assault, from a variety of sources including family members, friends, and strangers (Miller & Dyk, 1993). Dating violence mirrors trends in domestic violence (Sousa, 1999). These unwanted experiences are clearly not a normal or desirable part of adolescent sexuality.

## Sexual Abuse

Sexual experiences among young adolescents are often forced. At age 13 and younger, more than 60% of sexually experienced girls report forced intercourse. That rate drops to 25% at age 15 and 10% at age 16 (Alan P. Guttmacher Institute, 1994). Although the legal definitions of rape and sexual assault vary from state to state, they usually include nonconsent of the victim, penetration, and the use of threat, force, deception, or intimidation. Difficulties that victims might have in or ambivalence that they may feel about reporting rape further complicate situations.

Adolescents are typically abused by someone they know and trust (Miller & Dyk, 1993). It is often just a continuation of abuse that started during childhood. The victim is often manipulated into believing it is all her fault, and this manipulation serves to maintain both silence and abuse. Sadly, adolescents who are victims of sexual abuse may run away, and adolescent runaways are then at risk for many other forms of victimization, including prostitution. Sexual victimization before adolescence also contributes to the risk for delinquency as well as other risks for other emotional and physical difficulties in adolescence (Elders & Albert, 1998; Widom, 1994). Elders and Albert (1998) believe that improved identification by health care professionals of victims and those at high risk of victimization could help us better understand and intervene to help victims receive professional attention earlier, which may alter the long-term effects of abuse.

## Dating Violence

According to Sousa (1999), dating violence is "The Hidden Epidemic" and can be defined as physically or emotionally aggressive behavior that occurs within the context of a single date or dating relationship. Dating violence often goes unreported, and, as a result, occurrence statistics are difficult to compile. Dating violence is much more common than most adults like to believe and, unfortunately, is often ignored and/or minimized (Sousa, 1999). Sadly, many teen victims feel that they will not be believed or that they will be blamed for their victimization and therefore do not seek help. Some researchers suggest that both male and female adolescents are equally at risk for dating violence (Molidor & Tolman, 1998). However, females are much more likely than males to be victims of severe violence. Females also report more serious physical and emotional consequences of dating violence (Molidor & Tolman, 1998). Teen dating violence tends to mirror adult domestic violence and can include emotional and verbal abuse, physical assault, rape, and murder (Sousa, 1999).

There is a pressing need for more training of parents, educators, health care providers, and court officers around the recognition and treatment of victims of teen dating violence. Although dating violence may be difficult to recognize because it may be covert (emotional rather than physical) and because the individuals involved may go to great lengths to hide the truth, there are warning signs. Certainly any sign of physical maltreatment should be carefully investigated. In addition, possessive behavior, which teens sometimes mistake as a sign of caring, can be a warning sign of an abusive dating relationship or a dating relationship that is escalating toward violence. Teens who have been threatened by a date or partner may be afraid to come forward to ask for help and may also dismiss or refuse offers for help. Adults must be sensitive and insightful about possible situations of dating violence.

## Date/Acquaintance Rape

Acquaintance rape generally occurs within the context of adolescent social activities. The aggressor is typically a boyfriend or a more casual acquaintance of approximately the same age. Because this type of rape often occurs within a dating relationship, it is sometimes referred to as date rape. Being raped by a dating partner or friend is no less damaging psychologically than being raped by a stranger (Davis, Peck, & Storment, 1993). In most cases, females are the victims, but there are incidents of male victimization as well (Miller & Dyk, 1993). Acquaintance rape occurs with disturbing frequency among high school students. Davis and colleagues (1993) obtained questionnaire data from 237 9th- to 12th-grade high school students in three metropolitan Louisiana high schools, with 20% reporting that they had been involved in a situation where sex was forced. This was more common among girls (26%) than boys (11%). Only half of the teenagers reporting the experience of forced sex had told anyone of their experience. In another high school survey, Feltey, Ainslie, & Gleib (1991) found similarly that 20% of high school students had engaged in sex when they did not want to.

Because so many adolescents do not disclose their abuse experience, professionals working with teens should be alert to behavioral signs of sexual victimization. Some adolescents showing symptoms of depression, psychosomatic illness, irritability, avoidance of men, loss of confidence, nightmares, fears of going outside or inside, or anxiety may be reacting to an acquaintance rape. Cultural beliefs and myths about the appropriate sexual behavior are partially blamed for the prevalence of acquaintance rape (Workman & Freeburg, 1999). Many of these myths likely contribute to the incidence of date rape.

Boys and men are more likely to agree with rape-tolerant attitudes than are girls and women (Holcomb, Holcomb, Sondag, & Williams, 1991). Sixty percent of the high school boys surveyed by Davis and associates (1993) indicated that it is acceptable for a boy to force sex on a girl in some situations, such as when the couple had been dating

for a while or had had sex in the past. Other common reasons given by high school students for justifying sexual coercion include the girl's behavior (she has done this with other guys; she is wearing sexy clothes; she says no but does not push him away), use of drugs or alcohol, and opportunity for the sexual relationship to take place (she goes to his house when his parents are not home or she invites him to her house when her parents are not home) (Feltey et al., 1991).

The beliefs used to justify sexual coercion reflect traditional sexual stereotypes regarding the uncontrollable sexual urges of males and an entitlement to sex based on length of dating relationship or amount of money spent. Girls are blamed for seducing boys and not recognizing the power of male sexuality. Among college-age men, almost one-half have reported that some women ask for and enjoy rape, one-third agreed that sexual aggression is closely tied to masculinity, and one-quarter agreed that rape is often provoked by women (Holcomb et al., 1991). Date rape prevention programs have been designed to alter the beliefs that perpetuate date rape. But true change will only come as the myths and beliefs in our broader society change.

# Adolescent Stress and Resilience

There are many stressors that can be present challenges for adolescents. Among the challenges adolescents face are coping with the bodily changes of puberty, adjusting to cognitive changes, developing new ways of relating with peers and family, dealing with sexual and other moral dilemmas, completing academic requirements, and planning for a future occupation. Although these are normal developmental tasks, they can be sources of stress for most adolescents.

In addition to developmental stressors, many adolescents also experience additional conflict because of changes in the family such as parental divorce, illness, or death. Hartos and Power (1997) believe that parents are not necessarily aware of the stress that adolescents feel. Studying mothers and adolescents, they found that teens reported more stress than their mothers reported for them. Adults often underestimate the stress of children and adolescents by suggesting that it will all pass. Open parent–child communication is an important factor when considering healthy development and adolescent stress is one more example.

In a longitudinal study of 10th-grade students, McFarlane, Bellissimo, Norman, & Lange (1994) found that stressful life events were both a risk and consequence of depression, suggesting a reciprocal interaction between the individual and the environment. This study suggests that some stressful life events are as much a consequence as a cause of behavioral and adjustment problems (Masten & Neeman, 1994). For example, the stressful life events of getting a poor grade in school, getting in trouble with the law, and becoming pregnant may be a consequence of antisocial behavior and learning or adjustment problems. Those events might also be explained by impulsive and aggressive personality characteristics, which are symptoms of mental disorders. When adolescents who are already troubled experience more negative life events, their stress levels and problems only increase.

We are all aware of short-term physical upsets such as fainting, rapid heartbeat, stomach aches, and nausea caused by the strains of everyday life. Many of these reactions are impairing. Daniels and Moos (1990) found that depressed youths reported more major stressors and daily hassles than healthy youths. Biederman and Spencer (1999) found that a history of stress is common with depressed young people. However, the researchers believe that the relationship between depression and stress is still unclear. Stress may precipitate depression in some people but depression itself may be a stressor. Youths with behavioral problems reported more parent and school stressors than healthy youths.

What makes one person handle difficult life stress better than another person? One answer is practice. Success with similar situations leaves a person with some experience and confidence to draw on in coping with a new stressful situation. The person is less rattled and is able to think more clearly and respond more logically to the situation. Social support has also been found to be an important factor in a person's ability to remain composed and to adapt successfully to stressful situations (DuBois et al., 2002).

Some people handle stress better than others, and researchers have been looking at the methods and the coping strategies that people use to cope with stress. Differences in coping may determine whether stress has negative psychological effects. Coping is defined as any effort used in response to stressful events (Compas, 1987). Coping can involve healthy productive behaviors as well as unhealthy behaviors (e.g., substance use). Coping may also be approach oriented, that is, dealing directly with the source of stress or its consequences, or avoidance oriented, denying or withdrawing from the source of stress and its consequences.

According to Ebata and Moos (1995), problem-focused coping efforts are generally approach oriented. Some emotion-focused coping strategies, such as trying to see the bright side of a problem, are approach oriented, whereas other emotion-focused strategies, such as trying to forget the situation, are avoidance oriented. Approach-oriented strategies generally produce better solutions or outcomes than do avoidance-oriented strategies. Ebata and Moos also found that older adolescents use more approach-oriented coping than younger adolescents. Adolescents who use approach-oriented strategies also believe they have some control over the stressors and have good sources of social support.

Patterson and McCubbin (1987) interviewed high school students to ask about common coping startegies. The most common coping strategies mentioned were relaxing (listening to music), developing independence, being optimistic, and making close friends. Females more often than males mentioned seeking social support, turning to family members to solve problems, making close friends, and being self-reliant. Ventilating feelings (swearing, blaming others for what's going wrong, and getting angry and yelling at people) and investing in close friends (being with a girlfriend or boyfriend and being close to someone you care about) were the most frequent coping strategies of adolescents who use drugs and alcohol. Friendships were probably related to substance abuse because most teens use drugs and alcohol with friends. Friends may also be important in persuading a teen to experiment with drugs.

Turning to family to solve problems, seeking spiritual support, and engaging in demanding activity appear to be coping strategies that help adolescents keep away from drug use. Recklitis and Noam (1999) found that avoidance and ventilation were associated with more behavior problems, whereas problem solving and the use of interpersonal skills were associated with fewer problem behaviors. They also found that girls were more likely to use interpersonal coping strategies, and boys were more likely to engage in physical activity as a coping strategy. Frydenberg and Lewis (1999) also found some gender differences in coping with girls using more self-blame and boys using physical activity to avoid dealing with a problem. McFarlane and colleagues (1994) found that teens who viewed their parents and siblings as sources of support were at low risk for the development of depression in adolescence.

Supportive family environments that provide feelings of warmth and closeness are often a protective factor for at-risk adolescents. Parents of resilient adolescents combine support and understanding with supervision of their children's activities and consistent discipline (see Chapter 4 on resilience). Most resilient adolescents have been able to establish a close relationship with at least one family member, either a parent, grandparent, aunt, brother, or sister. That family member is es-

pecially important in providing care, attention, and guidance when there is marital conflict or parental psychopathology (Werner, 1990; 1995). Werner and Johnson (1999) believe that we must make use of what we have learned about resilience to inform our practice with vulnerable children.

Resilient adolescents are also able to obtain support through the social network outside the family. A school in which teachers and counselors are closely involved with students can contribute to resilience. Relationships with caring adults including health care providers, older friends, and peers can provide the support needed by adolescents in coping with stress in their lives.

# Conclusion

The developmental tasks of adolescence are numerous. Issues of self and identity overlap with negotiating family and peer relationships. Changes in physical development present challenges, and cognitive changes are associated with growth in the ways that adolescents think about themselves and their relationships with others. Despite adolescent desire for greater independence, research suggests that continued connection to meaningful adults is important for healthy development. With greater understanding of adolescent development, health care providers can better meet the needs of adolescents. It is important for us, as adults, to listen carefully when we talk with adolescents. It is also important for us to ask appropriate questions when talking with adolescents. Most importantly, we must and consider the many developmental challenges faced by adolescents in light of their idiosyncratic way of thinking when we develop education, prevention, and intervention programs.

# References

Ainsworth, M. D. S., Blehar, M. C., Walters, E., & Wall, S. (1978). *Patterns of attachment: A psychological study of the strange situation.* Hillsdale, NJ: Erlbaum.

The Alan P. Guttmacher Institute. (1994). *Sex and America's teenagers.* New York: The Alan P. Guttmacher Institute.

Allen, J. P., Hauser, S. T., Bell, K. L., & O'Connor, T. G. (1994). Longitudinal assessment of autonomy and relatedness in adolescent-family interactions as predictors of adolescent ego development and self-esteem. *Child Development, 65,* 179–194.

Armsden, G. C., & Greenberg, M. T. (1987). The inventory of parent and peer attachment: Individual differences and their relationship to psychological well-being in adolescence. *Journal of Youth and Adolescence, 16,* 427–454.

Arnett, J. J. (1999). Adolescent storm and stress, revisited. *American Psychologist, 54,* 317–326.

Baumrind, D. (1991a). Effective parenting during the early adolescent transition. In P. A. Cowan & M. Hetherington (Eds.), *Family transitions* (pp. 111–163). Hillsdale, NJ: Erlbaum.

Beaty, L. A. (1999). Identity development of homosexual youth and parental and familial influences on the coming out process. *Adolescence, 34,* 597–601.

Bellah, R., Madsen, R., Sullivan, W., Swidler, A., & Tipton, S. (1985). *Habits of the heart: Individualism and commitment in American life.* Berkeley: University of California Press.

Besharov, D., & Gardiner, K. (1997). Trends in teen sexual behavior. *Children and Youth Services Review, 19,* 341–367.

Biederman, J., & Spencer, T. (1999). Depressive disorders in childhood and adolescence: A clinical perpsective. *Journal of Child and Adolescent Psychopharmacology, 9,* 233–237.

Blau, G. M., & Gullotta, T. P. (1993). Promoting sexual responsibility in adolescence. In T. P. Gullotta, G. R. Adams, & R. Montemayor (Eds.), *Adolescent sexuality, advances in adolescent development: An annual book series, Volume 5* (pp. 181–203). Newbury Park, CA: Sage.

Blos, P. (1979). *The adolescent passage.* New York: International Universities Press.

Bogenschneider, K., Wu, M., Raffaelli, M., & Tsay, J. (1998). "Other teens drink, but not my kid": Does parental awareness of adolescent alcohol use protect adolescents from risky consequences? *Journal of Marriage and the Family, 60,* 356–373.

Bogenschneider, K., Wu, M., Raffaelli, M. & Tsay, J. C. (1998). Parent influences on adolescent peer orientation and substance use: The interface of parenting practices and values. *Child Develoipment, 69,* 1672–1688.

Bowlby, J. (1969). *Attachment and loss. Volume I: Attachment.* New York: Basic Books.

Boxer, A. M., Cohler, B. J., Herdt, G., & Irvin, F. (1993). Gay and lesbian youth. In P. H. Tolan & B. J. Cohler (Eds.), *Handbook of clinical research and practice with adolescents* (pp. 249–280). New York: John Wiley.

Boxer, A. M., Cook, J. A. & Herdt, G. (1999). Experience of coming out among gay and lesbian youth: Adolescents alone? In J. Blustein, & C. Levine (Eds.), *The adolescent alone: Decision making in health care in the United State* (pp. 121–138). New York: Cambridge University Press.

Brooks-Gunn, J. (1991). How stressful is the transition to adolescence for girls? In M. E. Colten & S. Gore (Eds.), *Adolescent stress: Causes and consequences* (pp. 131–149). Hawthorne, NY: Aldine de Gruyter.

Brooks-Gunn, J., & Paikoff, R. L. (1993). Sex is a gamble, kissing is a game: Adolescent sexuality and health promotion. In S. G. Millstein, A. C. Petersen, & E. O. Nightingale (Eds.), *Promoting the health of adolescents: New directions for the twenty-first century* (pp. 180–208). New York: Oxford University Press.

Brown, L. M., & Gilligan, C. (1992). *Meeting at the crossroads: Women's psychology and girls' development.* Cambridge, MA: Harvard University Press.

Campbell, J. D., & Lavallee, L. F. (1993). Who am I? The role of self-concept in understanding the behavior of people with low self-esteem. In R. F. Baumeister (Ed.), *Self-esteem: The puzzle of low self-regard* (pp. 3–20). New York: Plenum Press.

Carnegie Council on Adolescent Development. (1995). *Great transitions: Preparing adolescents for a new century.* New York: Carnegie Corporation.

Carpenter, L. (1998). From girls into women: Scripts for sexuality and romance in Seventeen magazine, 1974–1994. *Journal of Sex Research, 35,* 158–168.

Clark, K., & Clark, M. (1947). Racial identification and preference in Negro children. In T. Newcomb & E. Hartley (Eds.), *Readings in social psychology* (pp. 551–560). New York: Holt.

Compas, B. (1987). Coping with stress during childhood and adolescence. *Psychological Bulletin, 101,* 393–403.

Daniels, D., & Moos, R. (1990). Assessing life stressors and social resources among adolescents. *Journal of Adolescent Research, 5,* 268–289.

D'Augelli, A. R. (1993). Gay men in college: Identity processes and adaptation. In R. A. Pierce and M. A. Black (Eds.), *Life-span development: A diversity reader* (pp. 190–208). Dubuque, IA: Kendall/Hunt.

D'Augelli, A. R., & Rose, M. L. (1990). Homophobia in a university community: Attitudes and experiences of heterosexual freshmen. *Journal of College Student Development, 31,* 484–491.

D'Augelli, D. A. (1988). The adolescent closet: Promoting the development of the lesbian or gay male teenager. *The School Psychologist, 42,* 2–3.

Davis, T. C., Peck, G. Q., & Storment, J. M. (1993). Acquaintance rape and the high school student. *Journal of Adolescent Health, 14,* 220–224.

Dekoric, M., Noom, M. J. & Meeus, W. (1997). Expectations regarding development during adolescence: Parental and adolescent perceptions. *Journal of Youth and Adolescence, 26,* 253–272.

Dittus, P., Jaccard, J., & Gordon, V. (1999). Direct and nondirect communication of maternal beliefs to adolscents: Adolescent motivations for premarital sexual activity. *Journal of Applied Social psychology, 29,* 1927–1963.

DuBois, D., Burk-Braxton, C., Swenson, L., Tevendale, H., Leckerd, E., & Moran, B. (2002). Getting by with a little help from self and others: Self-esteem and social supports as resources during early adolescents. *Developmental Psychology, 38,* 822–839.

Ebata, A., & Moos, R. H. (1994). Personal, situational, and contextual correlates of coping in adolescence. *Journal of Research on Adolescence, 4,* 99–125.

Eccles, J., Barber, B., Jozefowicz, D., Malenchuck, O., & Vida, M. (1999). Self evaluations of competence, task values and self esteem. In N. Johnson, M. Roberts, & Worell, J. (Eds.), *Beyond appearance: A new look at adolescent girls.* Washington, DC: APA.

Elders, J., & Albert, A. (1998). Adolescent pregnancy and sexual abuse. *Journal of the American Medical Association, 280,* 648–649.

Erikson, E. (1958). *Young man Luther: A study in psychoanalysis and history.* New York: W.W. Norton.

Erikson, E. (1959). Identity and the life cycle. *Psychological Issues, 1,* 18–164.

Erikson, E. (1963). *Childhood and society* (2nd ed.). New York: W.W. Norton.

Erikson, E. (1968). *Identity: Youth and crisis.* New York: W.W. Norton.

Erikson, E. (1969). *Gandhi's truth: On the origins of militant nonviolence.* New York: W.W. Norton.

Erikson, E. (1975). *Life, history and the historical moment.* New York: W.W. Norton.

Elkind, D. (1978). Understanding the young adolescent. *Adolescence, 13,* 127–134.

Elkind, D., & Bowen, R. (1979). Imaginary audience behavior in children and adolescents. *Developmental Psychology, 15,* 38–44.

Erikson, E., & Coles, R. (2000). *The Erik Erikson reader.* NY: W.W. Norton.

Feldman, S. S., & Rosenthal, D. A. (2000). The effect of communication characteristics on family members' perceptions of parents as sex educators. *Journal of Research on Adolescence, 10 (2),* 119–150.

Feldman, S. S., Turner, R. A., & Araujo, K. (1999). Interpersonal context as an influence on sexual timetables of youth: Gender and ethnic differences. *Journal of Research on Adolescence, 9,* 25–52.

Feltey, K. M., Ainslie, J. J., & Gleib, A. (1991). Sexual coercion attitudes among high school students. *Youth & Society, 23,* 229–250.

Flannery, D. J., Williams, L. L., & Vazsonyi, A. T. (1999). Who are they with and what are they doing? Delinquent behavior, substance abuse and early adolescents' after school time. *American Journal of Orthopsychiatry, 69,* 247–253.

Freud, A. (1958). Adolescence. In R. Eissler, E. Glover, E. Kris, H. Hartmann, P. Greenacre, and W. Hoffer (Eds.), *The psychoanalytic study of the child.* New York: International Universities Press.

Freud, A. (1968). Adolescence. In A. E. Winder and D. L. Angus (Eds.), *Adolescence: Contemporary studies.* New York: American Book.

Freud, A. (1969a). Adolescence as a developmental disturbance. In G. Kaplan and S. Lebovici (Eds.), *Adolescence: Psychosocial perspectives.* New York: Basic Books.

Freud, A. (1969b). Adolescence as a psychological disturbance. In G. Kaplan & S. Lebovici (Eds.), *Adolescence: Psychosocial perspectives.* New York: Basic Books.

Frydenberg, E., & Lewis, R. (1999). Things don't get better just because you are older: A case for facilitating reflection. *British Journal of Educational Psychology. 69,* 81–94.

Furstenberg, F. F. (1994). Fathering in the inner city: Paternal participation and public policy. In W. Marsiglio (Ed.), *Fatherhood: Contemporary scholarship* (pp. 118–147). Newbury Park, CA: Sage.

Furstenberg, F. F. (1994). History and current status of divorce in the United States. *Future of Children, 4,* 29–43.

Ge, X., Conger, R., & Elder, G. (2001). Pubertal transition, stressful life events, and the emergence of gender differences in adolescent depressive symptoms. *Developmental Psychology, 37,* 404–417.

Gilligan, C. (1982). *In a different voice. Psychological theory and women's development.* Cambridge, MA: Harvard University Press.

Gilligan, C., Lyons, N. P., & Hanmer, T. J. (1990). *Making connections: The relational worlds of adolescent girls at Emma Willard School.* Cambridge, MA: Harvard University Press.

Grotevant, H. D., & Cooper, C. R. (1986). Individuation in family relationships. *Human Development, 29,* 82–100.

Harter, S. (1990a). Self and identity development. In S. Feldman & G. Elliott (Eds.), *At the threshold: The developing adolescent.* Cambridge, MA: Harvard University Press.

Harter, S. (1990b). Processes underlying adolescent self-concept formation. In R. Montemayor, G. R. Adams, & T. P. Gullotta (Eds.), *From childhood to adolescence: A transitional period? Advances in adolescent development, Volume 2* (pp. 205–239). Newbury Park, CA: Sage.

Harter, S. (1993). Causes and consequences of low self-esteem in children and adolescents. In R. F. Baumeister (Ed.), *Self esteem: The puzzle of low self regard* (pp. 87–116). New York: Plenum Press.

Harter, S. (1999). *The construction of the self: A developmental perspective.* NY: Guilford.

Hartos, J., & Power, T. (1997). Mothers' awareness of their early adolescents' stressors: Relation between awareness and adolescent adjustment. *Journal of Early Adolescence, 17,* 371–389.

Hauser, S. T., & Bowlds, M. K. (1990). In S. Feldman and G. Elliot (Eds.), *At the threshold: The developing adolescent.* Cambridge, MA: Harvard University Press.

Holtzen, D. W., Kenny, M. E., & Mahalik, J. R. (1995). Contributions of parental attachment to gay or lesbian disclosure to parents and dysfunctional cognitive processes. *Journal of Counseling Psychology, 42,* 350–355.

Jacobson, K., & Crockett, L. (2000). Parental monitoring and adolescent adjustment: An ecological perspective. *Journal of Research on Adolescence, 10,* 65–97.

James, W. (1890/1950). *The principles of psychology.* New York: Dover.

Janus, C. J., & Janus, S. S. (1993). *The Janus Report on Sexual Behavior.* New York: John Wiley.

Johnson, B., Shulman, S., & Collins, W. A. (1991). Systemic patterns of parenting as reported by adolescents: Developmental differences and implications for psychosocial outcomes. *Journal of Adolescent Research, 6,* 235–252.

Jorgensen, S. R. (1993). Adolescent pregnancy and parenting. In T. P. Gullotta, G. R. Adams, & R. Montemayor (Eds.), *Adolescent sexuality, advances in adolescent development: An annual book series, Volume 5* (pp. 103–140). Newbury Park, CA: Sage.

Kenny, M. E. (1987). The extent and function of parental attachment among first-year college students. *Journal of Youth and Adolescence, 16,* 17–27.

Kenny, M. E., & Donaldson, G. (1991). Contributions of parental attachment and family structure to the social and psychological functioning of first-year college students. *Journal of Counseling Psychology, 38,* 479–486.

Kenny, M. E., Moilanen, D., Lomax, R., & Brabeck, M. M. (1993). Contributions of parental attachments to view of self and depressive symptoms among early adolescents. *Journal of Early Adolescence, 13,* 408–430.

Kinney, D. (1999). From "headbangers" to "hippies": Delineating adolescents' active attempts to form an alternative peer culture. In McLellan, J. & Pugh, M. J. (Eds.), *The role of peer groups in adolescent social identity: Exploring the importance of stability and change. New directions for child and adolescent development,* Volume 84 (pp. 21–35). CA: Jossey-Bass.

Kling, K., Hyde, J., Showers, C., & Buswell, B. (1999). Gender differences in self-esteem: A meta-analysis. *Psychological Bulletin, 125,* 470–500.

Kobak, R., & Sceery, A. (1988). Attachment in late adolescence: Working models, affect regulation, and representation of self and others. *Child Development, 59,* 135–146.

Kuttler, A., La Greca, A. & Prinstein, M. (1999). Friendship qualities and social emotional functioning of adolescents with close, cross-sex friendships. *Journal of Research on Adolescence, 9,* 339–366.

Lammers, C., Ireland, M., Resnick, M., & Blum, R. (2000). Influences on adolescents' decision to postpone onset of sexual intercourse: A survival analysis among youths aged 13 to 18 years. *Journal of Adolescent Health, 26,* 42–48.

Larose, S., & Boivin, M. (1998). Attachment to parents, social support expectations and socioemotional adjustment during the high school-college transition. *Journal of Research on Adolescence, 8,* 1–27.

Lasch, C. (1979). *The culture of narcissism: American life in an age of diminishing expectations.* New York: Warner.

Laursen, B. (1995). Conflict and social interaction in adolescent relationships. *Journal of Research on Adolescence, 5,* 55–70.

Laursen, B., Coy, K. C., & Collins, W. A. (1999). Reconsidering changes in parent-child conflict across adolescence: A meta-analysis. *Child Development, 69,* 817–832.

Lock, J., & Steiner, H. (1999). Gay, lesbian and bisexual youths risks for emotional and social problems: Results from a community based survey. *Journal of the American Academy of Child and Adolescent Psychiatry, 38,* 297–304.

Markstrom, C. (1999). Religious involvement and adolescent psychosocial development. *Journal of Adolescence, 22,* 205–221.

Martin, A. D., & Hetrick, E. S. (1988). The stigmitization of the gay and lesbian adolescent. *Journal of Homosexuality, 15,* 163–183.

Masten, A. S., Neeman, J., & Andenas, S. (1994). Life events and adjustment in adolescents: The significance of event independence, desirability, and chronicity. *Journal of Research on Adolescence, 4,* 71–98.

McCabe, M. P., & Collins, J. K. (1984). Measurement of depth of desired and experienced sexual involvement at different stages of dating. *Journal of Sex Research, 20,* 377–390.

McFarlane, A. H., Bellissimo, A., Norman, G. R., & Lange, P. (1994). Adolescent depression in a school-based community sample: Preliminary findings on contributing social factors. *Journal of Youth and Adolescence, 23,* 601–620.

Miller, B. C., & Dyk, P. A. (1993). Sexuality. In P. H. Tolan & B. J. Cohler (Eds.), *Handbook of clinical research and practice with adolescents* (pp. 95–123). New York: John Wiley.

Molidar, C., & Tolman, R. M. (1998). Gender and contextual factors in adolescent dating violence. *Violence Against Women, 4,* 180–194.

Money, J., & Ehrhardt, A. (1972). *Man & woman/boy and girl.* New York: New American Library.

Montgomery, R., Haemmerlie, F., & Zoellner, S. (1996). The imaginary audience. *Psychological Reports, 79(3),* 783–786.

Montgomery, M. J., & Sorell, G. (1998). Love and dating experience in early and middle adolescence: Grade and gender comparisons. *Journal of Adolescence, 21,* 677–689.

Muir, J. (1993, March 31). Homosexuals and the 10 percent fallacy. New York: The New York Times.

Nolen-Hoeksema, S., Girgus, J., & Seligman, M. P. (1991). Sex differences in depression and explanatory style in children. *Journal of Youth and Adolescence, 20,* 233–245.

Ohye, B., & Henderson Daniels, J. (1999). The "other" adolescent girls: Who are they? In N. Johnson, M. Roberts, & J. Worell (Eds.), *Beyond appearance: A new look at adolescent girls.* Washington, DC: APA.

Paikoff, R., & Brooks-Gunn, J. (1991). Do parent-child relationships change during puberty? *Psychological Bulletin, 110,* 47–66.

Parham, T., & Helms, J. (1985). Attitudes of racial identity and self-esteem of black students: An exploratory investigation. *Journal of College Student Personnel, 26,* 143–147.

Patterson, J., & McCubbin, H. I. (1987). Adolescent coping style and behaviors: Conceptualization and measurement. *Journal of Adolescence, 10,* 163–186.

Petersen, A. C. (1985). Pubertal development as a cause of disturbance: Myths, realities and unanswered questions—genetic, social, and general. *Psychology Monographs, 111,* 205–232.

Petersen, A., Kennedy, R., & Sullivan, P. (1991). Coping with adolescence. In Cohen, M., and Gore, S., *Adolescent Stress.* NY: Aldine.

Phinney, J. (1989). Stages of ethnic identity in minority group adolescents. *Journal of Early Adolescence, 9,* 34–49.

Phinney, J. (1990). Ethnic identity in adolescents and adults. *Psychological Bulletin, 108,* 499–514.

Phinney, J. S., & Alipuria, L. L. (1990). Ethnic identity in college students from four ethnic groups. *Journal of Adolescence, 13,* 171–183.

Phinney, J. S., & Chavira, V. (1995). Parental ethnic socialization and adolescent coping with problems related to ethnicity. *Journal of Research on Adolescence, 5,* 31–54.

Phinney, J. S., & Rosenthal, D. (1992). Ethnic identity in adolescence: Process, context, and outcome. In G. R. Adams, T. P. Gullotta, & R. Montemayor (Eds.), *Adolescent identity formation: Advances in adolescent development* (pp. 145–172). Newbury Park, CA: Sage.

Pipher, M. (1994). *Reviving Ophelia: Saving the souls of adolescent girls.* New York: Ballantine Books.

Pollack, W. (1998). *Real Boys.* NY: Henry Holt.

Pugh, M., & Hart, D. (1999). Identity development and peer group participation. In J. A. McLellan & M. Pugh (Eds.), *The role of peer groups in adolescent social identity: Exploring the importance of stability and change. New directions for child and adolescent development,* Volume 84 (pp. 55–70). San Francisco: Jossey-Bass.

Raffaelli, M., Bogenschneider, K., & Flood, M. F. (1998). Parent-teen communication about sexual topics. *Journal of Family Issues, 19,* 315–333.

Recklitis, C., & Noam, G. (1999). Clinical and developmental perspectives on adolescent coping. *Child Psychiatry and Human Development, 30,* 87–101.

Remafedi, G. (1988). Homosexual youth. *Journal of the American Medical Association, 258,* 222–225.

Roberts, R. E., Phinney, J., Masse, L., Chen, Y., Roberts, C. R., & Romero, A. (1999). The structure of ethnic identity of young adolescents from diverse ethnocultural groups. *Journal of Early Adolescence, 19,* 301–322.

Rogers, C. (1971). Facilitating encounter groups. *American Journal of Nursing, 71,* 275–279.

Rosenberg, M. (1985). Self-concept and psychological well-being in adolescence. In Robert L. Leahy (Ed.), *The development of self.* Orlando, FL: Academic Press.

Roye, C. (1998). Condom use by Hispanic and African American adolescent girls who use hormonal contraception. *Journal of Adolescent Health, 23,* 205–211.

Rycek, R., Stuhr, S., McDermott, J., Benker, J., & Schwartz, M. (1999). Adolescent egocentrism and cognitive functioning during late adolescence. *Adolescence, 33,* 745–749.

Sadker, M., & Sadker, D. (1991). The gender gap in self-esteem, achievement and instruction. *Communique, 4,* 27.

Sagrastano, L., McCormick, S., Paikoff, R., & Holmbeck, G. (1999). Pubertal development and parent-child conflict in low-income, urban, African American adolescents. *Journal of Research on Adolescence, 9,* 85–107.

Santelli, J., Brener, N., Lowry, R., Bhatt, A., & Zabin, L. (1998). Multiple sexual partners among U.S. adolescents and young adults. *Family planning perspectives. 30,* 271–275.

Savin-Williams, R. C. (1994). Verbal and physical abuse as stressors in the lives of lesbian, gay male, and bisexual youths: Associations with school problems, running away, substance abuse, prostitution, and suicide. *Journal of Consulting and Clinical Psychology, 62,* 261–269.

Savin-Williams, R. C. (1998). The disclosure to families of same-sex attractions by lesbian, gay and bisexual youth. *Journal of Research on Adolescence, 8,* 49–68.

Savin-Williams, R. C., & Berndt, T. J. (1990). Friendship and peer relations. In S. Feldman and G. Elliot (Eds.), *At the threshold: The developing adolescent.* Cambridge, MA: Harvard University Press.

Savin-Williams, R. C., & Rodriguez, R. C. (1993). A developmental, clinical perspective on lesbian, gay male and bisexual youths. In T. P. Gullotta, G. R. Adams, & R. Montemayor (Eds.), *Adolescent sexuality, advances in adolescent development: An annual book series, Volume 5* (pp. 77–101). Newbury Park, CA: Sage.

Scaramella, L. V., Conger, R. D., & Simons, R. L. (1999). Parental protective influences and gender-specific increases in adolescent internalizing and externalizing problems. *Journal of Research on Adolescence, 9,* 111–141.

Selman, R. L. (1976). Social-cognitive understanding. In T. Lickona (Ed.), *Moral development and behavior.* New York: Holt, Rinehart & Winston.

Selman, R. L. (1980). *The growth of interpersonal understanding: Developmental and clinical analysis.* New York: Academic Press.

Shulman, S., & Scharf, M. (2000). Adolescent romantic behaviors and perceptions. *Journal of Research on Adolescence,* 10(1), 99–118.

Siegel, D., Aten, M., & Roghmann, K. (1998). Self-reported honesty among middle and high school students responding to a sexual behavior questionnaire. *Journal of Adolescent Health, 23,* 20–28.

Siegel, J. M., Aneshensel, C. S., Taub, B., Cantwell, D., & Driscoll, A. K. (1998). Adolescent depressed mood in a multi-ethnic sample. *Journal of Youth and Adolescents, 27,* 413–427.

Sim, T. (2000). Adolescent psychosocial competence: The importance and role of regard for parents. *Journal of Research on Adolescence, 10,* 49–64.

Smetana, J., Yau, J., Restrepo, A., & Braeges, J. (1991). Conflict and adaptation in adolescence: Adolescent-parent conflict. In M. F. Colten & S. Gore (Eds.), *Adolescent stress: Causes and consequences.* New York: Aldine de Gruyter.

Smith, F., & Udry, J. R. (1985). Coital and non-coital sexual behaviors of white and black adolescents. *American Journal of Public Health, 75,* 1200–1203.

Smith, E., Udry, J. R., & Morris, N. (1985, September). Pubertal development and friends: A biosocial explanation of adolescent sexual behavior. *Journal of Health and Social Behavior, 26,* 183–192.

Sousa, C. (1999). Teen dating violence: The hidden epidemic. *Family and Conciliation Courts Review, 37,* 356–374.

Steinberg, L. (1981). Transformations in family relations at puberty. *Developmental Psychology, 17,* 833–840.

Steinberg, L. (1987). Impact of puberty on family relations: Effects of pubertal status and pubertal timing. *Developmental Psychology, 23,* 451–460.

Steinberg, L. (1988). Reciprocal relation between parent-child distance and pubertal maturation. *Developmental Psychology, 24,* 122–128.

Steinberg, L. (1990). Autonomy, conflict, and harmony in the family relationship. In S. Feldman and G. Elliot (Eds.), *At the threshold: The developing adolescent.* Cambridge, MA: Harvard University.

Talwar, R., Nitz, K., & Leruer, R. (1990). Relations among early adolescent temperament, parent and peer demands, and adjustment: A test of the goodness of fit model. *Journal of Adolescence, 13,* 279–298.

Theis, K. (1996). A developmental perspective on stress appraisal: How children understand the everyday challenges of living with a chronic health condition. In L. Powers, G. Singer, & J. Sowers (Eds.), *Making our way: Building self competence among youth with disabilities* (pp. 97–114). Baltimore: Paul Brookes Publishing.

Theis, K., & Walsh, M. E. (1999). A developmental analysis of cognitive appraisal of stress in children and adolescents with chronic health conditions. *Children's Health Care, 28,* 15–32.

Tolman, D. (1999). Female adolescent sexuality in relational context: Beyond sexual decision making. In N. Johnson, M. Roberts, & J. Worell (Eds.), *Beyond appearance: A new look at adolescent girls* (pp. 227–246). Washington, DC: APA.

Treboux, D., & Busch-Rossnagel, N. (1990). Social network influences on adolescent sexual attitudes and behaviors. *Journal of Adolescent Research, 5,* 175–189.

Trotter, J. (1999). Lesbian and gay issues in work with young people: Are schools "out" this summer? *British Journal of Social Work, 29,* 955–961.

Vartanian, L. (1997). Separation-individuation, social support, and adolescent egocentrism: An exploratory study. *Journal of Early Adolescence, 17,* 245–270.

Werner, E. E. (1990). Protective factors and individual resilience. In S. Meisels & J. Shonkoff (Eds.), *Handbook of early intervention.* New York: Cambridge University Press.

Werner, E. E. (1995). Resilience in development. *Current Directions in Psychological Science,* 4 (3), 81–85.

Werner, E. E., & Johnson, J. L. (1999). Can we apply, resilience? In *Resilience and development, positive life adaptation: Longitudinal research in the social and behavioral sciences* (pp. 259–268). NY: Kluwer Academic. In Glantz, M. and Johnson, J. (Eds.), Plenum Publishers.

Westney, O., Jenkins, R., Butts, J., & Williams, I. (1984). Sexual development and behavior in black preadolescents. *Adolescence, 99* (75), 557–568.

Whitaker, D., & Miller, K. (2000). Parent-adolescent discussions about sex and condoms: Impact of peer influences of sexual risk behavior. *Journal of Adolescent Research, 15,* 251–273.

Widom, C. (1994). Childhood victimization and adolescent problem behaviors. In R. D. Ketterlinus & M. E.

Lamb (Eds.), *Adolescent problem behaviors* (pp. 127–164). Hillsdale, NJ: Erlbaum.

Williams, C., & Vines, S. W. (1999). Broken past, fragile future: Personal stories of high risk adolescent mothers. *Journal of the Society of Pediatric Nurses, 4,* 15–23.

Workman, J., & Freeburg, E. (1999). An examination of date rape, victim dress and perceiver variables within the context of attribution theory. *Sex Roles, 41,* 261–277.

Youniss, J. (1989). Parent-adolescent relationships. In W. Damon (Ed.), *Child development today and tomorrow* (pp. 379–392). San Francisco: Jossey-Bass.

# Chapter 11

# Psychosocial Development: Challenges of Adulthood

John Dacey

Lisa Fiori

*As a college student, I once had a conversation with my 68-year-old German professor about how quickly time seems to pass. He smiled and provided me with some thoughts on the matter, reflecting on how when a person is 4 years old, 1 year may pass and it seems to go slowly because that 1 year equals one-fourth of that person's lifetime. As we get older, 1 year becomes a smaller and smaller fraction of our lives, until years seem to go by in the space of what once seemed like months. I've often remembered his words at times when I find myself saying, "Where did the time go?" It is interesting to think about how lives are changing for men and women every day, and although we may be adults biologically, we may still think and feel much like the children we were not many years ago.*

—Lisa Fiore

For health practitioners, it is important to recognize that much of the theory that has been written and debated about human development in adulthood focuses on the period typically known as "middle adulthood," approximately ages 35 to 65 years. For the purposes of this chapter, we will consider adulthood in terms of *general adulthood* and *later adulthood*. As life expectancy continues to increase, 79.4 years for women and 73.9 years for men (National Vital Statistics Report, 2002), early adulthood appears as a prolonged adolescence in many instances. The time that could be designated as early adulthood represents a transition from late adolescence into this category of adulthood, and the research literature does not necessarily reflect or acknowledge early adulthood as distinct from adulthood proper.

When we consider adulthood in terms of general adulthood and later adulthood, these periods entail many of the same benefits, concerns, and developmental applications. Yet, these periods are also unique and must be considered as distinct times in the lives of individuals whom you may meet and treat in the course of your professional and personal lives. Web sites and research information abound with regard to how long we may expect to live and how we can hope to enhance the lives we have (*http://www.nmfn.com/tn/learnctr—lifeevents—longevity*). Table 11.1 presents statistical information from the National Vital Statistics Report (2002). As depicted in the chart, the average life expectancy has increased 27.6 years for males and 31.1 years for females since the beginning of the 20th century. Much of the research emphasizes diet, exercise, and other lifestyle

*Table 11.1*   Disorders Linked to Over- and Underproduction of Cortisol

| Overproduction | Underproduction |
| --- | --- |
| Cushing's syndrome | Atypical/seasonal depression |
| Melancholic depression | Chronic fatigue syndrome |
| Diabetes | Fibromyalgia |
| Sleep deprivation | Hypothyroidism |
| Anorexia nervosa | Nicotine withdrawal |
| Excessive exercise | Rheumatoid arthritis |
| Malnutrition | Allergies |
| Obsessive-compulsive disorder | Asthma |
| Panic disorder | |
| Chronic active alcoholism | |
| Childhood physical and sexual abuse | |
| Functional gastrointestinal disease | |
| Hyperthyroidism | |

*From: McEwen, B. (2002).* The end of stress as we know it *(p. 64). Washington, DC: John Henry Press.*

factors as keys to a longer life, but much of what adults deal with on a daily basis revolves around the less tangible psychosocial factors that we discuss in detail in this chapter, particularly stress.

## Stress in Adulthood

If adolescence is considered the transition from childhood to adulthood, it is no wonder people feel the impact of stress in adulthood when they are faced with challenges that revolve around family, career, and the self. As children, we can look to others for help in times of crisis, but as adults we are expected to be competent and independent enough to handle life's difficulties with grace. It is, of course, important to ask for help when warranted, but many families today are confronted with stress on multiple levels, and crises often overlap in a seemingly endless cycle. For example, many families include a single parent, and this parent may not have a steady and comfortable source of income. If the family is below the poverty level, and the children have difficulties in school, this also affects the family dynamic.

Family members may experience stress in different ways, but it is largely due to the amount of change we endure on a daily basis. As human development progresses, we adapt to changing environments, expectations, and challenges. As young adults or teenagers, we have the support of other adults to help us navigate through the turbulent times, and our physical selves are much more resilient. More stress tends to occur as we get older, whether we are simply more aware of our situations and the reality of those situations, or the stress is basically an unavoidable by-product of our adult environments. If stress is unavoidable, then we need to develop knowledge about how stress affects us, as well as strategies to help avoid suffering ill effects of stress.

## *Physical Adaptation to Stress*

Known as the father of stress research, Hans Selye discovered what he called the *general adaptation syndrome* (Selye, 1956, 1975). His work is familiar to most health care providers. While conducting research on ovarian hormones, Selye injected hormones from cattle ovaries into rats to see what changes, if any, would occur. The experiment revealed some surprising results:

- The cortex of each rat became enlarged and hyperactive.
- Numerous glands shrank.
- Deep bleeding ulcers occurred in the rats' stomach and upper intestines.

Upon further investigation, Selye found that these reactions occurred in response to toxic substances, regardless of their source. Later research and experimentation showed the results occurring, to a lesser degree, as a reaction to harmful stimuli, such as infections, hemorrhage, and nervous irritation. Selye called this entire syndrome an *alarm reaction.*

He likened this reaction to a rallying cry to the body's defensive forces. To gain a better understanding of this syndrome, he questioned how the reaction would be affected if stress were present for a longer period of time. He found that another interesting thing occurs. If the organism survives the initial alarm, it enters a second stage—*a stage of resistance.* In this second stage, an almost complete reversal of the alarm reaction occurs. For instance, swelling and shrinkages subside; the adrenal cortex regains any secretions lost in the alarm stage; and various other shock-resisting forces are assembled. During this second stage, the organism appears to acquire strength and to have adapted successfully to the stressor.

This phenomenon changes, however, if the stressor continues. A gradual reduction in the organism's adaptational energy occurs (Selye, 1982). This eventually leads to the final stage—*the stage of exhaustion.* In this stage the physiological responses return to their condition during the initial stage of alarm. The ability to cope with the stress declines, the level of resistance is lost, and the organism ultimately dies.

Selye's work assumed that the human body seeks to achieve *homeostasis,* that is, a stable base-line of physiological functioning. More recent research suggests the relationship between the stress response and optimal physiology is more complex than Selye was able to appreciate. The newer interpretation is *allostasis,* which emphasizes variability as a means to stability.

Allostatic systems include the familiar role of the sympathetic/parasympathetic nervous system in the fight or flight/relaxation response. Allostasis also recognizes how the interactions among neuroendocrine, cardiovascular, and immune systems both maintain health and respond to stress. For example, getting out of bed in the morning requires a normative rise in cortisol—the so-called stress hormone—because we are making demands on the body to do so. In other words, allostasis refers to a range of normal variation in physiological functioning (McEwen, 2002).

*Allostatic load* occurs when the allostatic systems no longer work effectively. Allostatic load refers to four different scenarios (McEwen, 2002):

1. Unremitting stress, that is, the allostatic systems fail to adapt to a repeated stressor (e.g., threat becomes a normal constant); chronically activate allostatic systems inappropriately, "causing them to turn on themselves and eventually break down," (McEwen, 2002, p. 9) lowering resistance to illness (e.g, getting a cold);

2. Inability to adjust, that is, an inappropriate response to stress becomes the norm (e.g., chronic anxiety);

3. Not hearing the "all clear," that is, continuing to mount an allostatic response long after the stressor has passed, leading to an overdose of stress hormones, such as cortisol (e.g., high blood pressure) ;

4. Insufficient or uncoordinated response, that is, the stress response is sluggish, causing other systems to go into overdrive (e.g., allergies and autoimmune disorders).

The over- and underproduction of cortisol plays an important role in allostatic load. Table 11.1 lists diseases associated with inappropriate production of cortisol. Obesity, cardiovascular disease, high blood pressure, and depression—among the most common health disorders of adulthood—are all associated with allostatic load.

The stress response varies among individuals across the life span, accounted for by differences in experience, the meaning of stress, and physiology. Normative changes in aging, as well as disease processes and medications, will affect the production of stress hormones, for example. Health care providers will encounter patients or clients who are battling their own forms of stress, and it is interesting to note how some individuals rise above many obstacles, whereas others surrender to the stress (Klohnen, Vandewater, & Young, 1996).

## Risk and Resilience

There are many individuals who cope well with stress and who experience few psychological, behavioral, or other problems as a result. These individuals are said to possess resilience (Chapter 4 by Thies). News stories, for example, may feature a man who survived for 6 days, trapped in his car, despite freezing temperatures and lack of food and water; or the unwed mother who was able to feed and clothe her five children, work three jobs, and still create an after-school program for neighborhood children. Researchers have been interested in examining the characteristics of resilient individuals for various reasons. The stressors that we all encounter are called risk factors. Risk factors include poverty, chronic illness, parental mental illness and drug abuse, exposure to violence through war or other tragedies, and the family experiences such as divorce and teen parenthood.

In light of such factors, researchers have attempted to identify protective factors that combat the risks. Three kinds of protective factors have been identified frequently: family environments,

support networks, and personality characteristics (Hauser & Bowlds, 1990). Recent research indicates that women tend to suffer more frequently from domestic violence than men. Umberson, Anderson, Glick, & Shapiro (1998) found that women who experienced domestic violence reported feeling much less personal control over their lives, whereas men did not report any diminished sense of self-control. As is the case with any self-report measure, however, it is possible that the men in the study were hesitant to reveal their true feelings because of societal pressures or expectations. In a similar vein, Ratner (1998) found that women also experienced health problems if they developed psychopathology or drug addiction as a result of domestic abuse.

### PREVENTION

Physical and mental health professionals have been eager to identify risk and protective factors so that present knowledge can contribute to the prevention of future physical and psychological difficulties. Successful prevention programs seek to reduce the occurrence of disturbance and clinical dysfunction in two ways: first, by reducing the number of risk factors that an individual must contend with; and second, enhancing protective factors and effective coping strategies and tactics. Primary prevention programs are those that strive to eliminate problems before they begin. Secondary prevention programs intervene during the early phases of a problem to reduce its severity or the length of time it will last.

Differences in prevention programs initially revolve around the groups they are designed to assist. Some groups are directed toward all people in a particular city or community, whereas in some cases only those identified as at particular risk are invited to participate. Among adults, prevention programs are most often delivered in the workplace, places of worship, hospitals, or community centers. Effective programs have been designed to address the development of social skills and to reduce at-risk behaviors such as overeating, alcoholism, smoking, and gambling. To deliver the most powerful prevention programs, families, community organizations, and corporations must work together to reduce risks, expand protective factors, and promote healthy development.

# Relationships in Middle Adulthood

Regrettably, current prevention programs are still imperfect and are therefore unable to prevent the occurrence of mental disturbance. In some cases, psychotherapy, psychiatric hospitalization, and/or medications are needed to improve dysfunction for those individuals already suffering from mental disturbance. In the absence of all-powerful prevention programs, individuals most often turn to their families and friends for needed support. For this reason, we examine relationships in adulthood, particularly how they reflect the change that adults experience at this stage of human development. Later in the chapter, relationships are discussed with particular attention paid to the role of relationships in later adulthood (Blieszner & Adams, 1998).

## *Marriage*

Middle age is often a time when husbands and wives reappraise their marriage and overall relationship. Interestingly, research findings tend to apply primarily to relationships of relatively young couples, usually in their first decade of marriage (Gottman & Notarius, 2000). Contributing to the reappraisal of the marriage, the midlife transition is known as a period during which people critically evaluate their individual lives up to that point. Often, this causes people to reflect upon current relationships and consider changes they would like to make for the future. In many cases, tension that may exist in a marriage is masked while children continue to live at home. As children leave the home to attend college, work, or start families of their own, middle-aged couples may reveal and openly address their conflicts.

Experts in the field of marriage seem to support the idea that marital satisfaction over time may be represented by a U-shaped pattern (Van Laningham, Johnson, & Amato, 2001). The U-shaped pattern illustrates a period of early decline in satisfaction, followed by a leveling out during the parenting years, and subsequent improvement when children leave the home. Sources of dissatisfaction vary from couple to couple and person to person, but lasting relationships appear to have a knack for handling stress and conflict as it arises. Stressful life events include situations, transitions, or events experienced by a couple that impose upon their relationship and generate tension or stress (Parker, 2001).

Sometimes couples learn to endure each other rather than live with each other in a reciprocal manner. The only activities they might share are those that revolve around the children, and when the children leave, they are forced to confront the fact that they have drifted apart—sometimes very far apart. The effect of such a relationship is essentially an emotional divorce. The experience of divorce itself, in retrospect, can often be considered as a cluster of small divorces (Steefel, 1992).

Findings based on retrospective reports of marital satisfaction have been viewed with caution because much time has passed. However, some researchers argue that retrospective reports may actually be more accurate because the distance created by the passing of time provides a less biased perspective (Mackey & O'Brien, 1995). Most couples who have long-lasting marriages have built the type of relationship that can withstand evaluation and reappraisal, and this pattern continues for the rest of their lives. Statistics taken from the U.S. census (1996) indicate that the highest separation and divorce rates occur after approximately 5 years of marriage. The period after the children leave home is like a second honeymoon for many couples. Commonly referred to as the empty nest syndrome, the initial adjustment to the new home dynamics does not necessarily involve only negative emotions. Married couples can evaluate their accomplishments with their children and relax now that a major life goal has been achieved. The couple may realize that they now have fewer worries, and more privacy, freedom, and money to enjoy themselves. Due to the increase in life expectancy, couples can now look forward to spending approximately 20 to 30 years together as a couple, rather than only as a family unit.

## SUCCESSFUL MARRIAGE

There are a number of factors that figure in a happy, or at least an enduring, marriage. Gottman and Krokoff (1989) conducted a longitudinal study examining the types of interactions between spouses and the related effects on marital satisfaction. Earlier research tended to suggest that there was always more negative interaction in unhappy marriages than in happy marriages. The authors chose to look at the effect of different types of interactions rather than one global category or interaction. They found that certain types of conflict may in fact be positive components of a lasting, happy marriage. They also found that certain types of conflict, particularly defensiveness, stubbornness, and withdrawal on the part of the husband, indicated that a marriage was potentially unstable. Gottman and Krokoff assigned the role of manager to wives, with regard to confronting marital disagreements. They suggested that wives get their husbands to "confront areas of disagreement and to openly vent disagreement and anger" (Gottman & Krokoff, 1989, p. 50). Many husbands tend to try to avoid confrontations within relationships. Therefore, overcoming reluctance on the part of husbands may have significantly beneficial, long-lasting effects on a marriage.

Klagsburn (1985) reported on interviews with 87 middle-class couples who had been married at least 15 years. From these interviews she was able to identify eight characteristics of couples in long-lasting marriages:

- Ability to change and adapt to change
- Ability to live with the unchangeable
- Assumption of permanence
- Trust
- Balance of power
- Enjoyment of each other
- Cherished, shared history
- Luck

Klagsburn stated that the happier couples she interviewed had remained together because of the emotional benefits they gained through the marriage, but also in spite of the stress they may have experienced.

## ADULTS WHO DO NOT MARRY

Approximately 1 in 20 people in middle age have never been married (U.S. Census, 1996). Generally speaking, a person who has never been married by middle age will not get married. Demographic findings indicate that unwed, middle-aged people tend to have very low or very high levels of education. For example, of those people with fewer than 5 years of schooling, one person in seven has never married. Factors that may keep these individuals out of school may include mental illness or other disabilities and are likely the same ones that make them less likely to get married. At the other extreme, 13% of middle-aged women with 17 or more years of education have never been married.

There are a number of possible explanations for this. These women may choose higher education and career over marriage. Social and cultural factors may influence their positions because some men might feel threatened by women with more education than they have. Another possibility is that women who delay marriage in order to pursue education or career end up having a smaller pool of men to choose from, compounded by the fact that men die, on average, at an earlier age than women. Societal pressure to get married may often take its toll on people and manifest itself in depression, eating disorders, and alcoholism.

## Divorce in Adulthood

Divorce among middle-aged adults has been a particular focus of researchers. For example, the relationship between divorce and women's economic status is acknowledged as being more complicated than initially believed (Knoester & Booth, 2000; Smock, Manning, & Gupta, 1999). A woman's financial status may or may not change as a result of divorce and depends on several factors. Researchers have also argued that divorce rates are higher for second or subsequent marriages, for African Americans, and for those with less education and less learning potential. However, divorce at midlife is less likely to occur. As mentioned previously, most divorces occur during the first 5 years of marriage, and the numbers decline sharply after that. Because many people who divorce early do not remarry, the proportion of divorced individuals in midlife is relatively high.

In terms of a standard of living, women are often identified as being hit harder by divorce. The National Longitudinal Survey found that women experience significant declines in income as well as dramatic lifestyle changes upon separation, divorce, or widowhood, and increased rates of poverty (Hoffman & Duncan, 1988). Because most women who divorce at midlife are already working, they have few options for obtaining higher income after divorce.

Additional stress factors affect divorced women and their families. The absence of a father at home is becoming more and more common,

and more than half of single-parent mothers are not receiving full child support. Half of those women do not receive any child support. In the past, child support was awarded mainly because of mothers' limited income. Currently, most states use a specific formula to calculate reasonable child support payments in light of parents' incomes. Both parents must therefore provide sufficient financial support to the child, regardless of which parent has custody of the child (Cancian & Meyer, 1996).

### RECENT DIVORCE LAWS

More recent divorce laws are generally considered to have had a liberating effect on women. Before the revision of divorce laws, women sometimes felt that they had no choice but to endure a difficult and sometimes abusive marriage. In the past, it was necessary to establish "reasonable grounds" for divorce, such as physical abuse. Women were consistently awarded larger alimony settlements than today, to compensate for presumed loss of income. In 1970, divorce laws were loosened in California, and the repercussions were felt across the country. This change, called a "no-fault" divorce, holds that women and men are treated equally under the divorce law. Men and women did not live in an economically equitable system in 1970, nor is it equal today. Men continue to possess an edge in earning potential, and society still holds women responsible for raising children and managing the household. Middle-aged women, who have been running their households for years while their husbands invested time in their careers, cannot be expected to compete with others who have been gaining experience in the workforce.

No-fault divorce laws also mandate an equal division of property, which often means the house must be sold. Besides being a source of economic stress, the loss of the family home has psychological consequences for parents and children alike. Compound this with the stress of the divorce itself, and this becomes an extreme burden for all involved.

It is unlikely that divorce will ever be a civilized process, as the supporters of no-fault legislation would hope. However, some indications show that reform is on the way. Spousal responsibilities and burdens may be shared more equitably, and the suffering of children may be reduced. Having a sibling to turn to and commiserate with in times of stress is a source of strength when individuals are young, but even more so in adulthood. As we confront changes in our daily lives, relationships with siblings become more complex and challenging.

## Relationships with Siblings

The field of human development has acknowledged the importance of sibling relationships for a child's cognitive and social growth, but how do these unique relationships factor into development in adulthood? Does the relationship lose some of its importance as we grow older and more independent? Are the characteristics of the relationship the same in adulthood as they were in childhood? Psychological research has attempted to shed light on some of these questions.

Sibling relationships are potentially the most lasting relationships a person will have. Partners or spouses don't usually meet each other until young adulthood, or at least adolescence. Parents tend to pass away before their children, and those children tend to pass away before their own children. Yet most siblings are born within a few years of each other, therefore the relationship can last even 100 years!

Most adult siblings are faced with more important and serious tasks than childhood siblings. For example, most middle-aged siblings must make mutual decisions concerning the care of elderly parents and, ultimately, the consequences of their death.

The effects of changing family patterns on sibling relationships are also important to consider.

As couples choose to have fewer or no children, there will be fewer children available to parents for companionship and psychological support as people age. Needless to say, parents and their siblings will be able to live longer, active lives. Sibling relationships will continue to gain in importance in the future. Strategies for coping with stress and conflict help sustain the sibling relationship in later life (Schulman, 1999).

## Aging Parents

Middle age is also a time when relationships with parents tend to improve. Middle-aged children, many experiencing parenthood themselves, gain a new appreciation for the responsibility and energy required. They therefore reevaluate the behavior of their own parents. It is increasingly common, however, that the relationship begins to reverse itself. As elderly parents grow older, they sometimes become as dependent on their middle-aged children as those children once were on them. The longevity that is a blessing for some individuals is the enemy of others. Middle-aged children who see their parents frequently are often less aware of the toll that time is taking on them. When a parent does become sick or injured, the stress associated with such high-demand attention exacts a toll on the immediate family, as well as friends and the work environment.

Most people fail to consider the emotional and monetary costs that aging parents exact. This can ultimately lead to increased tension and resentment in the relationship. Frequently, earlier family experiences may have a positive or negative effect on the later relationship between adult children and their aging parents (Whitbeck, Hoyt, & Huck, 1994). It follows that young children who experience close relationships with their parents, and whose parents provided unconditional, consistent care, will have more positive later relationships.

As women enter middle age, the most commonly cited problem is not menopause or aging itself, but caring for aging parents and parents-in-law (James, 1990). Research has shown that the daughter(s) in a family most often assume the responsibility for care of elderly parents (Kendig, Hashimoto, & Coppard, 1992). Green (1991) suggested that the daughter who is the primary caretaker tends to rely on siblings, especially sisters if she has any, for emotional support. These sisters often feel guilty for not doing enough. Brothers tend to provide less help and feel less guilty about it. Recent research has maintained the idea that social support is of chief importance to daughters who are the primary caregivers for aging parents (Pohl, Given, Collins, & Given, 1994). Social support includes emotional, financial, or other support provided by friends and family. Daughters may feel more positive about assuming the caregiving role when they have secure income, health, and marriage. Some would argue that the demands on women to fulfill the role of family nurturer are deeply rooted and powerful. It is important to note, however, that as more women enter and remain in the workplace, this pattern may change, with men being expected to assume more of the load.

Caserta, Lund, & Wright (1996) examined caring for elderly parents or in-laws and proposed a multifaceted view of this responsibility. The authors proposed several aspects of the caregiving task, such as emotional strain, time constraints, and physical health of the caregiver. The well-being of the caregiver is undoubtedly important to the person receiving the care. Each aspect of the caregiving responsibility should be considered as having a potential effect on the child–parent relationship, as well as the child's relationships with others.

## Friendships

Middle age is a time in our lives when friendships become fewer and more valuable. Research conducted by Cartensen (1992) indicates that people begin narrowing their range of social partners well before middle age. The most dramatic reduction occurs between the ages of 18 and 30. Whereas frequent interaction with acquaintances and close friends tends to decline during this period, it increases with spouses, partners, and siblings. It appears that at approximately age 30, people choose a select few relationships from which they obtain support, self-confidence, and a sense of identity. Emotional closeness with relatives and close friends, however, increases throughout adulthood. These relationships with a select few tend to become increasingly close and satisfying, particularly during the middle-age years. Additionally, the notion that face-to-face contact is required for closeness is not supported. On the contrary, close proximity is not necessary to sustain a friendship. Friendship is multifaceted, and involves structure and context as well as cognitive and behavioral factors (Blieszner & Adams, 1998).

# Personality in Adulthood

Another multifaceted aspect of human development is personality. This concept has been debated in scientific research for decades: Is personality a set of stable, continuous traits, or rather a collection of changing characteristics? As mentioned earlier, the many changes adults face in their lives can be stressful. However, adapting to the numerous changes we are confronted with on a daily basis looks different for every individual. Some people seem to navigate through the stressful mire successfully, whereas others tend to get stuck and weighed down by spontaneous, sometimes unpleasant events. One's personality, then, might be the distinguishing factor that determines how one copes with stress, for example. The heading for the debate over this topic is summed up as continuity versus change. Do human beings change very much over the course of their lives, or do we basically stay the same? The search for answers to this question is important to the field of human development because of the implications.

If we agree that people remain the same despite what happens to them over the course of their lives, then the period of early childhood acquires significant meaning because that is the time known as the "formative years." Several developmental theorists, such as Sigmund Freud and Jean Piaget, focused their attention on the early years of childhood because they believed that what happens to a person during childhood largely determines what will happen to the person in the future. Other theorists, such as Erikson (whom we discuss later), believe that because people are constantly changing and developing, all life experiences must be considered formative and important. This brings the periods of adolescence and adulthood into greater focus. It also implies that a happy childhood isn't enough to sustain a person's success throughout the entire life span.

## Continuity Versus Change

In the study of adulthood, the debate over continuity versus change gets even more complex. In general, two clear theoretical positions affect the study of adult personality. On one hand, theorists believe that adults remain essentially the same and that the adult's personality is stable. This is the essence of continuity in adult development. Other theorists consider the adult as in a constant process of change and evolution.

The study of continuity versus change in adulthood is complicated by the various ways the issue is studied. Researchers who examine the pieces of the personality (personality traits) are known as trait theorists. Detailed questionnaires are usually included as one measure of an individual's overall ability and overall personality. Others argue that adult personality is far more complicated than a general list of personality traits. These researchers are interested most in how certain traits fit with the whole of one's personality, and how the adult's personality interacts with the world around him or her. These researchers are known as stage theorists because they argue that we must look at the stages of change that a person experiences before we can draw any conclusions about personality.

### CONTINUOUS TRAITS THEORY

Differences in opinion about how best to measure adult personality further complicate the study of personality, in terms of continuity versus change. Generally, trait theorists have reported that adult personality remains stable—the same. This supports continuity (Costa & McCrae, 1995). These researchers argue that personality remains stable over the years, and that personality traits are organized hierarchically. Narrow traits combine to define broader factors (Costa & McCrae, 1994). In this light, life circumstances such as divorce, job loss, menopause, or the so-called "midlife crisis" wouldn't significantly alter a person's personality. A different opinion has formed among stage theorists, who posit that change in adulthood is inevitable. These theorists take into account the life span as a whole and examine the stages each person goes through.

The work of Costa and McCrae (1991) reveals that certain personality traits characterize the adult personality: neuroticism, extrovertism, openness to experience, agreeableness, and conscientiousness. These five traits comprise the NEOAC model of personality:

- Neuroticism is the predisposition toward breakdown under stress; the tendency to experience physical and psychiatric problems, to drink or smoke, and to experience more general dissatisfaction with life.

- Extroversion is the tendency to be outgoing and social; individuals tend to possess an overriding interest in people and social connections.

- Openness to experience is the tendency to embrace new ideas, actions, values, and feelings; individuals are creative and imaginative.

- Agreeableness is the tendency toward trusting others; individuals are generally altruistic and modest.

- Concientiousness is the tendency toward self-discipline; individuals are competent and achieving.

Although these general traits would remain stable as a whole over the years, it is important to note that dramatic changes (e.g., physical illness, psychiatric disorder) can alter one's personality. Health professionals are in excellent positions to help adults who might be experiencing changes in their lives. A variety of settings, such as health clubs and outpatient clinics, facilitate an examination of one's life and health. Programs are offered that promote self-awareness and motivation and that monitor individuals' progress, for example, eating sensibly and exercising regularly. Benefits may affect mental and physical health (e.g., depression, diabetes). Theorists who believe that personality development is a natural, continous process support this type of proactive change.

## Levinson—Seasons of a Man's Life

The work of Daniel Levinson, though somewhat dated, offers insight into the development of the adult personality. Based on intensive interviews with 40 men (1978) and 40 women (1990), aged 35 to 45 years, Levinson developed his own theory of human development, which has at its core a concept he called the *life course.* This is fundamental to Levinson's theory because it incorporates the notion of life (every aspect of living that has significance to our lives) and the flow of that life over time (cycle). Life course refers to the complexity of one's life over time. Levinson proposed that although each human being is unique, "there is an underlying order in the human life course" (Levinson, 1986, p. 4) that he referred to as the *life cycle.* Within each life cycle, Levinson noted that there are separate eras that incorporate the biological, psychological, and social factors that affect an individual. Each era is separated by transition periods, and in any person's life there will therefore be periods of relative stability, followed by change. In adulthood, the settling-down phase and midlife transition apply to middle age.

### SETTLING DOWN

According to Levinson's theory, the settling-down phase typically extends from age 33 to 40. At this time in their lives, most men have decided upon a career or occupation that they assume will involve a relatively strong commitment. During this period, the primary tasks men attempt to achieve are 1) to establish a niche in society and 2) to advance up the occupational ladder. The man tends to think less about what others want him to do and think, and more about what his own views dictate. Once men have arrived at these conclusions, they are ready to enter the next phase of adulthood—the midlife transition.

### THE MIDLIFE TRANSITION

Usually lasting approximately 5 years, the midlife transition generally extends from age 40 to 45. It incorporates three major developmental tasks: 1) review, appraisal, and termination of the early adult period; 2) decisions on how the period of middle adulthood should be conducted; and 3) dealing with the polarities that tend to cause deep division in the man's life at this stage. These polarities are 1) young/old, 2) destruction/creation, 3) masculinity/femininity, and 4) attachment/separation.

**Young/Old**   The young/old polarity is the major one to be confronted during the midlife transition. Levinson acknowledged the ideas of Carl Jung (1933), suggesting that there is a shared experience from generation after generation of thousands of human beings, over time, that has gradually produced deeply rooted ideas that we each must deal with. The major idea is that we begin to grow old the moment we are born; however, we are also concerned with maintaining our youth, if only to avoid the ultimate outcome of our mortality: death.

In symbolic terms, the word *young* represents fertility, growth, energy, potential, birth, and spring. *Old,* on the other hand, embodies termination, death, completion, fruition, winter, and ending. Before age 40, a man has been able to maintain his youthful self-image. Through the process of being productive, whether in terms of raising children or through a creative product such as a book, invention, or painting, he has been able to envision himself as part of a new and youthful recycling of life. Whether intentional or processed on a subconscious level, the man has sustained the myth of immortality.

When this man approaches his 40th birthday, he is confronted with evidence of his own declining powers. He is no longer able to swim, play softball, or shoot basketballs as effectively as he could 20 years earlier. He sometimes forgets things, and his eyesight may not be as sharp. Even more detrimental to his hopes of immortality is the illness of friends. Among men in their 40s, heart attacks, strokes, and other serious problems are not uncommon. His parents might suffer serious illness, or even die. These events propel him toward the inevitable conclusion: he is going to die, and perhaps sooner than later. Even the time left him (approximately 36 years, on average) is small consolation, because over half of his life is now behind him.

The desire to leave a legacy now surfaces. Most individuals want to feel that their life has made some difference, and they want to leave something behind them that will be remembered. It is therefore typical at this time for the individual to become more creative, working harder than he has in the past. He wants to make a contribution that is considered worthwhile by others.

**Destruction/Creation**    The male experiencing a midlife transition realizes the potential of the world to destroy, as well as his own capacity for destruction. He recognizes his own vices and his own ability to harm, damage, and injure himself and others. If he is truly honest with himself, he realizes that he has sometimes hurt people inadvertently, but also with clear intent. He perceives himself as both victim and villain.

The more he sincerely reflects upon his own abilities, the more he realizes how great is his ca-

pacity to destroy. The upside to this honesty, however, is that he also realizes his potential for creation. He begins to see that he may be truly powerful in creating new and useful forms of life. As with the previous polarity of young/old, he now attempts to strike a balance between his destructive and creative sides.

**Masculinity/Femininity**    Levinson again acknowledged the work of Jung, adapting the concept that all people have a masculine and feminine side, and that they emphasize one more than the other due to societal demands. This emphasis often costs us dearly, and many people attempt to compensate, in adulthood, for the side that was denied during childhood. In most males, the feminine side has typically been undernourished and must now emerge if the man wants to be all he is capable of being.

According to Levinson, femininity has numerous undesirable connotations for the male in young adulthood. To the young man, masculinity connotes strength, toughness, achievement and ambition, power, and intellectuality. On the other hand, femininity represents weakness, incompetence and lack of ambition, and emotionality. Midlife is the time when the polarity between these perceptions must be acknowledge and reconciled.

The male who is to achieve Levinson's idea of individuation most successfully now recognizes that these dichotomies are false and that he indeed possesses a feminine side that must also be nourished. The mature male is able to indulge in what he previously belittled as feminine aspects of his personality. Such a male feels secure enough in his masculinity to enjoy his ability to feel, nurture, and be dependent when warranted. Levinson suggests such men are more likely to assume independent relationships with their mothers, to develop more intimate love relationships with female friends, and to become mentors to younger men and women.

**Attachment/Separation**    In terms of the attachment/separation process, Levinson meant that each of us needs to be attached to others in society, but also to be separate from them. Throughout human development, people waver between these needs. In childhood, a clear-cut attachment to mother and family exists. Children need support because of their lack of skill in dealing with the complex world around them. Nevertheless, children do begin the separation process by forming attachments to their peers.

During adolescence an adjustment is made emphasizing separateness from family along the quest for identity. Most adolescents tend to need to separate themselves not only from their parents but also from the entire society around them in order to try out new ways of being. This need switches back toward attachment during early adulthood, although the ultimate goal is interdependence.

Men in their 20s and 30s are most often involved in the world of career and family and have a strong attachment to those who can help them achieve their goals. In the midlife transition a new separateness, almost a second adolescence, occurs. The man, particularly the successful man, becomes reflective and gains a greater awareness of his feelings. He becomes more in touch with himself by being temporarily less in touch with others.

Because the men interviewed so thoroughly by Levinson and his colleagues were between the ages of 35 and 45, their study of adult development ends at the midlife transition. Levinson acknowledged, however, that much is yet to be learned about development after this stage.

## Seasons of a Woman's Life

More recently, Levinson (1990) focused on female maturation. He selected three groups of women for his research, all between the ages of 35 and 45. One-third of the participants were homemakers whose lives followed a traditional family-centered pattern, one-third were teachers at the college level, and one-third were working in a business environment. Levinson considered these women to represent a continuum from the domestic orientation to the public orientation, with the college teachers situated somewhere in-between. Each of the participants was interviewed 8 to 10 times by the researchers (half of whom were female) for a total of 15 to 20 hours.

Likely the most significant finding was that females go through a series of stages similar to the stages experienced by males who were studied. Each gender may be described as proceeding through an alternating series of structure-building and structure-changing phases. For example, Levinson determined that a man in his late 30s wants to become "his own man." He also found that a woman at this same point in her life wants to become "her own woman." Both sexes seek greater affirmation from themselves as well as people around them.

While the progress toward maturity for both males and females may occur in similar stages, Levinson and his associates also believed that major differences exist for the genders within these similar stages. For women, the primary themes of these differences are *gender splitting,* the *traditional marriage,* and the *perpetual gender revolution.*

### GENDER SPLITTING

Virtually all societies support the idea that clear differences should and do exist in terms of what is considered appropriate for males and females. The term *gender splitting* refers to this division, and it appears to be a universal phenomenon. Women's lives have traditionally revolved around the domestic arena, whereas men's lives are aimed at the public sphere. Human societies have perceived a need for females to stay at home to protect the offspring while the male goes about being the so-called "provider."

### TRADITIONAL MARRIAGE

Regardless of the roles that evolve between partners, people tend to enter into a marriage because they believe that their lives will be enriched as a result of the union. Although exceptions do occur, the main goal of a traditional marriage is to create and maintain a family. Gender splitting is seen as contributing to this goal.

Some women perceive a significant part of their role in the family as being supportive of their husbands' role. When the wife goes to work, this role is not measurably altered. Levinson reported that it is still a source of conflict when a female becomes the boss, both at home and at work. Some women feel that there is a heavy price paid for the financial security afforded by a successful career. Many also find it potentially dangerous to develop a strong sense of self outside the traditional role. Health professionals will likely encounter research on depression and anxiety related to women's experiences at midlife. The transition is more challenging for women, who receive vastly conflicting messages from society at large about what constitutes appropriate behavior and expectations.

### GENDER REVOLUTION

The meanings and understandings of gender are changing, which has a tendency to cause some comfort and others stress. Young and middle-aged adults have much more work to do today than in years past. Increased life expectancy has created a large group of consumers: the elderly. This group consumes more than they produce, which has contributed to more women leaving the home environment to join the workforce. Other factors contributing to the on-going gender revolution are divorce rate and educational levels of women. Women therefore face the challenge of balancing career and family, and nurturing both accordingly. For many women, the attempt at this balance brings on overload and conflict, and renewed self-assessment.

Related to the findings of Levinson's studies, Reinke, Ellicott, Harris, & Hancock (1985) found important transitions in the lives of women. Similar methodology revealed transitions that are not exclusively clustered around the midlife period of 35 to 45, but rather occur around ages 30, 40, and 60. Researchers will likely examine the division between men and women closely, and the effects and implications of the changing gender divide.

## Erikson — Generativity versus Stagnation

Whereas Levinson's viewpoint was psychological in nature, Erik Erikson's theory is rooted in a psychiatric vein. A student of Freud, Erikson's classic theory attempts to explain development in adulthood as the reconciliation of the crisis known as *generativity versus stagnation*. This theory incorporates personality development as well as social experience and identity.

*Generativity* refers to the ability to be useful to ourselves and society as a whole. The goal of this stage, occurring between the ages of 25 and 65, is to be productive and creative. In this stage, productivity is aimed at being helpful to others. This is self-rewarding, regardless of recognition or reward. Erikson stated that generativity is

*That middle period of the life cycle when existence permits you and demands you to consider death as peripheral and to balance its certainty with the only happiness that is lasting: to increase, by whatever is yours to give, the good will and the higher order in your sector of the world (1978, p. 124).*

Erikson recognized that for many people, procreation is an important part of generativity, yet he did not believe that everyone must be a parent in order to be generative. For example, some people cannot apply their generative energies to offspring of their own, so instead apply their gifts and motivation in other directions. They find other ways to be altruistic and creative.

At this stage of adulthood some people find themselves bored and are unable to contribute to society and the welfare of others. They experience stagnation. Such individuals behave as though they were their own only child. If they have children of their own, they may come to resent the natural demands of their offspring.

Wacks (1994) suggested that each individual has an "inner elder-child," which incorporates shame and fear of aging with a childlike appreciation of life and wisdom. In terms of generativity,

Wacks found that the elder-child phenomenon occurs during the middle years of adulthood. A person can gain maturity by nurturing this elder-child and learning from experiences, even ones that are uncomfortable or frightening. In a sense, there is an integration of the young self with the older self at midlife, which promotes more generativity.

Although generativity is satisfying to those who accomplish it, some theorists have suggested that there are alternate experiences. McAdams, de St. Aubin, & Logan (1993), for example, examined generativity across age groups in a cross-sectional study. They looked at four separate facets of generativity: *generative concern, commitments, action,* and *narration.* They found some support for Erikson's hypothesis that generativity is relatively low in young adulthood, peaks at midlife, and declines in the later years. However, they also reported findings of other studies that suggest differences between men's and women's experiences in this generativity stage.

# Later Adulthood

All of the theories discussed in this chapter indicate that we go through many important changes as we age. These changes sometimes contribute to individuals experiencing stress, which affects all aspects of life, particularly relationships with family and others. As we examine in the following sections, later adulthood presents unique challenges related to that particular time of life.

## Erikson—Integrity Versus Despair

The final stage in Erikson's theory of human development emphasizes the crisis denoted as *integrity versus despair.* Erikson proposed that successful resolution of each of the previous seven crises in his theory should lead adults to achieve a sense of personal integrity—a feeling that life had been well lived. Older adults who have this sense of integrity believe that decisions made and actions taken throughout life seem to make sense and fit together. Their lives are integrated. They may feel saddened that time seems to be running out and that they have limited opportunity to make a lasting impact on their world, yet they feel quite satisfied with their accomplishments. They often have a sense of having helped to achieve a more dignified life for humankind. Fundamental to this sense of integrity is the acceptance of human progress. This is the path to wisdom, defined by Erikson as, "the detached and yet active concern with life itself in the face of death itself" (1978, p. 26).

When individuals reflect on their lives and feel that they have made many poor decisions, or that they have failed to make any decisions at all, they tend to view life as lacking integrity. They feel despair, which is the second half of this last stage of crisis. These people resent that there can never be another chance to make sense of their lives. They often disguise their fear of death as contempt for humanity in general, particularly those of other races, religions, or socioeconomic groups. Erikson (1968) stated, "Such despair is often hidden behind a show of disgust" (p. 140).

It is difficult to understand what it feels like for an individual to reach late adulthood. This is of particular interest for health care providers because one of the fastest-growing age groups in the country is the over-85 category. These older adults generally experience changes in physical, cognitive, and psychosocial abilities, as well as increasing illness. Maintaining quality of life becomes a central theme in late adult development. This presents a challenge for this age group, as they are simultaneously adjusting to the changes in their societal roles.

## Changing Roles—Care of Elderly Parents

The field of human development has become increasingly interested in caregiving to elders in recent years. Studies have examined various factors, such as stress caused by living alone or in nursing homes (Naleppa, 1996; Ponder & Pomeroy, 1996; Tirrito, 1996; Stephens & Townsend, 1997) and coping strategies (Davis et al., 2000; DeVries, Hamilton, Lovett, & Gallagher-Thompson, 1997; Kramer & Lambert, 1999; Mok & Mui, 1996). Caring for elderly parents affects the caregivers as well as those for whom care is being provided.

## Care by Family Members

Elderly people consider their adult children, if they have them, as the primary helpers in their lives. When elders have both an adult son and an adult daughter, elderly people most often declare the son is the primary helper (Kramer & Lambert, 1999). This seems contradictory because we pointed out earlier that the care of elderly parents is almost always undertaken by daughters, when there are daughters in the family. The role that men play in caregiving should therefore not be taken for granted because they certainly contribute to the care of their elder parents in significant ways (Marks, 1996).

In years past, care of the elderly was almost always done by unmarried daughters in a family. It was assumed that the work would be easier for them because they had no responsibilities to husband or children. On the contrary, married women tend to find that marriage and family make the caregiving easier because of the support they receive.

It is not only biological daughters of elderly parents who provide caretaking support, however. Davis and colleagues (2000) found no differences between care provided by biological daughters and by daughters-in-law. The researchers suggest that it is the quality of the interactions with the elderly, not the relation to the person, that is most significant.

Many risk factors for the caregivers have been acknowledged in related research. Depression and stress are the two most common risk factors cited in the literature. Interestingly, the degree of depression and stress has been connected with specific caregiver characteristics. For example, Meshefedjian, McCusker, Bellavance, & Baum-garten (1998) proposed that the closer the relationship of the caregiver to the elderly person, the higher the caregiver scored on a test of depression. Also, the less education the caregivers have, the more likely they are to be depressed. These findings are supported by the work of Lawrence and associates (1998), who found that having a close relationship with the elderly person resulted in increased perceptions of overload by the caregiver.

The quality of the associations between caregiver and elderly parent is as important as the closeness of the relationship (i.e., parent/child). Unfortunately, poor interactions between caregivers and those in their care may result in verbal and physical aggression in adults (Cohen-Mansfield & Werner, 1998). Researchers have also found that the number of difficulties experienced in one's caregiving role is related to stress and responsibility. For example, Riedel, Fredman, & Langenberg (1998) argued that caregivers who reported more types of difficulty in their role experienced higher levels of burden than caregivers who reported only one type of difficulty.

## Risks to Caregivers

It is apparent that there are clear risks for depression and stress for the adult placed in the caregiving role. Many researchers have attempted to find ways in which the burden of such a responsibility may be eased. Recent research by Chang, Noonan, & Tennstedt (1998) indicates that spiritual and religious beliefs are beneficial for coping with caregiving responsibilities. Caregivers who utilized such beliefs reported better relationships with those in their care, as well as fewer feelings of resentment in coping with caregiving for disabled elders. Shared responsibility has also been found to be beneficial for caregivers. Lower stress levels and levels of depression were reported by family members who used adult day care to assist with caregiving responsibilities (Zarit, Stephens, Townshend, & Greene, 1998).

Research suggests that elderly people with no relatives tend to substitute a close friend whom they persuade to take the place of the absent family members. Most family and close friends still believe that they should take care of the elderly in their own homes if possible. Racial and ethnic variations exist in terms of who should be responsible for caring for the older generations. However, Lee, Peek, & Coward (1998) found that African American elderly were more likely to expect to be cared for by their children than elderly Anglo-American parents. Burr and Mutchler (1999) found that elderly Latinos shared similar expectations—they would be cared for by the younger generation.

The younger generation is not always the caregiving provider for elderly persons. The spouse or partner of the elderly person often assumes this role. Kramer and Lambert (1999) studied older husbands who cared for their ailing wives. They found that, in many aspects, these men fared less well than men married to healthy wives. Marital interactions, social integrations, household responsibilities, and well-being were all affected negatively. This confirms that it is more stressful to be in a relationship with an infirm person than a healthy person. Caring for an elderly person with dementia has been found to be the most stressful condition of all. Ory, Hoffman, Yee, Tennstedt, & Schulz (1999) found that caregivers of dementia patients spend significantly more time in the caregiving role than other types of caregivers. Dementia caregivers experience more caregiver strain and report higher levels of physical and mental health problems.

### CARE OUTSIDE THE FAMILY

Another option for elder care is a nursing home facility or retirement community. This option presents unique challenges. For example, how does a family choose an appropriate home for the parent? Numerous studies have investigated positive and negative characteristics of nursing homes. Castle and Fogel (1998) compared nursing homes that utilize restraint to those that are restraint-free. In general, the restraint-free facilities were smaller with a lower occupancy rate, had a more diverse nursing staff, and were more likely to employ more full-time equivalent registered nurses. Cohen-Mansfield and Werner (1998) found that, as expected, nursing homes that had enhanced environments, such as an outdoor nature environment, produced more positive evaluations by both residents and their families.

## Grandparenting

Family systems have been affected in other ways by the increased life expectancy; for many grandparents, this is a unique experience (Pruchno, 1999; Drew & Smith, 1999; King & Elder, 1998). The grandparenting experience has been positively linked to mental health and morale of elderly individuals. For example, in a classic study, Neugarten and Weinstein (1964) examined styles of grandparenting and devised categories for five general styles: "formal," "the fun seeker," "the surrogate parent," "the reservoir of family wisdom," and "the distant figure." A noteworthy finding was that the fun seeker and the distant figure appeared to be the most popular styles of grandparenting. Both styles reject an emphasis on authority. This reflects the finding that many grandparents preferred a grandparent–grandchild relationship in which their role was simply to enjoy spending time with their grandchildren, rather than feeling responsible as coparents with their adult children.

More frequently, however, many grandparents in today's world play a more integral part in the lives of their grandchildren. A survey conducted by the American Association of Retired Persons (AARP, 2000) concluded that the state of American grandparenting is strong. More than 80% of grandparents in the study had seen a grandchild in the previous month. Eleven percent of those participants were regular caregivers.

Recent research by Pruchno (1999) indicates that an increasing number of grandparents are raising their grandchildren alone. The parents of these children, the middle generation, are typically absent. Reasons for their absence include substance abuse, death, or incarceration. Pruchno found that African American and Anglo-American grandmothers differed in two important ways. First, it is more common for African American grandmothers to have peers who are sharing similar situations, raising the grandchildren. Second, a household containing several generations living under one roof is more common for African American grandmothers. These two findings may explain why black grandmothers experienced fewer emotional burdens from their caregiving roles than did white grandparents.

Grandparents are also playing a bigger role as day-care providers for their grandchildren. Most grandparents hope to have a positive effect on their grandchildren. King and Elder (1998) identified various factors that predicted how effective grandparents believed they were in the lives of their grandchildren. Some factors that were predicted to be effective were participation in church, living nearby, having a small number of grandchildren, and having known one's own grandparents.

Erikson's (1968) concept of generativity provides an explanation for the significance of grandchildren to grandparents. Erikson believed that generativity incorporated providing a better life for future generations and that not having reached the stage of generativity would lead to stagnation and self-absorption in the individual. Grandparents' personal development is fostered by their close rapport with younger generations and vice versa. When this essential relationship is disrupted, as in the case of divorce, the suffering of grandparents can be unbearable (Gray & Geron, 1995).

## Working in Later Adulthood Versus Retirement

A small percentage of all older adults—approximately 11%—remain in the labor force past the typical retirement age. Many older adults simply choose to stop working past age 65, whereas some careers require individuals to retire because of age. For example, airline pilots and public safety workers (e.g., fire fighters and police) can be forced to retire due to age. Of those adults who choose to remain in the workforce, most appear able to continue to successfully meet their job requirements (Clay, 1996).

### JOB PERFORMANCE

Some of the stereotypes about aging are being questioned, due to the increased life expectancy, aging of the baby boom generation, and decrease in birth rates. The stereotype that old age translates into declining performance is receiving more research attention recently because the number of workers in the last two decades of their careers will increase by 41%, while the number of workers 16 to 35 years old will decline slightly (Johnston, 1987).

This stereotype is supported by research on aging that indicates a decline in abilities such as dexterity, speed of response, agility, hearing, and vision. If all of these abilities decline, then one may conclude that job performance must also decline with age. McEvoy and Cascio (1989) compiled and analyzed the results of 96 studies and found no relationship between age and job performance. Regardless of type of performance measure (ratings or productivity) and type of job (professional or nonprofessional), no connection between age and job performance was evident.

A possible explanation for these results is experience. There may be no substitute for it, and it is extremely valued by employers. Older employees also tend to have lower absenteeism and accident rates, and less turnover and illness (Kacmar & Ferris, 1989; Martocchio, 1989). They also tend to report higher job satisfaction and more positive work values than younger workers. These qualities seem to offset any decreases in abilities caused by older age.

### RETIREMENT

For many older adults, retirement is a welcome relief from a less-than-enjoyable and unfulfilling job. For others it is very difficult and similar to being unemployed. Retirement requires changing habits that have formed over the adult lifetime. This likely explains why the aforementioned 11% of elderly people remain in the workforce.

Regardless of the reasons, most elderly people choose not to work. Smith and Moen (1998) suggest that the decision to retire is influenced by the retiree's spouse. Although most retirees consider their spouse's opinion a major factor, the spouses frequently believe that their opinions have little effect. The decision to retire is a complicated one, but many people believe that they have enough financial security to leave work. Health is likely the biggest factor. Retirement seems to be harder for males than females. Many men feel that they now have nothing to do, while their wives are often still working. Most older women have already adjusted to the reduction in their roles because the children have left the home, whereas for men the change seems to occur all at once.

**Leisure and Retirement**  How an older adult views retirement tends to vary depending on the work and leisure experiences an individual has before retirement. The leisure activities enjoyed throughout life play a vital role in later social adjustment. Type of work also affects how a person spends leisure time.

For example, work schedule affects when and how leisure time is available. A person who works night shifts will likely be unable to participate in typical evening activities, such as dancing or dining. Also, the specific type of work one does may influence leisure activities. People with physically draining jobs may be too tired to do anything except take a nap at the end of the day. On the other hand, a person with a desk job might choose physically challenging activities during leisure time.

When leisure is merely an extension of work experiences and attitudes, it performs what leisure theorists call a spillover function. For example, some people try to relax by performing some easier work tasks at home. Conversely, when leisure time is used to compensate for disappointment and stress at work, it is described as a compensatory function. An example would be excessive partying at the end of the workday or work week.

**Enjoying Retirement**  The belief that retired persons are an asset to the community is growing. Various efforts have been made recently to tap into this powerful resource. Many national programs now make an effort to involve retired people in volunteer and paid service to society.

Recent surveys seem to indicate that the "golden years" are not so golden for many retired individuals. However, this may change due to improving health conditions, improved understanding of the nature of life after age 65, and a considerable increase in government involvement. The lives of retirees may have a better chance at being rich and fulfilling. Getting old does not mean being lonely, despite stereotypes. In fact, most of the elderly have a good deal of free time, which they use to develop their social lives.

## Personal Development

In the field of personality development, two perspectives have received the most attention: the *activity theory* and the *disengagement theory*. According to the activity theory, human beings thrive through interaction with others and by keeping physically active. People are unhappy when, as the older years approach, their contacts with others diminish as a result of death, illness, and societal limitations. Individuals who are able to maintain the social activity of their middle adult years are considered the most successful.

Disengagement theory contradicts this notion. The disengagement theory proposes that the most mature adults are likely to gradually disengage themselves from fellow human beings in preparation for death. They become less interested in social interaction and more concerned with internal issues. They accept the decreasing attention of a society that considers them to be losing power.

This does not mean to imply that disengagement is more common than the tendency toward activity. It is believed by some that what has appeared to be disengagement is instead a transition from the highly active role of the middle-age adult to the more sedate, spiritually oriented role of the elderly person. Most individuals truly enjoy social contact, so disengagement from fellow adults may be the result of traumatic experience or mental disturbance, such as clinical depression.

On the other hand, activity theory may be considered too general, in terms of its stance on social contact (Marshall, 1994). For example, many people may reduce social contacts, yet keep active with solitary hobbies. Activity, per se, has not been found to correlate with a personal sense of satisfaction with life. Carstensen (1995) proposed a resolution of the debate by suggesting that humans use social contact to obtain physical survival, information they need, maintenance of a sense of self, and pleasure and comfort. Although these goals exist throughout one's life, the relative importance of each changes. For elderly people, the need for emotional support grows, while the needs for physical survival and information from others decreases. They tend to get support from relatives and close friends, and less frequently from casual acquaintances, such as coworkers.

Furthermore, the challenges faced in later life are quite unique. For example, Kling, Seltzer, & Ryff (1997) investigated elderly coping with loss of home, community relocation, and caring for a mentally ill adult child. Heckhausen (1997) and Tabourne (1995) have also evaluated coping skills of older adults. The elderly appear to be disengaging, but in fact they may be simply becoming more selective about with whom they wish to spend their social time.

## Relationships

The family system undergoes changes in membership, organization, and roles throughout human development. Because individuals may expect to live longer, due to improved health care, married couples will have more years together after children leave home. Though exceptions exist, most couples go through similar stages in the life cycle:

1. Child-rearing stage
2. Childlessness before retirement stage
3. Retirement stage
4. Widowhood and widowerhood

### CHANGES IN FAMILIES

The duration of each life stage and the ages of the family members vary from family to family. Childbearing patterns have much to do with quality of life in the later stages. Couples who complete their families in their early years will have a different lifestyle when the children leave home than couples who have children at home when they are ready to retire. This can present economic challenges for those retirees on fixed incomes, trying to meet the overwhelming costs of higher education. It also makes saving for retirement more difficult.

Retirement may bring about changes for both spouses, but wives who have not prepared themselves emotionally and financially for retirement may find it particularly stressful. Retirement typically includes a decrease in income and a lowering of the standard of living, but it may be awhile before some of these problems are noticed. Household responsibilities may change, with husbands generally contributing more.

Although many changes affect the elderly family, for some marriages, the saying "the more things change, the more they stay the same" may hold true. Studies have shown that among elderly married couples, certain factors contribute to the well-being of the relationship that, in turn, promote a stable, satisfying relationship. It has been found, however, that couples in which one partner suffers a long-term illness tend to have more problems (Wickrama, Lorenz, Conger, & Elder, 1997). As couples change over time, it will be interesting to learn whether interactions in the long-term marriage also change or if they remain stable despite individual development.

Conflict is an inevitable factor in any relationship that lasts over time. The relationship between elderly parents and their adult children is no exception. Clarke, Preston, Raksin, & Bengtson (1999) conducted a study of aging parents and their middle-aged children. They specifically investigated the emergence of common conflict themes. They found six types of conflict:

1. Communication and style of interaction
2. Lifestyle choices and habits
3. Religion, ideology, and politics
4. Work habits
5. Standards of household maintenance

Generational differences were indeed revealed. For example, older parents more often reported conflicts over habits and lifestyle choices than did their adult children. The children more often reported communication conflicts and interaction style conflicts.

Additionally, gender differences were found between older married husbands and wives as to the importance of support from family and friends (Lynch, 1998). Support from children was considered by women as most positive, whereas spousal support was considered most important by men.

### WIDOWHOOD

With women outliving men by large margins, the wife is most often the survivor. Only half of women over 65 are living with a partner. Many widows must assume additional duties, including managing household finances and janitorial tasks, and some will need to find employment. Widowhood affects social relationships with family and friends. Often a widow feels she is a "fifth wheel" in social settings, and previous relationships may dissipate. Fortunately, new social activities and friends emerge and replace old ones.

Howie (1992) proposed that we consider widowhood to be a normal part of aging for women. Thus, the ideal focus is shifted from bereavement to concern with the social implications of the extended years of the women's lives. Women should consider widowhood as yet another passage in the process of aging and dying.

Remarriage is an alternative to the loneliness most widows and widowers feel. However, remarriage rates for senior citizens are low, and most do not consider remarriage an option. Reasons for not remarrying include the following:

- Many elderly consider it to be improper.
- Children may be opposed to remarriage.
- Social Security laws penalize widows who remarry.
- There are three single women for every single man over age 65.

In her study of older widows' attitudes toward remarriage, Talbot (1998) learned that two-thirds of the participants said they were interested in and attracted to men. However, 55% were strongly opposed to remarriage. Only 15% felt favorably toward remarriage. Senior citizens who choose to remarry, however, enjoy much success if the ingredients of love, companionship, financial security, and consent of their children are present.

## Conclusions and Implications

Health care providers share a unique perspective on the periods of life generally known as adulthood and late adulthood. In a variety of ways, working in many different settings, health care providers have an opportunity to work with one of the fastest-growing age groups in the country. This opportunity entails a range of challenges that include psychological and counseling concerns as well as nutritional guidance.

In all aspects of adulthood, human beings experience the stresses that accompany life events, such as marriage, caring for aging parents, retirement, and declining physical health. Research literature may shed some light on particular issues in adulthood, but there is no one theory or model that encompasses the breadth or depth of this distinct time of life. Drawing from specific models, such as those presented in this chapter, may provide some guidance in terms of understanding the complexity of the human adult. Whether you are interested in learning more about spirituality or biopsychosocial factors involved in development, for example, the health care profession lends critical support to clients of all ages.

# References

A.A.R.P. (2000). Grandparents and kids: Getting along fine. *AARP Bulletin, 21.*

Blieszner, R., & Adams, R. G. (1998). Problems with friends in old age. *Journal of Aging Studies, 1,* 223–248.

Burr, J. A., & Mutchler, J. E., (1999). Race and ethnic variation in norms of filial responsibility among older persons. *Journal of Marriage and the Family, 61,* 674–687.

Cancian, M., & Meyer, D. R. (1996). Changing policy, changing practice: Mothers' incomes and child support orders. *Journal of Marriage and the Family, 58,* 618–627.

Carstensen, L. L. (1992). Social and emotional patterns: Support for socioemotional selectivity theory. *Psychology and Aging, 7,* 331–338.

Carstensen, L. L. (1995). Evidence for a lifespan theory of socioemotional selectivity. *Current Directions in Psychological Science, 4,* 151–156.

Caserta, M. S., Lund, D. A., & Wright, S. D. (1996). Exploring the caregiver burden inventory (CBI): Further evidence for a multidimensional view of burden. *International Journal of Aging and Human Development, 43* (43), 21–34.

Castle, N. G., & Fogel, B. (1998). Characteristics of nursing homes that are restraint free. *The Gerontologist, 38,* 181–188.

Chang, B. H., Noonan, A. E., & Tennstedt, S. L. (1998). The role of religion/spirituality in coping with caregiving for disabled elders. *The Gerontologist, 38,* 463–470.

Clarke, E., Preston, M., Raksin, J., & Bengtson, V. (1999). Types of conflicts and tensions between older parents and adult children. *The Gerontologist, 39,* 261–270.

Clay, R. (1996). Some elders thrive on working into later life. *APA Monitor, 35,* 12.

Cohen-Mansfield, J., & Werner, P. (1998). Predictors of aggressive behaviors: A longitudinal study in senior day care centers. *Journal of Gerontology, 53B,* P300–P310.

Costa, P. T., & McCrae, R. R. (1991). Trait psychology comes of age. In T. Sonderegger (Ed.), *Psychology and aging* (pp. 169–204). Nebraska symposium on motivation 1991. Lincoln: University of Nebraska.

Costa, P. T., & McCrae, R. R. (1994). Set like plaster? Evidence for the stability of adult personality. In T. F. Heatherton and J. L. Weinberger (Eds.), *Can personality change?* Washington, DC: American Psychological Association.

Davis, K. J., Sloane, P. D., Mitchell, C. M., Pressier, J., Grant, L., Hawes, M. C., et al. (2000). Specialized dementia programs in residential care settings. *Journal of Applied Biobehavioral Research, 4,* 139–156.

DeVries, H. M., Hamilton, D. W., Lovett, S., & Gallagher-Thompson, D. (1997). Patterns of coping preferences for male and female caregivers of frail older adults. *Psychology and Aging, 12,* 263–267.

Drew, L., & Smith, P. (1999). The impact of parental separation/divorce on grandparent/grandchild relationships. *International Journal of Aging and Human Development, 49,* 61–78.

Erikson, E. (1968). *Identity: Youth and crisis.* New York: Norton.

Gottman, J., & Krokoff, L. J. (1989). Marital interaction and satisfaction: A longitudinal view. *Journal of Consulting and Clinical Psychology, 57,* 47–52.

Gottman, J. & Notarius, C. (2000). Decade review: Observing marital interaction. *Journal of Marriage and the Family, 62,* 927–947.

Gray, C. A., & Geron, S. M. (1995). The other sorrow of divorce: The effects on grandparents when their adult children divorce. *Journal of Gerontological Social Work, 23,* 139–159.

Green, C. P. (1991). Clinical considerations: Midlife daughters and their aging parents. *Journal of Gerontological Nursing, 17* (11), 6–12.

Hauser, S. T., & Bowlds, M. K. (1990). In S. Feldman & G. Elliot (Eds.), *At the threshold: The developing adolescent.* Cambridge, MA: Harvard University Press.

Heckhausen, J. (1997). Developmental regulation across adulthood: Primary and secondary control of age-related challenges. *Developmental Psychology, 33,* 176–187.

Hoffman, S., & Duncan, G. (1988). What are the economic consequences of divorce? *Demography, 25,* 641–645.

Howie, L. (1992–93). Old women and widowhood: A dying status passage. *Omega, 26,* 223–233.

James, M. (1990). Adolescent values clarification: A positive influence on locus of control. *Journal of Alcohol and Drug Education, 35* (2), 75–80.

Johnston, W. B. (1987). *Workforce 2000: Work and workers for the 21st Century.* Indianapolis, IN: Hudson Institute.

Jung, C. (1933). *Modern man in search of a soul.* New York: Harcourt, Brace, and World.

Kacmar, K. M. & Ferris, G.R. (1989). Theoretical and methodological considerations in the age-job satisfaction relationship. *Journal of Applied Psychology, 74,* 201–207.

Kendig, H., Hashimoto, A., & Coppard, L. (1992). *Family support for the elderly: The international experience.* Oxford: Oxford University Press.

King, V. & Elder, G. H. (1998). Perceived self-efficacy and grandparenting. *Journal of Gerontology, 53,* 249–257.

Klagsburn, F. (1985). *Married people: Staying together in the age of divorce.* Toronto: Bantam Books.

Kling, K., Seltzer, M., & Ryff, C. (1997). Distinctive late-life changes. *Psychology and Aging, 12,* 288–295.

Klohnen, E., Vandewater, E., & Young, A. (1996). Negotiating the middle years. *Psychology and Aging, 11*(3), 431–442.

Knoester, C., & Booth, A. (2000). Barriers to divorce: When are they effective? *Journal of Family Issues, 21,* 78–99.

Kramer, B. J., & Lambert, J. D. (1999). Caregiving as a life course transition among older husbands: A prospective study. *Gerontologist, 39,* 658–667.

Lawrence R., Tennstedt, S., & Assmann, S. (1998). Quality of the caregiver–care recipient relationship. *Psychology & Aging, 13*(1), 150–158.

Lee, G. R., Peek, C. W., & Coward, R. T. (1998). Race differences in filial responsibility expectations among older parents. *Journal of Marriage and the Family, 60,* 404–412.

Levinson, D. (1978). *The seasons of a man's life.* New York: Knopf.

Levinson, D. (1986). A conception of adult development. *American Psychologist, 41,* 3–13.

Levinson, D. (1990). *Seasons of a woman's life.* Presented at the 98th annual convention of the American Psychological Association, Boston.

Lynch, S. (1998). Who supports whom? How age and gender affect the perceived quality of support from family and friends. *The Gerontologist, 38,* 231–238.

Mackey, R. A., & O'Brien, B. A. (1995). *Lasting marriages: Men and women growing together.* Westport, CT: Praeger.

Marks, N. F. (1996). Caregiving across the lifespan: National prevalence and predictors. *Family relations: Journal of Applied Family & Child Studies, 45,* 27–36.

Marshall, J. R. (1994). The diagnosis and treatment of social phobia and alcohol abuse. *Bulletin of the Menninger Clinic, 58* (2A), A58–A66.

Martocchio, J. J. (1989). Age-related differences in employee absenteeism: A meta-analysis. *Psychology and Aging, 4,* 409–414.

McAdams, D. P., de St. Aubin, E., & Logan, R. L. (1993). Generativity among young, midlife, and older adults. *Psychology and Aging, 8,* 221–230.

McEvoy, G. M., & Cascio, W. F. (1989). Cumulative evidence of the relationship between employee age and job performance. *Journal of Applied Psychology, 74,* 11–17.

McEwen, B. (2002). *The end of stress as we know it.* Washington, DC: John Henry Press.

Meshefedjian, G., McCusker, J., Bellavance, F., & Baumgarten, M. (1998). Factors associated with symptoms of depression among informal caregivers of demented elders in the community. *The Gerontologist, 38,* 247–253.

Mok, B., & Mui, A. (1996). Empowerment in residential care for the elders: The case of an aged home in Hong Kong. *Journal of Gerontological Social Work, 27* (1/2), 23–25.

Naleppa, M. (1996). Families and the institutionalized elderly. *Journal of Gerontological Social Work, 27,* (1/2), 87–111.

*National Vital Statistics Report, 50* (6). (2002).

Neugarten, B. L., & Weinstein, K. K. (1964). The changing American grandparent. *Journal of Marriage and the Family, 26,* 199–206.

Ory, M., Hoffman, R. R., Yee, J. L., Tennstedt, S., & Schulz, R. (1999). Prevalence and impact of caregiving: A detailed comparison between dementia and nondementia caregivers. *Gerontologist, 39,* 177–185.

Parker, R. (2001). Making marriages last: Why do some marriages dissolve in a relatively short space of time, while others go on for as long as 75 years or more, still vibrant happy relationships enjoyed by both partners? *Family Matters, 10,* 80–100.

Pohl, J. M., Given, C. W., Collins, C. E., & Given, B. A. (1994). Social vulnerability and reactions to caregiving in daughters and daughters-in-law caring for disabled aging parents. *Health Care for Women International, 15,* 385–395.

Ponder, R., & Pomeroy, E. (1996). The grief of caregivers. *Journal of Gerontological Social Work, 27,* (1/2), 3–21.

Pruchno, R. (1999). Raising grandchildren: The experiences of black and white grandmothers. *The Gerontologist, 39,* 209–221.

Ratner, P. A. (1998). Modeling acts of aggression and dominance as wife abuse and exploring their adverse health effects. *Journal of Marriage and the Family, 60,* 453–465.

Reinke, B., Ellicott, A., Harris, R., & Hancock, E. (1985). Timing of psychosocial change in women's lives. *Human Development, 28,* 259–280.

Riedel, S. E., Fredman, L., & Langenberg, P. (1998). Associations among caregiving difficulties, burden, and rewards in caregivers to older post-rehabilitation patients. *Journal of Gerontology, 53B,* 165–174.

Schulman, G. L. (1999). Siblings revisited: Old conflicts and new opportunities in later life. *Journal of Marital and Family Therapy, 25,* 517–518.

Selye, H. (1956). *The stress of life.* New York: McGraw-Hill.

Selye, H. (1975). Implications of stress concept. *New York State Journal of Medicine, October,* 2139–2145.

Selye, H. (1982). History and present status of the stress concept. In L. Goldberger & S. Breznitz (Eds.), *Handbook of stress: Theoretical and clinical aspects*. New York: The Free Press.

Smith, D. B. & Moen, P. (1998). Spousal influence on retirement: His, her, and their perceptions. *Journal of Marriage and the Family, 60,* 734–744.

Smock, P., Manning, G., & Gupta, S. (1999). The effect of marriage and divorce on women's economic well-being. *American Sociological Review, 64,* 794–812.

Steefel, N. M. (1992). A divorce transition model. *Psychological Reports, 70,* 155–160.

Stephens, M., & Townsend, A. (1997). Stress of parent care. *Psychology and Aging, 12,* 376–386.

Tabourne, C. (1995). The effects of a life review program on disorientation, social interactions and self-esteem of nursing home residents. *International Journal of Aging & Human Development, 41,* 251–266.

Talbot, M. (1998). Older widows' attitudes towards men and remarriage. *Journal of Aging Studies, 12,* 429–449.

Tirrito, T. (1996). Mental health problems and behavioral disruptions in nursing homes. *Journal of Gerontological Social Work, 27* (1/2), 73.

Umberson, D, Anderson, K., Glick, J., & Shapiro, A. (1998). Domestic violence, personal control, and gender. *Journal of Marriage and the Family, 60,* 442–452.

Van Laningham, J., Johnson, D. R., & Amato, P. (2001). Marital happiness, marital duration, and the U-shaped curve: Evidence from a 5-wave panel study. *Social Forces, 78,* 1313–1341.

Wacks, V., Jr. (1994). Realizing our inner elder-child. *Journal of Humanistic Psychology, 34* (4), 78–100.

Whitbeck, L., Hoyt, D. R., & Huck, S. M. (1994). Early family relationships, intergenerational solidarity, and support provided to parents by their adult children. *Journal of Gerontology: Social Sciences, 49* (2), S85–S94.

Wickrama, K. A. S., Lorenz, F. O., Conger, R. D., & Elder, G. H. (1997). Marital quality and physical illness: A latent growth curve analysis. *Journal of Marriage and the Family, 59,* 143–155.

Zarit, S., Stephens, M., Townshend, A., & Greene, R. (1998). Stress reduction for family caregivers: Effects of adult day care use. *Journal of Gerontology, 53B,* 267–277.

# Part Three

# Alternative Routes Along the Development Path

# Chapter 12

# Prenatal Development: Fetal Alcohol Spectrum Disorders

Paul D. Connor

Janet Huggins

Why would you, as a nurse, nurse-practitioner, physical or occupational therapist, or other primary care provider, need to know about prenatal alcohol exposure and the long-term impact of prenatal alcohol exposure on development? As a front-line provider of services, you may encounter individuals, children, adolescents, or adults who have been prenatally exposed to alcohol and have therefore been exposed to a teratogen that has lifelong developmental consequences. These individuals may come to you with a formal diagnosis of fetal alcohol syndrome (FAS) or a related diagnosis (e.g., partial fetal alcohol syndrome, alcohol-related neurodevelopmental disorder, or fetal alcohol effects). They will present with a complex developmental profile and will require interventions suited to this profile.

It is also likely that you will encounter patients who have been prenatally exposed to alcohol but not evaluated for FAS. These individuals may be completely unaware of their exposure history, have a multiple-problem history, and carry other diagnostic labels. Depending on your clinical environment, you may also work with women of childbearing age who are at risk for having prenatally alcohol-exposed children. These women may

have a serious drinking problem, but, more commonly, they may drink episodically at moderate or more socially acceptable levels, which also carries risk for the developing fetus (Jacobson & Jacobson, 1999). This chapter is designed to help practitioners identify individuals with FAS, understand appropriate interventions, and help prevent future births of alcohol-affected children.

## Historical Perspective

Although modern understanding of the damaging effects of prenatal alcohol exposure is relatively new, beginning with Lemoine's (Lemoine, Harrousseau, Borteyru, & Meneut, 1968) description of the offspring of alcoholic mothers, there are numerous historical reports of warnings about the dangers of alcohol consumption during pregnancy. The Bible demonstrates this warning by stating "Behold thou shalt conceive and bear a son: and now drink no wine or strong drink." (Judges 13:7). Further notations can be found throughout classical Greek and Roman mythology, suggesting that maternal alcoholism could lead to deleterious outcomes in offspring. In ancient Carthage, bridal couples were prohibited from drinking on their wedding night, for fear of producing a defective child (Haggard & Jellinek, 1942). In 1834, a committee of the British House of Commons indicated that maternal alcoholism was implicated in children who sometimes had a "starved, shriveled, and imperfect look."

It wasn't until 1900 that the first empirical study of the offspring of alcoholic mothers occurred (Sullivan, 1900). Sullivan studied incarcerated female alcoholics and noted an increase in the rate of stillbirths and infant death in the offspring. The rate of infant death from alcoholic mothers was more than double that of nonalcoholic female relatives. He further noted that as the mothers' alcoholism progressed, the outcomes of subsequent pregnancies were progressively worse. From his study, Sullivan determined that maternal drinking was the primary cause of this damage to the fetuses.

After the report by Sullivan in 1900 there was virtually no further research on the topic until 1968, when an article was published in a French journal (Lemoine et al., 1968). In this article, Lemoine and colleagues reported on 127 children of alcoholic mothers and found striking similarities in the children. All of them were small in stature, had psychomotor retardation, and had a specific pattern of facial anomalies. Lemoine concluded that these children were so similar that the cause of their anomalies must be due to the mothers' alcoholism. Unfortunately, this article was not translated into English, wasn't widely disseminated, and was thus not recognized for its importance at the time.

Five years later, a dysmorphologist at the University of Washington had similar experiences to Lemoine's when seeing the offspring of mothers who were alcoholics (Jones & Smith, 1973). Jones and Smith reported three cases of children exposed to alcohol in utero. They found that these children had a distinct pattern of facial malformation, were growth deficient, and showed a number of functional abnormalities. In addition to describing the children's anomalies, Jones and Smith coined the term *fetal alcohol syndrome* (FAS), a term that persists today.

Since these first reports of FAS in offspring of alcoholic mothers, research has progressed in human studies and animal models, gaining further understanding of the effects of prenatal alcohol exposure in the offspring of alcoholic and nonalcoholic women who drink during pregnancy. Furthermore, several prospective longitudinal dose-response studies were undertaken, first at the University of Washington and then in Detroit and Pittsburgh, to assess the effects of varying amounts of alcohol throughout pregnancy on offspring development. These studies have documented increased alcohol exposure associated with increased cognitive impairments persisting through adolescence and into adulthood.

# Teratogenesis of Prenatal Alcohol Exposure

The teratogenic effects of prenatal alcohol exposure reflect an interaction between the amount and the timing of exposure. It is often difficult to determine the amount of exposure to alcohol given the size of drinks and the variability of self-report. However, Table 12.1 offers general guidelines for categorizing drinking levels into four categories: abstainer, light, moderate, and heavy drinking patterns (NIAAA, 1997). Research employing these criteria, and using animal models of FAS, has confirmed that alcohol is a teratogen.

## Definition of Teratogen

For a substance to be considered teratogenic it must:

1. cause cell death, malformations, retardation of growth, and functional deficits;

2. be dose-dependent;

3. have critical periods of susceptibility; and

4. be affected by the interaction between genetics and environment (Wilson & Warkany, 1972).

*Table 12.1*  Guidelines for the Level of Drinking by Number of Drinks Consumed Per Day

| Drinking Level | Number of Drinks Per Day* |
|---|---|
| Abstain | 0 |
| Light | 0.02–0.99 |
| Moderate | 1.00–1.99 |
| Heavy | 2.00–3.99 |

*One drink = 1 oz. 100 proof liquor, 12 oz. beer, or 5 oz. of wine.

## Evidence of Teratogenic Effects

High doses of alcohol administered during gestation produced structural malformations such as eye defects (Cook, Nowotny, & Sulik, 1987); microencephaly (Pierce & West, 1986); cardiac and neural abnormalities (Ellis & Pick, 1980); defective neuronal migration, atypical cell proliferation (Miller, 1992); delayed myelination of the fetal brain (Phillips, 1992); and hippocampal and cerebellar cell loss (Goodlett, Bonthius, Wasserman, & West, 1992; Goodlett & West, 1992). Increased prenatal exposure to alcohol has lead to concomitant decreases in weight and increases in the rate of spontaneous abortions and malformations in animal models (Chernoff, 1977; Randall & Taylor, 1979).

Other studies have shown that the timing of the alcohol exposure impacts the subsequent type of damage to the brain. Although facial dysmorphology associated with FAS occurs with alcohol exposure very early in gestation (the equivalent of the first 6 to 8 weeks of pregnancy [Sulik, Johnston, & Webb, 1981], the central nervous system (CNS) develops throughout the entire gestation period and is therefore vulnerable to alcohol exposure at any time during pregnancy (Moore & Persaud, 1993). Brain weights were decreased and cellular migrations in the neocortex, hippocampus, cerebellum, and sensory nucleus were altered in rats exposed to alcohol during the second half of gestation (equivalent to the second trimester in humans) (Miller, 1992). Alcohol exposure during the animal equivalent of the third trimester revealed brain weight reductions, decreased head circumference, and reduction of cerebellar and hippocampal cells (Bonthius et al., 1996; West & Goodlett, 1990).

The final criterion of teratogenicity is that there is genetic susceptibility. This was confirmed by studies showing that specific genetic strains of mice are more susceptible to the effects of prenatal alcohol exposure than others (Chernoff, 1977).

## Diagnosis of Prenatal Alcohol Damage

The diagnostic term FAS was introduced in 1973 (Jones & Smith, 1973). Three diagnostic criteria were required in the presence of confirmed maternal alcohol use during pregnancy:

1. growth deficiency (low birth weight, lack of weight gain over time, disproportional low weight to height);

2. CNS disorders (small brain size at birth, structural brain abnormalities, neurological hard or soft signs such as impaired fine motor skills, neurosensory hearing loss, poor tandem gait, poor eye–hand coordination, mental retardation, and other cognitive impairments); and

3. a distinctive pattern of abnormal facial features or facial phenotype (short palpebral fissures, thin upper lip, flattened philtrum, and flat midface).

Since 1973, research and clinical experience revealed the need for additional diagnostic terminology to classify people who did not completely fulfill the criteria for a diagnosis of FAS but who had been significantly and adversely affected by prenatal alcohol exposure. The term *fetal alcohol effects* (FAE) was often used to describe these individuals whose facial dysmorphology were not sufficient for a full FAS diagnosis but whose central nervous systems were compromised. However, this term was not used uniformly, creating problems for clinicians, researchers, and policy makers trying to establish service guidelines.

## Diagnostic Categories

In an attempt to better codify the diagnosis of prenatal alcohol damage, the Institute of Medicine (IOM) reviewed the scientific literature and developed five diagnostic categories (Figure 12.1) (Stratton, Howe, & Battaglia, 1996).

Astley and Clarren (2000) note that although the IOM committee guidelines provided diagnostic clarification by creating additional categories to capture the range of people with prenatal alcohol exposure, the guidelines are not sufficiently specific to assure diagnostic accuracy or precision.

They propose a four-digit diagnostic code to reflect the magnitude of expression of the four key diagnostic features of FAS: *growth deficiency, FAS facial phenotype, CNS damage/dysfunction,* and *gestational alcohol exposure.* The magnitude of expression of each feature is ranked independently on a four-point Likert scale, and the resulting four-digit code is used for diagnosis (e.g., 4-4-4-4 = FAS).

### DIFFICULTIES WITH DIAGNOSIS

There is some controversy surrounding the emphasis that is placed on the FAS facial phenotype in standard diagnostic procedures due to concerns that it produces too many false negatives (Moore et al., 2002; Sampson, Streissguth, Bookstein, & Barr, 2000). As mentioned previously, facial dysmorphology only occurs from alcohol exposure very early in gestation. Several studies have demonstrated that neuroanatomic dysmorphology exists in patients with prenatal alcohol exposure in the absence of facial dysmorphology sufficient for the diagnosis (Bookstein, Sampson, Streissguth, & Connor, 2001; Sowell et al., 2001). In addition, the facial features of FAS are not static and can change to become much more normalized as children with FAS reach adolescence

---

*Figure 12.1*   Diagnostic Categories of Prenatal Alcohol Damage

- Category 1 (FAS with confirmed maternal alcohol exposure) retains many criteria originally proposed by Jones and Smith (Jones & Smith, 1973) and Clarren and Smith (Clarren & Smith, 1978).
- Category 2 (FAS without confirmed maternal alcohol exposure), as the title implies, utilizes the full criteria of FAS but is applied in cases where the alcohol exposure cannot be confirmed.
- Category 3 (partial FAS with confirmed maternal alcohol exposure) is for individuals who have confirmed exposure to substantial amounts of alcohol in utero; some (but not all) of the facial features of FAS; and evidence of either growth deficiency, CNS neurodevelopmental abnormalities, or a complex pattern of behavior and cognitive abnormalities.
- Category 4 (alcohol-related birth defects [ARBD]) is used for individuals who have confirmed alcohol exposure and evidence of physical anomalies that have been linked to maternal ingestion of alcohol.
- Category 5 (alcohol-related neurodevelopmental disorder [ARND]) characterizes individuals with confirmed alcohol exposure who have no physical manifestations of FAS but do have the CNS neurodevelopmental abnormalities that clinical and animal research have found to be related to prenatal alcohol exposure.

*Source:* Stratton, Howe, & Battaglia (1996), Institute of Medicine.

(Streissguth et al., 1991). Recently, in attempts to deemphasize the perceived importance of facial features in prenatal alcohol damage, researchers have proposed using the term *fetal alcohol spectrum disorders* (FASD), suggesting there is a wide range of effects due to prenatal alcohol damage (Streissguth & O'Malley, 2000).

Correctly diagnosing someone who has been heavily prenatally exposed to alcohol is a complex task. May and Gossage succinctly describe this difficulty: "FAS, ARBD, and ARND, . . . are complex, involving multiple indicators of physiology, development, and behavior, many of which are not obvious at all or are at least more difficult to identify at particular ages (e.g., birth)." (p. 161). An additional difficulty is confirming whether the biological mother drank during pregnancy. When available, this information is based on the mother's self-report or the reports of family members and friends. Detailed information about the number of drinks and the timing of exposure is difficult to obtain, and many children with heavy prenatal alcohol exposure are in foster care or are adopted and do not have access to even the most general self-report information. However, even with the difficulties inherent in obtaining an FASD diagnosis, as will be seen in the following sections, it is important to seek a diagnosis for those suspected of prenatal alcohol damage to ensure appropriate intervention and establish realistic treatment goals.

## Neuroanatomical Findings

This section describes the damage to the brain that is associated with heavy prenatal alcohol exposure. Subsequent sections demonstrate how researchers have linked this information with behavioral outcomes. It is important to understand the CNS damage found in patients with FASD because it underlies the cognitive, neuropsychological, and behavioral deficits seen by front-line health care providers working with these patients and impacts treatment efficacy.

### EFFECTS ON THE DEVELOPING BRAIN

Prenatal alcohol exposure damages organs and cells in the fetus with the most sensitive organ being the brain. Some of the first studies to investigate this type of damage involved autopsies of deceased infants with FAS. These autopsy cases involved the most severe cases of FAS, where the level of damage was not compatible with life. Although the brain anomalies found in these extreme cases may be more severe than those found in most patients with FASD, many of the same brain regions are affected. Jones and Smith ( Jones & Smith, 1973) described the first autopsied brain from a 32-week gestational age infant who died 5 days after birth. The brain was small (equivalent to 25 weeks gestation) and had massive gray matter displacement covering the left hemisphere, a thin and disorganized cortex, and enlarged lateral ventricles. There was dysgenesis (underdevelopment) of the cerebellum and agenesis (complete lack of development) of the corpus callosum. More autopsy studies followed showing similar damage due to heavy prenatal alcohol exposure (Clarren, 1981; Clarren, Alvord, Sumi, Streissguth, & Smith, 1978; Coulter, Leech, Schaefer, Scheithauer, & Brumback, 1993; Peiffer, Majewski, Fischbach, Bierich, & Volk, 1979; Wisniewski, Dambska, Sher, & Qazi, 1983).

The emergence of neuroimaging studies coupled with quantitative analyses of images have vastly improved our understanding of how prenatal alcohol exposure alters brain structures in individuals that survive early childhood. It has laid the groundwork for studies that measure the relationship between structural changes in the brain and behavioral outcomes. Reports of MRI and CT scans with samples of alcohol-affected individuals revealed complete or partial agenesis and underdeveloped corpus callosum along with a high incidence of midline anomalies; reductions in cerebral and cerebellar volumes as well as increased cortical and subcortical fluid; reductions of the basal ganglia, particularly the caudate; and reduction of white matter volume relative to gray matter volume, especially in the left hemisphere (Archibald et al., 2001; Johnson, Swayze, Sato, & Andreasen, 1996; Mattson et al., 1994, 1996; Mattson, Jernigan, & Riley, 1994; Mattson & Riley, 1996; Mattson et al., 1992; Riley et al., 1995; Sowell et al., 1996, 2001; Swayze et al., 1997). The majority of these studies have used traditional methods of measuring the volume and size of various brain regions. However, another method of analysis is to measure the shape of these regions. One such study found that patients with heavy prenatal alcohol exposure demonstrated a hypervariability of the thickness of the corpus callosum (either too thick or too thin) with respect to nonexposed subjects (Bookstein, Sampson, Connor, & Streissguth, 2002; Bookstein et al., 2001).

### NEUROIMAGING FINDINGS

These autopsy and neuroimaging studies have demonstrated that heavy prenatal alcohol exposure leads to damage in many regions within the brain. Understanding this connection is an important first step in appreciating the complexity of FASD. The next step is understanding the complicated relationship between this damage and neuropsychological and behavioral functioning throughout the life span.

# Neuropsychological and Clinical Profile

Prenatal alcohol exposure is associated with a broad spectrum of neuropsychological and behavioral deficits. These deficits are manifested in a number of cognitive impairments, personality traits, problem behaviors, adaptive function deficits, and learning difficulties that have been observed by parents, teachers, researchers, and clinicians (see Table 12.2). Not all these characteristics are seen in every individual who has been prenatally exposed to alcohol, but the range of behaviors and difficulties reported at different developmental levels is striking, showing the complexity of the clinical profile, and is related to the diversity of CNS damage. The precise relationship between CNS damage in a specific brain region, neuropsychological and behavioral testing performance, and their clinical presentation is sometimes unclear. This topic is an area of active research.

However, an example of this linkage is the finding that hypervariability of the corpus callosum thickness was found to be related to a specific pattern of neuropsychological performance in patients with heavy prenatal alcohol exposure. Those with an overly thin callosa demonstrated deficits in motor functioning with relative sparing of executive function abilities. Conversely, those with the overly thick callosa demonstrated deficits on executive function performance with relative sparing of motoric functioning (Bookstein, Streissguth, Sampson, Connor, & Barr, 2002). Therefore, those with the overly thick callosa and thus executive function deficits may present to the front-line practitioner with failures to keep appointments or troubles following recommendations or applying information inappropriately. In addition, these impairments in executive function could contribute to mental health problems and lead to adverse life outcomes such as troubles with employment, difficulty or inability to function independently, and troubles with the law, often referred to as secondary disabilities (Streissguth, Barr, Kogan, & Bookstein, 1996).

Often, practitioners rely on screening tools such as the Mini Mental Status Exam to assess the patient's gross neurological intactness. Although these tools can be useful in patients with other conditions such as dementias or an acute trauma, they have not been found to be clinically relevant in patients with FASD who have brain damage of prenatal origin.

A traditional neuropsychological report includes information garnered from a battery of tests assessing intellectual ability (IQ), academic achievement, learning and memory skills, executive function skills, attention, motor coordina-

*Table 12.2*  Personality and Learning Traits That May Be Associated with Fetal Alcohol Exposure

| Kindergarten– Sixth Grade | Middle School/ Junior High | High School | Post-High School and Early Adulthood |
|---|---|---|---|
| • Easily influenced by others; gets into trouble by following, or is "put up to it" by others who recognize their vulnerability<br>• Difficulty separating reality from fantasy. A "What did you do this weekend?" question might get this as an answer: "We flew to Hawaii on my Daddy's jet."<br>• Temper tantrums; different perception of either reality or environment<br>• Lying, stealing, disobedience<br>• Delayed physical/ academic/social development<br>• Memory loss or retrieval problems; may seem selective<br>• Impulsive<br>• Inappropriate social behavior<br>• Regression/retreat from the situation (or teacher)<br>• Silence<br>• Needs constant and consistent reteaching and repeating | • Passive response when asked to do a task<br>• Lying, stealing, without any reason for it, or because of a different perception of reality<br>• Poor reasoning skills<br>• "Me" centered<br>• Poor motivation<br>• Low self-esteem<br>• Academic impairments especially in math<br>• Depression<br>• Unwanted pregnancy/ STD's<br>• Possible loss of living facility<br>• Lacks a concept of time and time management<br>• Needs constant reteaching<br>• Possible alcohol and drug involvement<br>• Memory loss or retrieval problems | • Poor sequencing<br>• Lying, stealing, cheating, different perception of reality<br>• Poor reasoning<br>• Memory loss or retrieval problems<br>• Self-centered<br>• High level of frustration<br>• Unwanted pregnancy/STDs<br>• Low self-esteem<br>• Poor motivation<br>• Poor concept of time and time management<br>• Depression<br>• Need for constant reteaching<br>• Need for a different living facility; homeless<br>• Alcohol and drug involvement | • Constant retraining<br>• Need for patience and praise<br>• Poor logic and reasoning<br>• Poor concept of time and time management<br>• Unwanted pregnancy/STDs<br>• Inappropriate "showing off"<br>• Inability to sort information and set priorities<br>• Withdrawal<br>• Isolation<br>• Alcohol and drug involvement<br>• Lack of concept of cause and effect<br>• Unpredictable behavior<br>• Difficulty with finances<br>• Depression<br>• Suicide risk |

*Adapted from National Institute of Health—NIAAA (1999a). Publication No. 99-4369, p. 33.*

tion, and psychosocial functioning. The next section summarizes neuropsychological deficits associated with prenatal alcohol exposure within each of these domains and the implication of these deficits for daily functioning.

## Intellectual and Academic Function

Research over the past 30 years has shown that prenatal alcohol exposure is associated with general reductions in intellectual functioning. There is, however, a wide variation of intellectual functioning in this population. The first clinical reports of FAS predominantly described individuals whose intellectual abilities fell in the mentally retarded range (Streissguth, Herman, & Smith, 1978). Mattson and Riley (1998) reviewed studies from 1973 to 1996 that contained individual case reports of individuals with FAS. The average IQ score for all 79 collective cases was 66 (which falls in the mentally retarded range) with scores ranging from 20 to 120. When they reviewed retrospective studies of groups of children who had been diagnosed with FAS or had documented prenatal alcohol exposure, the average weighted IQ was 72 with scores ranging from 47 to 98.

In the Fetal Alcohol Follow-up Study, Streissguth and colleagues (Streissguth et al., 1996) report the intellectual abilities of a broad spectrum of individuals (age 6–51 years) diagnosed with FAS, FAE, PFAE, or ARND (between 1973 and 1996). The 178 individuals with FAS had an average IQ of 79 with scores ranging from 20 to 120, while those with FAE (295 cases) had an average IQ of 90 with scores ranging from 49 to 142. In other words, there is considerable variability in IQ across the spectrum of prenatal alcohol exposure; reduction in intelligence is not restricted to individuals with the facial phenotype. This study challenged the commonly held notion that all or most patients with FAS/FAE are mentally retarded. In fact, only 27% of the individuals with FAS and 9% of those with FAE had

an IQ score that fell in the mentally retarded range. Thus, it is the minority of cases that would be classified as mentally retarded. Therefore, when front-line practitioners are given a report that their patient has an IQ of 85, which is low-normal, this does not rule out the possibility that the patient has been affected by prenatal alcohol exposure.

The Fetal Alcohol Follow-up Study also assessed academic functioning in subjects with FAS and FAE. Individuals with FAS functioned roughly close to their intellectual ability in reading and spelling but below their intellectual ability in arithmetic. However, for those diagnosed with FAE, academic achievement in all three areas was below their measured intellectual level (Streissguth et al., 1996). Mathematics deficits are common in FASD populations and may help explain the chronic difficulties they seem to have managing money. Therefore, even though they may not be mentally retarded, as adults they may need a protective payee to help them administer finances appropriately and avoid being financially victimized.

## Learning and Memory (Verbal and Visual Spatial)

Learning impairments have also been noted in patients with FASD. Children with FAS and control subjects were administered a list learning test (Mattson, Riley, Delis, Stern, & Jones, 1996). When compared to control subjects, on average, the children with FAS had difficulty learning and recalling the words after a delay period and tended to make an increased number of intrusion and perseveration errors. They also had difficulty discriminating target words from distracter words and made more false-positive errors on recognition testing.

In addition to verbal learning impairments, patients with FASD often have deficits in spatial memory and visual spatial organization and planning. However, these deficits have not been well characterized (Mattson & Riley, 1998). Uecker and Nadel (1996, 1998) assessed children with FAS and matched control subjects on a task of spatial and object memory. On average, the FAS group demonstrated difficulties remembering the spatial location of objects but remembered the objects themselves. Carmichael Olsen and colleagues found that FAS patients had particular difficulties with spatial memory and visual-spatial processing ability (Carmichael Olson, Feldman, Streissguth, Sampson, & Bookstein, 1998). Sowell and colleagues report that a group of children, adolescents, and adults with prenatal alcohol exposure performed significantly worse than nonexposed controls on a measure of visuospatial organization and planning (Sowell et al., 2001).

These memory impairments can have direct implications for the provision of services. Persons with prenatal alcohol exposure may have difficulty remembering verbal instructions and thus may not follow through on recommendations. Due to spatial memory impairments they may get lost coming to the office, even if they have been there in the past, resulting in missed appointments.

## Executive Function

Executive functions are a group of crucial cognitive abilities that include self-regulation of behaviors, sequencing of behaviors, cognitive flexibility, response inhibition, planning, and organizing of behavior. They are essential for adaptively functioning within a complex world. Children and adults with FASD often demonstrate deficits in executive function abilities. A study by Kodituwakku and colleagues showed that, on average, children with FAS and FAE performed more poorly on a card-sorting test, with fewer categories correctly identified and more perseverative errors. They also demonstrated poorer verbal fluency and had poorer performance on a tower-planning test than did control subjects (Kodituwakku, Handmaker, Cutler, Weathersby, & Handmaker, 1995).

In another study, children with prenatal alcohol damage performed more poorly, on average, than control subjects, with specific impairments in planning, response inhibition, abstract thinking, and flexibility (Mattson, Goodman, Caine, Delis, & Riley, 1999). In this study no difference was found between subjects with the FAS facial features and those without the features but exposed to significant amounts of alcohol prenatally. Coles and colleagues found that, on average, children with FAS and FAE completed fewer categories on a card-sorting test than did either control subjects or children without prenatal alcohol exposure who were diagnosed with ADHD (Coles et al., 1997). Adolescents and adults with FAS and FAE made many more bizarre responses (reporting the length of a dollar bill as 12 inches) than did control subjects on a cognitive estimation task (Kopera-Frye, Dehaene, & Streissguth, 1996). Connor and colleagues found that many subjects with heavy prenatal alcohol exposure who were administered a battery of executive function tests performed more poorly than predicted based on IQ, suggesting that in a prenatal alcohol-damaged population, executive function deficits are a more direct result of the alcohol damage than an indirect result of alcohol damage on poorer intellectual functioning (Connor, Sampson, Bookstein, Barr, & Streissguth, 2000).

## Attention

Attentional functioning, either visual or auditory, is a common area of neuropsychological deficit in both children and adults with FASD. Visual attention is perhaps the most commonly assessed form by neuropsychologists. One study found that children of mothers who were alcoholics had higher rates of visual concentration impairments than either normal subjects or children of mothers with epilepsy (Steinhausen, Nestler, & Huth, 1982). Other studies have compared visual attention functioning of children with FASD to those with ADHD. Nanson and Hiscock (1990) found that children with FAS/FAE and children with

ADHD, on average, made more impulsive errors on attention tasks than did a group of control subjects. Another study found that children with ADHD had trouble focusing and sustaining attention, whereas children with FAS did not appear to have this difficulty as often (Coles et al., 1997). However, in this study subjects who were unable to complete the practice trials were not given the attention tasks, thus potentially eliminating children with FAS/FAE who had the most severe attentional problems. In a different study of adolescents and adults, patients with FAS were much more impulsive than the comparison group on tasks of letter cancellation and sustained visual attention (Carmichael Olson, Feldman, & Streissguth, 1992).

Auditory attention has been studied less frequently, especially in an FASD population. In one of the few studies, adolescents and adults with FAS performed more poorly, on average, than the normative sample on tasks of auditory attention (Kerns, Don, Mateer, & Streissguth, 1997). Another study utilized both auditory and visual attention tasks in assessing patients with FAS and FAE compared with control subjects (Connor, Streissguth, Sampson, Bookstein, & Barr, 1999). In comparison to control subjects, patients with FAS/FAE, on average, had deficits in both auditory and visual attention, but auditory attention deficits appeared to be greater.

The concept of attention seems simple at first blush. However, it is a fundamental skill that affects many areas of functioning. Poor attention can impact the patient's ability to learn new information, recognize early warning signs of problems, and attend to important safety cues in the environment.

## Motor Control

Although sometimes overlooked in neuropsychological evaluations, motor deficits have been reported in a number of studies. Evaluation of motor coordination is especially important in this population because this skill impacts their voca-

tional and recreational options. Individuals with FASD who have other cognitive impairments may typically be steered toward vocational training and careers, but if their motor coordination is impaired, this could pose difficulties for their employment success. One study examined the ability to maintain postural balance (Roebuck, Simmons, Mattson, & Riley, 1998). The examiners found that when visual and environmental cues were reliable, the alcohol-exposed group could remain balanced as well as the control group. However, when these cues were manipulated to be inaccurate or contradictory, the alcohol-exposed group performed more poorly than did control subjects, suggesting that they were more dependent on visual and environmental cues for balance than controls. In South Africa (Adnams et al., 2001) researchers found that although there were no significant mean differences between FAS and control children on the gross motor locomotion tasks, FAS subjects, on average, performed more poorly on tasks of eye-and-hand coordination.

Studies in children exposed to various levels of drinking in utero have shown dose-dependent increases in fine and gross motor deficits with increased levels of prenatal alcohol consumption (Barr, Streissguth, Darby, & Sampson, 1990). They found that the greater the prenatal alcohol exposure, the poorer the fine motor performance. The relationship was linear and not attributable to other prenatal ingestants or conditions. Fine motor steadiness (tremor) and latency to correct errors were related to both early and midpregnancy exposure. Balance, fine motor performance, and ratings of the quality of motor performance were related to early pregnancy exposure.

## Psychosocial Deficits and Problem Behaviors

Deficits in psychosocial skills and behavioral functioning related to prenatal alcohol exposure have been found at every developmental level. Prenatal alcohol exposure predicted aggressive behaviors in 4- to 6-year-olds (Griffith, Azuma, & Chasnoff, 1994). In 4-year-olds, moderate prenatal alcohol exposure was related to decreased attention and compliance compared to unexposed children (Landesman-Dwyer, Ragozin, & Little, 1981). Six-year-olds with moderate to heavy prenatal alcohol exposure were found to have increased impulsivity and hyperactivity versus unexposed controls (Fried, Watkinson, & Gray, 1992). Carmichael Olsen and colleagues, when studying 11-year-olds exposed to varying amounts of prenatal alcohol, reported dose-dependent alcohol-related behavioral differences in teacher ratings of such classroom behaviors as distractibility, restlessness, lack of persistence, and reluctance to meet challenges (Carmichael Olson, Sampson, Barr, Streissguth, & Bookstein, 1992).

Another study found that heavily alcohol-exposed children between the ages of 6 and 12 had, on average, higher elevations on several problem scales than nonexposed controls and that alcohol-exposed children, regardless of facial dysmorphology or diagnosis, had strikingly similar behavioral profiles with significant attention, social, and aggressive problems (Mattson & Riley, 2000). In another sample of 12-year-old children with prenatal alcohol exposure, Autti-Ramo (2000) found a relationship between the length of intrauterine alcohol exposure and the severity and frequency of behavioral problems. Behavior disturbances related to prenatal alcohol exposure do not appear to be due to reduced intellectual functioning, demographic factors, or full diagnosis of FAS (Mattson & Riley, 2000; Roebuck, Mattson, & Riley, 1999).

Behavioral problems of childhood that are related to prenatal alcohol exposure persist into adolescence and adulthood and may worsen, possibly resulting in an increased rate of mental health disorders (NIAAA, 2000). Carmichael Olsen and colleagues (1997), in a 14-year follow-up of children with varying amounts of prenatal alcohol exposure ranging from abstention to heavy, reported a relationship between greater prenatal alcohol exposure and increased behavior and learning difficulties in adolescence. In addition, a binge-like pattern (five or more drinks on an occasion) of maternal drinking and exposure early in pregnancy were related to antisocial and delinquent behaviors.

In a long-term follow-up of patients with FAS into adolescence, Steinhausen (1996) reported that 63% of the patients had psychiatric abnormalities, and there was an increase in emotional disorders and stereotypic behaviors across time. Streissguth and colleagues (1991) examined a group of adolescents and adults (age 12–40) with an FASD diagnosis and found that 62% had significant levels and 38% had intermediate levels of maladaptive behaviors. The most frequently reported problem behaviors were poor concentration and attention, stubbornness/sullenness, social withdrawal, dependency, teasing/bullying, impulsivity, periods of high anxiety, and a tendency to lie, cheat, and/or steal.

Adults with FASD appear to be at risk for mental health problems. Streissguth and colleagues (1996) note that over half of the adults in their large clinical sample were reported to have problems with depression. Another study examining the psychiatric history of 25 adults with FAS and FAE found that 44% reported a past or present major depressive episode (Famy, Streissguth, & Unis, 1998). Of particular concern is the high rate of suicide attempts; 23% are reported to have attempted suicide in their lifetime (Streissguth et al., 1996). The rate of adult suicide attempts in this alcohol-exposed sample is higher than the general population rate of 4.6% reported in the National Comorbidity Study (Kessler, Borges, & Walters, 1999).

### SECONDARY DISABILITIES

The neuropsychological and mental health problems described previously represent the primary disabilities associated with prenatal alcohol exposure. Secondary disabilities are those that a client is not born with that can be prevented or ameliorated with appropriate intervention. Secondary disabilities associated with FASD include disrupted school experiences, trouble with the law, confinement, inappropriate sexual behavior, substance abuse problems, and, in adults, difficulty with independent living and vocational problems (Streissguth et al., 1996). The incidence of each secondary disability varies depending on age but ranges from 30% for alcohol and drug problems to 60% for disrupted school experiences and trouble with the law. In adults, 78% were reported to have problems with employment (e.g., trouble getting hired or holding a job and losing a job without understanding reasons), and 82% had problems with independent living (e.g., needing help with daily living activities, managing finances, and organizing personal affairs).

Environmental factors interacting with the child's CNS damage can minimize or exacerbate the severity of secondary disabilities. For example, a child with CNS damage leading to poor impulse control, being raised by a parent who has poor frustration tolerance and limited parenting skills or supports, is at risk for problems at school, troubled peer relationships, mental health problems (e.g., conduct disorder, depression), and early substance abuse. However, evidence suggests that individuals who are raised in a stable and nurturing home, receive appropriate support services, and are diagnosed at an early age have fewer secondary disabilities than those who do not receive such services (Streissguth et al., 1996). Early intervention and diagnosis has generally been found to maximize the potential of children prenatally exposed to substances (Coles, Kable, Drews-Botsch, & Falek, 2000; Smith, 1993; Weiner & Morse, 1994).

## Intervention

The adverse outcomes of alcohol exposure during development have been well characterized as a result of 30 years of research, but interventions have not been systematically developed and evaluated (Carmichael Olson & Burgess, 1997; Coles & Lynch, 2000; Randall, 2001; Stratton et al., 1996). This lack of systematic research resulting in evidence-based interventions is unfortunate given that the incidence of FAS is estimated at 0.5 to 2 cases per 1,000 births, while the incidence and prevalence of FAS and ARND is estimated at nearly 1 per 100 (May & Gossage, 2001; Sampson et al., 1997).

Without evidence-based interventions, parents, clinical practitioners, and educators have come to rely upon the "wisdom of practice," the valuable knowledge drawn from the collected experience of those who work with individuals with FASD (Kleinfeld, 2000). Wisdom of practice has shown that working with FASD patients is not hopeless. However, it is difficult to predict the long-term outcomes of these interventions in adulthood given the number of variables that impact outcome, such as the variable effects of prenatal alcohol exposure, the quality of the postnatal family environment, the limited number of professionals knowledgeable about FASD, and the quality and availability of services (DeVries, Waller, & McKinney, 1999; Kleinfeld, 2000; Stratton et al., 1996).

The recommended intervention for FASD is a family-based, individualized, and multimodal management approach throughout the life span (Carmichael Olson & Burgess, 1997; Clarren, 2002; Hagerman, 1999; Smith & Coles, 1991; Stratton et al., 1996; Streissguth, 1997). Multimodal management involves coordinating several interventions: diagnostic assessments, special education, parenting training, individual therapy, medication therapy, family therapy, advocacy, group therapy and/or group support, medical and dental care, vocational training, and respite care. The areas of intervention included in a management plan will vary depending on the age, strengths, and weaknesses of the individual and the needs of the family.

## Levels of Prevention

Front-line providers often conceptualize treatment into three interrelated levels. Primary interventions promote healthy behaviors to prevent problems. Secondary interventions focus on the early identification and treatment of problems. Finally, tertiary interventions entail ongoing treatment and support services that ameliorate and/or accommodate the primary disabilities. The type of intervention varies depending on the FASD patient's developmental stage.

For women of childbearing age, primary interventions to avoid drinking during pregnancy help prevent the birth of alcohol-damaged children. During infancy and early childhood, secondary interventions include early screening and diagnosis, developmental monitoring, and early intervention programming. Tertiary interventions would include referral to parent and family support groups and respite care. During adolescence and adulthood, tertiary interventions include mental heath treatment, special education, vocational planning, and social skills training. Treatment involves a careful balancing of individual and family interventions. Also, the focus returns to primary intervention to prevent future births of alcohol-affected children.

## Examples of Interventions

This section briefly describes the interventions needed for prospective mothers and alcohol-exposed children at each developmental level (Clarren, 2002; DeVries et al., 1999; Hagerman, 1999; Kleinfeld, 2000; Kleinfeld & Wescott, 1993). These interventions lay a foundation for the next developmental stage, helping to reduce the risk of future problems (Streissguth, 1997). For example, if an adolescent receives appropriate treatment for a mood disorder, he or she is less likely to self-medicate with illegal substances or alcohol and develop a substance abuse disorder in adulthood.

### WOMEN OF CHILDBEARING AGE

Drinking during pregnancy remains a significant public health problem (Hankin, 2002). According to the Centers for Disease Control and Prevention (CDC), 3.3 % of pregnant women interviewed in 1999 reported frequent drinking and 2.7% reported binge drinking (CDC, 2002). Given such statistics and the fact that alcohol use among women of reproductive age is common, primary care appointments and family-planning visits provide an excellent opportunity to screen women of childbearing age for alcohol problems and to educate them about the risks of alcohol use during pregnancy or during the time they are considering becoming pregnant. Because there is no known safe amount of alcohol consumption during pregnancy, the Surgeon General and the American Academy of Pediatrics recommend abstinence from alcohol for women who are pregnant or who are planning a pregnancy (AAP, 2000; USDHHS, 1981).

The National Institute on Alcohol Abuse and Alcoholism has produced an important practical guide for primary-care providers to assist them with identifying at-risk drinking and intervening effectively with women of childbearing age (NIAAA, 1999c,). Several brief, self-administered screening questionnaires are available (e.g., TWEAK, T-ACE, Audit, CAGE) that demonstrate sensitivity and specificity for detecting problem drinking (Chang, 2001). If screening indicates that a woman is having problems with drinking, appropriate referrals for further assessment and interventions can be made. Brief interventions delivered in the primary care office setting or motivational interviewing techniques may be helpful because these strategies have been shown to reduce drinking levels (Handmaker & Wilbourne, 2001; NIAAA, 1999a). Brief interventions vary but typically involve one to three patient consultations incorporating personalized feedback on health problems, risks of drinking, setting drinking limits, problem-solving about how to avoid drinking, and/or discussing options for treatment and self-help. Women who are actively drinking should be counseled to use a reliable family planning method to prevent the birth of an alcohol-exposed child (Astley, Bailey, Talbot, & Clarren, 2000). Early detection of alcohol-exposed infants to facilitate early intervention is an area of current research. BARC+, a newly constructed screening scale, has shown promise for detecting individuals at risk for FASD (Barr & Streissguth, 2001). Coles and colleagues (2000) found that it was possible to identify infants at risk for alcohol-related developmental delay using a cumulative risk index.

## INFANCY

Infancy is a time to identify, monitor, and protect a child with prenatal alcohol exposure (Coles et al., 2000; Hagerman, 1999). The infant should receive consistent medical monitoring, evaluation, and treatment for any alcohol-related birth defects and referral to a high-risk infant-monitoring program if necessary. Infancy is also a time for intensive family intervention. If the family has a member with an active substance abuse problem, it is obviously difficult for the family to provide the calm and predictable environment that an infant with FASD requires. If one or both of the child's caretakers has a substance abuse problem, they should be referred for a substance abuse evaluation and subsequent treatment. If her substance abuse problem was detected when she was receiving prenatal care, the mother may have already completed treatment. In this case, it is important to directly support her abstinence or reduction in drinking. Be alert for signs of relapse and prepared to provide support services and respite care to help reduce overall family stress. The mother, in particular, will need parenting education to help her respond appropriately to the CNS dysfunctions common in alcohol-exposed children, such as tremulousness, irritability, weak suckle and feeding difficulties, disrupted sleep/wake cycle, and poor habituation (Coles, Smith, Fernhoff, & Falek, 1984).

Some infants may have been removed from the care of biological parents and may therefore be living in foster care or with relatives. Foster parents or relatives unfamiliar with the impact of prenatal alcohol exposure need education regarding the consequences of prenatal alcohol exposure and appropriate caregiving techniques. Such education helps caregivers to establish realistic expectations for the child, develop skills for responding to the child's special needs, and prevent caregiver "burn out" that can lead to multiple placements, a risk factor for secondary disabilities (Streissguth et al., 1996).

## TODDLER/PRESCHOOL YEARS

Prenatally exposed children at this age need continued medical evaluation and follow-up for any alcohol-related birth defects, monitoring for any signs of developmental delay and problem behaviors, and referral for necessary evaluations and intervention. These evaluations provide the information needed for an FAS diagnostic evaluation by a dysmorphologist, medical geneticist, or pediatrician who specializes in neurodevelopmental disorders. Because some of the physical and neurobehavioral features of FAS are similar to those found in other genetic, metabolic, toxicologic, and neurodevelopmental syndromes and conditions (e.g., Aarskog syndrome, Williams syndrome, Noonan syndrome, maternal phenylketonuria fetal effects) differential diagnosis is important (Thackray & Tifft, 2001). The role of primary care providers in the early identification and care of children with fetal alcohol exposure is so important that the National Institute on Alcohol Abuse and Alcoholism has produced a helpful guide (NIAAA, 1999b). The guide outlines steps for establishing an office-based intervention practice with connections to specialty services in the community.

Recommended interventions during this developmental period include speech-language therapy, enrollment in a Head Start program or an early intervention preschool, sensory-integration therapy, and/or occupational therapy (Carmichael

Olson & Burgess, 1997; Carmichael Olson, Morse, & Huffine, 1998; Morse & Weiner, 1996). During this time, the child continues to need a stable, calm environment with predictable responses from caregivers; therefore, referring caregivers for behavior management training is strongly recommended, as is referral to a support group for families raising children with FASD. These groups provide emotional support, information about services, and education regarding successful intervention strategies.

Even parents with children who have no developmental problems need a break from parenting, and this need is even greater for the parents of children with prenatal alcohol exposure who have complex developmental needs. Helping caregivers locate respite care is therefore an important intervention. A care provider who has ongoing contact with the child's family or caregivers is in a knowledgeable position to monitor family functioning and assess the need for further services. Additional support services that may be needed include psychiatric assessment and treatment for family members, housing assistance, vocational training, and couple/family therapy.

## SCHOOL AGE

Early diagnosis has been identified as a possible protective factor against multiple secondary disabilities associated with FASD (Streissguth et al., 1996). Ideally, a child with prenatal alcohol exposure should have received an FAS diagnostic evaluation by school age, so if this has not occurred, the child should be referred for assessment. Restructuring the environment to regulate sensory stimulation, teaching the child skills, and maintaining a consistent environment are three primary intervention goals during the school age years (Weiner & Morse, 1994). Participation in specialty therapies such as speech language therapy, occupational therapy, sensory-motor integration therapy, social skills training, and ongoing psychoeducational evaluation are critical for monitoring and maintaining progress.

Appropriate educational placement is a major intervention and challenge during the school age years, especially if teachers and school personnel are unfamiliar with FASD and its complexities. Continued monitoring and advocacy by parents is required, which can be a time-consuming and frustrating task. The impulsivity, attentional difficulties, and mood instability of an FASD child may be partly managed through medication, so referral for a medication consultation by a child and adolescent psychiatrist with particular expertise in neurodevelopmental disorders is often necessary.

## ADOLESCENCE

Clinical experience and the reports of families raising children with FASD indicate that adolescence is a particularly difficult period; however, there has been little scientific work to study these issues (Coles & Lynch, 2000). Kleinfeld suggests that this stage is difficult because it brings expectations for independence and achievement beyond what is possible for an individual with the neurobehavioral and cognitive deficits associated with prenatal alcohol exposure (Kleinfeld, 2000). The adolescent with FASD is unable to cope with the same level of independence as a typical teenager. Common problems encountered during this developmental phase include poor judgment (that requires caregivers to provide greater supervision than is typical of adolescents), difficulty finding friends due to poor social skills (that renders the adolescent vulnerable to the wrong peer group), psychiatric disorders (e.g., mood disorders, anxiety disorders, and PTSD), emotional distress as the child realizes that he or she is different, difficulty managing sexuality appropriately, problems with anger control, and poor academic achievement leading to decreased interest in school and risk of dropping out.

Psychiatric medications can help ameliorate the mood, anxiety, impulsivity, and attentional problems of the adolescent with FASD (Hagerman, 1999). Careful educational and vocational planning, which can include home schooling, special education placement, school-based vocational training, and/or social skills training can be beneficial. Participation in intentional groups (e.g., recreational groups, church-related activities, and summer programs) provides social contact, develops social and leisure skills, and provides opportunities for building self-esteem. Social skills training, sex education, and individual therapy adapted to the visual and experiential learning style of an adolescent with FASD can be valuable interventions (Baxter, 2000; Miranda & Levine, 2000).

An older child or teenager known to have been prenatally exposed to alcohol, who demonstrates longstanding behavioral problems, poor school performance, impulsivity, attentional difficulties, and mood lability, should be screened for FASD (Thackray & Tifft, 2001). Accurate identification, even at later ages, is still important so that appropriate treatment and intervention can occur. Most importantly, the diagnosis will help everyone, both the individual and those around him or her, to understand the individual's behavior. Instead of the behavior being viewed as an indicator of willful opposition, for example, it can be appropriately understood as reflecting neurobehavioral deficits.

### ADULTS

FASD adults, even if they have been receiving prior intervention, may reach adulthood with relatively normal intellectual abilities but with significant deficits in adaptive behavior and neuropsychological functioning, combined with psychiatric problems. These deficits may make it difficult for them to independently and routinely manage their own affairs, such as maintaining stable employment, remembering appointments, following through with instructions (including medications), managing financial obligations, and answering questions about past history (including medical). Therefore, adults with FASD may require continued support services, including psychiatric medication management, individual counseling, sheltered/supervised living arrangements such as group homes and supervised apartment programs, vocational training and/or coaching, assistance with life management, and, in particular, help with money management. The extent of the support and who provides the service—a family member, a social service agency, or a health practitioner—varies depending on the needs of the individual. However, the experience of families who have raised FASD individuals indicates that they need external support and structure even into adulthood (DeVries et al., 1999). Without such support and even in spite of this support, the adult with FASD is at risk for multiple secondary disabilities as well as various forms of victimization (DeVries et al., 1999; Kleinfeld, 2000; Streissguth & O'Malley, 2000).

## Conclusions

Although there is a dearth of systematic research resulting in evidence-based interventions for individuals with FASD, considerable information is available suggesting that "wisdom of practice" strategies can lead to good outcomes across the life span. Formal *diagnosis* of FAS requires a specialist; however, initial *identification* often occurs when an alert front-line service provider who is knowledgeable about FASD recognizes early risk indicators. Optimum care of individuals with FASD involves the custodial parent(s) along with a multidisciplinary team of providers, including occupational therapists, speech therapists, physical therapists, mental health professionals, teachers and educational specialists, and medical personnel. Front-line service providers are also in an ideal position to initiate prevention strategies with women at risk for bearing a child with FASD. We hope this chapter, by providing current information about the identification, diagnosis, and care of individuals with FASD, will serve as a resource and a foundation for your work with such patients and their families.

# Resources

## Practitioner Resources

NIAAA. (1999a). Brief intervention for alcohol problems. *Alcohol Alert, no. 43.* Available from *www.niaaa.nih.gov/publications/alalerts.*

NIAAA. (1999b). *Identification and care of fetal alcohol-exposed children: A guide for primary-care providers* (Volume 99-4369). Rockville, MD: National Institute of Health. Available from *www.niaaa.nih.gov/publications.*

NIAAA. (1999c). *Identification of at-risk drinking and intervention with women of childbearing age: A guide for primary-care physicians.* (Volume 99-4368). Rockville, MD: National Institute of Health. Available from *www.niaaa.nih.gov/publications.*

Kleinfeld, J. (2000). *Fantastic Antone grows up: Adolescents and adults with fetal alcohol syndrome.* Fairbanks, AK: University of Alaska Press.

Kleinfeld, J., & Wescott, S., (Eds.). (1993). *Fantastic Antone succeeds!* Alaska: University of Alaska Press.

Hagerman, R. (1999). Fetal alcohol syndrome. In R. Hagerman (Ed.), *Neurodevelopmental disorders: diagnosis and treatment.* New York: Oxford University Press.

## Further Web-Based Resources

- National Organization on Fetal Alcohol Syndrome (NOFAS): *www.nofas.org*
- Fetal Alcohol Spectrum Disorders Center for Excellence: *www.fascenter.samhsa.gov*
- National Institute on Alcohol Abuse and Alcoholism (NIAAA): *www.niaaa.nih.gov*
- FAS Family Resource Institute (FASFRI): *www.fetalalcoholsyndrome.org*
- Fetal Alcohol and Drug Unit (FADU): *http://depts.washington.edu/fadu*
- National Clearing House for Alcohol and Drug Information (NCADI): *www.health.org*

# References

AAP (2000). Fetal alcohol syndrome and alcohol-related neurodevelopmental disorders. *Pediatrics, 106,* 358.

Adnams, C. M., Kodituwakku, P. W., Hay, A., Molteno, C. D., Viljoen, D., & May, P. A. (2001). Patterns of cognitive-motor development in children with fetal alcohol syndrome from a community in South Africa. *Alcoholism: Clinical and Experimental Research, 25,* 557–562.

Astley, S. J., Bailey, D., Talbot, C., & Clarren, S. K. (2000). FAS primary prevention through FAS diagnosis: Part II. A comprehensive profile of 80 birth mothers of children with FAS. *Alcohol & Alcoholism.* 35(5), 498–508.

Astley, S. J., & Clarren, S. K. (2000). Diagnosing the full spectrum of fetal alcohol exposed individuals: Introducing the 4-Digit Diagnostic Code. *Alcohol & Alcoholism, 35*(4).

Autti-Ramo, I. (2000). Twelve-year follow-up of children exposed to alcohol in utero. *Developmental Medicine and Child Neurology, 42,* 406–411.

Barr, H., Streissguth, A., Darby, B., & Sampson, P. (1990). Prenatal exposure to alcohol, caffeine, tobacco, and aspirin: Effects on fine and gross motor performance in 4-year old children. *Developmental Psychology, 26,* 339–348.

Barr, H. M., & Streissguth, A. P. (2001). Identifying maternal self-reported alcohol use associated with fetal alcohol spectrum disorders. *Alcoholism: Clinical and Experimental Research, 25,* 283–287.

Baxter, S. (2000). Adapting talk therapy for individuals with FAS/E. In J. Kleinfeld (Ed.), *Fantastic Antone grows up: adolescents and adults with fetal alcohol syndrome* (pp. 169–192). Anchorage, AK: University of Alaska Press.

Bonthius, D. J., Bonthius, N. E., Napper, R. M., Astley, S. J., Clarren, S. K., & West, J. R. (1996). Purkinje cell deficits in nonhuman primates following weekly exposure to ethanol during gestation. *Teratology, 53,* 230–236.

Bookstein, F., Sampson, P., Connor, P., & Streissguth, A. (2002). Midline corpus callosum is a neuroanatomical focus of fetal alcohol damage. *The Anatomical Record (New Anatomist), 269,* 162–174.

Bookstein, F., Streissguth, A., Sampson, P., Connor, P., & Barr, H. (2002). Corpus callosum shape and neuropsychological deficits in adult males with heavy fetal alcohol exposure. *NeuroImage, 15,* 233–251.

Bookstein, F. L., Sampson, P. D., Streissguth, A. P., & Connor, P. D. (2001). Geometric morphometrics of corpus callosum and subcortical structures in the fetal-alcohol-affected brain. *Teratology, 64,* 4–32.

Carmichael Olson, H., & Burgess, D. M. (1997). Early intervention for children prenatally exposed to alcohol and other drugs. In M. J. Guralnick (Ed.), *The Effectiveness of early intervention.* Baltimore, MD: Paul H. Brookes Publishing Company.

Carmichael Olson, H., Feldman, J., & Streissguth, A. P. (1992). Neuropsychological deficits and life adjustment in adolescents and adults with fetal alcohol syndrome. *Alcoholism: Clinical and Experimental Research, 16,* 380.

Carmichael Olson, H., Feldman, J. J., Streissguth, A. P., Sampson, P. D., & Bookstein, F. L. (1998). Neuropsychological deficits in adolescents with fetal alcohol syndrome: Clinical findings. *Alcoholism: Clinical and Experimental Research, 22,* 1998–2012.

Carmichael Olson, H., Morse, B., & Huffine, C. (1998). Development and psychopathology: Fetal alcohol syndrome and related conditions. *Seminars in Clinical Neuropsychiatry, 3,* 262–284.

Carmichael Olson, H., Sampson, P. D., Barr, H., Streissguth, A. P., & Bookstein, F. L. (1992). Prenatal exposure to alcohol and school problems in late childhood: A longitudinal prospective study. *Developmental Psychopathology, 4,* 341–359.

Carmichael Olson, H., Streissguth, A. P., Sampson, P. D., Barr, H. M., Bookstein, F. L., & Thiede, K. (1997). Association of prenatal alcohol exposure with behavioral and learning problems in early adolescence. *Journal of the American Academy of Child and Adolescent Psychiatry, 36,* 1187–1194.

CDC. (2002). Alcohol use among women of childbearing age—United States, 1991–1999. *Morbidity and Mortality Weekly Reports, 51*(13), 273–276.

Chang, G. (2001). Alcohol screening instruments for pregnant women. *Alcohol Research & Health, 25,* 204–209.

Chernoff, G. F. (1977). The fetal alcohol syndrome in mice: an animal model. *Teratology, 15,* 223–229.

Clarren, S. (2002). Matrices track problems and interventions. *Iceberg, 12*(3), 3–5.

Clarren, S., & Smith, D. (1978). The fetal alcohol syndrome. *New England Journal of Medicine, 298*(8), 1063–1067.

Clarren, S. K. (1981). Recognition of fetal alcohol syndrome. *Journal of the American Medical Association, 245,* 2436–2439.

Clarren, S. K., Alvord, E. C., Jr., Sumi, S. M., Streissguth, A. P., & Smith, D. W. (1978). Brain malformations related to prenatal exposure to ethanol. *Journal of Pediatrics, 92,* 64–67.

Coles, C. D., Kable, J. A., Drews-Botsch, C., & Falek, A. (2000). Early identification of risk for effects of prenatal alcohol exposure. *Journal of Studies on Alcohol, 61,* 607–616.

Coles, C. D., & Lynch, M. (2000). Adolescents with disabilities: Insights for individuals with FAS/E. In J. Kleinfeld (Ed.), *Fantastic Antone grows up: Adolescents and adults with fetal alcohol syndrome* (pp. 247–258). Anchorage, AK: University of Alaska Press.

Coles, C. D., Platzman, K. A., Raskind-Hood, C. L., Brown, R. T., Falek, A., & Smith, I. E. (1997). A comparison of children affected by prenatal alcohol exposure and attention deficit, hyperactivity disorder. *Alcoholism: Clinical and Experimental Research, 21,* 150–161.

Coles, C. D., Smith, I. E., Fernhoff, P. M., & Falek, A. (1984). Neonatal ethanol withdrawal: characteristics in clinically normal, nondysmorphic neonates. *Journal of Pediatrics, 105,* 445–451.

Connor, P. D., Sampson, P. D., Bookstein, F. L., Barr, H. M., & Streissguth, A. P. (2000). Direct and indirect effects of prenatal alcohol damage on executive function. *Developmental Neuropsychology, 18,* 331–354.

Connor, P. D., Streissguth, A. P., Sampson, P. D., Bookstein, F. L., & Barr, H. M. (1999). Individual differences in auditory and visual attention among fetal alcohol-affected adults. *Alcoholism: Clinical and Experimental Research, 23,* 1395–1402.

Cook, C. S., Nowotny, A. Z., & Sulik, K. K. (1987). Fetal alcohol syndrome. Eye malformations in a mouse model. *Archives of Ophthalmology, 105,* 1576–1581.

Coulter, C. L., Leech, R. W., Schaefer, G. B., Scheithauer, B. W., & Brumback, R. A. (1993). Midline cerebral dysgenesis, dysfunction of the hypothalamic-pituitary axis, and fetal alcohol effects. *Archives of Neurology, 50,* 771–775.

DeVries, J., Waller, A., & McKinney, V. (1999). *FAS/E: A standard of care for toddlers, children, adolescents and adults.* Lynnwood, WA: FAS Family Resource Institute.

Ellis, F. W., & Pick, J. R. (1980). An animal model of the fetal alcohol syndrome in beagles. *Alcoholism: Clinical and Experimental Research, 4*(2), 123–134.

Famy, C., Streissguth, A. P., & Unis, A. S. (1998). Mental illness in adults with fetal alcohol syndrome or fetal alcohol effects. *American Journal of Psychiatry, 155,* 552–554.

Fried, P., Watkinson, B., & Gray, R. (1992). A follow-up study of attention and behavior in six-year-old children exposed prenatally to marijuana, cigarettes, and alcohol. *Neurotoxicology and Teratology, 14,* 299–311.

Goodlett, C. R., Bonthius, D. J., Wasserman, E. A., & West, J. R. (1992). An animal model of CNS dysfunction associated with prenatal alcohol exposure: Behavioral and neuroanatomical correlates. In E. A. Wasserman (Ed.), *Learning and memory: behavioral and biological processes* (pp. 183–208). Inglewood NJ: Lawrence Erlbaum.

Goodlett, C. R., & West, J. R. (1992). Fetal alcohol effects: rat model of alcohol exposure during the brain growth spurt. In T. A. Slotkin (Ed.), *Maternal substance abuse and the developing nervous system* (pp. 45–75). San Diego, CA: Academic Press.

Griffith, D. R., Azuma, S. D., & Chasnoff, I. J. (1994). Three-year outcome of children exposed prenatally to drugs. *Journal of the American Academy of Child and Adolescent Psychiatry, 33,* 20–27.

Hagerman, R. (1999). Fetal alcohol syndrome. In R. Hagerman (Ed.), *Neurodevelopmental disorders: diagnosis and treatment.* New York: Oxford University Press.

Haggard, H., & Jellinek, E. (1942). *Alcohol explored.* New York: Doubleday.

Handmaker, N., & Wilbourne, P. (2001). Motivational interventions in prenatal clinics. *Alcohol Research & Health, 25,* 219–229.

Hankin, J. (2002). Fetal alcohol syndrome prevention research. *Alcohol Research & Health, 25,* 219–229.

Jacobson, J. L., & Jacobson, S. W. (1999). Drinking moderately and pregnancy. Effects on child development. *Alcohol Research & Health, 23,* 25–30.

Johnson, V. P., Swayze, V. W., II, Sato, Y., & Andreasen, N. C. (1996). Fetal alcohol syndrome: craniofacial and central nervous system manifestations. *American Journal of Medical Genetics, 61,* 329–339.

Jones, K. L., & Smith, D. W. (1973). Recognition of the fetal alcohol syndrome in early infancy. *Lancet, 2*(7836), 999–1001.

Kerns, K. A., Don, A., Mateer, C. A., & Streissguth, A. P. (1997). Cognitive deficits in nonretarded adults with fetal alcohol syndrome. *Journal of Learning Disabilities, 30,* 685–693.

Kessler, R., Borges, G., & Walters, E. (1999). Prevalence of and risk factors for lifetime suicide attempts in the National Comorbidity Survey. *Archives of General Psychiatry, 56,* 617–626.

Kleinfeld, J. (2000). *Fantastic Antone grows up: Adolescents and adults with fetal alcohol syndrome.* Fairbanks, AK: University of Alaska Press.

Kleinfeld, J., & Wescott, S. (Eds.). (1993). *Fantastic Antone Succeeds!* Alaska: University of Alaska Press.

Kodituwakku, P. W., Handmaker, N. S., Cutler, S. K., Weathersby, E. K., & Handmaker, S. D. (1995). Specific impairments in self-regulation in children exposed to alcohol prenatally. *Alcoholism: Clinical and Experimental Research, 19,* 1558–1564.

Kopera-Frye, K., Dehaene, S., & Streissguth, A. P. (1996). Impairments of number processing induced by prenatal alcohol exposure. *Neuropsychologia, 34,* 1187–1196.

Landesman-Dwyer, S., Ragozin, A. S., & Little, R. E. (1981). Behavioral correlates of prenatal alcohol exposure: A four-year follow-up study. *Neurobehavioral Toxicology and Teratology, 3,* 187–193.

Lemoine, P., Harrousseau, H., Borteyru, J. P., & Meneut, J. C. (1968). Les enfant des parents alcooliques: Anomalies oberveés, à propos de 127 cas. *Ouest Medical, 21,* 476–482.

Mattson, S., Riley, E. P., Jernigan, T. L., Garcia, A., Kaneko, W. M., Ehlers, C. L., et al. (1994). A decrease in the size of the basal ganglia following prenatal alcohol exposure: a preliminary report. *Neurotoxicology and Teratology, 16,* 283–289.

Mattson, S. N., Goodman, A. M., Caine, C., Delis, D. C., & Riley, E. P. (1999). Executive functioning in children with heavy prenatal alcohol exposure. *Alcoholism: Clinical and Experimental Research, 23,* 1808–1815.

Mattson, S. N., Jernigan, T. L., & Riley, E. P. (1994). MRI and prenatal alcohol exposure: Images provide insight into FAS. *Alcohol Health and Research World, 18,* 49–52.

Mattson, S. N., & Riley, E. P. (1996). Brain anomalies in fetal alcohol syndrome. In E. L. Abel (Ed.), *Fetal alcohol syndrome: From mechanisms to prevention.* Boca Raton, FL: CRC Press.

Mattson, S. N., & Riley, E. P. (1998). A review of the neurobehavioral deficits in children with fetal alcohol syndrome or prenatal exposure to alcohol. *Alcoholism: Clinical and Experimental Research, 22,* 279–294.

Mattson, S. N., & Riley, E. P. (2000). Parent ratings of behavior in children with heavy prenatal alcohol exposure and IQ-matched controls. *Alcoholism: Clinical and Experimental Research, 24,* 226–231.

Mattson, S. N., Riley, E. P., Delis, D. C., Stern, C., & Jones, K. L. (1996). Verbal learning and memory in children with fetal alcohol syndrome. *Alcoholism: Clinical and Experimental Research, 20,* 810–816.

Mattson, S. N., Riley, E. P., Jernigan, T. L., Ehlers, C. L., Delis, D. C., Jones, K. L., et al. (1992). Fetal alcohol syndrome: A case report of neuropsychological, MRI and EEG assessment of two children. *Alcoholism: Clinical and Experimental Research, 16,* 1001–1003.

Mattson, S. N., Riley, E. P., Sowell, E. R., Jernigan, D. F., Sobel, D. F., & Jones, K. L. (1996). A decrease in size of the basal ganglia in children with fetal alcohol syndrome. *Alcoholism: Clinical and Experimental Research, 20,* 1088–1093.

May, P., & Gossage, J. (2001). Estimating the prevalence of fetal alcohol syndrome: A summary. *Alcohol Research & Health, 25,* 159–167.

Miller, M. (1992). Effects of prenatal exposure to ethanol on cell proliferation and neuronal migration. In M. Miller (Ed.), *Development of the central nervous System: Effects of alcohol and opiates* (pp. 47–69). New York: Wiley-Liss Inc.

Miranda, S., & Levine, K. (2000). Sexuality and young adults with FAS/E. In J. Kleinfeld (Ed.), *Fantastic Antone grows up: Adolescents and adults with fetal alcohol syndrome* (pp. 203–217). Anchorage, AK: University of Alaska Press.

Moore, E., Ward, R., Jamison, P., Morris, C., Bader, P., & Hall, B. (2002). New perspectives on the face in fetal alcohol syndrome. *American Journal of Medical Genetics, 109,* 249–260.

Moore, K., & Persaud, T. (1993). *The developing human: Clinically oriented embryology.* Philadelphia: W.B. Saunders Co.

Morse, B., & Weiner, L. (1996). Rehabilitation approaches for fetal alcohol syndrome. In H. C. Steinhausen (Ed.), *Alcohol, pregnancy, and the developing child* (pp. 249–267). New York: Cambridge University Press.

Nanson, J. L., & Hiscock, M. (1990). Attention deficits in children exposed to alcohol prenatally. *Alcoholism: Clinical and Experimental Research, 14,* 656–661.

NIAAA. (1997). *Alcohol and health: Ninth special report to the U.S. Congress* (Volume Publication Number: 97-4017). Bethesda, MD: National Institutes of Health.

NIAAA. (1999a). Brief intervention for alcohol problems. *Alcohol Alert, no. 43.*

NIAAA. (1999b). *Identification and care of fetal alcohol-exposed children: A guide for primary-care providers* (Volume 99-4369). Rockville, MD: National Institute of Health.

NIAAA. (1999c). Identification of at-risk drinking and intervention with women of childbearing age: A guide for primary-care physicians. (Volume 99-4368). Rockville, MD: National Institute of Health.

NIAAA. (2000). Prenatal exposure to alcohol. *Alcohol Research & Health, 24,* 32–41.

Peiffer, J., Majewski, F., Fischbach, H., Bierich, J. R., & Volk, B. (1979). Alcohol embryo- and fetopathy. Neuropathology of 3 children and 3 fetuses. *Journal of the Neurological Sciences, 41*(2), 125–137.

Phillips, D. E. (1992). Effects of alcohol on the development of glial cell and myelin. In R. R. Watson (Ed.), *Alcohol and neurobiology: Brain development and hormone regulation* (pp. 83–108). Boca Raton: CRC Press.

Pierce, D. R., & West, J. R. (1986). Alcohol-induced microencephaly during the third trimester equivalent: Relationship to dose and blood alcohol concentration. *Alcohol, 3*(3), 185–191.

Randall, C. (2001). Alcohol and pregnancy: Highlights from three decades of research. *Journal of Studies on Alcohol, 62,* 554–558.

Randall, C. L., & Taylor, W. J. (1979). Prenatal ethanol exposure in mice: teratogenic effects. *Teratology, 19*(3), 305–311.

Riley, E. P., Mattson, S. N., Sowell, E. R., Jernigan, T. L., Sobel, D. F., & Jones, K. L. (1995). Abnormalities of the corpus callosum in children prenatally exposed to alcohol. *Alcoholism: Clinical and Experimental Research, 19,* 1198–1202.

Roebuck, T., Simmons, R., Mattson, S., & Riley, E. (1998). Prenatal exposure to alcohol affects the ability to maintain postural balance. *Alcoholism: Clinical and Experimental Research, 22,* 252–258.

Roebuck, T. M., Mattson, S. N., & Riley, E. P. (1999). Behavioral and psychosocial profiles of alcohol-exposed children. *Alcoholism: Clinical and Experimental Research, 23,* 1070–1076.

Sampson, P. D., Streissguth, A. P., Bookstein, F. L., & Barr, H. M. (2000). On categorizations in analyses of alcohol teratogenesis. *Environmental Health Perspectives, 108*(Suppl 3), 421–428.

Sampson, P. D., Streissguth, A. P., Bookstein, F. L., Little, R. E., Clarren, S. K., Dehaene, P., et al. (1997). Incidence of fetal alcohol syndrome and prevalence of alcohol-related neurodevelopmental disorder. *Teratology, 56,* 317–326.

Smith, G. (1993). Intervention strategies for children vulnerable for school failure due to exposure to drugs and alcohol. *International Journal of the Addictions, 28,* 1435–1470.

Smith, I., & Coles, C. (1991). Multilevel intervention for prevention of fetal alcohol syndrome and effects of prenatal alcohol exposure. In M. Galanter (Ed.), *Recent developments in alcoholism: Children of alcoholics* (Volume 9, pp. 165–180). New York: Plenum Press.

Sowell, E. R., Jernigan, T. L., Mattson, S. N., Riley, E. P., Sobel, D. F., & Jones, K. L. (1996). Abnormal development of the cerebellar vermis in children prenatally exposed to alcohol: size reduction in lobules I-V. *Alcoholism: Clinical and Experimental Research, 20,* 31–34.

Sowell, E. R., Mattson, S. N., Thompson, P. M., Jernigan, T. L., Riley, E. P., & Toga, A. W. (2001). Mapping callosal morphology and cognitive correlates: Effects of heavy prenatal alcohol exposure. *Neurology, 57,* 235–244.

Sowell, E. R., Thompson, P. M., Mattson, S. N., Tessner, K. D., Jernigan, T. L., Riley, E. P., et al. (2001). Voxel-based morphometric analyses of the brain in children and adolescents prenatally exposed to alcohol. *Neuroreport, 12,* 515–523.

Steinhausen, H. C. (1996). Psychopathology and cognitive functioning in children with fetal alcohol syndrome. In H. C. Steinhausen (Ed.), *Alcohol, Pregnancy and the Developing Child* (pp. 227–248). Cambridge, UK: Cambridge University Press.

Steinhausen, H. C., Nestler, V., & Huth, H. (1982). Psychopathology and mental functions in the offspring of alcoholic and epileptic mothers. *Journal of the American Academy of Child and Adolescent Psychiatry, 21,* 268–273.

Stratton, K., Howe, C., & Battaglia, F. (1996). *Fetal alcohol syndrome: Diagnosis, epidemiology, prevention, and treatment.* Institute of Medicine, U.S. National Academy of Sciences Washington DC: National Academy Press.

Streissguth, A. (1997). *Fetal alcohol syndrome: A guide for families and communities.* Baltimore: Paul H. Brookes.

Streissguth, A. P., Aase, J. M., Clarren, S. K., Randels, S. P., LaDue, R. A., & Smith, D. F. (1991). Fetal alcohol syndrome in adolescents and adults. *Journal of the American Medical Association, 265,* 1961–1967.

Streissguth, A. P., Barr, H., Kogan, J., & Bookstein, F. L. (1996). *Understanding the occurrence of secondary disabilities in clients with fetal alcohol syndrome (FAS) and fetal alcohol effects (FAE). Final report to the Centers for Dis-*

ease Control and Prevention. Grant #R04/CCR008515. Seattle: University of Washington School of Medicine.

Streissguth, A. P., Herman, C. S., & Smith, D. W. (1978). Intelligence, behavior, and dysmorphogenesis in the fetal alcohol syndrome: A report on 20 patients. *Journal of Pediatrics, 92*, 363–367.

Streissguth, A. P., & O'Malley, K. (2000). Neuropsychiatric implications and long-term consequences of fetal alcohol spectrum disorders. *Seminars in Clinical Neuropsychiatry, 5*, 177–190.

Sulik, K. K., Johnston, M. C., & Webb, M. A. (1981). Fetal alcohol syndrome: Embryogenesis in a mouse model. *Science, 214*(4523), 936–938.

Sullivan, W. (1900). The children of the female drunkard. *Med. Temp. Rev., 1*, 72–79.

Swayze, V. W., 2nd, Johnson, V. P., Hanson, J. W., Piven, J., Sato, Y., Giedd, J. N., et al. (1997). Magnetic resonance imaging of brain anomalies in fetal alcohol syndrome. *Pediatrics, 99*, 232–240.

Thackray, H., & Tifft, C. (2001). Fetal alcohol syndrome. *Pediatrics in Review, 22*(2), 47–55.

Uecker, A., & Nadel, L. (1996). Spatial locations gone awry: object and spatial memory deficits in children with fetal alcohol syndrome. *Neuropsychologia, 34*, 209–223.

Uecker, A., & Nadel, L. (1998). Spatial but not object memory impairments in children with fetal alcohol syndrome. *American Journal of Mental Retardation, 103*, 12–18.

USDHHS. (1981). Surgeon general's advisory on alcohol and pregnancy. *FDA Drug Bulletin, 11*(2), 9–10.

Weiner, L., & Morse, B. (1994). Intervention and the child with FAS. *Alcohol Health and Research World, 18*, 67–72.

West, J. R., & Goodlett, C. R. (1990). Teratogenic effects of alcohol on brain development. *Annals of Medicine, 22*, 319–325.

Wilson, J., & Warkany, J. (1972). *Teratology: Principles and techniques.* Chicago, IL: University of Chicago Press.

Wisniewski, K., Dambska, M., Sher, J. H., & Qazi, Q. (1983). A clinical neuropathological study of the fetal alcohol syndrome. *Neuropediatrics, 14*, 197–201.

# Chapter 13

# People with Mental Retardation and the Developmental Disabilities Philosophy

George Singer

This chapter is designed to provide the reader with key information about working with individuals with mental retardation and their families. The focus is on the way views about people with mental retardation (MR) and their life outcomes have changed dramatically over the past 20 years and the implications of these changes for the practice of medicine, nursing, and occupational/physical therapy. It is very important that health professionals have an up-to-date understanding about this population because there are many long-standing assumptions about individuals with developmental disabilities and their families that have been challenged and replaced with a new vision. There has, however, been a lag between the promotion of new ideas about dignity, self-determination, and innovative human service models and common views within the medical professions (Hahn, 2003). The purpose of this chapter is to bring to light these discrepancies and suggest ways that the newer thinking can impact nursing services for this important population of citizens and their families. This chapter then provides examples of ways that nurses can act on more recent values and options.

## Relevance for Health Care Professionals

Between 0.9% to 2.5% of people in the United States experience mental retardation, roughly 2.6 to 7.2 million people (Biasini, Grupe, Huffman, & Bray, 1999). Health care providers will inevitably work with people with mental retardation during their careers. All but a small percentage of people with mental retardation live in our communities either with their families or in apartments, group homes, and larger community facilities. Mental retardation is a developmental condition that is usually, but not always, identified in early childhood, and it has lifelong impacts. There is no single cause of the condition. The American Association on Mental Retardation's (AAMR) 2002 handbook on assessing mental retardation lists over 300 identified causes, and the number increased in the 2002 edition (AAMR, 2002). In fact, recent developments in the etiology of mental retardation have revealed multiple causes that can occur during each stage of childhood development, beginning with genetic anomalies at conception, exposure to environmental toxins during pregnancy, birth trauma, very low birth weight, and head injury. Many of the syndromes linked to mental retardation also disrupt other biological systems so that some individuals with mental retardation require unusual levels of medical support. In 2002 the Surgeon General issued a report on the health of people with mental retardation. The report explains that people with mental retardation from early childhood through the life span have poorer health and less access to care than the general population. (U.S. Dept. of Health and Human Services, 2002).

MR occurs in all social classes and in all ethnic groups. MR is more prevalent among low-income families because they are exposed to dangerous environmental conditions that cause mental retardation. Poverty and minority ethnic status overlap extensively in the United States. Consequently, individuals of color with mental retardation have even less access. There are many reasons for this problem, including the limited number of health care providers who have received training in care for people with MR. Individuals with mental retardation may have difficulties in identifying when they need to seek help, in reporting their symptoms, and in understanding recommended care. They may require more time for medical appointments and more patient education. The lack of trained health professionals and these extra demands may be explanations for the fact that people with MR have reported that they have been treated rudely by medical professionals (Hahn, 2003).

The latter of these concerns is based on many anecdotal reports by parents and people with mental retardation. For example, Hart (1998) interviewed 13 in-patients with mental retardation in a British general hospital and found that they expressed fears about their care, felt they were treated rudely and even abusively, and expressed concerns about not giving consent for treatments. Communication problems with doctors and nurses were also a major problem for these individuals.

Limited access to medical care for people with mental retardation includes difficulties in obtaining the services of dentists and medical specialists. A recent study found that one in five parents of children with MR had a great deal more difficulty in finding and getting access to medical specialists compared to parents of nondisabled individuals (Krauss, Gully, Sciegaj, & Wells, 2003).

Unfortunately, the curriculum for student nurses at all levels has traditionally included only brief attention to mental retardation (Hahn, 2003). Many health professionals receive little or no educational and clinical experience serving people with mental retardation during their preservice education. In a survey of 583 nurses in New Jersey, 60% reported that they had little or no training in how to serve individuals with mental retardation either during their formal education or through continuing education (Walsh, Hammerman, Josephson, & Krupka, 2000). Without specific education and supervised clinical experience, health care providers are likely to base their views about people with mental retardation on common stereotypes. Students enter their health professional education programs with attitudes from their own previous experiences and from socialization (Brillhart, Jay, & Wyers, 1990). Regrettably, attitudes toward people with disabilities in school and general society are often based on a lack of knowledge, fear of the unknown, an overemphasis on difference rather than sameness, and negative stereotypes learned from others (Thompson, Emrich, & Moore, 2003). Pfeiffer and colleagues (2003) reviewed the literature on attitudes toward people with disabilities in many nations, cultures, and religious traditions and concluded that people with disabilities are often viewed in the most pejorative of terms.

Studies suggest, for example, that physicians and nurses tend to overestimate the impact of impairments on people with disabilities and their families (Pfieffer et al. 2003). Brillhart and colleagues (1990) compared the attitudes of people with disabilities with those of nursing faculty, entering nurses, graduating nurses, and registered nurses. They found that people with disabilities had much more favorable attitudes than any of the nursing groups, with nursing faculty and graduating nurses having the most negative attitudes. Such negativity is not inevitable. When students are given information and provided with clinical experience, their attitudes become significantly more favorable (Thompson et al. 2003).

# A History of Traditional Views About Mental Retardation

Our culture is permeated with negative assumptions about people with mental retardation. These views are readily assimilated as part of the socialization process, so that it is possible to have absorbed negative views without conscious knowledge. Negative cultural stereotypes grow out of a long history of stigmatization, exclusion, and social marginalization of people with intellectual disabilities. During many centuries of recorded history, the way Western societies have officially cared for individuals with disabilities has been one of benign neglect, at best, and cruelty at the worst (Winzer, 1997). There have, sadly, been many atrocities directed at this vulnerable population, representing the worst in our collective past.

## Ancient Greece Through the American Civil War

In ancient Greece, children who were born with visible disabilities were abandoned to starve to death in the wilderness or, as in Sparta, executed by order of the rulers. One late Roman emperor literally staged hunts ending in slaughter of individuals with disabilities. Parents often abandoned children with disabilities in the forests of Medieval Europe or placed them in public places where strangers acquired them as slaves or servants. As early as the 14th century there is a record of a parent who sold her child with multiple disabilities to a band of traveling merchants. They put her on public display for a fee (Boswell, 1987). The practice of displaying people with disabilities for public entertainment was common in this country as recently as 50 years ago (Bodgan, 1988). A Renaissance Florentine prince served rotten meat to his court fool for the entertainment of his guests (Scheerenberger, 1987). In major cities in 18th century Europe, many unwanted children with disabilities, along with children from poor families, were placed in hospitals where most died from infectious diseases (Boswell, 1987).

In the United States during much of our history, people with disabilities were kept at home and joined in household or farm labor when possible. The English Poor Laws were transported to the American colonies and guided the minimal community care available for people with mental retardation (Braddock & Parrish, 2001). Towns were responsible for preventing starvation and homelessness in some instances, although other towns developed practices to warn away people who might become public wards. There are accounts of public whippings to discourage people from staying in a town. In keeping with the English legal tradition, some families were provided with outdoor relief, a minimal payment of town funds. Individuals with disabilities were considered to be a member of a wider class of people—the poor. Town councils would grant subsidies to keep indigent families from starvation or homelessness. For the most part, the family was seen as the sole provider of help to vulnerable individuals.

In the first half of the 19th century, several states and cities built alms houses where a small number of people with mental retardation were housed at public expense along with vagabonds, indigents, the mentally ill, and prostitutes (Braddock & Parrish, 2001). They resided there along with people who were extremely poor, those with mental illness, prostitutes, and those who were homeless. This whole group was classified together as the poor. The reformer, Dorothea Dix, traveled by horseback around Massachusetts in 1841 to investigate the living conditions of people with mental illness and mental retardation (Winzer, 1993). She presented her famous Memorial to the Massachusetts State Legislature in 1843. This document was the first of many over the ensuing two centuries to paint a picture of inhumane treatment of mentally retarded and mentally ill individuals under the care of cities and states. Dix's advocacy paved the way for the creation of the first public institutions for these individuals.

After the American Civil War the main state policies toward individuals with MR, reflecting reformist efforts in France and England, centered on the creation of public residential institutions. Although originally designed to educate and rehabilitate people with mental retardation, by the 1880s, most institutions became places where people were given minimal custodial care instead of preparation to live and work in the community (Trent, 1995). Residents were often treated worse than prize animals. In some places these conditions existed as recently as the late 1970s and beyond (Blatt, 1974). Despite very expensive reform efforts, large residential institutions for people with MR are now considered regressive examples of a social policy aimed at extreme segregation and isolation.

## The Eugenics Movement of the 19th and 20th Centuries

Beginning at the end of the 19th century and enduring until the end of World War II, a movement to purify the U.S. genetic pool led to harsh treatment of people with disabilities and their families. Under the influence of nationalist and Darwinian ideologies, some of the most influential intellectual and political leaders in the

United States viewed mental retardation as a social threat. People with mental retardation were particularly highlighted as dangers to the competitiveness and strength of the nation (Selden, 1999). The eugenics movement was not just the work of extremists. Many of the country's most prominent citizens were in the grip of the Darwinian idea that people with intellectual disabilities were a social menace (Trent, 1995).

Through campaigns in many state legislatures, the eugenics movement resulted in the legalization of forced sterilization as well as involuntary placements in state residential institutions for thousands of people with mental retardation. In 1927 the Supreme Court upheld a Virginia state law that allowed the state to forcibly sterilize individuals who were seen as pollutants to the country's gene pool. Many victims of this policy are still alive. As recently as December of 2002, the Governor of Oregon publicly apologized to the survivors and their families for the 2,648 forced sterilizations that took place without knowledge or consent of the victims and their families between 1917 and 1983 in Oregon's state institution for people with mental retardation. The practice was discontinued in this country only after the tragic results of Nazi Germany's mad obsession with racial purity and its resultant horrors came to light (Black, 2003).

In Nazi Germany the murders that led to genocide were carried out on individuals with mental illness, MR, and other disabilities. Many were children. Families were told their children were moved to better hospitals which were, in fact, the location of the first gas chambers and mass crematoriums. The Nazi government referred to these vulnerable human beings as "useless eaters," along with other dehumanizing language (Mostert, 2002). There is substantial evidence that the Nazi obsession with racial purity and the plan for purging of the gene pool through genocide were influenced by the U.S. eugenics movement that was disseminated with an evangelical fervor to Europe by people funded by the Carnegie Foundation and prominent wealthy donors (Black, 2003).

## Social Ostracism

There have been other less horrendous but nonetheless damaging ways that our society has treated individuals with developmental disabilities. These include a general exclusion from community life. Most individuals with developmental disabilities historically have been cared for by their families and were until recently kept out of public view. Many children with mental retardation were not able to attend a public school until the passage of the federal legislation that became the Individuals with Disabilities Education Act (IDEA) in 1975 (Winzer, 1993). However, some states and cities had been providing segregated day classes of children with developmental disabilities since the late 19th century.

A majority of people with MR have been excluded from regular employment even though there is substantial evidence that individuals with MR can be dependable and productive employees in competitive work settings when given the right forms of support (Wehman, 2003). Those who do work are paid well below the minimum wage and usually have few or no benefits.

It is not inevitable that society mistreats people with disabilities. There have been bright spots in history. For example, in the latter Middle Ages in Europe, monastic orders often took in individuals with disabilities, and provided care and even membership in the religious communities (Boswell, 1987). Accounts also survive from the Middle Ages of people with severe disabilities who were looked after in supportive way by friends, families, and sometimes strangers. The mother, mentioned earlier, who sold her 16-year-old daughter did so after she had taken her on a dangerous pilgrimage to a holy site and failed to receive a miracle. Historians have shown that Medieval parents of children with physical disabilities took great risks to bring them on pilgrimages to holy sites where it was believed saints could cure them (Shahar, 1992).

## Reform Initiatives

Major advances in the treatment of individuals with mental retardation took place during the Enlightenment. Physicians were the first modern professionals to contribute to reform. In the years immediately after the French Revolution, the medical profession contributed to an increasingly more humane and enlightened understanding of mental retardation and other developmental disabilities (Scheerenburger, 1987). Special education services were first offered in the United States after the Civil War as the main mission of residential institutions. Later in the 19th century, public schools began to offer special classes and specially trained teachers for children with mental retardation. The term *special education* first came into use in 1898 in the United States (Winzer, 1993). During the Progressive Era from 1900 to the early 1920s, the same reformers who were active in establishing public health nursing, settlement houses, juvenile courts, and mandatory high schools also advocated for special education programs (Winzer, 1993). By 1920, Columbia College provided the first teacher preparation program for special educators. These efforts had to compete with the eugenics movement that favored segregation and saw individuals with mental retardation as uneducable. Public services for people with mental retardation were largely limited to particular special education services in communities and to large residential institutions away from communities.

After World War II the hidden and segregated status of people with mental retardation began to erode. Parents and family members of individuals with MR began to organize and advocate for services and civil rights for their loved ones (Trent, 1995). Parent-led organizations such as the Association for Retarded Citizens, now known at the ARC, advocated for public education for all children with disabilities at the state level during the 1960s and early 1970s. The era from the 1960s to the present day has been marked by successive waves of reform, the creation of a community-based service system, the availability of special education to all children with disabilities, and the growing participation by people with mental retardation in our communities (Braddock & Parrish, 2001).

The move from segregation to inclusion has required the medical profession to address the needs of this population of citizens in regular community clinics, public health programs, and hospitals. The disability rights movement will continue to inject energy and bring to light the needs for further reform. In 2002 the Surgeon General of the United States issued a report on the need for expanded care, open access, and equal medical treatment for people with mental retardation (U.S. Dept. of Health and Human Services, 2002). Nurses and other providers are playing an essential role in this movement.

As a result of these reforms, the numbers of people housed in large public institutions has been steadily dropping since the late 1950s, so that in 2003 only a small percentage of adults with mental retardation resided in them. Eighty-five percent of adults with MR live in their families' homes in communities (Fujiara & Braddock, 1992). Of the remaining 15%, the great majority live in community residences of under 16 people (Lakin, Anderson, Prouty, & Polister, 1999). Thus a primary goal for nurses and other support providers is to assist people with MR to become as fully participative as possible in home living, work, recreation, worship, education, and loving relationships.

# New Vision of Mental Retardation: Self-Determination

The new vision of mental retardation includes an emphasis on maximum participation in all of the valued activities and lifestyles available to citizens of the United States. A major emphasis in this new vision of support is the idea that medical services should be delivered in ways that promote self-determination in individuals with MR. Best practices that promote self-determination include the following:

- Recognize that people with mental retardation are people first and foremost.
- Make full inclusion and high quality of life a goal.
- Understand that MR is not about IQ but about fitting into the environment.
- Build strong partnerships between people with MR, families, and health care providers.
- Understand the role of the family in adaptation to MR.

## People with Mental Retardation are People First and Foremost

One of the best ways to learn about mental retardation is to talk to parents and siblings who see their son or daughter, brother or sister, as a person first and foremost. Such descriptions will likely not include IQ test scores or lists of adaptive behavior skills. If asked, family members speak of strengths, interests and preferences, endearing characteristics, educational progress, and contributions these individuals make to their families and communities. You may also hear about challenges and stresses related to raising and supporting family members with intellectual disabilities. Here is a description a mother of a young woman with mental retardation gave in a recent seminar:

*Ella is a beautiful woman with long brown hair and striking blue eyes. She is aware of her attractiveness and it is important to her. She is a very social and winning person who loves to converse with people who take the time. She has a great sense of humor, and it is important to her that she makes up her own mind about her life. She is much more interested in people her own age now than in her family, especially young men. We are very proud that she lives in her own apartment and has her own life. She has nursing care around the clock. We had to work hard with local agencies to see that she could live in her own apartment rather than a nursing home or intermediate care facility. We're really pleased about the quality of her life.*

This parent did not mention some other facts about Ella. She did not begin by talking about her need for supports and accommodations. For example, Ella uses a wheelchair, communicates by pointing to a communication board with pictures on it, and requires frequent nursing support in order to enjoy her life in the community. She needs daily nursing assistance because of a recurring lung infection and a renal disease. This mother did not mention that her daughter is typically labeled by service providers as having severe mental retardation and cerebral palsy. Nor did she mention that her daughter is nonverbal.

She also did not mention the many battles she has had to fight to obtain the necessary supports for her daughter, nor did she mention the battles ahead that she knows are inevitable. Because of a centuries-old tradition of prejudice and discrimination toward people with mental retardation, parents often have to work hard to obtain access to even basic services like medical care for their family members with mental retardation. When asked, however, she will also talk with enthusiasm about those professionals who have been her allies over the years in supporting her daughter. Often

professionals who have taken a long-term interest in their child become important allies for parents.

This mother is not in denial, she is not unrealistic, and she is not ignorant of the scientific explanations of mental retardation. As a woman with a graduate degree and a high-status job, she knows about the formal, professional terms in which physicians and nurses are trained to think and talk. Rather, she has chosen to put her lived experience of her daughter first as her way of thinking about her young adult child. When asked about which professionals have made an important difference in her daughter's life, she speaks of people who "get who Ella is," "know their stuff," "tune-in to her," and "take the time to listen and learn about her from her family." She has high praise for two nurses who have worked with Ella over the past 5 years. They understand Ella's ways of communicating, enjoy her sense of humor, and find ways to help her participate in the activities that she chooses in her town. They offer Ella choices about her daily care and find ways for her to participate in her medical care routines. The nurses keep Ella's family well informed about her medical needs. On more than one occasion the nurses have advocated on Ella's behalf to insurance companies and state agencies.

## Full Inclusion and High Quality of Life as a Goal

Over the past 30 years it has become clear that people with mental retardation, regardless of their level of functioning, can participate in the full array of daily routines, pleasures, and responsibilities available to all citizens in the United States. Individuals with mental retardation, when provided with the right kinds of supports, can own their own homes, work at regular jobs in the community, develop friendships and long-term healthy relationships with their families, be active in their churches, and enjoy the many forms of recreation available in typical communities.

For people who require more intensive levels of support, the goal is for them to participate as fully as possible in those aspects of community life with the accommodations needed to maximize their engagement, independence, and self-determination.

Newly emerging systems of support for people with mental retardation in the community aim to base supports on person-centered plans in which services are individually designed and delivered according the preferences of people with disabilities and their families. This form of individualization places the preferences of the people served at the center of service provision. The approach emphasizes flexibility, responsiveness to changing needs, and ongoing efforts to empower and promote self-determination in the lives of people with MR and their families. Self-determination includes the ability to make choices about one's life, to set goals, make plans, assert preferences, and advocate for one's self. This new emphasis requires nurses and other providers to make every effort to explain medical choices, to actively and thoroughly seek informed consent even when people have guardians, and to actively teach individuals with MR self-care, health promotion behaviors, and medical self-management skills.

## New Understandings of Mental Retardation

One of the many changes in this area is in the way that MR is defined. Traditionally, people with intellectual disabilities were assigned a label indicating levels of severity in mental retardation. These labels were mild, moderate, severe, and profound, and were often based on IQ testing. The problem with this approach is two-fold. First, it is a deficit model of retardation; that is, the person with MR is considered to be less capable compared to people without intellectual disabilities. Second, it does not account for the relationship between the person and the environment, a concept increasingly accepted as fundamental to all human development. A person who scores below a cut-off score on an IQ test may succeed very well in everyday settings where people are supportive and accommodations are applied. The same person in an unsupportive setting could appear to be quite impaired. Because of the recent recognition of the importance that the environment makes to a person's level of functioning, the AAMR definition has done away with these categories and instead, it partly describes people in terms of the levels of support they need for major activities of life.

The main professional association determining the definition is the AAMR (2004). In 2000, the association issued a new definition that incorporated new thinking in the field. Here are some statements by the AAMR that evoke these newer views:

*Mental retardation is not something you have, like blue eyes, or a bad heart. Nor is it something you are, like short, or thin. It is not a medical disorder, nor a mental disorder. Mental retardation is a particular state of functioning that begins in childhood and is characterized by limitation in both intelligence and adaptive skills. Mental retardation reflects the "fit" between the capabilities of individuals and the structure and expectations of their environment (AAMR, 2004).*

The emphasis here is different from the deficit model that health professionals often use to think about medical conditions. Instead of being solely centered in a person, as is an infection or an injury, MR is created by the interactions of a person's present abilities and his or her social and physical environment. A person can function in one setting very differently than in another, and, consequently, their functioning level cannot be simply characterized with a global label based on testing alone.

## THE ROLE OF ENVIRONMENTAL SUPPORT

A person's state of functioning can change according to what is expected of her and what kinds of supports are available. Supports are a central feature of the new outlook and new definition. For example, the inability to work is often considered an indicator of a disability. For most people, the ability to work effectively is dependent on a variety of supports such as transportation, day care, and even eyeglasses and key holders. A nearsighted person without prescription lenses can be excluded from many kinds of work. A secretary, for example, who cannot read a computer screen without reading glasses cannot perform her job without corrective lenses. These simple, widely available forms of support are taken for granted in our society. But in many developing countries, people with easily correctable visual problems function at far less than their optimum because of the prohibitive costs of eyeglasses. The presence or absence of this simple support can radically change a person's state of functioning. The requirements of the environment also partly determine state of functioning. In the airline industry, people who require eyeglasses are not allowed to work as pilots even though they function the same as anyone with normal eyesight when wearing glasses.

Over the past 50 years a large variety of supports have been developed and tested to assist people with intellectual disabilities to improve their functioning. These can be as simple as a nurse speaking in plain language, asking questions in a friendly way to make sure a patient understands how to take a course of antibiotics. Or the supports can be more elaborate, including behavioral and/or educational supports that allow a person with MR to participate in the typical activities, routines, and pleasures afforded by our society. It is clear from research and the experience of many successful service programs that people with MR can work successfully at community jobs with the help of a job coach or some

extra assistance when needed from coworkers. This applies even to people with severe MR. The new definition of MR asks us to understand that a job coach and a pair of glasses are both ways to improve a person's state of functioning, because both help determine the fit between the person and their environment.

The AAMR has provided a model for understanding supports that categorizes them according to their function. These support functions are

- Teaching
- Befriending
- Financial planning
- Employee assistance
- Behavioral support
- In-home living assistance
- Community access and use
- Health assistance

(AAMR, 1992, p. 104.)

One of the essential categories of support is *medical assistance*. Nurses can and do play a key role in accommodating medical practice to meet the needs of people with MR. It is important to note that several forms of supports may be necessary in addition to *medical assistance*. Several additional support functions play a key role in providing health assistance effectively to this population: teaching, befriending, behavioral support, and community access. The implication is that nurses who work with this population need to collaborate with other professionals often from several different agencies. Support for individuals with intellectual disabilities is an interdisciplinary team effort requiring networking, sharing of information within the bounds of confidentiality, coordinating care with other professionals, and advocating for services from other agencies.

## A NEW DEFINITION OF MR

Because the nature of supports and accommodations for people with mental retardation makes such a large difference in how they think, feel, and act in different environments, the definition of MR was changed in 2002. The AAMR (2002) has revised its definition of MR so that environmental supports, rather than individual differences, are the basis for classification into subcategories. Traditional levels of MR have been replaced with descriptions of the amount and intensity of supports required to allow individuals to participate in community life. The tenor of these changes has been to understand MR as a contextualized state of functioning. It is no longer simply a matter of scores on IQ tests and measures of adaptive behavior (skills of everyday living). In the new way of thinking, MR cannot be adequately described without study of the social environments in which an individual lives and the supports afforded in these settings.

The formal AAMR 2002 definition of MR is presented below. It is important to notice the central place that supports are given in the definition as well as interaction with the environment across several central life domains.

*Mental retardation is a disability characterized by significant limitations both in intellectual functioning and in adaptive behavior as expressed in conceptual, social, and practical adaptive skills. This disability originates before the age of 18. A complete and accurate understanding of mental retardation involves realizing that mental retardation refers to a particular state of functioning that begins in childhood, has many dimensions, and is affected positively by individualized supports. As a model of functioning, it includes the contexts and environment within which the person functions and interacts and requires a multidimensional and ecological approach that reflects the interaction of the individual with the environment, and the outcomes of that interaction with regards to independence, relationships, societal contributions, participation in school and community, and personal well-being. (AAMR, 2004)*

A person with MR may function with competence when given the right kinds of nursing support and at a less adaptive level when these supports are lacking. Here is an example from a clinic providing community health services to people in an urban neighborhood.

Edward, a young man with MR, attends an asthma outpatient clinic in a metropolitan-area hospital. When one particular nurse and physician team work at the clinic, Edward does very well with his visits and benefits. On a recent visit, Ed was friendly and talked about his recent vacation. He readily participated in testing his lung capacity, used a nebulizer correctly in the office, demonstrated to the nurse that he understood how to use it and left with written and line-drawing instructions as reminders. His brother Hank observed the nurse's instruction on how and when to use the inhaler and avoiding environmental allergens. During the next 6 months, Ed, accompanied by his brother, visited the clinic only once to have his lungs checked after developing bronchitis.

At his 6-month regular visit to the clinic, however, Ed encountered a different health care team at the clinic. Ed refused to answer questions after a nurse talked to him like a child, passively resisted the medical examination, became confused about how to breathe deeply and slowly while using the nebulizer, and left the clinic confused about how to administer a new dosage from his inhaler. The nurse did not allow Hank to observe the patient education session, so he left feeling less able to assist his brother. During the next 6 months, the brothers attended the clinic on four occasions because Ed's asthma was not as well controlled as previously. Although Ed's profile on intelligence and adaptive behavior tests were the same on both visits, his ability to work with his health care providers and benefit from their care differed because their approach to him differed. However, they might report that *he* was the one who was different on each visit. There are many ways to modify a typical provider–patient with mental retardation encounter that can enhance the patient's ability to participate in and benefit from the interaction.

## AGE- VERSUS STAGE-APPROPRIATE CARE

Mental retardation is a set of developmental phenomena. A long-standing debate in the study of MR has focused on the question of whether children and adults with MR move through the same stages of development as typically developing individuals. A synthesis of this literature suggests that the biggest group of people with MR, those who only need intermittent supports to participate in school and community life, do experience the typical stages of development (Hodapp, Burack, & Zigler, 1990). They move more slowly through these stages and usually do not move as far along as is typical. A now-outdated way of interpreting MR was to assign individuals a chronological and a mental age. This approach has been abandoned because it contributed to the cultural assumption that people with MR somehow remain as perpetual children who should be supported in the same way as young children.

The emphasis over the past 30 years has gradually shifted to the assumption that the way supports are provided should be age-appropriate based on the individual's chronological age. This means that it is inappropriate to talk to person with MR in a tone of voice that is ordinarily used with infants and young children. It would, for example, be equally inappropriate to offer a patient a lollipop or suggest that an older child play with toys for preschoolers in the waiting room. The central concept in this regard is dignity. The ways that health care professionals provide care should demonstrate respect and support for human dignity, as well as vigilance to suppress ways of treating citizens with MR as if they are permanent children. For example, it can be very helpful to speak to patients with mental retardation in concrete, jargon-free language and to check frequently to make sure the person has understood. But it can be counterproductive and demeaning to do these things with attitudes and actions typically reserved for young children.

Although the majority of people with MR go through typical stages of childhood development, individuals who require sustained and intensive forms of support for daily living often have conditions that not only delay but also alter normal development. Similarly, these individuals may not move uniformly through all stages of development, and, consequently, their adaptive behavior may have a profile of peaks and valleys in which several domains of daily living may be performed with much less independence than is typical of same-age nondisabled individuals. At the same time, they may have typical levels of performance in other domains. For example, some persons with MR may have difficulty managing money but are capable of doing very well earning it through competitive employment. Understanding the stages of typical development when working with individuals with MR is most useful in deciding how to give information in clear, understandable ways. By contrast, it is not helpful to assume that a person with MR must be treated paternalistically or that his or her views should be discounted.

## Partnerships as Key to Effective Support

The new approach to supporting people with MR requires professionals to develop relationships with patients, their families, and caregivers based on the spirit of teamwork and equality. Recent research on partnerships between parents of children with disabilities and professionals has revealed some of the key elements necessary to becoming a reliable ally (Blue-Banning, Summers, Frankland, Nelson, & Beegle, 2003; Turnbull & Turnbull, 2000). Blue-Banning and colleagues (2003) conducted focus groups and interviews with parents and professionals in three communities to learn how to precisely describe parent/professional statements characterized by genuine working partnerships. Both parents and professionals agreed on all of the major elements that make up a productive relationship. As would be expected, communication was central to the creating partnerships. There are two related concerns here: 1) how to communicate with the patient with mental retardation; and 2) how to communicate with the family or caregivers.

The same principles that guide effective partnerships with parents and caregivers also apply directly to individuals with MR, provided that health professionals make some modifications to take into account the patient's cognitive functioning. These principles include

- Listening
- Respect
- Communication
- Valuing the uniqueness of the person with MR
- Commitment to patient, family, and caregivers

### LISTENING

Blue-Banning and colleagues (2004) found that parents and professionals believed that listening was a key. They quote one father as saying

*The first thing is to listen to us . . . because we know our kids better than anybody . . . I think some of these people have preconceived notions about everything. So if I tried to say—to tell them (the professionals) something, it'd be LISTEN TO ME. (Blue-Banning et al., 2003, p.18)*

In interviews conducted by Singer (1991), parents of children with disabilities including MR discussed the differences between pediatricians who were helpful and those who were not. All parents discussed the importance of listening. One mother recounted the way a doctor refused to listen to her when she explained that the best way to remove her son's sutures from a surgery for cleft palate was to allow him to sit in her lap during the procedure. She had arrived at this conclusion through trial and error with her son's previous physician. The doctor ignored her advice and had to use force to hold her son on the examining

table. The child had a tantrum, resisted the doctor, and the whole procedure became stressful for everyone concerned.

### RESPECT

The principle involved in the previous example is the importance of seeking and respecting parents' or caregivers' knowledge (Singer, 1991). Family members have long-term knowledge they have gained from living together, seeking care, and working with many professionals. These experiences give them a knowledge base regarding the patient that formal professional training cannot. Medical professionals who form effective alliances with family members make a serious effort to tap into this expertise with the same respect they would afford to any other expert. Respect is an indispensable attitude (Blue-Banning et al., 2004). Equally important is to respect the suggestions and preferences of patients with MR. Most individuals with MR are able to tell you what they prefer in regard to care procedures. Because individuals with MR are often not accustomed to being listened to respectfully, health care providers need to create opportunities for them to state their preferences and make choices.

### COMMUNICATION

Communication in a partnership requires honesty. Parents reported to Blue-Banning and her colleagues (2003) that they wanted professionals to be straightforward and not mask their findings. At the same time they appreciated tactful communication. Parents did not want information to be "sugar coated." They also did not want to be treated as if they were somehow participating in a tragedy. One mother recently reported on her experience in a regional hospital where she gave birth to a daughter with Down syndrome, a chromosomal disorder that is associated with mental retardation. When her baby was delivered in the hospital, the nurses acted as if something terrible had happened, they turned off the lights in the delivery room, whispered among themselves, and did not make eye contact with the mother. Her baby was whisked away to the newborn intensive care unit, and it was many hours before a doctor explained to her that her daughter had Down syndrome. An event that she had expected to be joyous was treated by others as if a calamity had occurred. This mother commented "Why didn't anyone bring balloons for my baby?" She went on to say that she now felt sorry for people who had such a misunderstanding of her child. Nurses and other health professionals must be careful not to contribute to stigmatization of individuals with MR and their families.

## VALUE THE UNIQUENESS OF THE PERSON WITH MR

Many parents and family members of people with MR would like to work with nurses who can also appreciate their insider's view of the person they love. In an interview study, parents of children with developmental disabilities were asked to describe medical care providers who were especially supportive. One single mother of a child with a rare genetic disorder was asked what she would like pediatricians to know about her child. She responded, "I want them to know that this is my only child and she is precious to me and she needs the best care possible" (Singer, 1991).

In studies of what parents want from professionals, they commonly express the desire that the professionals see their child the way they do—as a full person with many positive traits and as a person who can learn and become more competent with the right kinds of supports. Parents value professionals who appreciate their children, take pleasure in their accomplishments, and take time to interact in friendly and supportive ways with their child or sibling with mental retardation.

## COMMITMENT

Commitment was a major theme in Blue-Banning and colleagues' research (2003). Parents wanted to develop partnerships with professionals who showed they were dedicated to their work.

Parents reported that the most helpful professionals viewed their work as "more than a job" and communicated in ways that let parents know that their child was "more than just a case" (Blue-Banning et al., 2003, p. 19). In other words, such health professionals view individuals with developmental disabilities as people first and foremost, while also providing the best professional and technical assistance they can. A single mother of a child with a rare genetic disorder recounted how much she was encouraged and validated when a geneticist gave her young child a hug and said "she looked like a perfectly wonderful child to her" (Singer, 1991). Parents also, of course, want professionals to be very good at their particular professional roles, provide clear understandable information, take the time to answer questions, and provide encouragement and a sense of hope (Singer & Nixon, 1996).

## New Understandings of Family and Disability

Accommodating medical care to meet the needs of people with MR usually requires partnerships between medical care providers, the person with MR, and either a family member or paid caregiver. Approximately 85% of adults with MR continue to reside in their parents' homes until their parents become elderly (Fujiara & Braddock, 1992). Thus partnerships with parents and/or siblings or extended family members are an essential part of medical practice with this group of people. Unfortunately, many parents continue to be stigmatized by health professionals and thus require efforts on the part of providers to build trust to overcome their expectations of professional devaluation based on past experience. Again there is a long historical precedent for negative attitudes toward parents and family members of people with disabilities. Parents have been blamed for their children's disabilities for centuries. In Medieval and early modern Europe, parents, usually mothers, were accused of sinful behavior and their children judged as proof of God's displeasure. Unfortunately, this tradition in new forms has survived into contemporary times. Some parents of children with disabilities continue to blame themselves for their children's impairments and continue to be treated as if they are at fault. Further, until the late 1980s most scholarly research on families took for granted the assumption that children with developmental disabilities damaged their families (Ferguson, 2001).

## IMPACT ON FAMILY

For much of the past century, it was assumed that the impact of children with MR on their families was negative, resulting in parental sorrow and even psychological disorder. It has taken researchers that past two decades to sweep away such myths. The most radical critique of tragic view derives from research on parent's positive perceptions of the impact of a child's disability. The development of measures of adaptation that measure positive aspects of the parenting experience has begun to add another dimension to our understanding of how mothers and other family members are impacted in a manner that directly contradicts the tragedy assumption.

Hastings & Taunt (2002) reviewed five published studies on parent's perceptions of the positive impacts of their children with disabilities on themselves and their families. Although in an early stage, this literature strongly suggests that not only do many families adapt well, but also an unknown percentage of parents also benefit from the experience. Parents have reported many positive effects including personal growth, expansion of tolerance for human differences, valuable life lessons learned, strengthened families, the child as a source of joy, and appreciation of their children's contributions to the quality of family life (Hastings & Taunt, 2002; Poston et al., 2003).

Other studies attest to the fact that parents cherish their children with disabilities and perceive the locus of problems to be societal rather than in their sons and daughters (Harry,

Kalyanpur, & Day, 1999). Recent meta-analyses show that the negative impact of children with MR on their families has been exaggerated in the research literature. These reviews indicate that the great majority of families of children with MR are not more troubled, roughly 70% of mothers do not have unusual levels of depressive symptoms, and differences in divorce and marital distress between these families and the general population are small (Singer, 2003; Risdal & Singer, 2004). Although parents and siblings may experience times of stress, in the long term most families do as well as the general population. Parents, brothers, sisters, and extended family members often benefit from serving as lifelong sources of support for people with MR.

# Promoting Medical Self-Management in Individuals with MR and Their Families or Caregivers: Implications for Health Care Professionals

Recent trends in the treatment and management of chronic illness in children and adults are compatible with the new values about people with MR. Increasingly, nurses in particular are acting as educators, instructing and encouraging their patients to learn and maintain medical self-management routines, ranging from monitoring blood glucose levels to using nebulizers and inhalers, taking medication at correct times, self-monitoring of nutrition and exercise, and other preventive health care measures.

With support, most people with MR are capable of managing medical regimens such as maintaining special diets, taking their own temperatures, taking a course of medication, and using an inhaler. Even those individuals who require the most intensive forms of support can learn to participate and cooperate in their own care. To be an effective nurse to patients with MR, it may be necessary to make modifications to the typical way nurses teach medical self-management. These educational supports include

- modifying self management routines to simplify them;
- teaching these procedures in a systematic way;
- giving extra prompts and encouragement;
- setting up ways to transfer learning from the clinic to the patient's home; and
- enlisting the help of families and caregivers.

The kinds of supports that are needed vary with each individual's adaptive functioning in regard to the skills that are needed for self-care. In the next discussion, guidelines are presented for teaching and supporting medical self-management skills in people with MR in partnership with their families and/or care providers.

## Teaching Medical Self-Care Skills to Patients with MR

Often a family member or caregiver will accompany a person with MR to a medical setting. It is essential to talk to them first about how the patient responds to instruction and learning. Ask if there are any tips they can give you on how to teach best and what to avoid doing. Invite them to observe when you demonstrate and teach a self-care routine. Many individuals who only need intermittent help will be able to travel to the appointment and join in the instructional session without help from others.

In either case it is always important to build rapport with the patient. Because teaching individuals with MR often requires more care and more repetition than usual, it is important to schedule extra time with the patient. It may be necessary to schedule exta visits. Follow-up scheduling is required for most individuals to assist them to retain the skill and to refine the way they perform the routines.

### POSITIVE INSTRUCTION

The positive instructional method has been supported by a large number of studies on teaching individuals with MR how to do practical skills. It is also called *systematic instruction* and sometimes *task analytic instruction* (Westling & Fox, 2000). This positive approach minimizes patients' frustration at performing a new skill and gives patients the level of assistance that they need to succeed at the task. The first rule in doing this kind of teaching is to be positive and supportive of the patient during the instruction. Use frequent praise while describing what the patient is doing correctly. For example, a nurse teaching a patient how to use a thermometer might say, "That's just right! You put the thermometer under your tongue." It is important not to scold, become impatient, or criticize. There should be a ratio of praise to correction of at least four praises for every correction.

Most people with MR enjoy learning and will respond well to kindness and a positive attitude. For some individuals it will be very helpful to tell them or show them something they will earn if they learn and practice the self-care routine. Usually health care providers can learn what patients prefer from the family members or caregivers who may accompany the patient to the medical appointment. Contingency agreements worked out with a parent or caregiver can be helpful for individuals who need higher levels of support. For example, a nurse and parent together might strike a simple deal with a patient: "I understand from your sister that if you let me show you how to use a thermometer, you're going out to eat when you leave here." In using praise and rewards, it is important not to treat adult patients as a young child. Adults compliment one another in ways that are subtler than for children. Maintaining the patient's dignity includes speaking with age-appropriate words and in a normal, positive tone of voice.

People with MR are at higher risk of having behavioral problems than the general population.

Some may fear the medical setting and procedures, or the person may have difficulties with following instructions. In many cases, by using reassurance and making the visit positive for the patient, this resistance will go away. If a patient refuses to join in the self-care instruction by trying to leave, pushing the materials away, or objecting strongly, give the patient a short break and try again gently. If the patient still resists, then it may be necessary to teach a family member or caregiver how to help the patient with the task. People who know the individual with MR well can be extremely helpful if they are enlisted as allies in helping their family member or friend with self-care.

## POSITIVE BEHAVIOR SUPPORT

There are very effective ways to work with individuals with MR who resist instruction, but unless a nurse has had training in *positive behavioral support* (PBS), it may be necessary to team up with a psychologist, special education teacher, or some parents who have been trained in these methods. PBS grew out of a school of psychology known as *applied behavior analysis.* It focuses on developing a careful understanding of the conditions in which problem behaviors arise and the functions that these behaviors play regarding what they yield for persons with problematic behavior. It emphasizes the importance of teaching positive alternative skills and behaviors to replace the maladaptive behavior, and it emphasizes using gentle and positive methods rather than punishment. These services are increasingly available around the United States through agencies that serve individuals with developmental disabilities.

## SIMPLIFY TASKS

There are several ways to simplify medical self-care tasks. To understand these modifications, it is necessary to look at the elements of a self-care task. Any task can be broken down into steps and taught one step at a time. Typically, nurses will give a patient written directions about how to monitor blood pressure or how to inhale medications dispensed with aerosol methods. A common way to teach the skill is to demonstrate it. Many people can watch the whole procedure and learn it from one demonstration. But people with mental retardation may not learn from one demonstration. Instead, a nurse may need to break the self-care task into smaller steps and teach one step at a time. Sometimes several demonstrations are needed. It is strongly recommended that a nurse create a data sheet that contains the steps in the task and spaces for marking what steps are difficult for the patient. Figure 13.1 gives an example of a task analysis for teaching the use of an in-

---

*Figure 13.1*    An Example of a Task Analysis for Teaching a Medical Self-Care Skill

1. Patient notices he is having trouble breathing.
2. Take inhaler out of pocket.
3. Remove the cover, put it in pocket.
4. Orient the nozzle toward body.
5. Grip the inhaler between the first two fingers on top and thumb on the bottom.
6. Place nozzle in mouth.
7. Inhale deeply through mouth.
8. While still breathing in, push the aerosol unit down from the top with the first and second fingers.
9. Hold the breath for 20–30 seconds.
10. Retrieve the cover from pocket.
11. Replace the cover.
12. Return the unit back to the pocket.

## Figure 13.2  Teaching Techniques for People with Mental Retardation

A. **Modeling:** Show the patient how to do the routine by performing the whole task sequence so she can watch.

B. **Explain:** While demonstrating the routine, use short simple statements to describe the step: "Now I'm putting this part in my mouth" (point to the nozzle) and demonstrate.

C. **Test:** Ask the patient to perform the task.

D. **Descriptive praise:** For each step that the patient performs correctly or partially correct, praise her enthusiastically and describe what she did correctly: "Excellent! You put the nozzle in your mouth."

E. **Verbal prompt:** As the patient tries to do each step of the task, use easy words to tell her what to do. ("Take the cover off.")

F. **Time delay:** It is very important to give the patient a chance to do each step or respond to each prompt before giving more assistance. For example, if the nurse says "Hold it like this," while demonstrating how to hold the inhaler, he should wait 4 or 5 seconds before giving more help with that step.

G. **Physical prompt:** The nurse guides the patient through the step by putting his hands on the patient's hands.

H. **Repetition:** Patients with mental retardation are likely to need to practice more than others. Allow time to practice the task four or five times until the patient performs it correctly at least twice.

I. **Pulling out difficult steps:** Some steps in a task may be more difficult than others. Practicing these steps separately and then placing them back into the whole task is one way to overcome difficulty in learning specific parts of a task.

halent for asthma. There are several tools for teaching this kind of task. Figure 13.2 lists these simple techniques. Figure 13.3 gives an example of how to put these techniques together in a lesson.

The idea of supporting self-care by simplifying tasks is one that is already well known to nurses. The most common form of illness self-management is self-administration of pills. Most patients simply need the instructions on the medicine bottle. However, studies indicate that without reminders, many people do not finish a course of medicine unless special efforts are made to encourage compliance. (Russell, Daly, & Hoog, 2003). Some patients need a simple, widely available modification, a pill organizer. Even with this way to make the task easier, nurses have to make careful judgments about how best to support a patient.

There are a variety of organizers available in most drug stores. It is common for nurses to help patients chose the one that works best for them.

One very helpful way to look at the array of choices is to rank them by ease of use: from the easiest to the hardest. Another way to rank them is by how much support from other people is needed for the patient to use a modification. For example, pill organizers range from complex ones with small compartments that hold a month's worth of pills, to those with only a few large compartments and large print. With this variety of options, nurses try to match the right kind of device to the needs of the patient and the kinds of support available. A patient who can readily count and organize pills might use the most complex pill organizer once a month. Another person might require a caregiver to fill the organizer and provide a reminder to take the medications. One individual will require the help of a caregiver to use the organizer, while another may need an organizer with fewer and larger compartments, with days of the week marked on them in larger print.

Approximately one-half of individuals with MR require only intermittent assistance to live

*Figure 13.3*   Systematic Instruction of a Medical Self-Management Routine

1. Demonstrate the self-care routine.
   A. Model each step in its normal sequence.
   B. Describe what you are doing with each step: "Watch, I'm taking the cover off the inhaler."
   C. Repeat the demonstration.
2. Test.
   A. Ask the patient to do the routine.
   B. Notice what steps are difficult, and mark them on a data form.
   C. Praise the patient for trying. Never use a harsh tone of voice or criticism.
3. Repeat Steps 1 and 2 again.
4. Break out the difficult steps.
   A. By looking at your data sheet, identify steps requiring more instruction.
   B. Pull out the difficult step by starting at the beginning of that step and demonstrating it two times.
   C. Ask the patient to do the step. If he continues to have difficulty, give additional prompts until he does the step independently or with as little help as possible.
5. Teach the difficult step using additional prompts (see Figure 13.2).

ordinary lives in the community. These individuals are able to read instructions as long as they are written at roughly a sixth-grade level. Individuals with need for more extensive supports may need simplified written checklists instead of full instructions. Others may benefit from photos of a person doing each step of self-care or line drawings. Just as most patients require clear explanations and demonstration of some procedures, so do individuals with MR, but they may need more cognitive supports to understand the information.

## Conclusion

In summary, people with MR are currently attending school, living, working, and participating in the lives of ordinary communities to an extent never before permitted or realized in the United States. The central values in this movement are self-determination, full societal inclusion, and a dynamic balance of independence and interdependence within a network of support. A key to delivering the best health care for people with MR

is effective partnerships among these individuals, their family members, and care providers. When health care professionals are provided with knowledge and experience in working with individuals with MR, their attitudes and feelings about this important group of people change in positive ways.

A willingness to break with the past and with unspoken negative assumptions about individuals with MR can help build alliances between providers and patients. A combination of clear and friendly communication and the use of structured skills training can help many individuals with MR and/or their caregivers to promote health and treat chronic illnesses that can occur with syndromes that cause some forms of MR. Giving information and linking individuals to formal and informal sources of support is a major means of assisting people with MR and their families. Effective partnerships in serving this important group of citizens can be extremely rewarding for physicians, nurses, and other health care professionals as part of their larger health care mission.

# References

American Association on Mental Retardation. (2002). *Mental retardation: definition, classification, and systems of supports* (10th ed.).Washington DC: AAMR.

American Association on Mental Retardation. (n.d.). *Mental retardation fact sheet.* Retrieved January 29, 2004 from *http://www.aamr.org/Policies/faq_mental_retardation.shtml.*

Biasini, F. J., Grupe, L., Huffman, L., & Bray, N. W. (1999). Mental retardation: A symptom and a syndrome. In S. Netherton, D. Sandra, & D. Holmes (Eds.), *Child and adolescent psychological disorders: A comprehensive textbook* (pp. 6–23). London: Oxford University Press.

Black, E. (2003). *War against the weak: Eugenics and America's campaign to create a master race.* New York: Four Walls Eight Windows.

Blatt, B., & Kaplan, F. (1974) *Christmas in purgatory: A photographic essay on mental retardation.* Syracuse, NY: Human Policy Press.

Blue-Banning, M., Summer, J. A., Frankland, H. C., Nelson, L. L., & Beegle, G. (2004). Dimensions of family and professional partnerships: Constructive guidelines for collaboration. *Exceptional Children.* 70(2), 167–184.

Bogdan, R. (1988). *Freak show: Presenting human oddities for amusement and profit.* Chicago: University of Chicago Press.

Boswell, J. (1987). *The kindness of strangers: The abandonment of children in western Europe from late antiquity to the Renaissance.* New York: Pantheon Books.

Braddock, D. L., & Parish, S. L. (2001). An institutional history of disability. In G. L. Albrecht, K. D. Seelman, & M. Bury (Eds.), *Handbook of disability studies* (pp. 11–68). Thousand Oaks, CA: Sage Publications.

Brillhart, B. A., Jay, H., & Wyers, M. E. (1990). Attitudes toward people with disabilities. *Rehabilitation Nursing, 15,* 80–82.

Ferguson, P. M. (2001). Mapping the family: Disability studies and the exploration of parental response to disability. In G. L. Albrecht, K. D. Seelman, & M. Bury (Eds.), *Handbook of Disability Studies* (pp. 373–395). Thousand Oaks, CA: Sage Publications.

Fujiara, G. T., & Braddock, D. (1992). Fiscal and demographic trends in mental retardation services: The emergence of the family. In L. Rowitz (Ed.), *Mental retardation in the year 2000* (pp. 316–338). New York: Springer.

Krauss, M. W., Gulley, S., Sciegaj, M., & Wells, N. (2003). Access to speciality medical care for children with mental retardation, autism, and other special health care needs. *Mental Retardation, 41,* 329–339.

Lakin, K. C., Anderson, L., Prouty, R., & Polister, B. (1999). Community residential services wouild require expansion of 72% to serve everyone in community settings. *Mental Retardation, 37,* 251–253.

Hahn, J. E. (2003) Addressing the needs for education: Curriculum development for nurses about intellectual and developmental disabilities. *The Nursing Clinics of North America, 38,* 185–204.

Hart, S. L. (1998). Learning-disabled people's experience of general hospitals. *British Journal of Nursing, 13,* 470–477.

Hastings, R. P., & Taunt, H. M. (2002). Positive perceptions in families of children with developmental disabilities. *American Journal on Mental Retardation, 107,* 116–127.

Harry, B., Kalyanpur, M., & Day, M. (1999). *Building cultural reciprocity with families: Case studies in special education.* Baltimore: Paul H. Brookes Publishing.

Mostert, M. P. (2002). Useless eaters: Disability as genocidal marker in Nazi Germany. *Journal of Special Education, 36,* 155–168.

Pfeiffer, D., Sam, A. A., Guinan, M., Ratliffe, K. T., Robinson, N. B., & Stodden, N. J. (2003). Attitudes toward disability in the helping professions. *Disability Studies Quarterly, 23,* 132–149.

Poston, D., Turnbull A. P., Park, J., Mannan, J., Marquis, J., & Wang, M. (2003). Family quality of life: A qualitative inquiry. *Mental Retardation, 41,* 313–328.

Risdal, D., & Singer, G. (2004). Marital adjustment in parents of children with disabilities: A historical review and meta-analysis. *Research and Practice for Persons with Severe Disabilities, 29(2),* 95–103.

Russell, S., Daly, J., & Hoog, C. C. (2003). Nurses and 'difficult patients': Negotiating noncompliance. *Journal of Advanced Nursing, 43,* 281–287.

Scheerenberger, R. C. (1987). *A history of mental retardation.* Baltimore: Brookes Publishing.

Selden, S. (1999). *Inheriting shame: The story of eugenics and racism in America.* New York: Teacher's College Press.

Shahar, S. (1992). *Childhood in the Middle Ages.* London: Routeledge.

Singer, G. H. S. (1991). *Parents and pediatricians: What does and doesn't work.* Givertz Graduate School of Education, University of California at Santa Barbara.

Singer, G. H. S., & Nixon, C. (1996). You can't imagine unless you've been there yourself: The parental experience of a child's brain injury, a qualitative inquiry. In G. H. S. Singer, A. Glang, & J. Williams, (Eds.), *Families and Children with Acquired Brain Injury: Focus on Family Support.* Baltimore, MD: Paul Brookes Publishing.

Singer, G. H. S. (2004). A meta-analysis of comparative studies of depression in mothers of children with and without developmental disabilities. Manuscript submitted for publication.

Surgeon General of the United States. (2002). *Closing the gap: A national blueprint to improve the health of persons with mental retardation.* Rockville, MD: Office of the surgeon. Retrieved January 29, 2004 from *http://www.nichd.nih.gov/publications/pubs/closing the gap/index.htm.*

Timothy, T. L., Emrich, K., & Moore, G. (2003). The effect of curriculum on the attitudes of nursing students toward disability. *Rehabilitation Nursing, 28,* 27–30.

Trent, J. W. (1995). *Inventing the feeble mind: A history of mental retardation in the United States.* Berkeley, CA: University of California Press.

Turnbull, H., & Turnbull, A. (2000). Accountability: Whose Job Is It, Anyway? *Journal of Early Intervention, 23*(4), 231–234.

U.S. Department of Health and Human Services. (2002). *The Surgeon General Report on Mental Health in the United States.* Washington, D.C.: U.S. Public Health Service.

Walsh, K., Hammerman, S., Josephson, F., & Krupka, P. (2000). Caring for people with developmental disabilities. *Mental Retardation, 38*(1), 33–41.

Walsh, K. K., Hammerman, S., & Krupka, P. (2002). Caring for people with developmental disabilities: Survey of nurses about their education and experience. *Mental Retardation, 38,* 33–41.

Wehman, P. (2003). Opening the community for persons with disabilities. *Journal of Vocational Rehabilitation, 19*(3), 121–122.

Westling, D. L., & Fox, L. (2000). *Teaching students with severe disabilities* (2nd ed.). Upper Saddle River, NJ: Merrill.

Winzer, M. A. (1993). *The history of special education: From isolation to integration.* Washington, DC: Gallaudet University Press.

Winzer, M. A. (1997). Disability and society before the eighteenth century. In L. J. Davis. (Ed.), *The Disability Studies Reader.* 75–109. New York: Routledge.

# Chapter 14

# Young Children with Developmental Disabilities and Their Families: Needs, Policies, and Services

Penny Hauser-Cram

During the past two decades we have witnessed an increase in the proportion of young children who are identified as having developmental disabilities and related special needs. Current figures indicate that approximately 13% of all children, and 5% of preschool-aged children, receive special education services (U.S. Department of Education, 1990; 2001). The largest increase in service provision over the past decade has occurred in the birth-to-kindergarten population (National Center for Education Statistics, 2001). The increase is attributable to several factors. First, although more children with very low birth weight are surviving due to medical technological advances, they often experience a range of complications, including hypoxic (inadequate oxygen) ischemic encephalopathy (inadequate blood supply) (Shonkoff & Marshall, 2000). Such deprivation can result in neuropathology and eventual developmental delays or disabilities (Hack, Wright, Shankaran, & Tyson, 1995). Stanton-Chapman, Chapman, and Scott (2001), for example, reported that the rate of learning problems among boys born with very low birth weight is 2.4 times greater than that among boys born full term.

Second, children are being identified with potential disabilities, such as learning disabilities, at increasingly younger ages (Lyon, 1996). This may be a result of early screening programs at or before school entry (e.g., Child Find), which have led to identifying children at a young age with suspected developmental problems (Meisels, 1991). Further, our understanding of early indicators of developmental difficulties has grown, and children with certain disorders, such as autism, are now diagnosed at younger ages (e.g., Baron-Cohen et al., 1996; Frith, 2003). Finally, the growth of early intervention programs, as a result of federal legislation (Part C of the Individuals with Disabilities Education Act) (IDEA), has made such services more visible and accessible (Kochanek & Buka, 1998). With increasing evidence of the value of early assistance (Guralnick, 1997; Shonkoff & Hauser-Cram, 1987), pediatricians and other health care providers are replacing former practices that involved seeing if children "grow out of" their delayed or unusual development with new practices that incorporate referrals to early intervention services.

Health care providers serve a central role in identifying children who have a developmental disability or delay. In the National Institute of Child Health and Development (NICHD) Study of Early Child Care, La Paro, Olsen, and Pianta (2002) found that the majority of very young children with special needs were identified by a medical professional. Increasingly, physicians and other health care professionals have become involved in the screening and referral processes for early intervention services (Soloman, 1995), yet many health care providers report they have a lack of familiarity with federal laws and the early intervention system (Soloman, Clougherty, Shaffer, Hofkosh, & Edwards, 1994). The purpose of this chapter is to provide an overview of policies related to young children with developmental disabilities and a review of research on the needs of their families and the effectiveness of early intervention services.

# Federal Policy About Young Children with Special Needs

Enormous policy changes related to services for young children with disabilities and their families have occurred over the past few decades in the United States. Indeed, as a nation we have moved from an implicit policy of institutionalizing children with special needs, especially children with Down syndrome and other forms of intellectual disabilities, to an explicit one of supporting families as they raise children at home (Meisels & Shonkoff, 2000). Legislation developed over the past three decades has required publicly supported services be provided to younger and younger children.

## *Legislation*

In the 1970s Congress passed landmark legislation for children with disabilities, Public Law 94-142 (the Education for All Handicapped Children Act of 1975), which established the right to a free and appropriate public education for school-aged children with disabilities. Although the law did not require states to provide services for children under school age, it did endorse the importance of such services. Over 10 years later, in 1986, Congress enacted Public Law 99-457, which encouraged (but did not mandate) states to provide services for infants and toddlers with disabilities and also strengthened incentives for states to provide services for preschoolers with disabilities.

This was soon followed by legislation in 1988 (P.L. 102-119, the Individuals with Disabilities Education Act) (IDEA), which required states to both 1) develop a system of early intervention services for children from 0 to 3 years old (referred to as Part C) and 2) provide free and appropriate public education and related services to children with disabilities beginning at age 3 (referred to as Part B). Although the public schools were to be responsible for services for children of preschool age, each state had discretion as to the state agency responsible for administering and implementing the system of early intervention (EI) services. Therefore, the lead agency for EI varies by state. About one-third of the states initially selected education as the lead agency, whereas slightly fewer chose public health, and fewer still selected mental health or human services (Garwood, Fewell, & Neisworth, 1988). Current trends indicate that more departments of health and fewer departments of education are taking the lead (Meisels & Shonkoff, 2000). The legislation requires that regardless of lead agency selected, the EI system should emerge from the coordination of health and education agencies at the state and local level. Such collaboration between the medical and educational communities is a unique feature of the early intervention system.

## *Eligibility*

One critical issue in providing EI services is in determining who is eligible to receive them. The law states that such services should be provided to children who are experiencing developmental delays and to those who have a diagnosed condition that results in a high probability of subsequent delays. States have the option of also providing services to children who are "at risk of having substantial delays if early intervention services are not provided" (20 U.S.C. # 1432). States have difficulty determining which children are "at risk" and vary substantially in the extent to which services are provided to these children (Hebbeler et al., 2001). A recent survey indicates that 58% of children enter EI due to developmental delay, 29% because of a diagnosed condition (e.g., Down's syndrome), and 13% because they are "at risk" for developing delays (Hebbeler et al., 2001). The most common reasons for receipt of EI services are listed in Table 14.1, and, as indicated in that table, most children who exhibit developmental delays do so because of speech or communication problems.

An important requirement of IDEA is the development of an individualized education plan (IEP) for children aged 3 or older and of an individualized family service plan (IFSP) for children in early intervention. Like the IEP, the IFSP delineates the needs and goals for the child, but unlike the IEP, the IFSP also specifies family strengths and needs. The importance of the family as the primary niche in which young children are nurtured and learn is clearly recognized in the legislative requirements relating to the IFSP. Although some concern has been expressed about the construction of the IFSP as a potential intrusion into family life (Krauss, 1990), the family focus inherent in the legislation reflects contemporary perspectives about the importance of the family in enhancing the optimal development of young children with disabilities.

# The Needs of Parents of Young Children with Developmental Disabilities

All families need to adjust to the birth of a child, but adjustments can be more pronounced when the infant experiences health or developmental problems. Much has been written about the grief and "chronic sorrow" that parents experience in learning that their infant has a developmental disability (e.g., Solnit & Stark, 1961). It is now widely recognized, however, that individuals vary considerably in their responses to this event, and that expectations that all parents experience "chronic sorrow" may be misguided. Some variation in parental responses relates to parents'

*Table 14.1*　Common Reasons for Receipt of Early Intervention Services[a]

| Reason | Percentage[b] |
| --- | --- |
| Speech/communication impairment or delay | 41 |
| Prenatal/perinatal abnormalities (e.g., low birth weight) | 19 |
| Motor impairment or delay | 17 |
| Delayed development (global) | 12 |
| Cognitive disorders (e.g., Down syndrome) | 9 |
| Intellectual/cognitive impairment or delay | 7 |
| Central nervous system disorders (e.g., cerebral palsy) | 7 |
| Social environment risk factors | 4 |
| Social/behavioral impairment or delay | 4 |
| Sensory impairment (e.g., vision, hearing impairment) | 3 |

[a]*Source: National Early Intervention Longitudinal Study (U.S. Department of Education, 2000).*
[b]*Percentages sum to more than 100 because children may have more than one reason for receipt of services.*

sociocultural beliefs about the etiology of the disability (e.g., the child is a gift to parents who can master the challenge, or the child's disability is a punishment for parents' past behaviors) (Garcia Coll & Magnuson, 2000). For most parents, the knowledge that their infant may exhibit unusual or delayed development requires an adjustment, but the assumption that all parents will endure "chronic sorrow" lacks empirical evidence.

In the 1960s and 1970s, a stage theory was proposed to health professionals as a way to predict parents' reactions to the birth or diagnosis of a child with disabilities (Blacher, 1984). The three proposed stages followed those reported for individuals coping with the illness or death of a close family member (Kubler-Ross, 1997). In the first stage, parents experience disbelief and "shop" for physicians and treatments. The second stage is characterized by guilt, anger, and disappointment. The third stage occurs when parents reorient themselves toward adjustment and acceptance of their child and take on an advocacy role. Although this stage theory may be appealing, the empirical evidence for these stages has been found to be weak (Blacher, 1984). Therefore, research has turned away from delineating stages toward understanding parents' adaptive functioning.

## Studies of Maternal Behavior

Much research has been conducted on caregivers, especially mothers, of young children with disabilities. Many studies on the mother–child dyad have been guided by the transactional model (Sameroff & Chandler, 1975), which emphasizes the bi-directional interactions between a mother and a child. This theoretical model does not assume that influences occur only from mother to child but instead focuses on the responses that each has to the other in complex changing patterns. Barnard and colleagues (1989) refer to these interactive patterns as a "mutually adaptive dance." Investigations of the mother–child dyad of typically developing children indicate that responsive reactions by mothers that are contingent

on children's behaviors promote positive cognitive and social-emotional development in children (Osofsky & Thompson, 2000). In contrast, mothers who repeatedly ignore children's responses or are highly controlling and intrusive into children's activities reduce children's opportunities for self-efficacy (Heckhausen, 1993).

Research on the mother–child dyad when the child has a developmental disability demonstrates that maternal contingent responsiveness during children's early years is an important predictor of development of positive cognitive and communication skills over time (Hauser-Cram, Warfield, Shonkoff, & Krauss, 2001). Such productive mother–child interaction appears to be more challenging in dyads where the child has a disability than in other dyads, however. Children with certain disabilities, such as those with Down's syndrome, may provide fewer, more delayed, or less appropriate signals to parents during interactions (e.g., Beeghly, Perry, & Cicchetti, 1989; Landry & Chapieski, 1990). Children with autism and related disabilities may rarely make eye contact with the mother or caregiver (Hoppes & Harris, 1990), which results in reduced opportunities for mutually responsive interaction and joint attention. Thus, the child with a developmental disability may display fewer or unusual cues, making it difficult for a caregiver to respond contingent to the child's actions.

Possibly as a result of children's unusual or unexpected cues, mothers of children with disabilities, in comparison to other mothers, appear to be more directive to children with disabilities (Marfo, 1990). For example, Mahoney, Fors, and Wood (1990) found that during free play activities, mothers of children with Down syndrome, unlike mothers of typically developing children, directed their child's attention away from the objects the child was using and toward more challenging tasks. Crawley and Spiker (1983) found that parents were more directive of children with Down syndrome who showed less interest in play and initiated fewer interactions with objects.

Such directiveness could result in either promotive or deleterious outcomes for children. Directiveness could diminish children's attempts at self-initiation as has been found in research on dyads where the child is developing typically (Lepper, 1981). Alternatively, directiveness could assist children in their interactions by providing necessary scaffolding (i.e., incremental support and guidance as the child works on a task), for example, by making materials easier for the child to reach or asking questions that will aid in problem solution. Tannock (1988) found that maternal directives assisted children with Down syndrome in more fully participating in the interaction. Roach, Barratt, Miller, and Leavitt (1998) reported that mothers of children with Down syndrome were both more directive *and* more supportive than were other mothers of both mental-age-matched and chronological-age-matched typically developing children. They found that the combination of maternal directiveness and support elicited more object play and vocalizations by the children with disabilities. Thus, it appears that although mothers tend to interact using a more directive style with young children with disabilities, benefits accrue to those children when that style is complemented by maternal support of children's actions.

## Parenting Stress

Maternal–child interaction occurs within a family system that may be functioning well or poorly (Minuchin, 1988). If individuals experience high levels of stress, their parental functioning is diminished. According to researchers who focus on the family system (McCubbin & Patterson, 1983), the adaptation of the family to the birth or diagnosis of a child with disabilities can be explained by several factors, including the meaning ascribed to the disability, and the internal and external resources of the family.

Of the many factors that comprise parental well-being, parenting stress appears to be the one most frequently studied in relation to parenting a child with a disability. Although many have claimed that parents of infants with disabilities have exceedingly high levels of stress, empirical work indicates otherwise. Studies indicate that, on average, parents report normative stress during their child's infant and toddler years (Shonkoff, Hauser-Cram, Krauss, & Upshur, 1992). Increasing stress levels occur during early childhood (Innocenti, Huh, & Boyce, 1992), with high stress levels during the middle childhood years (Hauser-Cram et al., 2001; Orr, Cameron, Dobson, & Day, 1993).

These findings are based on families who have received early intervention services, however. It is possible that such services provide sufficient support to parents to temper the levels of stress parents feel during the infant and toddler years. When the family support services of EI are withdrawn and children make the transition from EI to preschool and school services, parental stress levels increase. The child-focused services of the school years may offer some families respite from intense involvement in services and the concomitant demands made by such involvement but may also lack the means for providing support for the family system as a whole.

Mothers and fathers evince different patterns of parenting stress. Although mothers, in comparison to fathers, often provide more caregiving functions for children during the infant and toddler years, fathers in general report more stress at that time (Hauser-Cram et al., 2001). Fathers' increasing levels of stress appear to be moderated by problem-focused coping skills. Fathers who approach their stressful problems by selecting problem-solving strategies report less stress over time than fathers who lack such strategies. The stress levels of mothers, on the other hand, are moderated by the construction of satisfying social support networks (Hauser-Cram et al., 2001). Mothers who find their support networks, whatever the size, to be helpful show less increase in stress. These different patterns of stress and its moderators for mothers and fathers suggest that different types of assistance would be valuable to different family members.

## The Role of Fathers

We have little information about the service needs of fathers, however, because fathers have been relatively neglected in studies of children with disabilities (Lamb & Billings, 1997). Indeed, many studies have used the mother as a spokesperson for the family or viewed fathers only as adjuncts to mothers. In summarizing studies on fathers of children with disabilities, Hornby (1995) concludes that they paint "a negative picture" (p. 105). For example, Wikler, Wasow, and Hatfield (1981) suggest that fathers are more affected (than mothers) by the physical aspects of a child's disability. Schillinge, Schinke, and Kirkham (1985) contend that fathers have more difficulty accepting their sons with disabilities than accepting their daughters.

Many of the prior studies, however, are based on autobiographical accounts and clinical impressions, and most are dated in terms of contemporary family arrangements and roles. Because many mothers of young children with disabilities are now in the workforce (Landis, 1992), the roles of fathers in families have changed. Therefore, we need carefully constructed research on fathers' perspectives in today's family.

A few investigations have focused on the positive changes that have occurred in individuals' lives as a result of parenting a child with a disability. Abbot and Meredith (1986) interviewed parents of children with mental retardation and found that 88% reported positive outcomes, such as having greater compassion and developing stronger families. Based on survey research, Scorgie and Sobsey (2000) found that parents of children with disabilities reported personal growth, improved relations with others, and changes in their philosophical or spiritual values as a result of their parenting experiences. Such studies indicate the complex emotions associated with parenting a child with a disability, which have yet to be fully investigated.

As the core of the family system, parents set the emotional tone for the family and determine the opportunities available to children. Most families are composed of other members as well, and research attention is increasingly focused on the enduring importance of sibling relationships.

# Siblings of Children with Developmental Disabilities

Siblings share a powerful and complex emotional bond that is often the most abiding of familial relationships (Seligman, 1999). Early interactions between siblings provide a context for the development of social competencies and a significant influence on emotional, behavioral, and cognitive development (Dunn, 1999). When one sibling has a disability, the relationship may take on additional complexity. For the child with a disability, who may experience limited peer interaction and few friendships (Gresham & MacMillan, 1997), the sibling relationship may provide the primary context for positive socialization experiences with peers. Furthermore, the nondisabled sibling may assume the role of caretaker and companion in adulthood (Seltzer, Greenberg, Krauss, & Gordon, 1997; Seltzer & Krauss, 2001). Clearly, a child's disability has an impact on all members of the family, including siblings.

Just as early studies of parents of children with disabilities focused on negative outcomes, early investigations of siblings also assumed maladjustment. Traditionally, investigators hypothesized that the presence of a child with a disability is a source of developmental risk for other children in the family (e.g., Farber, 1959). Much early work indicated that sisters of children with developmental disabilities often assumed much greater caregiving and household responsibility than their peers. This disproportionate responsibility was considered to be related to increased levels of depression and anger (Farber, 1959), a higher incidence of antisocial behavior (Gath, 1973), and decreased coping effectiveness (Grossman, 1972). Researchers now suggest that these early studies may not reveal an accurate picture.

For example, these studies were conducted before the passing of IDEA, when few, if any, special services or supports were available to families of young children with disabilities. The presence of a child with a disability may well have been a source of stress for the entire family, which had to face the challenges of raising the child with little or no support from the community. Thus, these early studies may reflect an anachronistic understanding of the meaning of disability (Lamorey, 1999).

Furthermore, several methodological criticisms of this work exist. First, studies were largely retrospective reports based on patients referred for clinical assistance (Cuskelly, 1999). Thus, they failed to recognize the many siblings who did not suffer from psychological adjustment problems. Second, these reports were based largely on anecdotal evidence and self-report. They did not empirically investigate actual differences in responsibility between siblings of children with disabilities and siblings of typically developing children, nor did they demonstrate any correlation between responsibility and poor psychological outcomes through systematic measurement (Damiani, 1999).

## The Role of Siblings

More recent work has also focused on the roles that siblings of children with disabilities may play within the family. Research largely supports earlier findings that siblings, particularly sisters, of children with disabilities spend more time involved in caregiving activities, such as babysitting or helping with feeding, dressing, or bathing (McHale & Gamble, 1989), even when the typically developing sibling is younger (Stoneman, Brody, Davis, Crapps, & Malone, 1991). However,

generally speaking, female children appear to shoulder greater responsibility in the home, regardless of the presence of a sibling with a disability (McHale & Gamble, 1989; Stoneman, Brody, Davis, & Crapps, 1987). Gender aside, when other home responsibilities, such as household chores and self-care activities were considered, Cuskelly and Gunn (1993) found no difference in levels of responsibility between siblings of children with disabilities and those of nondisabled children. It appears that, regardless of gender, siblings of children with disabilities do assume more childcare responsibility in the family, but they are not expected to simultaneously take on more household chores or self-care responsibilities.

Although it is largely accepted that when there is a child with a disability in the family, siblings bear greater childcare responsibility in the home, it is not clear that this heightened responsibility leads to global adjustment problems. Although McHale and Gamble (1989) found a positive relation between amount of time spent in childcare activities and anxiety, they also reported that depression, self-esteem, and conduct problems were not related to home responsibilities. Others report a positive relation between responsibility and socioemotional functioning of siblings. For example, Cuskelly and Gunn (1993) found that sisters of children with disabilities exhibited fewer conduct problems when they had more responsibilities in the home. Finally, there is some indication that when typically developing siblings of children with disabilities have greater caregiving responsibility, these sibling relationships are characterized by low levels of conflict (Stoneman et al., 1991).

There is a belief that siblings of children with disabilities may be at increased risk for adjustment problems because they receive less attention from parents than their brothers and sisters (Stoneman, 2001). This is supported by the literature on typically developing siblings in which differential parental attention is often associated with deleterious sibling outcomes (Brody, Stoneman, & Burke, 1987). Nonetheless, evidence is mixed about whether siblings of children with disabilities actually receive less attention (Kaminsky & Dewey, 2001; McHale & Gamble, 1989; Stoneman et al., 1987). Furthermore, studies on siblings of children with disabilities do not clearly indicate that the effects of differential attention are detrimental. Corter and colleagues (Corter, Pepler, Stanhope, & Abromovitch, 1992) found no relation between maternal partiality and sibling interactions. Pit-ten Cate and Loots (2000) reported that although siblings perceived a difference in parental attention, they were accepting of it and largely recognized and appreciated their parents' attempts at justness.

## Sibling Interactions

Interactions between siblings when one has a developmental disability may differ appreciably from those in which both siblings are typically developing. Although McHale and Gamble (1989) found no difference in the amount of time sibling pairs spent in interaction with each other, the nature of the interactions and the type of activities were very different when one sibling had a disability. In addition to more caregiving, siblings of children with disabilities often display more managerial behavior and engage in less cooperative interaction with their brothers and sisters when compared to siblings of typically developing children (Dallas, Stevenson, & McGurk, 1993; Stoneman et al., 1987). Additionally, when compared to siblings of typically developing children, siblings of children with Down syndrome have been observed to be more nurturing towards their brothers or sisters, regardless of birth order (Abramovitch, Stanhope, Pepler, & Corter, 1987).

There is substantial evidence that the sibling relationship develops differently when one member has a disability. In dyads in which the typically developing sibling is older, there is a high

degree of role asymmetry in the relationship as the older sibling assumes a position of dominance (Abramovitch et al., 1987; Dallas et al., 1993; Stoneman et al., 1987). Although this is typical of any sibling relationship, when one sibling has a disability, the imbalance of power is not minimized over time but rather may become more pronounced (Stoneman, 2001).

When the child with a disability is the older sibling, the development of the sibling relationship may be even more atypical. Over time, the pair may experience a reversal of roles as the younger sibling catches up to, and bypasses, the older sibling in terms of cognitive ability and/or functional skills, eventually assuming the dominant role (Abramovitch et al., 1987; Brody, Stoneman, Davis, & Crapps, 1991; Dallas et al., 1993; Stoneman et al., 1991). Although the development of the relationship between children with disabilities and their siblings may not be normative, there is no evidence that this asymmetry is in any way detrimental to the development of the individuals or the relationship. Stoneman (2001) emphasizes that relationships that are atypical may be considered adaptive, rather than necessarily pathological or problematic.

Many current investigations regarding the siblings of children with disabilities consider the complexity of both the sibling relationship and the family context and recognize a range of possible psychological outcomes. It is important to understand the different processes and mechanisms by which these potential outcomes occur (McHale & Gamble, 1989). For example, Dyson (1989) compared older siblings of children with disabilities to older siblings of typically developing children and found no significant differences between the two groups on measures of self-concept, social competence, and behavior problems. She reported, however, significant within-group variation related to both child and family characteristics. In other words, Dyson found that for both groups, those with and without siblings with disabilities, there was great variability in adjustment and behavior. For all siblings, some demonstrated high levels of self-concept and social competence with few behavior problems, whereas some exhibited the opposite. This suggests that such distinctions have more to do with individual differences and differences in family functioning than with whether or not a child with a disability is present in the home. In a follow-up study, Dyson, Edgar, and Crnic (1989) indicated that family context variables, such as parental stress, family relationship, social support, and the family's emphasis on personal growth, were significant predictors of self-concept, social competence, and behavior problems in siblings of children with a variety of disabilities.

## Sibling Adjustment

Sibling adjustment is related to many factors, including the type and severity of the sibling's disability and the temperament of both siblings; however, evidence increasingly points to the importance of the family context. Parents' psychological well-being, interactions, and responses to stress affect the well-being of the individual children within the family. In a 3-year longitudinal study, siblings of children with pervasive developmental delay (PDD) exhibited more behavior problems than either the siblings of children with Down syndrome or those of typically developing children (Fisman, Wolf, Ellison, & Freeman, 2000). Sibling behavior problems in all groups, however, were related to parental stress, and parents of children with PDD were found to maintain the highest stress levels over time. McHale and Gamble (1989) found no direct connections between the characteristics of children with disabilities and the well-being of their older brothers and sisters, but they did find that siblings who experienced more negative interactions with their mothers exhibited more depression, anxiety, and low self-esteem. Thus, family environment is a critical factor in understanding sibling adjustment to childhood disability.

Some recent studies have found that the presence of a child with a disability has a positive impact on family climate and sibling adjustment. In one study, siblings of children with Down syndrome were collectively found to have above average scores on a measure of self-concept (Van Riper, 2000). Then again, higher self-concept scores were related to greater family resources and fewer stressful events experienced by the family. These family characteristics, as well as coping strategies and effective problem-solving communication techniques, also predicted the sibling's social competence.

Although family context is important in understanding the relationships that exist between siblings when one has a disability, focus on this topic is just emerging in the research literature (Stoneman, 2001). There is evidence that children regard their siblings with an intellectual disability more positively when they perceive their families as communicative and emotionally responsive (Weinger, 1999). This indicates that in families in which members are safely able to express a range of feelings, children express a greater acceptance of their siblings with disabilities. More investigation is needed, however, to determine the process by which the family climate influences the relationship between siblings when one has a disability.

In general, many children reflect positively on the experience of having a sibling with a disability (Eisenberg, Baker, & Blacher, 1998; Grossman, 1972; Kaminsky & Dewey, 2001; Pitten Cate & Loots, 2000; Roeyers & Mycke, 1995; Van Riper, 2000). These children tend to rate their sibling relationships more positively than do comparison children (Roeyers & Mycke, 1995), report fewer conflicts, and express greater admiration for their siblings (Kaminsky & Dewey, 2001). Many children acknowledge that they have benefited from having a sibling with a disability.

They credit their siblings with helping them gain virtues such as patience, tolerance, benevolence, and appreciation of health and family (Eisenberg et al., 1998; Van Riper, 2000).

## THE ROLE OF SUPPORT GROUPS

When children talk about the negative aspects of having a sibling with a disability, they often cite worry about health concerns and the future (Eisenberg et al., 1998). In one study, 75% of siblings reported that they sometimes worried about their sibling's health, or future, or both (Pit-ten Cate & Loots, 2000). Damiani (1999) suggests that worry is quite prevalent among the siblings of children with disability and that this might present one of the greatest risk factors for these children.

Given the worries of these siblings, such children may benefit from support groups that address the concerns and uncertainty that they feel about the future lives of their brothers and sisters and their place in it. Research also indicates that siblings have a need for information. Roeyers and Mycke (1995) found that brothers and sisters of children with autism rated their sibling relationships more positively when they had more knowledge about the nature of autism. In a sample of Dutch children, aged 10 to 19 years, with siblings with physical disabilities, many of the participants were unable to provide details regarding their siblings' disabilities, but when given the opportunity asked many questions about medical matters (Pit-ten Cate & Loots, 2000). This is a further indication that siblings may need a reliable and accessible source of information about disabilities outside of the family; health care professionals could be a source of such information.

Siblings may also benefit from services targeted at supporting their psychological well-being, particularly in the presence of multiple risk factors. A group of low-income children, all having a sibling with a developmental disability, demonstrated decreased levels of anxiety, depression, and stress, and improved self-esteem after participating in a 15-week after-school program (Phillips, 1999). The program consisted of recreational activities, assistance with homework, and discussion groups focused on issues of developmental disabilities. A comparison group of children, who received no intervention, showed no similar gains over the same time period.

Clearly, siblings of children with disabilities have much to gain from interventions focused on their unique needs. The importance of the family context, however, carries additional implications for intervention. Given the existing empirical evidence, interventions focused on reducing parental stress, anxiety, and depression and increasing family communication and coping strategies may provide benefits for all members of the family. Many EI programs aim to support families as they raise children with disabilities and, as discussed in the next section, do so by providing a range of highly individualized services.

# Early Intervention Services

Early intervention services are multidisciplinary services provided to children with developmental disabilities, delays, or risks during the first few years of life. The goal of these programs is to promote the health and optimal development of the children as well as to support adaptive parenting and positive functioning of their families (Shonkoff & Meisels, 2000). A wide range of disciplines are involved in providing such services, including public health, medicine, education, psychology, social work, child care, speech and language services, and occupational and physical therapy, and, therefore, a broad range of services are provided (Table 14.2). The specific services are usually highly individualized based on child and family needs and strengths.

Early intervention programs are serving almost 60% more children and families now than they were a decade ago when states were first mandated to provide such services (U.S. Department of Education, 2001). In addition to improved early

*Table 14.2*   Types of Early Intervention Services Commonly Provided to Children and Families[a, b]

| Type | Percentage[c] |
|------|------------|
| Service coordination | 80 |
| Speech/language therapy | 53 |
| Special instruction | 44 |
| Occupational therapy | 39 |
| Physical therapy | 38 |
| Developmental monitoring | 38 |
| Health-related services | 25 |
| Family training | 20 |
| Other family support (e.g., counseling) | 14 |
| Audiology | 14 |
| Social work services | 12 |

[a]*Services most commonly provided within the first 6 months of enrollment.*
[b]*Source: National Early Intervention Longitudinal Study (U.S. Department of Education, 2000).*
[c]*Percentages sum to more than 100 because children and families often receive multiple services.*

diagnostic methods, the increased demand for services seems to be driven by a strong advocacy movement for and by individuals with disabilities and a heightened public awareness of the importance of the first 3 years of life in shaping developmental outcomes (Guralnick, 1998).

Notwithstanding the growing emphasis on, and awareness of, EI as an important factor in promoting optimal development for young children with disabilities, several challenges to research on the EI system persist. First, researchers disagree about how to determine the effectiveness of EI. Debates exist about which child outcomes deserve to be studied; whether family outcomes also should be evaluated; how to measure and reliably record the types, intensity, and individualized nature of services themselves; and the extent to which both quantitative and qualitative approaches are needed to understand family processes (Hauser-Cram, Warfield, Upshur, & Weisner, 2000). Historically, evaluation research on EI focused almost exclusively on cognitive outcomes with a neglect of socioemotional functioning of children and families (Shonkoff &

Hauser-Cram, 1987). There appears to be considerable agreement that children with established disabilities who receive EI demonstrate less deterioration in their scores on standardized tests of intellectual ability than their peers who do not receive comprehensive services (Guralnick, 1998; Guralnick & Bricker, 1987; Hines & Bennett, 1996; Spiker & Hopmann, 1997). These advantageous effects, however, have generally been found only during the first 5 years of life; long-term gains remain to be examined (Guralnick, 1998).

Despite the focus of EI services on family strengths and needs as well as on the individual child, few evaluation studies have considered parental benefits of participation in EI. Examining parental benefits of EI services is important in its own right because positive adjustment to parenting a child with a disability has potential advantages for all family members. Furthermore, because the family context is central to the optimal development of children, including children with disabilities (Hauser-Cram et al., 2001), assisting families with maintaining a supportive context for parenting is an aim of most EI programs. In one of the few studies on parental outcomes associated with EI participation, Warfield and colleagues (Warfield, Hauser-Cram, Krauss, Shonkoff, & Upshur, 2000) found that at the end of the EI experience, mothers who had received more hours of EI services reported improved family cohesion and more helpful social support networks in comparison to other mothers in EI.

## Evaluating Early Intervention Programs

Most studies of EI effectiveness have focused on the program as a whole. In an attempt to determine which features of EI programs were most effective, researchers at the Early Intervention Research Institute conducted a series of longitudinal studies employing randomized experimental designs. These studies yielded little information about the relative effectiveness of various program components, however. For example, White et al. (1994) reported no outcome differences for children who received intensive, family-centered intervention services in comparison to those who received center-based services once per week. One reason why so few program variation effects were found may be that not all children and families benefit equally from equal amounts of intervention (Dunst & Trivette, 1997). Indeed, given the diversity of children enrolled in the system and the wide range of services provided, it is difficult, and perhaps not even particularly meaningful, to consider the effectiveness of EI at a macro level (McCollum, 2002).

Additionally, Marfo and colleagues (1992) found that factors such as a child's developmental competency at entry into EI and the home environment were stronger predictors of developmental outcomes than were specific program variables. In other words, children who entered EI with the greatest delays tended to show the least improvement in developmental scores, but the quality of the home environment and parental expectations

also contributed significantly to post-intervention developmental status. These are important findings for several reasons. First, that entry-level child characteristics were the most influential predictor of developmental outcomes highlights the need for parents and professionals to be realistic in their expectations of what EI can accomplish for young children with significant deficits. Second, the importance of family ecology in determining developmental outcomes underscores the necessity for EI services to focus not only on the child, but also on the family as a whole.

Guralnick (1997) makes a useful distinction between first-generation and second-generation research in EI. First-generation research focuses on investigating the general effectiveness of comprehensive EI programs. In contrast, second-generation research addresses more specific issues that are aimed at optimizing individual outcomes, informing program design, and increasing our understanding of the influence of individual child and family characteristics on intervention efficacy. Some researchers maintain that global efficacy of EI has been established by first-generation research, and second-generation studies are now needed to inform the development of services that are responsive to individual needs and will evoke the most advantageous outcomes (Guralnick, 1997; McCollum, 2002). Such studies are difficult to conduct, however, given the individualized nature of EI and the heterogeneous population of children and families served.

## Challenge of Inconsistency and Fragmentation

A related challenge to the evaluation of EI services is due to the inconsistency and fragmentation within the EI system. For example, EI programs vary widely from state to state. Not only does federal legislation allow the states latitude in choosing a lead agency, it also gives them considerable discretion in the determination of who is eligible for services. Although all states must serve children with established disabilities and developmental delays, these criteria are not clearly defined by the federal government for children under 3 years of age, and states are allowed to establish their own criteria. State definitions of "developmental delay" vary widely (Hebbeler et al., 1999).

For example, Massachusetts has specific guidelines about the minimal extent of delay required for a child to be eligible for EI based on the child's age (e.g., 1.5 months delay for children aged 6 months or less, 6 months delay for children aged 19–36 months) (Massachusetts Department of Public Health, 1998). In Utah, a significant delay is defined as 1.5 standard deviations at or below the mean or below the 7th percentile in one or more areas of development based on a standard assessment (Utah Department of Health, 1999). In Alabama, infants or toddlers must be delayed by at least 25% in their cognitive, communicative, social, emotional, or adaptive development to be eligible for EI services (Alabama Department of Rehabilitation Services, 2003). Additionally, states may also decide whether or not to provide services to children "at risk" for exhibiting delays. This has resulted in great inconsistency; many children who are eligible for services in one state are not in another. Hence, although there exists a federal mandate to serve infants and toddlers with disabilities, there is little equity with regard to who may participate in EI programs (Bailey, 2000).

Additionally, there is considerable variability among states along several other dimensions. Specifically, states differ with regard to the number and type of agencies that are involved in the provision of services and in the ways that services are coordinated among agencies. There is even significant disparity in the degree to which states manifest within-state differences in local systems (Hebbeler et al., 1999).

For example, in Illinois each local area has an entity called "Child and Family Connections" under contract from the state lead agency, which is responsible for intake and for connecting families with the local service provider. This system pro-

vides some uniformity across the state in terms of intake, referral, and services. In contrast, in Ohio each county has a collaborative group that is responsible for establishing an EI system. That system varies widely from county to county; one county may have a single entry point to EI services, and the adjacent county may offer several points of entry.

Any general discussion of EI and its effectiveness is made more difficult by the heterogeneous nature of the children and families who participate in EI services. State differences aside, children may be eligible for EI services for a variety of reasons. The heterogeneity of children entering EI is illustrated by early reports from the National Early Intervention Longitudinal Study (NEILS). Commissioned by the Office of Special Education Programs, NEILS involves a nationally representative sample of more than 5,000 children and their families (Hebbeler et al., 2001; U.S. Department of Education, 2000). Preliminary data include a total of 305 specific descriptors of reasons for participants' initial eligibility for EI services, such as visual impairment, Down syndrome, spina bifida, or homelessness, to name but four. These descriptors can be classified into diverse categories, such as sensory impairments, congenital disorders, central nervous system disorders, and social environment risk factors (Hebbeler et al., 2001; U.S. Department of Education, 2000).

Because EI serves children with a broad range of abilities and needs, systems nationwide offer a wide array of services to both children and their families. These services are provided by many different types of practitioners and professionals, frequently through multiple agencies. Services may be child focused, such as occupational therapy, physical therapy, or speech and language services; medical care or special education services may also be included. Parents may receive mental health counseling, social services, or attend parenting classes, information sessions, or support groups. EI services may also be provided in a range of environments, from the home, to community settings such as childcare centers, to segregated, self-contained programs. Goals may focus on improving cognitive outcomes, communication skills, physical functioning, or social and emotional competencies. A systemwide objective of EI is that children and their families receive a package of services that is individualized to meet their needs.

## Developmental Systems Model

Given the diversity of the participants, the range of goals, and the breadth of services provided, combined with the inconsistencies and fragmentation that characterize the system at the state and national levels, it is small wonder that questions about effectiveness have been difficult to address with scientific rigor, and a coherent framework in which to view and discuss the EI system has been elusive. However, despite this diversity, there are some unifying themes that emerge when EI is considered overall. Although service delivery models may differ from state to state, the federal legislation (Part C of IDEA) requires an interdisciplinary collaborative system of services and agencies that serve children and families with a wide range of abilities and needs.

When we look at the various models of EI that currently proliferate, two overarching principles emerge (McCollum, 2002). First, EI practices are guided by an ecological perspective of human development that recognizes that the child develops within multiple intersecting environments (Bronfenbrenner, 1979). Second, service delivery models adopt a "systems of service" framework that stresses coordination and collaboration among various agencies and professionals. Taken together, these guiding themes underlie the developmental systems model of EI (Guralnick, 2001).

### FAMILY

The developmental systems model recognizes that the family is the primary context of develop-

ment for the young child (Bronfenbrenner, 1986). Guralnick (1997) notes that within this context, families influence child development in three ways: through the quality of parent–child interactions, through the types of experiences that are made available to the child, and by ensuring the child's health and safety. These three patterns are largely determined by both personal characteristics of the family, such as psychological well-being and intellectual ability, as well as environmental characteristics, such as the availability of social support and the family's financial resources. Furthermore, this model adopts a transactional perspective (Sameroff & Fiese, 2000) by recognizing that these factors interact with child characteristics, such as the nature and severity of a child's disability and the child's individual temperament, to shape the family ecology and create a unique developmental context for every family.

Current configurations of EI emphasize family by providing a system of services aimed at supporting a family ecology that optimizes child development. EI programs routinely include services focused on providing support and information to family members, including mental health services, counseling, and educational programs focused on parenting a child with a disability. Furthermore, many child-focused therapeutic services take place in the home environment and/or involve family members actively.

### SCHOOL AND COMMUNITY

Present EI practices also recognize the importance of other, more distal, contexts of development beyond the family, most specifically, school and community. There is considerable emphasis in both EI theory and practice on encouraging participants in EI programs to engage in inclusive community settings and activities. Such practices promote peer relationships and enhanced social competence (Guralnick, 2000). It is understood that one role of EI is to enable young children with disabilities to participate in the same developmental contexts as their typically developing peers (McCollum, 2002), including daycare and preschool settings. Toward this end, practitioners make every attempt to provide EI services in inclusive *natural environments* (Walsh, Rous, & Lutzer, 2000). Thus, to the maximum extent possible, all services and therapies are provided in home, school, or community settings, as opposed to segregated settings. Indeed, Guralnick (2001) considers community inclusion to be one of the three core principles of a developmental systems model, along with a focus on families and integration at the systems level.

EI's focus on family and community contexts draws heavily on current theories of human development, recognizing that the factors that influence optimal development for children with and without disabilities are many and diverse, and often interact in complex ways. Clearly, no single provider or agency can address all of these factors or the wide array of developmental needs that may be presented by the heterogeneous community of children and families who participate in EI programs. To provide the comprehensive, individualized package of services that has become the hallmark of the EI system, an integrated, multidisciplinary system of services consisting of multiple practitioners and agencies is essential.

For such a system to operate smoothly, a high level of collaboration and cooperation among the various components is warranted. Additionally, a service coordinator is an important component to help successfully navigate the complexities of the system and smooth transitions for families. Family members also may be viewed as integral components of the system of service. The formation of parent–professional partnerships that recognize parents as cocoordinators and co-providers of services for their children is key to the success of EI services (Turnbull, Turbiville, & Turnbull, 2000).

The formation of such partnerships, however, requires EI service providers to be knowledgeable of and sensitive to the various ethno-theories that parents hold about intervention practices and about the nature of developmental disabilities. Parents' belief systems, and the cultural contexts in which such beliefs develop, are an often overlooked but important part of the provision of services (Garcia Coll & Maguson, 2000; Super & Harkness, 1997). The future of the EI system will depend on its ability to attend to the development of cultural competence of service providers (Hanson, 1998).

# Conclusion

In conclusion, research on the effectiveness of EI faces many challenges. Nevertheless, this system of services has much to offer young children with disabilities and their families. It is an evolving system that requires responsiveness to a heterogeneous range of children and families. Health care providers are important sources of information about such services, and they will serve families well by becoming knowledgeable not only about the particular needs of children with disabilities and their families but also about the various EI services provided in their local communities.

# References

Abbott, D., & Meredith, W. (1986). Strengths of parents with retarded children. *Family Relations, 35,* 371–375.

Abramovitch, R., Stanhope, L., Pepler, D., & Corter, C. (1987). The influence of Down's syndrome on sibling interaction. *Journal of Child Psychology and Psychiatry, 28,* 865–879.

Alabama Department of Rehabilitation Services. (2003). *Alabama's Early Intervention System: General information.* Retrieved August 6, 2003 from *http://www.rehab. state.al.us/home/services/AEIS/General+Inform.*

Bailey, D. B. (2000). The federal role in early intervention: Prospects for the future. *Topics in Early Childhood Special Education, 20*(2), 71–78

Barnard, K. E., Hammond, M. A., Booth,, C. I., Bee, H. L., Mitchell, S. K., & Spieker, S. J. (1989). Measurement and meaning of parent-child interaction. In F. J. Morrison, C. Lord, & D. P. Keating (Eds.), *Applied developmental psychology, Volume 3* (pp. 39–80). New York: Academic Press.

Baron-Cohen, S., Cox, A., Baird, G., Swettenham, J., Nightingale, N., Morgan, K., Drew, A., & Charman, T. (1996). Psychological markers in the detection of autism in infancy in a large population. *British Journal of Psychiatry, 168*, 158–163.

Beeghly, M., Perry, B. M., & Cicchetti, D. (1989). Structural and affective dimensions of play development in young children with Down syndrome. *International Journal of Behavioral Development, 12*, 257–277.

Blacher, J. (1984). Sequential stages of parental adjustment to the birth of a child with handicaps: Fact or artifact? *Mental Retardation, 22*, 55–68.

Brody, G. H., Stoneman, Z., & Burke, M. (1987). Child temperaments, maternal differential behavior, and sibling relationships. *Developmental Psychology, 23*, 354–362.

Brody, G. H., Stoneman, Z., Davis, C. H., & Crapps, J. M. (1991). Observations of the role relations and behavior between older children with mental retardation and their younger siblings. *American Journal of Mental Retardation, 95*, 527–536.

Bronfenbrenner, U. (1979). *The ecology of human development: Experiments by nature and design.* Cambridge, MA: Harvard University Press.

Bronfenbrenner, U. (1986). Ecology of the family as a context for human development: Research perspectives. *Developmental Psychology, 22*, 723–742.

Corter, C., Pepler, D., Stanhope, L., & Abramovitch, R. (1992). Home observations of mothers and sibling dyads comprised of Down's syndrome and nonhandicapped children. *Canadian Journal of Behavioural Science, 24*, 1–13.

Crawley, S., & Spiker, D. (1983). Mother-child interactions involving two-year-olds with Down syndrome: A look at individual differences. *Child Development, 54*, 1312–1323.

Cuskelly, M. (1999). Adjustment of siblings of children with a disability: Methodological issues. *International Journal for the Advancement of Counselling, 21*, 111–124.

Cuskelly, M., & Gunn, P. (1993). Maternal reports of behavior of siblings of children with Down syndrome. *American Journal of Mental Retardation, 97*, 521–529.

Dallas, E., Stevenson, J., & McGurk, H. (1993). Cerebral-palsied children's interactions with siblings - II. Interactional structure. *Journal of Child Psychology and Psychiatry, 34*, 649–671.

Damiani, V. B. (1999). Responsibility and adjustment in siblings of children with disabilities: Update and review. *Families in Society, 80*, 34–40.

Dunn, J. (1999). Siblings, friends, and the development of social understanding. In W. A. Collins & B. Laursen (Eds.), *Relationships as developmental contexts: The Minnesota symposia on child psychology* (Volume 30, pp. 263–279). Mahwah, NJ: Lawrence Erlbaum Associates.

Dunst, C. J., & Trivette, C. M. (1997). Early intervention with young at-risk children and their families. In R. T. Ammerman & M. Hersen (Eds.), *Handbook of prevention and treatment with children and adolescents: Interventions in the real world context* (pp. 157–180). New York: John Wiley & Sons.

Dyson, L. L. (1989). Adjustment of siblings of handicapped children: A comparison. *Journal of Pediatric Psychology, 14*, 215–229.

Dyson, L. L., Edgar, E., & Crnic, K. (1989). Psychological predictors of adjustment of siblings of developmentally disabled children. *American Journal of Mental Retardation, 94*, 292–302.

Eisenberg, L., Baker, B. L., & Blacher, J. (1998). Siblings of children with mental retardation living at home or in residential placement. *Journal of Child Psychology and Psychiatry and Allied Disciplines, 39*, 355–363.

Farber, B. (1959). The effects of severely retarded children on the family system. *Monographs of the Society for Research in Child Development, 24* (2, Serial No. 71).

Fisman, S., Wolf, L., Ellison, D., & Freeman, T. (2000). A longitudinal study of siblings of children with chronic disabilities. *Canadian Journal of Psychiatry, 45*, 369–375.

Frith, U. (2003). *Autism: Explaining the enigma.* Malden, MA: Blackwell.

Garcia Coll, C., & Magnuson, K. (2000). Cultural differences as sources of developmental vulnerabilities and resources. In J. P. Shonkoff & S. J. Meisels (Eds.), *Handbook of early childhood intervention* (2nd ed., pp. 94–114). New York: Cambridge University Press.

Garwood, S. G., Fewell, R. R., & Neisworth, J. T. (1988). Public Law 94-142: You can get there from here! *Topics in Early Childhood Special Education, 8*, 1–11.

Gath, A, (1973). The school age siblings of mongol children. *British Journal of Psychiatry, 123*, 161–167.

Gresham, F. M., & MacMillan, D. L. (1997). Social competence and affective characteristics of students with mild disabilities. *Review of Educational Research, 76*, 377–415.

Grossman, F. K. (1972). *Brothers and sisters of retarded children: An exploratory study.* Syracuse, NY: Syracuse University Press.

Guralnick, M. J. (1997). Second-generation research in the field of early intervention. In M. J. Guralnick (Ed.), *The effectiveness of early intervention* (pp. 3–20). Baltimore: Brookes.

Guralnick, M. J. (1998). Effectiveness of early intervention for vulnerable children: A developmental perspective. *American Journal on Mental Retardation, 102*, 319–345.

Guralnick, M. J. (2000). Early childhood intervention: Evolution of a system. *Focus on Autism and Other Developmental Disabilities, 15*(2), 68–79.

Guralnick, M. J. (2001). A developmental systems model for early intervention. *Infants and Young Children, 14*(2), 1–18.

Guralnick, M. J., & Bricker, D. (1987). The effectiveness of early intervention for children with cognitive and general developmental delays. In M. J. Guralnick & F. C. Bennett (Eds.), *The effectiveness of early intervention for at-risk and handicapped children* (pp. 115–173). San Diego, CA: Academic Press.

Hack, M. Wright, L. I., Shankaran, S., & Tyson, J. E. (1995). Very low birth weight outcomes of the National Institute of Child Health and Human Development Neonatal Network, November 1989 to October, 1990. *American Journal of Obstetrics and Gynecology, 172,* 457–464.

Hanson, M. J. (1998). Ethnic, cultural, and language diversity in intervention settings. In E. W. Lynch & M. J. Hanson (Eds.), *Developing cross-cultural competence: A guide for working with young children and their families* (2nd ed., pp. 3–22). Baltimore, MD: Brookes.

Hauser-Cram, P., Warfield, M. E., Shonkoff, J. P., & Krauss, M. W. (2001). Children with disabilities: A longitudinal study of child development and parent well-being, *Monographs of the Society for Research in Child Development, 66* (3, serial No. 266).

Hauser-Cram, P., Warfield, M. E., Upshur, C. C., & Weisner, T. S. (2000). An expanded view of program evaluation in early childhood intervention. In J. P. Shonkoff & S. J. Meisels (Eds.), *Handbook of early childhood intervention* (2nd ed., pp. 487–509). New York: Cambridge University Press.

Hebbeler, K., Spiker, D., Wagner, M., Cameto, R., McKenna, P., & SRI International. (1999). *State-to-state variations in early intervention systems.* Menlo Park, CA: SRI International.

Hebbeler, K., Wagner, M., Spiker, D., Scarborough, A., Simeonson, R., & Collier, M. (2001). *A first look at the characteristics of children and families entering early intervention services* (NEILS Data Report 1). Menlo Park, CA: SRI International.

Heckhausen, J. (1993). The development of mastery and its perception within caretaker-child dyads. In D. J. Messer (Ed.), *Mastery motivation in early childhood: Development, measurement and social processes* (pp. 55–79). London: Routledge.

Hines, S., & Bennett, F. (1996). Effectiveness of early intervention for children with Down syndrome. *Mental Retardation and Developmental Disabilities Research Reviews, 2,* 96–101.

Hoppes, K., & Harris, S. L. (1990). Perceptions of child attachment and maternal gratification in mothers of children with autism and Down syndrome. *Journal of Clinical Child Psychology, 19,* 365–370.

Hornby, G. (1995). Fathers' views of the effects on their families of children with Down syndrome. *Journal of Child and Family Studies, 4*(1), 103–117.

Innocenti, M. S., Huh, K., & Boyce, G. (1992). Families of children with disabilities: Normative data and other considerations on parenting stress. *Topics in Early Childhood Special Education, 12,* 403–407.

Kaminsky, L., & Dewey, D. (2001). Sibling relationships of children with autism. *Journal of Autism and Developmental Disorders, 31,* 399–410.

Krauss, M. W. (1990). A new precedent in family policy: The individualized family service plan. *Exceptional Children, 56,* 388–395.

Kochanek, T. T., & Buka, S. L. (1998). Influential factors in the utilization of early intervention services. *Journal of Early Intervention, 21,* 323–338.

Kubler-Ross, E. (1997). *On death and dying.* New York: Scribner.

Lamb, M. E., & Billings, L. A. (1997). Fathers of children with special needs. In M. E. Lamb (Ed.), *The role of the father in child development* (pp. 179–190). New York: Wiley.

Lamorey, S. (1999). Parentification of siblings of children with disability or chronic disease. In N. D. Chase (Ed.), *Burdened children: Theory, research, and treatment of parentification* (pp. 75–91). Thousand Oaks, CA: Sage Publications.

Landis, L. J. (1992). Marital, employment, and childcare status of mothers with infants and toddlers with disabilities. *Topics in Early Childhood Special Education, 12,* 496–507.

Landry, S. H., & Chapieski, M. L. (1990). Joint attention of six-month-old Down syndrome and preterm infants: I. Attention to toys and mother. *American Journal on Mental Retardation, 91,* 488–498.

LaParo, K. M., Olsen, K., & Pianta, R. C. (2002). Special education eligibility: Developmental precursors over the first three years of life. *Exceptional Children, 69,* 55–66.

Lepper, M. R. (1981). Intrinsic and extrinsic motivation in children: Detrimental effects of superfluous social controls. In W. A. Collins (Ed.), *Minnesota symposium on child psychology, Volume 14.* Minneapolis, MN: University of Minnesota Press.

Lyon, G. R. (1996). Learning disabilities. *The Future of Children, 6,* 54–76.

Marfo, K. (1990). Maternal directiveness in interactions with mentally handicapped children: An analytical commentary. *Journal of Child Psychology and Psychiatry, 31,* 531–549.

Marfo, K., Dinero, T., Browne, N., Gallant, D., Smyth, R., & Corbett, A. (1992). Child, program, and family ecological variables in early intervention. *Early Education and Development, 3,* 27–44.

Mahoney, G., Fors, S., & Wood, S. (1990). Maternal directive behavior revisited. *American Journal on Mental Retardation, 94,* 398–406.

Massachusetts Department of Public Health. (1998). *Massachusetts Early Intervention Operational Standards.* Retrieved on August 6, 2003 from *www.statema.us/dph/tch/eiopstnd.pdf.*

McCollum, J. A. (2002). Influencing the development of young children with disabilities: Current themes in early intervention. *Child and Adolescent Mental Health, 7*, 4–9.

McCubbin, H. I., & Patterson, J. M. (1983). The family stress process: The double ABCX model of adjustment and adaptation. *Marriage and Family Review, 6*, 7–37.

McHale, S. M., & Gamble, W. C. (1989). Sibling relationships of children with disabled and nondisabled brothers and sisters. *Developmental Psychology, 25*, 421–429.

Meisels, S. J. (1991). Dimensions of early identification. *Journal of Early Intervention, 15*, 26–35.

Meisels, S. J., & Shonkoff, J. P. (2000). Early childhood intervention: A continuing evolution. In J. P. Shonkoff & S. J. Meisels (Eds.), *Handbook of early childhood intervention* (2nd ed., pp. 3–31). New York: Cambridge University Press.

Minuchin, P. P. (1988). Relationships within the family: A systems perspective on development. In R. A. Hinde & J. Stevenson-Hinde (Eds.), *Relationships within families: Mutual influences* (pp. 7–26). New York: Oxford University Press.

National Center for Education Statistics. (2001). *Digest of educational statistics, 2001* (NCES number 2002130). Retrieved October 30, 2002 from *http://nces.ed/gov/pubs2002/digest2001*.

Orr, R. R., Cameron, S. J., Dobson, L. A., & Day, D. M. (1993). Age-related changes in stress experienced by families with a child who has developmental delays. *Mental Retardation, 31*, 171–176.

Osofsky, J. D., & Thompson, M. D. (2000). Adaptive and maladaptive parenting: Perspectives on risk and protective factors. In J. P. Shonkoff & S. J. Meisels (Eds), *Handbook of early childhood intervention* (2nd ed., pp. 54–75). New York: Cambridge University Press.

Phillips, R. S. C. (1999). Intervention with siblings of children with developmental disabilities from economically disadvantaged families. *Families in Society, 80*, 569–577.

Pit-ten Cate, I. M., & Loots, G. M. P. (2000). Experiences of siblings of children with physical disabilities: An empirical investigation. *Disability and Rehabilitation, 22*, 399–408.

Roach, M. A., Barratt, M., Miller, J. F., & Leavitt, L. A. (1998). The structure of mother-child play: Young children with Down syndrome and typically developing children. *Developmental Psychology, 34*, 77–87.

Roeyers, H., & Mycke, K. (1995). Siblings of a child with autism, with mental retardation and with normal development. *Child: Care, Health and Development, 21*, 305–319.

Sameroff, A. J., & Chandler, M. J. (1975) Reproductive risk and the continuum of caretaking casuality. In F. D. Horowitz, M. Hetherington, S. Scarr-Salapatk, & G.

Siegel (Eds.), *Review of child development research: Volume 4* (pp. 187–244). Chicago: University of Chicago Press.

Sameroff, A. J., & Fiese, B. H. (2000). Transactional regulation: The developmental ecology of early intervention. In J. P. Shonkoff & S. J. Meisels (Eds.), *Handbook of early childhood intervention* (2nd ed., pp. 135–159). New York: Cambridge University Press.

Schilling, R. F., Schinke, S. P., & Kirkham, M. A. (1985). Coping with a handicapped child: Differences between mothers and fathers. *Social Science and Medicine, 21*, 857–863.

Scorgie, K., & Sobsey, D. (2000). Transformational outcomes associated with parenting children who have disabilities. *Mental Retardation, 38 (3)*, 195–206.

Seligman, M. (1999). Childhood disability and the family. In V. L. Schwean & D. H. Saklofske (Eds.), *Handbook of psychosocial characteristics of exceptional children.* (pp. 111–113). New York: Kluwer Academic/Plenum Publishers.

Seltzer, M. M., Greenberg, J. S., Krauss, M. W., & Gordon, R. M. (1997). Siblings of adults with mental retardation or mental illness: Effects of lifestyle and psychological well-being. *Family Relations: Interdisciplinary Journal of Applied Family Studies, 46*, 395–405.

Seltzer, M. M., & Krauss, M. W. (2001). Quality of life of adults with mental retardation developmental disabilities who live with family. *Mental Retardation and Developmental Disabilities Research Reviews, 7*, 105–114.

Shonkoff, J. P., & Hauser-Cram, P. (1987). Early intervention for disabled infants and their families: A quantitative analysis. *Pediatrics, 80*, 650–658.

Shonkoff, J. P., Hauser-Cram, P., Krauss, M. W., & Upshur, C. C. (1992). Development of infants with disabilities and their families. *Monographs of the Society for Research in Child Development, 57 (6)*, (Serial No. 230).

Shonkoff, J. P., & Marshall, P. C. (2000). The biology of developmental vulnerability. In J. P. Shonkoff & S. J. Meisels (Eds), *Handbook of early childhood intervention* (2nd ed., pp. 35–53). New York: Cambridge University Press.

Shonkoff, J. P., & Meisels, S. J. (2000). Preface. In J. P. Shonkoff & S. J. Meisels (Eds), *Handbook of early childhood intervention* (2nd ed., pp. xvii–xviii). New York: Cambridge University Press.

Solnit, A. J., & Stark, M. H. (1961). Mourning and the birth of a defective child. *Psychoanalytic Study of the Child, 16*, 523–537.

Solomon, R. (1995). Pediatricians and early intervention: Everything you need to know but are too busy to ask. *Infants and Young Children, 7(3)*, 38–51.

Solomon, R., Clougherty, S. L., Shaffer, D., Hofkosh, D., & Edwards, M. (1994). Community-based developmental assessment sites: A new model for pediatric "child find" activities. *Infants and Young Children, 7,* 67–71.

Spiker, D., & Hopmann, M. R. (1997). The effectiveness of early intervention for children with Down syndrome. In M. J. Guralnick (Ed.), *The effectiveness of early intervention* (pp. 271–305). Baltimore: Brookes.

Stanton-Chapman, T. L., Chapman, D. A., & Scott, K. G. (2001). Identification of early risk factors for learning disabilities. *Journal of Early Intervention, 24,* 193–206.

Stoneman, Z. (2001). Supporting positive sibling relationships during childhood. *Mental Retardation and Developmental Disabilities Research Reviews, 7,* 134–142.

Stoneman, Z., Brody, G. H., Davis, C. H., & Crapps, J. M. (1987). Mentally retarded children and their same-sex siblings: Naturalistic in-home observations. *American Journal of Mental Retardation, 92,* 290–298.

Stoneman, Z., Brody, G. H., Davis, C. H., Crapps, J. M., & Malone, D. M. (1991). Ascribed role relations between children with mental retardation and their younger siblings. *American Journal of Mental Retardation, 95,* 537–550.

Super, C. M., & Harkness, S. (1997). The cultural structuring of child development. In J. W. Berry, Y. P. Poortinga, J. Pandey, P. R. Dason, & T. S. Saraswathi (Vol. Eds.), *Handbook of cross-cultural psychology: Volume 2. Basic processes and human development* (pp. 1–39). Boston, MA: Allyn & Bacon.

Tannock, R. (1988). Control and reciprocity interactions with Down syndrome and normal children. In K. Marko (Ed.), *Parent-child interaction and developmental disabilities: Theory, research, and intervention* (pp. 162–180). New York: Praeger.

Turnbull, A. P., Turbiville, V., & Turnbull, H. R. (2000). Evolution of family-professional partnerships: Collective empowerment as the model for the early twenty-first century. In J. P. Shonkoff & S. J. Meisels (Eds.), *Handbook of early childhood intervention* (2nd ed., pp. 630–650). New York: Cambridge University Press.

U.S. Department of Education. (1990). *Twelfth annual report to Congress on the implementation of The Education of the Handicapped Act.* Washington, DC: Author.

U.S. Department of Education. (2000). *Twenty-second annual report to congress on the implementation of the Individuals with Disabilities Education Act.* Washington, DC: Author.

U.S. Department of Education. (2001). *Twenty-third annual report to congress on the implementation of the Individuals with Disabilities Education Act.* Washington, DC: U.S. Department of Education.

Utah Department of Health (1999). *Utah State Plan: The Individuals with Disabilities Act Part C: Early Intervention for Infants and Toddlers with Disabilities.* Retrieved August 6, 2003 from *www.utahbabywatch.org/agencyinfo/eligibility.*

Van Riper, M. (2000). Family variables associated with well-being in siblings of children with Down syndrome. *Journal of Family Nursing, 6,* 267–286.

Walsh, S., Rous, B., & Lutzer, C. (2000). The federal IDEA Natural Environments Provisions: Making it work. *Young Exceptional Children, Monograph Series No. 2,* 3–15.

Warfield, M. E., Hauser-Cram, P., Krauss, M. W., Shonkoff, J. P., & Upshur, C. C. (2000). The effect of early intervention services on maternal well-being. *Early Education and Development, 11,* 499–517.

Weinger, S. (1999). Views of the child with retardation: Relationship to family functioning. *Family Therapy, 26(2),* 63–79.

White, K. R., Boyce, G. C., Casto, G., Innocenti, M. S., Taylor, M. J., Goetze, L., & Behl, D. (1994). Comparative evaluations of early intervention alternatives: A response to commentaries by Guralnick and Telzrow. *Early Education and Development, 5,* 56–68.

Wikler, L., Wasow, M., & Hatfield, E. (1981). Chronic stresses of families of mentally retarded children. *Family Relations, 30,* 281–288.

# Chapter 15

# Learning Disabilities and Attention Deficits

David Scanlon

## Introduction

Learning disabilities and attention deficits are not the same thing, although they are sometimes confused. They share many familiar traits, and may in fact share some familial traits. Both only came to be commonly recognized in the 20th century but have rapidly risen to be among the highest incidence disabilities, although many cultures and nations do not recognize either one. The legitimacy of both internal and external determinants of these conditions has been continually questioned by both professional communities and the public.

Both conditions are cognitive disorders considered to be incurable. Although not developmental in nature, neither is commonly detected in early childhood and each may manifest differently across childhood, adolescent, and adult life stages. They are not routinely screened for as are vision, hearing, and a variety of other health impairments.

Despite acknowledgement as lifelong conditions, neither is well understood or treated beyond the developmental stage of adolescence, nor are they as clearly protected by disabilities rights laws

and policies as are some other disabling conditions. Both are primarily recognized due to their impact on academic learning. Thus, although they have impact across all aspects of daily living, they are best understood as school-based or educational disabilities.

The two disorders are quite distinct in some regards, particularly in their detection, bearing almost no resemblance beyond a surface-level appearance that can result in confusing their identification. Although they sometimes occur concomitantly, they otherwise have nothing to do with one another. Still, schools often treat students with the two conditions similarly when providing special services and interventions. Although both are most commonly identified in early school-age years, attention deficit is far more likely than a learning disability to be manifested and observed in younger children. Only attention deficit is responded to with medication; however, both are commonly treated with cognitive academic interventions.

This chapter provides descriptions of the two conditions, providing links for each among their origins, manifestations, identification, and treatment.

# Learning Disabilities

From at least the late 1800s through the first 60 years of the 20th century, physicians, psychologists, neurologists, and educators attempted to label a unique group of individuals we today consider to have a learning disability (LD). The common thread of these varied efforts was to understand what distinguished individuals who seemed to process information "incorrectly," or different from the norm, but whose condition was not yet familiar to the sciences. Some of those attempts isolated types of mental retardation, reflected perceptual disorders, or led to other classifications such as minimal brain dysfunction (Hallahan & Mercer, 2001).

## Background

In the early 1960s, Samuel Kirk proposed the condition we commonly recognize today as learning disabled. Kirk was a well-known American psychologist working in the area of mental retardation. Delivering the keynote address in New York City to the Conference on Exploration into Problems of the Perceptually Handicapped Child, he spoke of a group of children he had come to recognize in his work who did not fit the categories of mental retardation or brain injury and whose differences in learning and performance could not be otherwise explained by sensory or other known impairments. Kirk proposed that he had observed a class of children who "have disorders in development in language, speech, reading, and associated communication skills" (Kirk, 1963). Response of the parents[1], educators, and advocates attending the conference was swift. The organization voted that same day to form the

Association for Children with Learning Disabilities (now the Learning Disabilities Association of America) and to promote study and recognition of this newly named condition.

The condition *learning disabled* began to be considered, and the term was also almost immediately pressed into use. Parents asked schools to provide services to this group of students, services distinct from those provided to students with mental retardation (MR). The rationale was that the learning needs and potential of the two groups differed. As might be expected, the new condition was also questioned, including some questions regarding the social implications of recognizing LD. Advocates of the "new" disability were criticized as being motivated to distinguish Caucasian and middle-class children from racial minority and low-income children labeled with MR, particularly Black children (see National Research Council, 2002).

The children initially labeled as having a learning disability were primarily transferred over from the ranks of those identified with MR (MacMillan, Gresham, & Bocian, 1998; MacMillan & Sipperstein, 2001; National Research Council, 2002; Tucker, 1980). Then, as is still true today, Black and low-income children were disproportionately represented as having MR (National Research Council, 2002). Compared to the percentage of the total school populations, they had considerably greater representation in the MR category than White children (see Table 15.1). By 2000 only minor positive corrections have been seen. Both in the 1970s and today, children from most racial and ethnic minority groups and from low-income environments are thought to be disproportionately highly represented across disability categories (National Research Council, 2002).

An equally fundamental questioning of the new LD category has concerned the scientific basis for the condition. Critics argued that the so-called condition is based on observations of learning behaviors and not of any organic

---

1. Wherever the term *parent* is used, it represents the person or persons with primary responsibility for raising the child and who may have legal responsibility for the child. It includes legal guardians, extended family members, siblings, case workers, and so on.

*Table 15.1*   Percentage Representation in MR and LD Categories by Race

| | Population | Percent of Population 1978[a,b] | 2000[c] |
|---|---|---|---|
| Black or African American | Total School | 16 | 17 |
| | MR[d] | 38 | 33.4 |
| | LD | 15 | 18.3 |
| Caucasian | Total School | 75 | 61.5 |
| | MR | 56 | 53 |
| | LD | 75 | 61.8 |

[a] *First full year of nation-wide special education.*
[b] *U.S. Department of Education Office of Civil Rights (1979).*
[c] *U.S. Department of Education Office of Civil Rights (2001).*
[d] *1978 percentages are for "educable mentally retarded" (EMR). The MR labels "educable" and "trainable" were collapsed for the census count by 2000.*

phenomenon (Aaron, 1997). That criticism continues to today, with critics noting that the definition of LD is one of exclusion; that is, when all other measurable explanations for below-expected learning performance are excluded, LD is what is left (Kavale & Forness, 2000). That charge negates the current practice of indirectly measuring the condition using psychometric measures, but nonetheless it has stuck. Kirk and others have defended the category of LD as possibly misapplied and in need of continued study, but certainly as something more than a mere social construction. Despite the debates, an estimated 4.5% of Americans (approximately 50% of school students enrolled in special education) have an LD (U.S. Department of Education, 2001). The debate over the nature of LD can be seen in how it is defined.

## The Definition of *Learning Disability*

In 1975 the Federal government passed into law Public Law 94-142, the *Education for All Handicapped Children Act*. This was the first national special education law, and among the categories of disabilities it recognized was learning disabilities. Passage of the law (since reauthorized as the *Individuals with Disabilities Education Act*) required a commonly agreed upon definition of the condition and replicable criteria for identifica-

tion. Having undergone minor revisions since 1975, the definition currently used for the IDEA states:

*specific learning disability" means a disorder in one or more of the basic psychological processes involved in understanding or in using language, spoken or written, that may manifest itself in an imperfect ability to listen, think, speak, read, write, spell, or to do mathematical calculations. The term includes such conditions as perceptual disabilities, brain injury, minimal brain dysfunction, dyslexia, and developmental aphasia. The term does not apply to children who have learning problems that are primarily the result of visual, of hearing, of motor disabilities, of mental retardation, of emotional disturbance, or of environmental, cultural, or economic disadvantages (U.S. Department of Education, 1992).*

The National Joint Committee on Learning Disabilities (NJCLD) (a coalition of major LD advocacy and service organizations) proposed an alternative definition in 1981 and updated that in 1988. They state:

*learning disabilities is a general term that refers to a heterogeneous group of disorders manifested by significant difficulties in the acquisition and use of listening, speaking, reading, writing, reasoning, or*

| *Figure 15.1* | Major Definitional Descriptors of the Condition LD | |
| --- | --- | --- |
| | Federal Definition[1] | NJCLD[2] |
| Condition: | Specific learning disability | Learning disabilities |
| Nature of disorder | Disorder in one or more basic psychological processes | Central nervous system dysfunction |
| Inclusive Criteria | Understanding in using spoken or written language; imperfect ability to listen, think, speak, read, write, spell, or to do mathematical calculations; includes perceptual handicaps, brain injury, minimal brain dysfunction, dyslexia, and developmental aphasia | Significant difficulties in the acquisition and use of listening, speaking, reading, writing, reasoning, or mathematical abilities |
| Exclusive Criteria | Not a result of: visual, hearing, or motor handicaps; mental retardation; emotional disturbance; or environmental, cultural, or economic disadvantage | Not a direct result of other handicapping conditions |
| Population | Children | May occur across the lifespan |

[1] *U.S. Department of Education, 1992.*

*mathematical abilities. These disorders are intrinsic to the individual, presumed to be due to central nervous system dysfunction, and may occur across the life span. Problems in self-regulatory behaviors, social perception and social interaction may exist with learning disabilities but do not by themselves constitute a learning disability.*

*Although learning disabilities may occur concomitantly with other handicapping conditions (for example, sensory impairment, mental retardation, serious emotional disturbance) or with extrinsic influences (such as cultural differences, insufficient or inappropriate instruction), they are not the result of those conditions or influences. (NJCLD, 1989, p. 1)*

Their definition clarified three components of the Federal IDEA definition (see Figure 15.1). The term *basic psychological processes* was deleted because these have yet to be specified. They suggested that the disorder is linked simply to "central nervous system dysfunction" instead of to named conditions that are themselves controver-

sially defined. They also noted that the condition may possibly occur across the life span, which is in contrast to the Federal definition use of the word "children." The NJCLD's definition is widely considered the more accurate definition among professionals (Hammil, 1990). Persistent criticisms of the two definitions include that they are overly focused on operationalizing identification criteria and that they are still academic based and child centered.

## DESCRIPTION OF THE CONDITION

As can be discerned from the major definitions, an LD is presumed to be a cognitive processing disorder. Theoretically isolated to the central nervous system, the condition has been looked for in the structure and functioning of the brain. Early LD-brain research using EEG[2] technology

2. Electroencephalogram (EEG) testing is used to identify regions of cortical activity and relative cognitive effort in the form of brain wave activity.

provided convincing evidence that individuals with LD did not process information as efficiently as their nondisabled peers. They process more slowly but also appear to use different regions of the brain than the general population for affected tasks. Far more conclusive evidence from brain-scanning research employing methods such as CT, MRI, and fMRI technology has served to suggest that there are neuroanatomical distinctions for LD (Rumsey, 1996; Shaywitz et al., 1996). This neurological processing research indicated that children with LD do not use their brains in effective ways (or they at least use them in nonnormative ways) to process information. Findings on the neurology of LD continue to be questioned due to limitations in sample sizes and representativeness, and limited replications of findings (Fletcher et al., 2001), but the overall body of neurobiological research is compelling.

Related research on the heritability of LD lends further support for claiming an intrinsic nature for the disorder. One-third to one-half of children with LD are found to have a parent who also has LD (Shaywitz, 2003). In studies of children born to a parent with LD, between one-quarter and one-half will also have LD (Pennington, 1995; Shaywitz, 2003). In the case of siblings, for those with LD there is a nearly 50% likelihood of having a sibling with LD (Shaywitz, 2003). This last finding has been claimed by some to suggest that the condition may be more the product of environment than heritability. Environment may play at least a significant role in the identification of LD. Identical twins have only a 65% to 75% chance of both having LD (instead of the expected 100% if the condition were purely genetic in cause) (DeFries & Alarcon, 1996; Shaywitz, 2003). Despite the correlational evidence for inheritance as one route to acquiring an LD, no genetic link or inherited pattern of unique brain structure or functioning has been satisfactorily determined. Criticisms of nature over nurture explanations for LD are strong. Similar to criticisms of the limited brain-imaging research database, heritability studies of LD are not adequate in number or sample size and diversity in comparison to the general population with LD.

Related task performance research has demonstrated that a common characteristic of those with LD is to skip over or misuse important information when processing tasks such as aural or reading comprehension, mathematical calculations, general problem solving, or when communicating (e.g., Wansart, 1990). Affected individuals also tend not to monitor and think about their own cognitive processes. Drawing from the body of performance research, Torgesen (2000) proposed that students with LD are characteristically "inactive" or "inefficient" learners who passively participate in learning (i.e., cognitive processing). The body of brain-imaging research on cognitive processing in children with LD has been consistent with Torgesen's now classic characterization.

Despite scientific evidence of the condition of LD, Poplin (1998) has argued that incidences of learning disabilities are equally well or better explained by social factors than by genetics. Dudley-Marling and Dippo (1995) and McDermott (1993) have observed the differential treatment of children that led to or sustained LD classification. They found that teachers asked these students less-engaging questions and held lowered expectations for them. Further support for a more social explanation for LD includes the disproportionate representation of Hispanic, Black and African American, and Native American students among the 8.3% of the resident population served in special education in 2000. Of those students aged 6 to 21 years, 50.5% were served for a learning disability: 16.6% were Hispanic (16.2% of the overall resident population), 18.4% were Black or African American (14.5%), and 1.4% were Native American students (1.0%) (U.S. Department of Education, 2001). By contrast, only 62.1% of Caucasian children (64.5% of the resident population), and 1.6% Asian Americans/Pacific Islanders (3.8%) were identified as having an LD.

Thus, despite efforts to isolate a neurobiological condition of LD, there is not yet evidence for any theory of ontology that has widespread acceptance. Social-based explanations for the existence of the condition are equally questionable, however. The problem in isolating the condition may be due to the profession's seeking to define an observed set of behaviors in terms of their causes. The search for the cause of LD has logically been based in competing theories of what it may be; however, the best the profession can agree on is that the condition has been observed (Scanlon, 2000).

## Learning Disabilities Across the Life Span

According to the preeminent definitions of LD (IDEA, 1997; NJCLD, 1989), it is a condition associated with learning. Although learning may begin as early as the fetal stages of human development, it is almost exclusively academic learning that is considered for recognition of an LD. Thus, despite being considered a lifelong condition, LD is rarely detected prior to a child having a history of academic difficulties. The condition is seldom identified until after the kindergarten year. Our knowledge of how it may begin to manifest itself earlier and of how we might identify it then is limited. In fact, much of what is known about the condition and its impact on individuals is known in relation to school-age populations, particularly elementary grade students. However, attention is increasingly being paid to how LD is manifested in and impacts adulthood. This is due in part to the first generations of diagnosed school children having matured into adult years, as well as to disability rights legislation that has raised the professions' and the public's conscience, especially the Americans with Disabilities Act. Thus, we are beginning to understand this relatively new category of disability across the life span.

### IMPACT ON LIFE

Despite the definitional focus on academics, an LD can profoundly impact the daily social and emotional realms of an individual's life as well. Difficulties in calculation and estimation influence not only mathematics learning but also grocery shopping and enjoying a game of cards with friends; difficulties with organization and interpretive skills can influence how well one performs in social settings and business meetings; difficulties in reading and writing can lead to avoiding situations that require filling out forms, like visits to emergency rooms or job interviews; a former student of the author's left an emergency room when he could not complete forms he was given (Scanlon, 2000).

Reading, memory, and organization problems can also result in improper use of medication. Studies of urban adolescents with LD show that even when they have knowledge equal with their nondisabled peers about prevention of transmission of the HIV virus, they are less likely to make decisions and take actions to reduce the chances of transmission (Bell, Feraios, & Bryan, 1991). Young adults with LD report having fewer friends than do their nondisabled peers (Donahue, Pearl, & Bryan, 1980; Mehring & Colson, 1990), a factor reciprocal with mental health problems.

In recent decades, adolescents with LD dropped out of school at average annual rates estimated to be between 17% and 42% (Lichtenstein & Zantol-Wiener, 1988; National Center for Education Statistics, 2000), when the rate for the total school population dropped from approximately 16% and then stably ranged between 12% and 14% for the 1990s (National Center for Education Statistics, 2000). As adults, those with LD are more likely to hold a series of entry-level positions than to hold a job and advance (Scanlon, 2000), which certainly has both self-affect and economic consequences. Adolescents with LD have been found no more likely than other adolescents and young adults to get in trouble with the law, but, as results of miscommunications and poor decision making, are less likely to conduct themselves in ways that get them out of such situations with only warnings or minimal sanctions

(Pearl & Bryan, 1994). Finally, estimates of the incidence of LD in the adult prison population in America range from 28% to 42% (Morgan, 1979; Rutherford, Nelson, & Wolford, 1985), estimates of the incidence among minors under supervision of correctional agencies soar even higher (Forbes, 1991).

Despite the social and emotional ramifications of the skill deficits associated with learning disabilities, the condition does not only result in negative consequences. Some individuals have minor cases of LD that cause them no significant difficulties. Others with more profound learning disabilities learn to effectively compensate. They do well in school, and the impacts on socialization and daily living skills are insignificant to their general quality of life. Indeed, well-known successful individuals with self-disclosed learning disabilities include Charles Schwab, Cher, Tom Cruise, David Rockefeller, P. Buckley Moss, and Greg Louganis; Albert Einstein and Thomas Edison are also widely presumed to have had learning disabilities in addition to their genius. Some have even reported benefiting from the challenges presented by their LD (e.g., Seftel, 2000; Lee & Jackson, 1992). In short, many individuals with LD lead successful lives in both material and emotional ways (Gerber, 1998; Raskind, Goldberg, Higgins, & Herman, 1999).

## A COGNITIVE DISORDER

Someone who has an LD has difficulties in receiving, processing, and/or expressing information. (As Kirk [1963] stated when he first proposed the condition, these are difficulties that are not due to retardation or sensory impairments such as vision or hearing difficulties; also, by definition, these are not difficulties due to language or cultural differences, nor to lack of opportunity to develop such skills.) Difficulties in receiving information include problems of attending and understanding; a child may hear or read a series of directions but be unable to discern their sequence, for example. Difficulties with processing include problems being able to think with or about information, such as relating it to other knowledge, judging its veracity, or recognizing all of its important qualities. Expressive difficulties of persons with LD include weaknesses in being able to explain what they know, instead using physical, verbal (including word choice and intonation), and facial gestures to communicate and presenting information in coherent organization.

Isolating observed skill deficits exclusively to the receptive, processing, or expressive domain is often difficult without cognitive testing designed to measure discrete skills and in practical terms may not be necessary to understanding the condition or developing an intervention. For example, whether a child's difficulty reading a word on a page is due to recognizing the text characters (letters) presented or to relating letter combinations to the sounds they form, a practical intervention must address the combination of these and other isolatable skills (Fowler & Scarborough, 1993). Most practical skills involve a combination of the three domains, for example, reading a list aloud or doing a subtraction problem.

## DEVELOPMENT, MANIFESTATIONS, AND IDENTIFICATION

The incidence of identified LD in early childhood is rare, and it is not even considered in infancy or prenatally. However, early warning signs of the condition are occasionally seen in some preschool-age children. Typically, these involve delays in recognizing and using oral language. These indicators may trigger an early identification but more likely are recalled in parent and physician interviews when a student is being evaluated later in childhood. Interestingly, the condition does not always manifest itself in a certain developmental phase. Adolescents, young adults, and adults are all susceptible to the condition first appearing in those stages of life.

Unlike routine screenings such as those for hearing and vision, the identification criteria for LD are only investigated when a parent, educator, or physician requests an evaluation, or possibly an individual herself/himself. Since first proposed by Kirk (1963), the condition is primarily identified only when academic learning suffers. Under current IDEA guidelines for special education eligibility, the request for evaluation must accompany a demonstrated deficiency in learning, either overall or in specific academic domains.

Although the condition is presumed to be a neurological disorder, neurological examination beyond psychometrically measuring task performance is unrealistic at this time. Availability of resources is the second of two reasons neurological structure and processing exams are impractical. Equipment such as CT scanners and fMRI imagers and the technology used to record and process their findings are expensive, require considerable space, and involve the work of skilled professionals. Even more fundamental to the impracticality of neurological evaluations is the paucity of information to substantially support any evaluative approach or the interpretation of its findings to document a case of LD with acceptable levels of validity and reliability. The evaluation of LD nonetheless is focused on cognitive processing, however in the form of performance on various cognitive skill tasks that are measured psychometrically.

**Accepted Identification Criteria.** Learning disabilities identification requires that the individual be of average intelligence and not have any other disability that primarily explains the observed difficulties. The "psychological processing disorder" cited in the Federal definition is determined in the identification process by documenting a cognitive discrepancy between potential, or intelligence, and achievement. This may be either an inter- or intracognitive discrepancy. For an intercognitive discrepancy, a "significant" discrepancy between cognitive potential, or intelligence, and achievement is determined. Intelligence is overwhelmingly based on an IQ score. Achievement is typically measured by standardized achievement tests in academic domains such as

reading, writing, or mathematical performance. Intelligence tests are administered by licensed psychologists; school-trained personnel deliver achievement tests.

A "significant discrepancy" is commonly based on an "arbitrary" (Kavale & Forness, 2000, p. 248) deviation between scores. Although the acceptable variance differs by state, this is the discrepancy criteria most commonly applied for identification of a learning disability. Observations and work samples supplied by teachers, parents, or the individual are also commonly reviewed as supplementary information in making an identification determination. Because of long-standing concerns with the accuracy of the intercognitive discrepancy formula to determine the presence of an LD (Aaron, 1997; Kavale & Forness, 2000), some states or school districts instead rely on significant discrepancies between (or even within) achievement domains (e.g., reading, writing, reasoning, mathematical calculations), called the *intracognitive discrepancy.*

That the individual must present academic difficulties in order to be identified is almost hidden in the formulae for identification of a learning disability. Lags in learning or general cognitive prowess signal the possible need for evaluation. Allowing for reasonable opportunities for the individual to develop and for the time to accrue a record of achievement below potential slow the beginning of the identification process (Fuchs, Fuchs, & Speece, 2002). Thus, the percentage of students being screened and identified makes a steady but gradual climb until approximately grade four, when the percentage of students identified with LD increases significantly. The common explanation for this population shift is that fourth grade is the American school grade in which the curriculum shifts from 'learning skills to learn' to 'using skills to learn'. Because LD identification tends to be related to provision of educational services, the identification criteria and process are closely tied to academics, with some variation for young adult and older populations.

**Early Childhood.** In all but rare cases, the identification of an LD in a child younger than age 5 should be met with suspicion. The academic school-based nature of the identification process limits our ability to be certain whether the condition is present but undetected in the preschool years. Observable delays in learning and skill performance at this stage are more likely representative of another disabling condition if they are outside of the expected range. Unscrupulous individuals may, nonetheless, secure identification for leverage against a medical professional or a service provider who is claimed to have injured the child, or the diagnosis may be provided to mollify overly anxious parents. With that caution in mind, relevant indicators of potential to develop LD include toxin exposure prior to birth, low birth weight, and hypoxia or anoxia during birth. The children most likely to be evaluated for an LD in early childhood are those who are referred for an evaluation through a preschool or social services provider. Physician-recommended evaluations account for a very small portion of cases at this age.

**Childhood.** In the kindergarten and lower elementary school years children typically make rapid developments in learning, which varies in rate and what is learned. Further, this variation occurs both within and between individual children. For example, some children come to elementary school knowing how to read, others pick up the skills quite quickly, and still others develop the same skills but at a slower pace, or rapidly but only after taking longer in the school year before they begin to "get it." All of these children may, nonetheless, finish the school year with approximately equal proficiency in reading. Any one of these children may develop mathematical or abstract reasoning skills at a pace similar to their reading development or at quite different paces but again end the school year at normatively expected levels of proficiency. Developmentally, these are all reasonable scenarios for within- and between-child learning development and do not

necessarily signal cause for concern. However, it is such general delays or uneven development patterns that signal the presence of an LD. These are the observed learning behaviors that were the original impetus for naming the condition. The distinction between normal development and disabled development is in the degree of the differences.

Children with LD have persistent difficulties in developing affected skills. Evidence of their difficulties with the learning process include difficulty grasping concepts, persistent use of inappropriate cognitive strategies despite their failure, needing to relearn previously mastered skills and cognitive strategies, and not being sure how to approach a task. They are demonstrating the trait of being inefficient learners, or some have more recently characterized them as "nonresponders" or "treatment resisters" (Fuchs, Fuchs, & Speece, 2002; Gresham, 2001; Torgesen, 2000) to describe their not benefiting from instruction (although, this author warns that such terms could be inferred to mean students with LD just need to try harder).

As has been noted, LDs are most commonly associated with reading and writing difficulties. In fact, 80% of learning disabilities are primarily in the area of reading; most often they affect the foundational skills of reading such as phonemic awareness and developing a repertoire of print words immediately recognized by sight. They can, however, impact higher-order skills such as reading comprehension and drawing inferences. They are second-most-commonly related to difficulties in mathematical and spatial skills and in reasoning. Here, they may be in the form of difficulty with fundamental skills such as appreciating the concept of number or being able to compare proportions, but might involve complex calculation and estimation skills or abstract reasoning necessary for calculus, physics, or geometry. Of course, although there is a conceptual focus on academic areas, these difficulties may be observed in home and community contexts as well.

Over time, the skills deficiencies of persons with LD cause them to fall behind in learning further and more complex skills, resulting in a "skills gap" (Baker, Gersten, & Scanlon, 2002; Bulgren & Scanlon, 1997/1998). That is, a child who does not develop proficiency in the basic skills of reading, for example, will be hampered in being exposed to and being able to fruitfully practice higher-order reading skills such as detecting main ideas and inferring meaning. Also, because reading is a primary form of gaining information in our schools and society (Snow, Burns, & Griffin, 1998), children who are poor readers miss out on information in a variety of other domains.

Children with LD may signal their disability in ways in addition to an evolving skills gap. Depending on the severity of the disability and their individual disposition, they may demonstrate a frustration with schooling or certain learning tasks. This sometimes includes acting out behaviors or school avoidance. Consistent with the nature of an LD, they may not know more proactive responses. Failing at a task, not being sure how to proceed, or anticipating rejection are all reasons to become frustrated, especially when they become a familiar routine and one does not know how to alter it. Many children with LD are distinguished as socially awkward and have even been rejected by their peers before any pattern of academic difficulty becomes apparent (Donahue et al., 1980). As is true of many individuals, children with LD may prefer to avoid frustrating tasks and instead concentrate on their skills in other areas. On the one hand, these overt warning signs should be taken seriously as potential indicators of an LD, even though the more formalized identification testing focused on academics and cognitive processing is required for a diagnosis. And on the other hand, children may exhibit some of these difficulties and reactions for reasons not related to an LD. They may also be indicators of a variety of other conditions such as another disability, giftedness, cultural differences, or maybe "normal" development.

The identification criteria for LD are ideally suited for children who have begun elementary education. Under IDEA regulations, when a teacher or other individual first considers the possible presence of an LD, prereferral interventions must be tried. These interventions require the teacher to make minor reasonable adjustments in instruction that may correct the learning problem. For example, the teacher may move the child's seat in the classroom to alleviate distractions or may provide instructions for assignments in alternative formats to aid clarity. If prereferral interventions resolve the problem, it was likely not a learning disability. If difficulties persist, however, a learning disability may be at play and evaluation should proceed.

The IDEA includes provisions for evaluations to be performed in a timely manner and without expense to parents. They are routinely administered by school district personnel. Some parents may seek evaluations outside of their school district. In these cases, the evaluation may be conducted by a licensed psychologist. Parents need to be aware, however, that in addition to establishing the presence of an LD, the student must be determined to need special education services before they can be provided under the IDEA. Thus, if the concern is with an appropriate public education, schools will eventually have to be provided with evaluation results and then participate in a placement decision. In this process, medical professionals may be requested to provide information on the birth and development of the child and to participate in determining whether other disabling conditions are present. Otherwise, they tend to not be involved in the identification process.

**Adolescence.** Adolescent development most notably includes the onset of puberty, which is associated with rapid growth and adjustments in neurological and body functioning and with social maturation. Many adolescents go through personality changes that are a consequence of both their biological and social development. These changes can impact an existing LD, including provoking an LD to manifest itself for the first time.

Children who mature into adolescence with an already-manifested LD more often than not continue to experience the LD in their adolescent years. As has been noted, they commonly develop an evolving skills gap between their proficient skills and what is expected of them in school, home, and social settings. In all of these settings, adolescents are expected to have mastered certain fundamental skills and are encouraged to take more responsibility for being independent and completing more complex tasks; for example, they are expected to make complex decisions about budgets and product options when shopping, they should be able to plan and then follow the plan for going to several places and completing a variety of functions (e.g., following class schedules, running errands), they are expected to initiate and maintain social relationships on a variety of levels, and they are expected to recognize their own needs and abilities and to self-advocate. A compounding skills gap can induce frustration and reliance on avoidance strategies at heightened levels from those the adolescents may have employed as children.

Teens are also driven to conform to some social group or groups' standards. Having an LD can contribute to expanding the ways in which a teen is socially different. As school children with LD they may have been segregated by routine placement in the low-level groups, being required to periodically demonstrate their skill deficiencies (e.g., being asked to read aloud in class or write on the board), or by being removed from the general education classroom for a portion of the school day. At home they may have been given less independence than siblings at play time and more menial chores. Even teens with LD who are generally well accepted socially find they are less valued in particular contexts such as study groups, work teams, or athletic or social situations, due to their skills gaps or lack of organization (Beaumont, 1999; Jenkins & O'Connor, 2003). As part of the adolescent experience, many teens experience minor social difficulties. This normal awkwardness may attenuate other awkwardness resulting from an LD. For example, teens with LD may have difficulty discerning the social expectations on them or not be aware of when they are and are not replicating acceptable behaviors; likewise, they may make poor decisions about social alliances they would like to form. Thus, those who as children managed their disability well can grow into adolescents who become frustrated and begin to avoid challenging tasks.

For some adolescents with LD, the academic, social, and personal adjustment skills they now are compelled to perform reveal an LD that was previously masked. The additional memory required, the need to predict and compare alternative outcomes, and the organization required to plan a coordinated plan of action may for the first time demonstrate that the adolescent has an LD that renders her or him inefficient at one or more of these functions. For those discovering these experiences for the first time, understanding that they could have an LD and coming to accept such a condition are both novel experiences (e.g., Seftel, 2000; Lee & Jackson, 1992).

The criteria for LD identification do not change between childhood and adolescence. The practicality of the established identification practices does become more questionable, however. Adolescents with LD are virtually bound to be behind academically. Stanovich (1986) coined the term *Matthew effect* to describe the cumulative consequences of an LD. Borrowing from the Bible passage Matthew 13:12, he described how students with LD fall further and further behind in both their cognitive processing skills and their accumulated knowledge as a consequence of their limited skills of learning. Thus, a student with deficits in reading, for example, may fall further behind in math because some of what she or he needed to learn for more advanced math skills relied on proficient skills in reading. Due to the skills gap and Matthew effect, it becomes difficult to distinguish whether they are behind in specific achievement areas due to the LD or as a secondary consequence of LD in other areas (e.g., reading). Theoretically, the Matthew effect would similarly impact general intelligence, thus falsely influencing IQ performance (Aaron, 1997). Thus, psychologists and others involved in diagnosing LD in adolescents must be particularly vigilant in applying the criteria.

Some adolescents with LD become increasingly frustrated as a consequence of the daily difficulties posed by their LD. They may be reticent to show off the knowledge and skills they do have, for fear of being embarrassed, or they may barely communicate at all. These adolescents could be mistaken for having a mild emotional disturbance or some other more profound cognitive disorder. Many who are frustrated by their LD resort to acting-out behaviors to both mask their limitations and as an unsophisticated form of expressing their frustration. They may become labeled as socially maladjusted. Adolescents with this label may be expelled from schools because they are, in essence, choosing to behave that way.

**Young Adult Years and Adulthood.** Although chronologically the young adult years begin at approximately age 18 and last to about age 23, there are no standardized indicators for the beginning or ending of this social developmental phase. This is, nonetheless, a crucial phase in the life span development of a person with LD. In typical American culture, most students finish their secondary education by age 18 and embark on the world of work, military service, or postsecondary education—all of which are options for young adults with LD. They also begin to enjoy certain rights of emancipation, legally as well as in familial and social arenas. This is to say, they become dramatically more independent at a time when radically new options become available to them. For most teens, becoming young adults is the most dramatic life change they have experienced since they first entered school (Dacey, Kenny, & Margolis, 2000). For young adults with

LD, this is a crucial stage for establishing a healthy adult life, as career paths are selected, new living arrangements are initiated, primary responsibility for their affairs begins, and adult personalities emerge. Indeed, the young adult phase is considered to end when the stability of the adult phase begins.

The same scenario of intensified and or novel skill demands that accompanied the transition from childhood to adolescence is again at hand. Therefore, the potential for an existing LD to magnify in intensity or to appear for the first time is also again present. With the onset of the young adult years, however, the unfamiliarity of new expectations, the change in nature and availability of supports, and the potential direct lifelong consequences seem even more dramatic than they did in the transition from childhood to adolescence. The nature of schooling shifts from the elementary to junior or middle school years, and again to the high school years; but the nature of learning expected on the job, in the military, or in most postsecondary education settings is dramatically different from high school, as are performance standards. Failure results in dismissal, not remediation. Thus, the expectation for independent performance may be the trigger for an LD to manifest itself. Also, expectations to apply academic, social, and cognitive skills to a variety of novel tasks may tax the individual's ability to transfer what was learned and supported at home or in school. Self-reliance tends to be valued over being provided support.

One's specific academic skill deficits are most likely to have appeared before this stage of development. However, it is possible that advanced tasks or skill application scenarios may be introduced in the young adult years that would tap new skill areas to reveal an LD for the first time. Still, if there is a change in cognitive profile, it is more likely to be due to the ramifications of the already known deficits. For example, a child-cum-adolescent who had persistent difficulties with spatial reasoning may have been in lower-track mathematics classes designed to systematically address that throughout school, and may have been able to avoid affected tasks such as drawing three-dimensional representations or driving in congested areas of a city. The cognitive deficits the adolescent carries to the young adult years will likely pose new challenges as they are called on for new tasks. In response, the young adult with an LD who previously coped with her or his limitations may now become cognitively overwhelmed and unable to coordinate once-effective coping mechanisms.

The young adults most likely to experience pronounced difficulties due to an LD are the ones who never learned to self-regulate their skill performance and to compensate for their deficit skills. Self-regulation involves being able to identify what a task demands (e.g., read for information, interpret social cues from a friend, problem-solve in response to receiving unclear directions from an employer), to identify a method to complete the task that 1) will work and 2) the individual is capable of performing, and to monitor and adjust performance of the method as need be (Lenz, Ellis, & Scanlon, 1996). Young adults who fail to do these things are exhibiting *inefficient learner* behaviors. In addition to self-regulating task performance, students must have a repertoire of appropriate skills to perform, of course. By the time they are adolescents, if they still lag significantly behind in fundamental skills, it is appropriate to teach them alternative or *compensatory* strategies for completing a task. For example, adolescents who have difficulty remembering and comprehending what they read may learn a combination of activities such as taking notes while reading, asking the self-questions during reading, paraphrasing, previewing the text, and establishing questions or key learning goals before reading. This does not preclude continuing to work on fundamental skills, but it will allow the young adult to progress in practical tasks in the meanwhile. Without progression at this stage of life, which may also be

thought of as *laying foundations,* the young adult is not going to have positive stability in social, emotional, and material ways of life.

Development in all aspects of living do not culminate when the young adult enters the adult years, although (thankfully) for many a degree of stability is reached. Assuming the adult phase of life has been entered with the foundations for stability, an LD can still challenge the person at any point across the adult years, as it did in earlier life phases, or it may appear for the first time. Typically, the LD poses a problem when either the adult has yet to develop effective compensatory strategies or when new contexts become present. For example, forming relationships, changing jobs, moving, or developing changes in health can all require new and different skills performance. Emotionally, the adult may be worn down by the years of frustration that may accumulate from having an LD (see Lee & Jackson, 1992).

The factors that complicate LD identification for adolescents also extend into young adult and adult life stages. The construct of achievement used in the aptitude–achievement discrepancy becomes even more suspect. Due to factors such as the Matthew effect, achievement is more a measure of the impact of the legacy of an LD than an accurate indicator of the skills and knowledge of an adult. Indeed, because achievement is assessed in relation to skills and concepts valued in schools, those who have left school are easily disadvantaged on such tests because they have moved on from that context. Many quickly forget some of the geometric formulae others once knew by rote; the same is true for recalling key historical events or being practiced at the rules of grammar and composition. Thus, in addition to being artificially large, the discrepancy simply may not be relevant to the contexts of adult life.

A critical question in the identification process for adults should be, "why conduct this assessment?" The process is not terribly time-consuming but can be quite expensive (some health insurance policies provide for assessment). As has been noted, some find relief and impetus for correction when they have the condition finally identified. It is also true that an official diagnosis can make an individual eligible for certain legal rights and protections afforded to persons with disabilities. The information may also be of use to the adult who would like to develop compensatory social, school, or work skills, or engage in remedial learning. Such potential benefits of identification should be weighed against the "let sleeping dogs lie" principle of leaving the condition undiagnosed if the individual has no strong interest in pursuing it or if she or he is not yet prepared for the outcomes of the process.

## PROBABLE HEALTH CARE–RELATED NEEDS *AND* IMPLICATIONS FOR COMMUNICATION

Being a cognitive disability, LD does not directly impose any health-related needs on the individual. It is not an impairment of brain functions related to health and is not typically associated with any health impairment or other condition impinging on health. Thus, an LD is more likely to concern health care when 1) a health care provider is consulted about the condition or 2) the impaired cognition associated with the condition affects comprehension or other aspects of communication having to do with other matters of health, health care, or personal safety.

Those who are concerned about cognitive performance may consult a physician or other health care service provider. This is especially likely for questions about individuals who are not of school age, those who have an adversarial relationship with a school, or those who coincidentally have other conditions that involve the health care provider. Thus, health care professionals need to be aware of symptoms of a learning disability so that they do not contribute to a misdiagnosis. For example, a preschooler who appears to be slow to achieve certain cognitive milestones may have an LD, may have a sensory impairment, may be slow

to thrive for reasons of some other disability, may lack adequate stimulation, or simply may not be meaningfully behind in development. An adolescent who loses interest in academics between one school year and the next and who becomes generally unsociable may just be developing the way many teens do, may be involved in substance abuse, or may be beginning to experience an LD for the first time. Young adults and adults may similarly complain about newfound problems of memory or concentration or may find that postsecondary education or the world of work poses challenges to their organizational, problem-solving, or specific academic skills. In all of these examples, an LD may be at play, and any of a variety of other factors may also be involved. Physicians confronted with concerns over such lowered motivations, increased frustration, or inabilities that might be initially attributed to coordination or concentration need to ask questions about cognitive–academic skills histories and other factors that may provide an opportunity for the LD to present itself, for example, transitioning from elementary to junior high school.

The health care provider will find it useful to remember three of the main ways to categorize learning disabilities: *language-based, mathematical/spatial-based,* and *general cognitive functioning.* Questions may be asked and evidence sought regarding each of these "subtypes" of learning disabilities. Mellard and Scanlon (1999) provide examples of the types of information that might be sought as part of a screening for a possible LD in young adults and adults. These questions include educational history, learning goals, materials, activities and groupings preferred for learning, current levels of skills and knowledge such as might be used for determining educational program placement, and disability history (choice to disclose a disability should be optional). Of course, this type of information seeking can be done as part of the many forms of information seeking the health care provider uses to isolate a health condition while ruling out abuse, neglect, developmental differences, psychosomatic explanations, and the like.

When the health care provider suspects a possible LD, she or he should be able to recommend appropriate resources for the individual or family to become better informed, as well as resources for pursuing a diagnosis. Information resources on LD are plentiful. Batshaw's (2001) book on disabilities, written for parents, has useful medical-oriented information about the condition. Public and academic libraries can provide a wide variety of information on the condition, and on the Internet professional organizations including the Learning Disabilities Association of America, Council for Exceptional Children, and Council for Learning Disabilities have information about the condition and education and service options. In addition, the National Adult Literacy and Learning Disabilities Center and the National Institute for Literacy have information specifically geared toward adult populations. Most of these organizations also have toll-free phone numbers and print literature available. Public school systems and state and federal departments of education have tremendous amounts of information on the condition, rights and services available, and contact information for local professionals and advocates whom families can contact.

The health care provider should also be prepared to provide information that will be useful to those evaluating for an LD. This information might include the health of the mother and fetus prior to birth, trauma at the time of birth, history of any genetic or medical conditions that may have induced brain injury or impaired the nervous system, and overall medical history (e.g., a closed head injury, prenatal seizures, a hearing impairment corrected after delayed language development in the toddler years, fetal alcohol syndrome, alcoholism, or a pattern of medical concerns that border on hypocondricism). This information can be helpful to the evaluators trying to interpret formal testing performance and observational information supplied by families, teachers, and others.

# Attention Deficit Disorder

## Background

### HISTORY AND DEFINITION

Attention deficit is well known within disability professions as a misunderstood condition. In the general culture it is popularly known as "a new disability" or as no disability at all but rather an excuse for parents who do not discipline their children—it is neither. It is sometimes confused with a learning disability, and although they do share several similarities, they are not the same thing. The confusion about attention deficit may be due in part to it and its possible subtypes being frequently renamed, as well as to differences between medical and education professions regarding the nature and legitimacy of the disability, and to high and rapidly increased prevalence rates at the end of the 20th century.

Recognition of the condition began early in the 20th century and evolved through all of it. In a speech to the Royal College of Physicians of London in 1902, the physician George Still identified a class of children who lacked impulse control and who, consequently, acted in "immoral" ways (Stubbe, 2000). The children he had worked with had mental retardation or had been survivors of influenza or encephalitis. In Still's opinion, the children behaved immorally because they lacked the volition to inhibit themselves from participating in impulsive behaviors. Still's subjects had in common an organic brain disorder. These children's conditions were the precursors to the conditions we now know as attention deficit.

After examining soldiers who had sustained brain injuries in World War I, Goldstein noted that they tended to be disorganized, hyperactive, and prone to perseveration, a condition similar to what Still had observed (Hallahan & Kauffman, 2003). He noted that in figure–ground tests the head-injured soldiers had difficulty perceiving figures from their backgrounds (ground). Later, after they fled Nazi Germany, Strauss and Werner continued Goldstein's investigations into figure–ground distinctions and noted the same distractibility and hyperactivity in children with mental retardation. The American William Cruickshank continued their work in the 1950s and established that children who did not have mental retardation could also exhibit these traits. These children were often referred to as having a "minimal brain injury" (Hallahan & Kauffman, 2003) Over time, that label changed as documentation of the condition in children uninjured and of average intelligence was established. Although speculation and scientific evidence still support the presence of a brain injury or difference, subsequent labels focused on hyperactivity and then on inattention. Currently, as was the case across these eras of specifying and naming the condition, definitions have focused more on the observed behaviors than on attention deficit's etiology (Hinton & Wolpert, 1998).

**The Definition of *Attention Deficit Hyperactivity Disorder*.** Relatively recent labels reflect professional confusion over the relationship of hyperactivity and inattention behaviors to each other and to the condition. In 1968 the DSM-II (*Diagnostic and Statistical Manual of Mental Disorders* of the American Psychiatric Association) identified the condition as "attention deficit disorder" (ADD). Critics of this label noted that hyperactivity was a frequent component of the condition and should be accounted for (see Table 15.2). When the third edition of the DSM was published in 1980, the label was expanded to allow use of either "attention deficit disorder" or "attention deficit disorder with hyperactivity" (ADDH). The distinction between the two labels was that an individual could have inattentiveness, impulsivity, and restlessness alone, or in combination with overactivity—which constituted the subtype ADDH. Confusion over distinguishing the two labels resulted in the 1987 revision (DSM-III-R) using only the inclusive label "attention deficit hyperactivity disorder" (ADHD), with an understanding that hyperactivity, or "restlessness," was not present in all with the condition.

Most recently, the DSM-IV (1994) continues to use the single label ADHD but notes that individuals may have one of three subtypes: *predominately inattentive, predominately hyperimpulsive,* or *combined.* The *inattention* subtype does not mean maintaining attending behaviors, rather it means an inability to focus on stimuli and to be slow in processing (Stubbe, 2000). Although the current

---

*Table 15.2*   Comparisons of Attention Deficit Definitions

| DSM[a] edition | Labels | Behavioral Characteristics |
|---|---|---|
| II (1968) | ADD | inattentive, impulsivity, restlessness |
| III (1980) | ADD | inattentive, impulsivity, restlessness, |
|  | ADDH | inattentive, impulsivity, restlessness, *plus* overactivity |
| III-R (1987) | ADHD | hyperactivity or restlessness not always present |
| IV (1994) | ADHD |  |
|  | Predominantly inattentive | inattentive |
|  | Predominantly hyperimpulsive | hyperactive and/or impulsive |
|  | Combined | inattentive *plus* hyperactive and/or impulsive |

[a]Diagnostic and Statistical Manual of Mental Disorders (*American Psychiatric Association*).

label with three subtypes is the most precise labeling system yet, it is not commonly used outside of the medical professions. Education professionals tend to identify persons as having either ADD or ADHD, intending these labels to represent whether the case is predominately inattentive or hyperactive. Medical and clinical professionals are more likely to use all three subtypes, which serves to distinguish those with hyperactivity as being predominant or combined.

## DESCRIPTION OF THE CONDITION

Whatever ADHD is, whatever it is called, and however it is commonly regarded, it is a common condition. Accounting for between 30% to 50% of referrals for child mental health services, 3% to 5% of school-aged children are diagnosed with it, making it the most commonly diagnosed childhood psychiatric disorder (Cantwell, 1996; Stubbe, 2000). Children who have the condition are often characterized as antisocial and are likely to experience peer rejection. ADHD has been found to be comorbid most commonly with conduct and oppositional defiant disorders. Indeed, school suspension and expulsion, criminal activity, and substance abuse are more common for this population (Biederman et al., 1995; LeFever, Villers, Morrow & Vaughn, 2002; Stubbe, 2000). There is reasonable question as to whether the symptoms of ADHD and these other characteristics merely overlap or are related, however. In fewer cases, ADHD is also sometimes found in combination with Tourette's syndrome or LD.

ADHD is most commonly identified in children who exhibit externalizing behaviors, and they are most often boys. Boys are four to five times more likely than girls to be identified with the disorder (Bender, 1997) and more than twice as likely to be identified specifically with hyperactive or aggressive behaviors (Gershon, 2002; Greenblatt, 1994). This difference in identification may reflect vagaries of the process by which children are recommended for evaluation more than actual gender-based probabilities for having

the disorder, however. Greenblatt (1994) found that girls and boys were approximately equally likely to be diagnosed for the inattentive subtype. Robinson and colleagues (2002) have studied trends in medical referrals for evaluation of a possible ADHD diagnosis and identification by gender throughout the 1990s, and they found that the increasing rates of referrals and identification for girls were greater than those for boys. Thus, although the gender gap remained significant at the end of the 1990s, there is evidence that girls are becoming more likely to be identified.

Individuals with ADHD tend to underachieve in both academics and vocations (Stubbe, 2000). The condition is similar to LD in that those who have it have difficulty receiving and expressing information. However, they have these difficulties for a different set of specific processing reasons. Those with ADHD tend to experience gaps in taking in and organizing information, due to their inattention. Similarly, expression is disrupted by disorganization of information, with, for example, the individual skipping social conventions for order and emphasis when speaking or writing. The individual with ADHD may be thought of as "too excited to get the information out." For those with hyperactivity, restless behaviors interfere with the sustained focus and concentration required by most learning situations.

Genetic explanations for the origin of ADHD are widely theorized but have not been clearly documented to date. A family history of ADHD is thought to indicate a higher probability of having the condition (Stubbe, 2000). Children of parents with ADHD have a greater than 50% probability of having the condition. Having a sibling with the condition corresponds to a five to seven times higher than average likelihood for ADHD, and these sibling studies indicate an even higher probability in the cases of monozygotic twins (Batshaw, 2001). Population prevalence studies have found that ADHD is disproportionately identified in male, ethnic and racial minority, and low-income populations (Grenblatt, 1994; Salend

& Rohena, 2003), and within families consistent with those factors. However, Joseph (2000) reports that studies of twins and adopted siblings yield inconsistent findings. She claims that in a nearly 50-50 ratio, any familial study that indicates a genetic basis is countered by another study that does not. This confusion reflects the limited number of studies that have been conducted on the neurobiological origins of ADHD. In addition, of the studies that have been done, most have investigated divergent theories of the disorder or used dissimilar sample populations. Still, there does seem to be a higher incidence of identified ADHD within certain families. Although these trends are possible indicators of a genetic basis, they are also highly likely representative of a social phenomenon regarding who gets identified with the disorder.

Beyond familial–behavioral observations, neurological explanations for ADHD have also been investigated. Evidence in support of a genetic ontology for the condition is that dopamine transporter (DAT), a neurotransmitter that facilitates message exchange across neurons, is found to be present at abnormally low rates in persons with ADHD, and to a lesser extent the transmitter norepinephrine may also be deficient (Austin, 2003; Johnsen, 2001). The insufficient levels of neurotransmitters serve to reduce activity in the frontal lobes. This reduced functioning has been isolated to the right hemisphere of the region, which is the site of inhibition, executive, and attention control. In addition to insufficient levels of neurotransmitters, those present are used inefficiently (reuptake) in affected regions. Thus, the general deficit of DAT, which is presumed to be genetically determined, may explain the observed behaviors used to define ADHD. The low levels of accessible DAT can be increased with certain medications. Other research indicates that there may be excessive DAT in the portions of the frontal region affecting hyperactivity and impulsivity (basal ganglia [which, technically, is deeper within the brain beneath the frontal region]), and

insufficient levels in the portion controlling executive functioning (prefrontal lobes) (Castellanos, 1997). Abnormal functioning in other brain regions, including the cerebellar regions, have also been proposed. The frontal and cerebellar regions have also been found to be smaller in persons with ADHD than in the general population (Hynd, Semrud-Clikeman, Lorys, Novey, & Eliopulos, 1990).

The phenomenon of neuroplasticity suggests that environmental experiences cannot be ruled out as at least contributing influences to neurological differences. This plasticity of brain functioning reflects that just as the brain can influence behaviors, so can patterns of behaviors influence (or "hardwire") brain activity. Neural networks are developed, strengthened, and decayed based on their usage over time. There is no speculation that DAT levels are subject to neuroplastic manipulation, however. Interestingly, hyperactivity among persons with ADHD has been suggested to diminish with age, particularly with later adolescence, likely due to common developmental factors, but inattention is not as likely to be reduced.

## Considerations Across the Life Span

### DEVELOPMENT, MANIFESTATIONS, AND IDENTIFICATION

Both the inattentive and hyperactive aspects of ADHD represent behavioral inhibition. Persons with ADHD have difficulty inhibiting behaviors, whether it be to not engage in a behavior that occurs to them or to cease one behavior and begin another. Whereas suppressed inhibition may be the basic nature of ADHD, the most common characteristic across the three subtypes is disorganization. Aspects of an individual's subtype may inform the nature or extent of disorganization, but all three are susceptible to it because of limited focusing and failing to process information in short-term memory.

A second characteristic common across subtypes is inattention, although there is not one generic form of inattention common across subtypes. Those with the predominately inattentive subtype tend to have difficulty in focusing attention. They are likely to not notice stimuli calling for their attention (e.g., a billboard that most everyone else notices, someone calling their name) and are often considered to be daydreaming or "in a world of their own." These individuals' own thoughts can be as compellingly distracting as can any external stimuli.

For persons with the combined subtype, the attending difficulty is primarily with sustaining attention. Likely due to the hyperactive–compulsive nature of their condition, they are easily distracted to attend to other things instead of staying focused. These affected persons are easily distracted, which means constantly shifting attention to attend to most everything. At the family dinner table, on the playground, in the classroom, or in a quiet room where seated to do coloring or reading, there are constant barrages of stimuli that the average person filters out or attends to selectively. Careful observation of those with the hyperactive–impulsive subtype should indicate a subtle distinction regarding inattention. For these individuals, a limited ability for attending is not so much a factor of the condition as are high activity levels that preclude sustained attention.

As is sometimes the case with learning disabilities, those seeking identification of ADHD have been described as seeking excuses. In this case, parents are claimed to be seeking an excuse for their own poor job of teaching their child to behave. A disability label pins the cause of the observed behaviors on the individual and suggests that the behaviors are beyond her or his own control (Fine & Asch, 2000), and as such, parents, teachers, or others can be exonerated. Similarly, the label can be mistakenly sought to explain the differences presented by persons who come from different cultural traditions (e.g., Poplin & Philips, 1993; Salend & Rohena, 2003). Disability labeling can also be fulfillment of a desire to categorize and name an observed set of characteristics; it can be a step in the process of responding to those characteristics, by providing special education, accommodations, medication, or pity (Scanlon, 2003). Depending on the perspective taken, the explanatory power of a disability label can also be empowering. The detection and identification of ADHD can vary for such reasons, dependent on the age of the child.

**Early Childhood.** If the predominant scientific theories and evidence are correct that ADHD has a genetic or neurobiological origin, it should be present in the early stages of life. Nonetheless, it is not commonly detectable in the early childhood years. This is not because it somehow lays dormant, yet to effect DAT levels or the like. Rather, it is because it has yet to manifest at significant levels or the child has yet to be consistently observed in contexts where the condition is apparent. Infants and young children typically have short attention spans and limited memory, and most parents will tell you that wakeful periods at this stage of life include considerable amounts of energy. Because these are developmentally appropriate characteristics, it can be difficult to know in any but severe cases whether these behaviors are unreasonable. Certainly infants and young children can be compared to norms, especially if they participate in clinical or social service settings such as medical checkups, daycare, and preschool where ready comparisons can be made (or are subjected to psychometric testing). However, actual significant differences may go unnoticed in favor of believing the child is not meaningfully behind.

Whether detected or not, the early effects of ADHD (from all three subtypes) can begin a cumulative effect in the early childhood years. The child who is inattentive can begin a tradition of missing out on cues necessary for learning information, ranging from associating shapes with their figure names (e.g., squares, triangles, or letters with the sounds spoken that represent them) to socially acceptable norms for behavior (e.g., turn taking, asking instead of grabbing). Thus, both communication literacy and social or cultural literacy can be impacted. Similarly, hyperactive children can be excused from learning activities in the early years because they squirm and have limited sitting tolerance for contexts where these literacies are shared (e.g., story reading, watching television, sustained conversations). In a reciprocal process of influence, these young children are developing both social and neurological patterns of functioning.

Young children with ADHD will receive different social expectations and tolerances. Ascribed labels such as "quiet," "shy," "bundle of energy," and "all boy" can represent how their differences become enculturated. Children learn routines from their experiences. They may learn to "get away" with certain behavior patterns as a consequence of how they are treated. When negative behaviors become part of a routine, a pattern of antecedents and consequences that involve parents, teachers, and playmates can often be found (Salend & Rohena, 2003). When such interaction patterns are observed, they easily can be assumed to be the sole and full explanation for the observed behaviors. In the case of ADHD, that observation may be starting in the middle of the true explanation; the stimulus and response patterns may have their origin in an organic state within the child. For example, a child may loudly rebuke a parent's authority in a house of worship, not because she or he "is in control of the parent," but because the setting challenges the child's need for rapid stimulation and the parent's comment is the only stimuli available for an impulsive response. However, it is true that less desirable behaviors are usually learned at the expense of more desirable behaviors. If the condition is truly neurobiological and not just learned behaviors, these routines do not develop solely because of how the child is responded to and, therefore, are not merely learned behaviors children get away with.

The distinctions between nature and nurture bases for ADHD may never be teased out to everyone's satisfaction, but evidence that both are factors in the condition cannot be easily denied. Despite confusion over which factor may lead to which, the neurological basis of ADHD has been reasonably established. Brain functioning develops at an astonishing rate in the prenatal through early childhood stages of life. Communications across neurons via axons (the fibers that transmit electrical impulses between the brain cells) become routinized as certain cognitive functions become routine (e.g., responding with pleasure at the sight of grandparents, associating the word "green" with that color, touching one's nose when asked to). As these neural functions become routine, neural pathways (bundles of connections of axons associated in the function) become solidified (Lyon, 1996). This is how certain functions become easier or automatic. Children with inattentiveness might develop neural-functioning routines associated with short attention but comparatively poor pathways for sustained attention. The cognitive skills involved in attending to distractions will be strengthened over those skills associated with postponing or ignoring such attention (Ernst, 1996). The DAT levels that promote certain cross-neuron communications contribute to these disproportionate cognitive behaviors becoming cognitive routines as well. As a consequence, these behaviors become part of a repertoire that is easily performed; defying these behaviors (e.g., by giving sustained and undivided attention) requires forceful cognition. So, in the early childhood years social and neurobiological factors interact to develop the manifestations of ADHD. These manifestations often increase the ADHD behaviors while suppressing opposite behaviors, and the manifestations are likely to be more noticeable as the child ages.

Observations made in early childhood are most likely to be recalled as evidence for identification in later childhood years. However, both attention and activity levels may be judged in early childhood based on social norms, such as other children in the family, preschool, or playgroup. Activity levels are typically high in preschool children, and attention spans do tend to be short with attention easily shifted. Thus, only extreme cases of ADHD are likely to be detected in these early stages. This may be why the hyperimpulsive subtype is both the most commonly identified subtype for this age group and most commonly identified at this age. When a friend of the author was asked by a stewardess if her rambunctious toddler "is ADD?" (sic), she correctly responded "No, he's two!"

Certain factors thought to contribute to the condition can be used to help detect true cases of ADHD in the early childhood years. Reports of prenatal insult such as lead, alcohol, and cocaine toxification have been found to be correlated with ADHD (Batshaw, 1997). Prematurity and complicated births, as well as chromosomal abnormalities are also known to be related to the presence of the condition in children (Batshaw, 1999). Certain toxins that may be ingested directly by the developing child can also be detrimental. Lead paint poisoning continues to be a factor in causing or exacerbating ADHD (Goldstein & Goldstein, 2000). Of course, in addition to induced cases of ADHD, the condition may be hereditary (Batshaw, 2001). Thus, knowing whether a sibling or parent(s) has the condition can also contribute to speculating about a diagnosis.

**Childhood.** As children transition out of the early childhood years, expectations for social and academic cognitive functioning increase. These expectations are roughly commensurate with typical social and cognitive development. Differences in attention and hyperactivity can now be noticed more readily, as can their negative influences on socialization and learning. Previously suspected cases of ADHD are more easily confirmed, and manifestations finally begin to emerge in prominence in some other cases. Children of early elementary school age with ADHD may find that they have limited tolerance for the increased ex-

pectations put upon them. Their easy distractibility or hyperactive levels may become sources of frustration. The responses they receive from others and that they form regarding themselves can trigger the negative impact of having a disability condition such as ADHD (Ratey, Hallowell, & Miller, 1997).

Initial signs of ADHD in childhood may be indirect indicators of the condition. Certainly evidence of frustration in a child (or frustration by others with a child) can reflect its presence. Sometimes actions based on frustration can confuse identification of the particular subtype of ADHD. A child with hyperactivity may commonly withdraw from group interactions, knowing that negative sanctions will result from her or his "different" interactions. Likewise, a child who is inattentive may engage in a lot of movement and out-of-seat behavior out of boredom or to pursue a rapidly changing focus of attention but not be hyperactive by clinical standards. In either case, the most observable signs associated with ADHD would reflect a different subtype than that which the child has.

A frustrated child may first receive attention for seemingly depressive characteristics or inappropriate social skills. Indeed, poor social skills are a common characteristic of children with all three subtypes of ADHD. Child self-reports and parent, peer, and teacher observations and ratings all confirm the presence of poor social skills (Merrell & Wolfe, 1998; Ratey et al., 1997). As is the case for LD, some research documentation of social skills deficits has even established that social differences may be detectable by others before any primary indicator of the condition (Magyary & Brandt, 2002). Merrell and Wolfe (1998), for example, found that kindergarten-age children with ADHD have significantly lower skills in cooperation, adhering to routines, and meeting the social expectations of peers and adults. Children with hyperactivity are more likely to be shunned by others because of their aggressive and unpredictable behaviors. They are often considered to be unsociable or immature because they do not sufficiently self-regulate their behaviors. Children with inattentiveness are more likely to be socially excluded because they are socially withdrawn and easily overlooked. Others may be less interested in interacting with them because of these characteristics as well. Even subtle differences that cause children with ADHD to be less aware of social cues and norms may cause them to be different enough to be socially undesirable.

Some children with ADHD, particularly those with a hyperactivity component, are prone to injury. These children have high rates of injuries, ranging from minor to severe. Hyperactive children are more prone to running and jumping, and to moving quickly without forethought. Thus, the typical reasons most children become injured are magnified for those with hyperactivity. Inattentive children are not quite as prone to injury, but their short attention span or lack of focus can also cause them to reach without looking, forget they are in a perilous pose, or the like.

Just as social skills suffer because of limited attention or activity impulse control, so do academics. Thus, lagging academic performance is another common indicator of ADHD (LeFever et al., 2002; Salend & Rohena, 2003). The condition is not the same sort of information-processing disorder that learning disabilities is presumed to be; however, it has similar consequences. Students with all three subtypes of ADHD are likely to miss segments of lessons and to shift their concentration without giving sufficient thought to a task or concept. So, academic difficulties become a common secondary effect of having ADHD. These students simply miss a lot of information, and as a consequence of what they miss, they fall further and further behind. Many of these students find the school routine torturous. Children who do not stay focused on tasks are often confused and bored. Those who are hyperactive are constantly having to challenge routine in order to be active, and they miss significant segments of content too.

Children with the hyperactivity component are likely to have behavioral clashes with the school routine that earn them sanctions, including detentions, segregated classrooms, suspensions, and even expulsions. Disruptive behavior is one of the most common reasons for removing students with high-incidence disabilities from the general education environment. They often fall into detrimental stimulus-response patterns with classmates and adult staff. These interruptions of the education process interfere with learning too.

Operational definition/identification criteria specified in the DSM-IV (American Psychiatric Association, 1994) indicate that the condition should have been initially noticed no later than in the early school-age years (age seven). Although this may be taken to suggest that detection is ideally made prior to school age, the above cautions regarding early identification are noted. School provides a viable venue for observing the condition because certain expectations for attention and behavior are integral to schooling; the setting also provides immediate social comparisons.

Noting that inattention and/or hyperactive and impulsive behavior are manifestations of the condition, nine examples of each of the two types of characteristics are noted in the definition criteria (see Figure 15.2). To identify inattention or hyperactivity/impulsivity, at least six of the nine behaviors, respectively, must be identified. These characteristics must be judged as being maladaptive and inconsistent with the overall developmental level of the child. These two factors speak to the seriousness of the impact of the observed factors and to developmental considerations such as cognitive ability and psychosocial development that may explain a child's behaviors. The judged factors must have been observed to occur for a period of at least 6 months and in two or more settings. These conditions are intended to distinguish semipermanent conditions from temporary states for the child. In addition, the observed behaviors must have begun before age seven.

---

*Figure 15.2* Inattentive and/or Hyperactive-Impulsive Behaviors in the DSM-IV (American Psychiatric Association, 1994) Diagnostic Criteria for ADHD

---

*Inattention*

a. Often fails to give close attention to details or makes careless mistakes in schoolwork, work, or other activities.
b. Often has difficulty sustaining attention in tasks or play activities.
c. Often does not seem to listen when spoken to directly.
d. Often does not follow through on instructions and fails to finish schoolwork, chores, or duties in the workplace (not due to oppositional behavior or failure to understand instructions).
e. Often has difficulty organizing tasks and activities.
f. Often avoids, dislikes, or is reluctant to engage in tasks that require sustained mental effort (such as schoolwork or homework).
g. Often loses things necessary for tasks or activities (e.g., toys, school assignments, pencils, books, or tools).
h. Is often easily distracted by extraneous stimuli.
i. Is often forgetful in daily activities.

*Hyperactivity*

j. Often fidgets with hands or feet or squirms in seat.
k. Often leaves seat in classroom or in other situations in which remaining seated is expected.
l. Often runs about or climbs excessively in situations in which it is inappropriate (in adolescents or adults, may be limited to subjective feelings of restlessness).
m. Often has difficulty playing or engaging in leisure activities quietly.
n. Is often "on the go" or often acts as if "driven by a motor".
o. Often talks excessively.

*Impulsivity*

p. Often blurts out answers before questions have been completed.
q. Often has difficulty awaiting turn.
r. Often interrupts or intrudes on others (e.g., butts into conversations or games).

---

*American Psychiatric Association (1994).* Diagnostic and statistical manual of mental disorders *(4th ed.).* Washington, DC: author.

**Adolescence.** All three ADHD subtypes can carry over from childhood into adolescence. When this is the case, social and biological factors may interact with the condition to change its manifestations from the childhood years. Adolescence is a milestone in both biological and social development. Adolescents may find themselves going through rapid spurts of biological development that are inconsistent in intensity and duration. In reaction to their own development, affective domain changes in personal confidence and self-attributes may be sudden and significant. Thus, the ADHD from childhood may take on a new profile, even switching dominant subtype, and cases that existed but went unnoticed can now become apparent.

It is more common for a case of ADHD in adolescence to have carried over from the childhood years. Thus, there will be some familiarity with the condition for the adolescent and her or his family. Typically, it is familiar to health care providers and the school as well. If the subtype remains the same, the specific inattentive and impulsive or hyperactive behaviors may change.

These changes would be due to setting demands as well as to developmental factors. For example, students who had difficulty staying seated or standing still may as an adolescent instead fidget while remaining seated or standing. Depending on the specific behaviors that evolve, the disability may be more or less significant to the individual and others. Coping or compensatory strategies the individual used as a child to self-regulate the behaviors may not work in the same way under new manifestations.

When ADHD is recognized for the first time in adolescence it tends to be after a recent but intense change in behaviors. Attitudinal changes, decreased academic performance, or increased "clumsiness" are all indicators of the condition. Without the knowledgeable input of an expert, imprecise conclusions may be drawn as to the reasons for these new behaviors. Much gets blamed on "typical teen moodiness," a condition for which there seems to be no cure or intervention. Thus, by the time the condition is suspected and explored, the adolescent has already suffered significant consequences. Indeed, many teens do react negatively to having ADHD, regardless of whether it is a new or ongoing condition. This negativity and frustration can compound the condition in the spirit of the Matthew effect (Stanovich, 1986), making it difficult to know which behaviors are representative of the core condition. This is how identification of the wrong subtype or of other conditions (e.g., psychological conditions, LD, social maladjustment) may occur. Not knowing which behaviors are primarily the result of the condition can also confound intervention attempts.

There is a common misconception that children grow out of ADHD as they mature into adolescents or young adults. This is not the case. Interestingly, hyperactivity does subside for a number of teens with the hyperactive–impulsive or combined subtypes, particularly in the later teen years (Stein & Batshaw, 2001). Thus, as the teen develops, the ADHD condition may transi-

tion to the predominately inattentive subtype. It is true that for some it may also stop being considered a disabling condition, and the ADHD label will be removed. But, whereas hyperactivity does subside for some, it merely changes in form for others, and inattentive and impulsive behaviors are not as likely to dissipate (only evolve as discussed above). Thus, those with the combined inattentive and hyperactive condition are found to still be left with the inattentive component.

Detecting ADHD in adolescence may require greater observation the older the individual gets. In the same regard, simply relying on periodically reviewing whether the adolescent has the same profile she or he always had will not be a safe way to get a current assessment of the condition. The same APA identification criteria apply for the condition regardless of age (see Hallowell & Ratey, 1994 for a proposed modified identification procedure for adults); however, with increasing age it will be useful to consider alternative contexts. Whereas in children we assess sustained attention during play activities, for adolescents more age-appropriate social activities may be, for example, social conversation groups or employee training meetings. Similarly, because the nature of hyperactivity may change as the adolescent ages, it may become more represented by restlessness than out-right activity.

**Young Adult and Adult Years.** Even in these more mature years, cases of ADHD can be newly identified or may carry over from previous stages of life. And, again, manifestations are likely to change in type and or intensity. Sixty percent of those who were identified as having hyperactivity in childhood have an identified ADHD in adulthood (Stubbe, 2000). The new routines and challenges encountered in the young adult and adult years place new demands on already-known or previously unrecognized conditions. Success across the adult years depends on coping with or compensating for the condition. Although it may still evolve in its manifestations, at this broad life stage in particular the individual should know what the condition is, how it manifests in daily routines, and how to manage professionally and socially.

Newly identified cases in the young adult and adult years are generally the result of conflicts or negative social–emotional states. Because of disorganization, missing out on social cues, and poor decision making, this population is at increased risk for conflicts in school, at work, with the law, and in social relationships. As adolescents, students with ADHD are at risk for dropping out of school. Dropping out of school is generally a poor entrance into the young adult years. Experiences in postsecondary education, the military, or work may be equally or even more dissatisfying, however. The structure demanded by these environments, and expectations for appropriate behaviors and independence, may be less tolerant of the typifying differences of the adult with ADHD. Yet some adults with disabilities have found that the less-structured routines of settings such as adult basic education are more conducive to their optimal patterns of interaction (Scanlon & Mellard, 2002). Adults with ADHD tend to hold lower-level jobs than others and to leave jobs more often. These factors contribute to their lower-than-average socioeconomic status (Ratey et al., 1997).

Because of both how they process information and are reacted to by others, the adult with ADHD will often be at odds socially. Having fewer social relationships and failing at intimate relationships are more common for this population (Ratey et al., 1997). Adults with ADHD have higher-than-average rates of divorce and separation (Ratey et al., 1997). Their partners can find them to be distant, and they may not be familiar with needs for conflict. Some adults, particularly those with the hyper-impulsive subtypes, report craving conflict. They find that conflictual situations provide stimulation consistent with their rapid processing levels (Ratey et al., 1997). Periods after conflictual or intense

episodes can be particularly cathartic for these adults.

The consequences of ongoing negative academic, employment, or social experiences can include damaged social–emotional states. Adults with ADHD are known to have higher rates of alcohol and substance abuse than the general population (Ratey et al., 1997). These adults also report problems with knowing themselves; for example, they have difficulty understanding their own thought processes and being able to predict their own behaviors. Correspondingly, they frequently report states of guilt and shame regarding their interaction patterns and state of being. Emotionally, they tend to be immature (Ratey et al., 1997).

In cases where ADHD is first identified in adulthood, it generally is the result of a long process of searching for explanations of behaviors or general quality of life. Most likely, the identification process will trigger recall of characteristic symptoms that occurred well before adulthood (the identification process still requires that the core symptoms of hyperactivity-impulsivity occurred before age seven). In addition to seeking an explanation for current circumstances, the identification process may result from new frustrations encountered by job changes or the demands of lifestyle changes, such as forming and breaking relationships and parenthood. The adult may suddenly find that she or he can no longer seem to cope with expectations they and others hold for them. Such events may cause the health care provider to ask about personal circumstances relevant to ADHD.

## Probable Health Care–Related Needs

Because ADHD is a cognitive disorder, it itself does not present specific health concerns. As is the case for LD, it instead has implications for how one maintains her or his health. Core characteristics, such as disorganization and inattention, that mimic forgetfulness can mean that important health regimens can be neglected. Due to inattentiveness, individuals with ADHD may not fully track and remember instructions given by a health care provider. Missed medications would be typical for a person with ADHD, both because of forgetting to take them and frequently misplacing them. In addition, as was noted previously, individuals with ADHD are prone to injury, especially those with a hyperactive–impulsive component. The high activity level combined with lack of attention and rash decisions can lead to ignoring safety procedures, misusing kitchen implements, or provoking violent responses from others. The potentially exhaustive impact of living with ADHD can also lead to mental health needs. Individuals with the condition are not generally oblivious to the condition or its impact. These individuals may need support to cope with their ongoing routines. Partners, families, and others close to the person with ADHD may also need mental health support to cope. Indeed, the high separation and divorce rate for persons with ADHD necessarily involves a partner.

Health care professionals should take note of factors that are symptomatic of ADHD. Likely both the primary manifestations such as inattention and the secondary implications concerning daily routine will be apparent. Without careful consideration of the possibility of the ADHD subtypes, a physician could identify a potential case of mental illness, parental neglect resulting in frequent injury, or low cognitive performance attributed to an LD or other condition, when in fact ADHD is at hand. Even though ADHD is most commonly identified in children and in relation to their school functioning, a physician is required to make official diagnosis in accordance with the DSM-IV (APA, 1994) procedures. Thus, medical professionals should become familiar with these procedures and how the necessary information is reliably collected.

Once a diagnosis has been made, the option of providing an intervention including, or consisting solely of, medication may be considered. The physician clearly has a central role to play in this process. When individuals do receive medication for ADHD, dosages and their timing need to be carefully monitored. This is especially true for children and adolescents who are going through near-constant biological development. The medical professional will need to coordinate observations and interpretations of medication effectiveness with the affected individual, parents, family, and school personnel.

## MEDICATION

Pharmacological responses to health and social problems are increasingly controversial in American society. The pros include that proper use of regulated medications can ease or reduce sources of problems, improving health and enabling greater participation in normative activities. The cons include that self-regulation ability can be diminished, life differences including disability are not honored, and that medications can have undesired consequences. Medication as a response to ADHD is particularly hotly debated within the overall controversy. Part of the reason for particular focus on ADHD is the drastic increase in use of medication-centered interventions in the late 20th and early 21st centuries. It is also due to the majority of recipients being children (Brown, 2000; Zito et al., 2000). Between 1991 and 1995 there was an approximately threefold increase in preschool-age children receiving the stimulant medication Ritalin; similar rates of increase occurred for other psychotropic medications as well (Zito et al., 2000). In the same time span, the preschool population receiving special education services increased annually by 1% to 3% (U.S. Department of Education, 2001)[3]. The

---

3. Because for IDEA regulations ADHD has always been considered to be a subtype of other disability categories (first LD and then Other Health Impairment), data do not exist specific to ADHD.

kindergarten through 12th grade population experienced proportionally similar increases in stimulant prescription, with those aged 15 to 19 experiencing the largest percentage increase (Zito et al., 2000). As Ghodse (1999) has reported, the concerns with possible overreliance on medication for ADHD are fueled by the realization that some school enrollments have as high as 30% to 40% of students medicated for ADHD and that children who receive medication typically continue to receive it into adulthood.

The most commonly prescribed medication for ADHD is Ritalin (methylphenidate). Ritalin is a stimulant that increases the availability levels of DAT and norepinephrine. Increased production and use of neurotransmitters allows for balanced brain functioning instead of over-stimulation or inhibition of certain functions. Other stimulants sometimes prescribed for ADHD include amphetamines (e.g., Adderall and Dexedrine) and pemoline (Cylert). Negative side effects of all three have been disputed; however, they may include appetite suppression, weight loss, periods of lethargy, sleeplessness, rapid heartbeat, and liver damage (Austin, 2003; Johnsen, 2001). Although considered to be generally less effective, antidepressant drugs are also sometimes prescribed to treat ADHD (Johnsen, 2001).

Concerns with medication as an intervention for ADHD include that it is used as an alternative to teaching appropriate behaviors and that it is a substitute for tolerance of individual differences. Children whose inattentive or hyperactive behaviors are regulated by medication have less responsibility for learning to regulate those behaviors themselves. However, medicinally reducing those behaviors to manageable states may enable the child to begin learning to regulate them behaviorally, while at the same time removing negative sanctions that accompany the unmedicated behaviors. As children develop skills of self-regulation, the level or spacing between dosages can be changed, shifting control from pharmacological to self. However, once a child is regulated via medi-cine, the problem may be considered sufficiently controlled and no more attention will be paid to correcting it. By the same token, knowing that undesired behaviors can be easily regulated by medication can reduce teachers', parents', and others' willingness to tolerate the behaviors.

Investigations into the effectiveness of pharmacological responses to ADHD typically do not account for the complexity of behavioral and psychological interventions, nor for social responses to the behaviors, beyond sometimes making comparisons to samples that do not receive medication (MTA Cooperative Group, 1999). One established finding is that approximately 70% of children who receive Ritalin for ADHD benefit from it in intended ways (Austin, 2003). However, Hinton and Wolpert (1998) observed that the medication would have the same effect of reducing distractibility and energy levels on populations without ADHD. Timing and level of dosages can impact the effectiveness of ADHD medications, but once those are correctly established and monitored, the desired effects are expectable.

In the largest-ever study of medication and behavior-based interventions (MTA Cooperative Group, 1999), the National Institute of Mental Health and U.S. Department of Education sponsored the Multimodal Treatment Study of Children with ADHD (MTA), effects of medication, behavioral therapy, the two treatments in combination, and of community care were compared. The study involved a national sample of children between 7 to 9.9 years old identified with the combined subtype. They were observed over a 14-month period. Medication was found to be more effective than behavior therapy alone (i.e., parent training, self-regulation strategies and reinforcement schedules for the child, and teacher training in the behavior management strategies along with paraprofessional support for employing the student's reinforcement schedules while in the classroom, as well as daily report cards to coordinate home and school interventions).

According to parent and teacher reports, both inattention and hyperactivity–impulsivity were more effectively managed via medication. The combined treatment was found to be no more effective than medication alone, but was more effective than behavioral therapy alone. Community care (i.e., child's family only received assessment results from researchers along with a list of local community mental health resources) was also found to be less effective than either medication or the combined treatment, but not statistically significantly different from behavioral therapy for these variables. (Specific usage of information provided in the community care treatment was not tracked.) Thus, for direct treatment of the primary characteristics of ADHD, medication alone or in combination with behavioral interventions was found as most effective. Of course, the overall intentions of treatment for any individual with ADHD are more complex than simply seeking to reduce the core symptoms of ADHD, raising in effect a cost-benefit question. That is, some would ask how meaningful the outcomes are if academic, vocational, and social status are not meaningfully impacted.

Medication and other interventions to reduce the core symptoms of ADHD have generally been found to not result in significant changes in academic achievement or social status (e.g., LeFever et al., 2002). Interventions that have been found successful for these domains have, perhaps logically, been directly targeted for those outcomes. Claims that these targeted interventions may in turn impact the core ADHD condition have not been rigorously and systematically studied with the same thoroughness as the MTA study. It seems unlikely that interventions targeting the secondary effects of the condition would alter neurobiological states, however. Thus, advocates of either approach might be vexed by the corpus of intervention findings. It would seem that the "most effective treatment" depends on the desired outcome(s).

# Conclusion

Learning disabilities and ADHD may not seem that much alike after reading this chapter. They do share general similarities in their histories, probable etiologies, subjectivity of identification, and even in the "treatments" that respond to manifestations instead of core conditions. However, there are specific differences in all of these regards. Their strongest likeness is in practice.

In the case of both conditions, the science that contributes to understanding the nature of the conditions is different from the science that is used to respond to them. That is to say, the neurological and biological understandings we have of either condition in some ways inform day-to-day identification and treatment practices, but mostly indirectly if at all. For example, in both conditions the identification criteria are psychometrically rigorous but do not directly assess the presumed neurological conditions, they instead assess manifestations assumed to stand in for those neurological constructs. There is hard science that helps to identify those same presumed neurological constructs, but neurological and genetic identification is only used in research, not in practice. The educational and psychological sciences that contribute to remedial and compensatory treatments are also based on manifestations of the conditions (and almost exclusively academic manifestations), not their underlying natures. This is even true of medication use to treat ADHD. We medicate to adjust the child's concentration and activity levels to conform to the school day, not to completely ameliorate the condition or to regulate cognitive processing across all contexts in the waking day.

Learning disabilities and ADHD are a lot alike in practice because we are primarily concerned with them as they impact academics. The reasons we seek to identify them and the subjective identification criteria we follow allow us to confuse them. Further, the outcomes from treatment that we seek are largely the same. Without careful attention, one condition can easily be mistaken for the other at any point along the continuum from identification to treatment. The future of understanding and responding to the two conditions will require careful examination of their unique characteristics. The present requires medical, educational, and other social service professionals to be informed about similarities and differences of the two conditions and to be vigilant in their distinguishing between the two.

# References

Aaron, P. G. (1997). The impending demise of the discrepancy formula. *Review of Educational Research, 67,* 461–502.

American Psychiatric Association. (1994). *Diagnostic and statistical manual of mental disorders* (4th ed.). Washington, DC: author.

Austin, V. L. (2003). Pharmacological interventions for students with ADD. *Intervention in School and Clinic, 38,* 289–296.

Baker, S., Gersten, R., & Scanlon, D. (2002). Procedural facilitators, cognitive strategies: Tools for unraveling the mysteries of comprehension and the writing process and providing meaningful access to the general curriculum. *Learning Disabilities Research & Practice, 17,* 65–77.

Batshaw, M. L. (1997). *Children with disabilities* (4th ed.). Baltimore, MD: Paul H. Brookes.

Batshaw, M. L. (2001). *When your child has a disability* (revised ed.). Baltimore, MD: Paul H. Brookes.

Beaumont, C. J. (1999). Dilemmas of peer assistance in a bilingual full inclusion classroom. *The Elementary School Journal, 99,* 233–254.

Bell, D., Feraios, A. J., & Bryan, T. (1991). Learning disabled adolescents' knowledge and attitudes about AIDS. *Learning Disabilities Research & Practice, 6,* 94–111.

Bender, A. (1997). Effect of active learning on student teachers identifications and referrals of attention deficient hyperactivity disorder. *Dissertion Abstracts International Section A, 57*(7-A).

Biederman, J., Wilens, T., Mick, E., Milberger, S., Spencer, J. J., & Faraone, S. V. (1995). Psychoactive substance use disorders in adults with attention deficit hyperactivity disorder (ADHD): Effects of ADHD and psy-

chiatric comorbidity. *American Journal of Psychiatry, 152,* 1652–1658.

Brown, M. B. (2000). Diagnosis and treatment of children and adolescents with attention-deficit/hyperactivity disorder. *Journal of Counseling & Development, 78,* 195–203.

Bulgren, J., & Scanlon, D. (1997/1998). Instructional routines and learning strategies that promote understanding of content area concepts. *Journal of Adolescent & Adult Literacy, 41,* 292–302.

Cantwell, D. P. (1996). Attention deficit disorder: A review of the past 10 years. *Journal of the American Academy of Child and Adolescent Psychiatry, 35,* 978–987.

Castellanos, F. X. (1997). Toward a pathophysiology of attention-deficit/hyperactivity disorder. *Clinical Pediatrics, 36,* 381–393.

Dacey, J., Kenny, M., & Margolis, D. (2000). *Adolescent development* (3rd ed.). Carrollton, TX: Alliance Press.

DeFries, J. C., & Alarcon, M. (1996). Genetics of specific reading disability. *Mental Retardation and Developmental Disabilities Research Reviews, 2,* 39–47.

Donahue, M., Pearl, R., & Bryan, T. (1980). Learning disabled children's conversational competence: Responses to inadequate messages. *Applied Psycholinguistics, 1,* 387–403.

Dudley-Marling, C., & Dippo, D. (1995). What learning disability does: Sustaining the ideology of schooling. *Journal of Learning Disabilities, 28,* 408–414.

Ernst, M. (1996). Neuroimaging in attention-deficit/hyperactivity disorder. In G. R. Lyon & J. M. Rumsey (Eds.), *Neuroimaging.* Baltimore, MD: Paul H. Brookes.

Fine, M., & Asch, A. (2000). Disability beyond stigma: Social interaction, discrimination, and activism. In M. Adams, W. J. Blumenfeld, R. Casenaneda, H. W. Hackman, M. L. Peters, & X. Zuniga (Eds.), *Readings for diversity and social justice* (pp. 330–339). New York: Routledge.

Fletcher, J. M., Lyon, G. R., Barnes, M., Stuebing, K. K., Francis, D. J., Olson, R. K., et al. (2001, October 1). *Classification of learning disabilities: An evidence-based approach.* Paper presented at the 2001 Learning Disabilities Summit — Building a Foundation for the Future. Executive summary retrieved October 1, 2001, from *www.air.org/ldsummit.*

Forbes, M. A. (1991). Special education in juvenile correctional facilities: A literature review. *Journal of Correctional Education 42,* 31–35.

Fowler, A., & Scarboroug, H. (1993). Should reading-disabled adults be distinguished from other adults seeking literary instruction? *Report NCAL-TR-83-7.*

Fuchs, L., Fuchs, D., & Speece, D. (2002). Treatment validity as a unifying concept for identifying learning disabilities. *Learning Disability Quarterly, 25*(1), 33–45.

Gerber, P. J. (1998). Characteristics of adults with specific learning disabilities. In B. K. Lenz, N. A. Sturomski, & M. A. Corley (Eds.), *Serving adults with learning disabilities: Implications for effective practice.* Washington, DC: National Adult Literacy and Learning Disabilities Center, Academy for Educational Development.

Gershon, J. (2002). A meta-analytic review of gender differences in ADHD. *Journal of Attention Disorders, 5,* 143–154.

Ghodse, A. H. (1999). Dramatic increase in methylphenidate consumption. *Current Opinion in Psychiatry, 12,* 265–268.

Goldstein, S., & Goldstein, M. (2000). *A parent's guide: Attention deficit hyperactivity disorder in children* (4th ed.). Salt Lake City, UT: The Neurology, Learning & Behavior Center.

Greenblatt, A. P. (1994). Gender and ethnicity bias in the assessment of attention deficit disorder. *Social Work in Education, 16,* 89–95.

Gresham, F. (2001, October 1). *Responsiveness to intervention: An alternative approach to the identification of learning disabilities.* Paper presented at the 2001 Learning Disabilities Summit — Building a Foundation for the Future. Executive summary retrieved October 1, 2001, from *www.air.org/ldsummit.*

Hallahan, D. P., & Kauffman, J. M. (2003). *Exceptional learners: Introduction to special education* (9th ed.). Boston, MA: Allyn & Bacon.

Hallahan, D. P., & Mercer, C. D. (2001, October 1). *Learning disabilities: Historical perspectives.* Paper presented at the 2001 Learning Disabilities Summit — Building a Foundation for the Future. Executive summary retrieved October 1, 2001, from *www.air.org/ldsummit.*

Hallowell, E. M., & Ratey, J. J. (1994). *Driven to distraction: Recognizing and coping with attention deficit disorder from childhood through adulthood.* New York: Touchstone.

Hammill, D. (1990). On defining learning disabilities: An emerging consensus. *Journal of Learning disabilities, 23,* 74–87.

Hinton, C. E., & Wolpert, M. (1998). Why is ADHD such a compelling story? *Clinical Child Psychology and Psychiatry, 3,* 315–317.

Hynd, G. W., Semrud-Clikeman, M., Lorys, A. R., Novey, E. S., & Eliopulos, D. (1990). Brain morphology in developmental dyslexia and attention deficit/hyperactivity. *Archives of Neurology, 47,* 919–926.

Jenkins, J. R., & O'Connor, R. E. (2003). Cooperative learning for students with learning disabilities: Evidence from experiments, observations, and interviews. In Graham, S., Harris, K., & Swanson, H. L. (Eds.),

*Handbook of learning disabilities* (pp. 417–430). New York: Guilford Press.

Johnsen, K. (2001). Psychobiology and psychopharmacology: Attention deficit/hyperactivity disorder. *Journal of the American Psychiatric Nurses Association, 7* (2), 45–48.

Joseph, J. (2000). Not in their genes: A critical view of the genetics of attention-deficit hyperactivity disorder. *Developmental Review, 20,* 539–567.

Kavale, K. A., & Forness, S. R. (2000). What definitions of learning disability say and don't say: A critical analysis. *Journal of Learning Disabilities, 33,* 239–256.

Kirk, S. A. (1963). Behavioral diagnosis and remediation of learning disabilities. In *Proceedings of the Conference on the Exploration into the Problems of the Perceptually Handicapped Child.* Evanston, IL: Fund for the Perceptually Handicapped Child.

Lee, C., & Jackson, R. (1992). *Faking it: A look into the mind of a creative learner.* Portsmouth, NH: Heinemann Press.

LeFever, B. G., Villers, M. S., Morrow, A. L., & Vaughn, E. S. (2002). Parental perceptions of adverse educational outcomes among children diagnosed and treated for ADHD: A call for improved school/provider collaboration. *Psychology in the Schools, 39,* 63–71.

Lenz, B. K., Ellis, E. S., & Scanlon, D. (1996). Teaching learning strategies to adolescents and adults with learning disabilities. Austin, TX: Pro-Ed.

Lichtenstein, S., & Zantol-Wiener, K. (1988). *Special education dropouts (ERIC Digest #451).* Reston. VA: ERIC Clearing house on Handicapped and Gifted Children. (ERIC Document Reproduction Service No. ED 295 395).

Lyon, G. R. (1996). Foundations of neuroanatomy and neuropsychology. In G. R. Lyon & J. M Rumsey (Eds.), *Neuroimaging.* Baltimore, MD: Paul H. Brookes.

MacMillan, D. L., Gresham, F. M., & Bocian, K. M. (1998). Discrepancy between definitions of learning disabilities and school practices: An empirical investigation. *Journal of Learning Disabilities, 31,* 314–326.

MacMillan, D. L., & Siperstein, G. N. (2001, August). *Learning disabilities as operationally defined by schools.* Paper presented at the LD Summit. Washington, DC: U. S. Department of Education.

Magyary, D., & Brandt, P. (2002). A decision tree and clinical paths for the assessment and management of children with ADHD. *Issues in Mental Health Nursing, 23,* 553–566.

McDermott, R. P. (1993). The acquisition of a child by a learning disability. In S. Chaiklin & J. Lave (Eds.), *Understanding practice: perspectives on activity and context* (pp. 269–305). Cambridge: Cambridge University Press.

Mehring, T. A., & Colson, S. E. (1990). Motivation and mildly handicapped learners. *Focus on Exceptional Children, 22* (5), 1–14.

Mellard, D., & Scanlon, D. (1999). *The comprehensive adult education planner: Providing education for adult learners including those with learning and behavioral disabilities.* Lawrence, KS: University of Kansas Institute for Adult Studies.

Merrell, K. W., & Wolfe, T. M. (1998). The relationship of teacher-rated social skills deficits and ADHD characteristics among kindergarten-age children. *Psychology in the Schools, 35,* 101–109.

Morgan, D. J. (1979). Prevalence and types of handicapping conditions found in correctional institutions: A national survey. *Journal of Special Education, 13,* 283–295.

MTA Cooperative Group. (1999). A 14-month randomized clinical trial of treatment strategies for attention-deficit/hyperactivity disorder. *Archives of General Psychiatry, 56,* 1073.

National Center for Education Statistics. (2000). *Dropout rates in the United States 1998.* Washington, DC: U.S. Department of Education.

National Research Council. (2002). *Minority students in special and gifted education.* National Academy Press: Washington, DC.

Pearl, R. T., & Bryan, T. (1994). Getting caught in misconduct: Concepts of adolescents with and without learning disabilities. *Journal of Learning Disabilities, 27,* 193–197.

Pennington, B. F. (1995). Genetics of learning disabilities. *Journal of Child Neurology, 10,* 69–77.

Poplin, M. S. (1998). The reductionistic fallacy in learning disabilities: Replicating the past by reducing the present. *Journal of Learning Disabilities, 21,* 389–400.

Poplin, M., & Philips, L. (1993). Sociocultural aspects of language and literacy: Issues facing educators of students with learning disabilities. *Learning Disability Quarterly, 16,* 245–255.

Raskind, M. H., Goldberg, R. J., Higgins, E. L., & Herman, K. L. (1999). Patterns of change and predictors of success in individuals with learning disabilities: Results from a twenty-year longitudinal study. *Learning Disabilities Research & Practice, 14,* 35–49.

Ratey, J. J., Hallowell, E., & Miller, A. (1997). Psychosocial issues and psychotherapy in adults with attention deficit disorder. *Psychiatric Annals, 27,* 582–587.

Robinson, L. M., Skaer, T. L., Sclar, D. A., & Galin, R. S. (2002). Is attention deficit hyperactivity disorder increasing among girls in the US?: Trends in diagnosis and the prescribing of stimulants. *CNS Drugs, 16,* 129–137.

Rumsey, J. M., (1996). Neuroimaging in developmental dyslexia: A review and conceptualization. In G. R. Lyon & J. M Rumsey (Eds.), *Neuroimaging.* Baltimore, MD: Paul H. Brookes.

Rutherford, R. B., Nelson, C. M., and Wolford, B. I. (1985). Special education in the most restrictive environment: Correctional/special education. *Journal of Special Education, 19,* 59–71.

Salend, S. J., & Rohena, E. (2003). Students with attention deficit disorders: An overview. *Intervention in School and Clinic, 38,* 259–266.

Scanlon, D. (2000). Learning disabilities. In R. L. Leahy (Series Ed.) & C. L. Radnitz (Vol. Ed.), *Cognitive-behavioral interventions for persons with disabilities* (pp. 265–289). Northvale, NJ: Jason Aronson.

Scanlon, D., & Mellard, D. F. (2002). Academic and participation profiles of school-age dropouts with and without learning disabilities. *Exceptional Children, 68,* 239–258.

Seftel, J. (Producer and Director) (2000). *Ennis' gift: A film about learning differences* [Videotape]. United States: Seftel Productions. (Available from Hello Friends/Ennis William Cosby Foundation, P.O. Box 4061, Santa Monica, CA 90411.)

Shaywitz, S. E., Shaywitz, B. A., Pugh, K. R., Skudlarski, P., Fulgright, R. K., Constable, et al. (1996). The neurobiology of developmental dyslexia as viewed through the lens of functional magnetic resonance imaging technology. In G. R. Lyon & J. M Rumsey (Eds.), *Neuroimaging.* Baltimore, MD: Paul H. Brookes.

Shaywitz, S. E. (2003). *Overcoming dyslexia.* New York: Knopf.

Snow, C. E., Burns, M. S., & Griffin, P. (1998). *Preventing reading difficulties in young children.* Washington, DC: National Academy Press.

Stanovich, K. E. (1986). Matthew Effects in reading: some consequences of individual differences in the acquisition of literacy. *Reading Research Quarterly, 21,* 360–406.

Stein, M. A., & Batshaw, M. L. (2001). Attention-deficit/hyperactivity disorder, in Batshaw, M. L. (Ed.), *When your child has a disability* (revised ed.). Baltimore, MD: Paul H. Brookes.

Stubbe, D. E. (2000). Attention-deficit/hyperactivity disorder overview: Historical perspective, current controversies, and future directions. *Child & Adolescent Psychiatric Clinics of North America, 9,* 469–479.

Torgesen, J. K. (2000). Individual differences in response to early interventions in reading: The lingering problem of treatment resisters. *Learning Disabilities Research & Practice, 15,* 55–64.

Tucker, J. A. (1980). Ethnic proportions in classes for the learning disabled: Issues in nonbiased assessment. *Journal of Special Education, 14,* 93–105.

U.S. Department of Education (2001). Twenty-third Annual Report to Congress on the Implementation of the Individuals with Disabilities Education Act. Washington, DC: author.

U.S. Department of Education, Office for Civil Rights (1979). *1978 Office for Civil Rights Elementary and Secondary School Survey.* Washington, DC: author.

U.S. Department of Education, Office for Civil Rights (2001). *2000 Office for Civil Rights Elementary and Secondary School Survey.* Washington, DC: author.

Wansart, W. L. (1990). Learning to solve a problem: A microanalysis of the solution strategies of children with learning disabilities. *Journal of Learning Disabilities, 23,* 164–170.

Zito, J. M., Safer, D. J., dosReis, S., Gardner, J. F., Boles, M., & Lynch, F. (2000). Trends in the prescribing of psychotropic medications to preschoolers. *The Journal of the American Medical Association, 283,* 1025.

# Chapter 16

# Adolescent Anxiety: Developmental Context and Cognitive Perspectives

George Ladd

Although scientific knowledge of the biological mechanisms and processes of human development is becoming well established, the direct or indirect associations of development to psychological health and dysfunction remain insufficiently illuminated. At the root of this deficiency is the daunting complexity of overall human development. The development of each human being involves a dynamic collection of biological, social, familial, cultural, parental, historical, and environmental characteristics that interact on many levels in dynamic ways. What is understood is that development and its associated implications involve complex patterns of change and the reciprocal interaction of a myriad of variables across the entire life span. The psychological health and functioning of humans, then, is likely associated within the behavioral competencies and age-related developmental tasks found at each moment or context of life.

# Development and Psychological Health

At first glance one might not easily make the connection between human development and clinical topics of anxiety and coping. However, to understand a patient's appraisals of threats and their emotional and physiological reactions to them, it is necessary to consider the context within which a patient lives and functions. Developmental contextualism provides a perspective of human functioning that allows the researcher or clinician to consider individual health phenomena (i.e., anxiety disorders) as parts (or factors) within a larger system of development. In doing so, a more complete "picture" of the challenges, risks, and resources may be acquired, leading to the most appropriate assessment and course of intervention.

## Interacting Forces of Development

Patients do not experience health challenges as isolated incidents or occurrences that exist apart from other domains of their lives and functioning. The contexts in which we all live and develop throughout our lives are changeable and include multiple levels. Developmental contextualism considers behavior, health, and development as the dynamic result of the integration of changeable associations among the various levels of an individual's context. These contextual levels range widely from biological through cultural and include temporal levels such as personal or societal history (Bronfenbrenner, 1979; Elder, 1980; Gottlieb, 1992). When considered in more detail, they would also include numerous sublevels of context, all interdependent and systematically changing over time (Lerner, 1986). The central feature among all levels of context is that they are embedded within each other to form a combinative system of development (Elder, Modell, & Parke, 1993). Further, change at any one level of context is reciprocally associated with change within other levels of context (Hetherington, Lerner, & Perlmutter, 1988; Lerner & Spanier, 1978). The cliché "the whole is greater than the sum of its parts" may be a helpful way of thinking about contextual levels and the factors found within them.

Similar in some ways to the "transactional" perspective in health care research (see Lazarus & Folkman, 1987), developmental contextualism can be helpful in understanding the variability of patient challenges as well as creative opportunities to apply individualized interventions in the interest of optimal patient functioning. Adolescents with primary or secondary psychiatric disorders such as anxiety may be impaired in several domains of functioning (i.e., emotional, cognitive, physical, and/or behavioral), thus the context of the family, school, community, and culture must always be considered.

Developmental contextualism views development as a systematic process of change over time that is inextricably embedded within an interdependent matrix of contextual levels (Ford & Lerner, 1992). Development is a 'systematic process' in that all of the factors involved in development, such as relationships, health, genetics, or education, all combine with a myriad of other factors as a system of development in which each factor serves an important role that can only be defined as it exists within the larger system. The developmental factors working as a system then facilitate a process of development that involves 'change over time'. The temporal nature of change is an important component of developmental contextualism because it highlights the idea that development is not a qualitative shift from one "stage" to another but rather is a continuous developmental process occurring over time. Finally, developmental change is inextricably embedded or impossible to consider apart from the associated factors within the larger system of development.

## Developmental Context and Health

As most health care professionals understand, comforting anxious patients and assisting them with their efforts to cope with health challenges is not a "one size fits all" endeavor. Individual patients experience health challenges differently depending on such important considerations as varied as age, ethnicity, gender, faith, family, and countless others. The anxiety of adolescent patients is no exception. A contextualist approach to adolescent anxiety seeks to capture the temporal interaction between an individual's functioning and the context in which that individual is operating including developmental as well as across biological, psychological, and sociocultural levels. As clinicians engage the psychological health challenges of adolescent patients, an understanding of the levels and complexities of development will serve as a sensitized perspective from which each patient can be evaluated and treated.

The value of a contextualist perspective emerges from the interpretation of diagnostic assessments. For instance, consider an adolescent patient's assessment scores on a measure of anxiety before entering treatment and then after treatment has concluded. Before treatment, that patient's anxiety score may have been at a severe level, and then after treatment it may be significantly lower. At face value, we would be confident in comparing the two assessment scores that the patient experienced an alleviation of anxiety severity. Nevertheless, that change in anxiety severity would be very difficult to accurately interpret and understand unless we considered the many factors at work within that patient's life (context). A patient's anxiety may have lessened as the result of a combination of factors such as treatment, self-awareness, increased parental involvement, or even better eating habits. In this case, focusing on treatment as the sole facilitator of change in anxiety severity is to rely on a likely necessary but not singly sufficient factor within a larger complex and individualized system. Indeed, relying on such prominent factors at the expense of deeper, more individualized perspectives may constrain our ability to thoroughly understand individual development or health phenomena.

Anxiety does not generally develop as a direct result of a single biological or psychological factor. Like most other health phenomena, anxiety is dynamically associated with a larger context within which biological, psychological, and social levels and factors interact in complex ways and are embedded within each other to form individual experience. For instance, an anxiety-disordered patient may be a member of a family and thus is both influencing and being influenced within that familial context. All contexts in which development or health phenomena exist involve reciprocal interactions among the factors (i.e., the people, the environment, etc.) therein.

# Adolescent Development: Competencies and Immaturity

Before adolescence, children are less able to manage the complexities of their own internal and external daily life and rely on their parents and other authority figures for support and guidance. As children move through adolescence they develop cognitive skills. They are increasingly able to balance multiple concepts, solve complex problems, and think abstractly. Along with their cognitive skills, adolescents are developing their sense of self—an identity of their own. They also begin to recognize, build, and use their own coping skills and perspectives to guide their emotional and psychological selves.

## The Struggle for Independence

All these growing competencies are an important step in the development of autonomy as adolescents gradually learn to think and behave independently. Although adolescents may have increased capacities for independence, they have a great deal of development ahead of them, so they still require parental support and guidance. It is actually not uncommon for adolescents to be placed in a difficult position where they are treated like young adults and yet their social, emotional, psychological, and biological functioning may still be immature. The paradox of adultlike competency versus residual immaturity among adolescents makes them particularly vulnerable to anxiety because they often find themselves facing more new situations and challenges than older, more experienced adults. Although adolescents may think they can handle themselves like adults, they usually have less practice doing so, a narrower repertoire of coping skills, and less confidence than adults, so they are more likely to become overwhelmed.

Adolescent patients face a wide range of complex physical and psychosocial challenges when dealing with illness, trauma, hospitalization, and rehabilitation. Adults must understand that adolescents can experience anxiety as powerfully as adults, can *behave* as autonomously as adults, and yet are often not developmentally able to effectively cope with the cognitive and emotional challenges of anxiety or anxiety-provoking situations. It is not uncommon for adolescents to have more difficulty managing their anxiety when faced with the combinative realities of illness and an unfamiliar and sometimes intimidating health care context.

This lack of capacity for effectively dealing with acute or chronic anxiety can make the normally challenging period of adolescence particularly difficult for some youths (Kendall, Chansky, & Kane, 1992; Kendall & Macdonald, 1993). The challenge for clinicians and developmental psychologists is to identify methods of assisting adolescents with the adoption of autonomous cognitive skills that can be incorporated and utilized within existing developmental capacities.

# Fear and Anxiety

Anxiety and fear are commonly thought of as interchangeable. They are both unpleasant emotional states, acute or chronic, involving similar physiological reactions. However, there are important differences between fear and anxiety. Most people, regardless of age or background, have experienced fear when confronted with a situation that they recognized as a real threat (e.g., a large growling dog). Fear is a response toward a specific recognized danger. Fear is a helpful response because it forces us to quickly recognize and act to avoid (or confront) a presently dangerous circumstance.

In contrast to fear, anxiety is not readily associated with a specific source and is referred to as a future-oriented mood state because it usually focuses on what could or might happen. Essentially, anxiety is a largely generalized distress response to a somewhat vague and less immediate threat. For example, an adolescent patient completing inpatient rehabilitation after a brain injury may experience anxiety in facing a home discharge. The patient in this case may not be able to identify the source of anxiety but is generally distressed by the prospect of facing the challenges of the postrehabilitation period such as re-entering school, sports, socially engaging with friends and family members, and so on. Similar to fear, anxiety can be a helpful emotional state, one that serves to heighten awareness and maintain vigilance within contexts that hold a potential albeit indeterminate threat. As in the previous example, a patient experiencing a degree of anxiety at the beginning of post-rehabilitation entry back into physical sports may take greater care until his skills and competencies are established, thus decreasing the risk of injury.

## Anxiety and Development

From a developmental perspective, anxiety is an important part of motivating actions and learning about the environment. For children and adolescents in particular, anxiety serves as a signal that care should be taken in considering a strange or potentially threatening situation and that a new or modified course of action may be required to deal effectively with it. Thus, anxiety may be thought of as a confirming feeling that accompanies an individual's recognition that a situation requires action or change in ways that may challenge existing attitudes or capacities.

A short-term, moderate amount of anxiety can motivate adolescents to learn new methods of adjusting to their environments (i.e., school, social networks) and to develop their capacities to cope with and/or solve problems. Whether the perceived threat takes the form of knee reconstruction surgery, the first day of high school, or a big exam, all adolescents encounter uneasiness, and these circumstances change as they develop through adolescence and into adulthood.

Anxiety-provoking situations may be actual or perceived, but they nevertheless offer opportunities for personal development as long as they do not overwhelm an individual's ability (or perceived ability) to manage them. Over time, individuals establish a confidence in their abilities to manage their anxiety and utilize their capacities and skills to cope effectively with a wide range of challenging or threatening circumstances. Infants begin to regulate their emotions by sucking fingers (or pacifiers), holding firmly to clothing or blankets, and repetitive movements (e.g., rocking, caressing, etc.). These somatic strategies of coping continue through to 6 years, accompanied by the development of other strategies for controlling themselves such as turning their heads or covering their eyes from overwhelming stimuli (Saarni, 1999; Thompson, 1998).

As children develop, so too do their capacities to use their minds (cognitive) and language skills to modify their experience to make it more emotional palatable. For instance, a child may be temporarily separated from a caregiver and focus on a statement such as, "Daddy will be right back, I'm a good boy. . .". These self statements are evidence of developing internal coping strategies, in this case self-reassurance and supportiveness. Here is a humorous example of child's capacity to learn to regulate his emotional distress as needed: Mom finds her 4-year-old with a minor cut on his hand that would have usually been accompanied by crying and says, "Why, honey, you've hurt yourself! I didn't hear you crying." The little boy replies, "I didn't know you were home." (Maccoby, 1980).

## EXPRESSING ANXIETY

Although the basic physiological features of anxiety are relatively consistent across individuals, what usually differs by age group is the way in which symptoms are displayed (Kendall, 1992; Ollendick & Cerney, 1989). Further, the circumstances that give rise to anxiety and the effectiveness at which one manages anxiety remain variable across individuals. The occurrence and experience of anxiety among all age groups can be individualistic and depend on a complex interaction of biological, psychological, and social variables.

However, anxiety is influenced by developmental patterns in predictable ways. For example, an infant's anxious arousal usually revolves around sensory stimuli (e.g., noise, light), appetitive or internal stimuli (e.g., hunger, temperature, digestive distress), or nurturing contact. Toddlers experience anxious arousal when confronted with strange situations or people and become distressed

in the absence of a primary caregiver (i.e., separation anxiety). During childhood, anxiety is provoked by things found in the child's environment (e.g., dogs, dark rooms) and by less concrete sources such as imaginary villains or monsters. Adolescent anxiety typically is associated with more complex scenarios that may involve social networks, academic performance, or issues of vulnerably or isolation (e.g., health or emotional, etc.).

The range of circumstances and degrees in which anxiety can be experienced are likely as diverse and varied as humanity itself. Thus, the nature of anxiety is difficult to accurately describe qualitatively (i.e., what it is or what it is associated with) or quantitatively (i.e., intensity or degree). However, researchers such as Susan Folkman (1982) have suggested that the extent to which anxiety asserts itself may be a function of the relationship between the importance of the challenging event (i.e., how personally important or serious) and the individual's perception of what coping strategies are available to bring to bear on the event.

As adolescents develop, they are increasingly able to explore the world independently and abstractly process their experiences in complex and creative ways. In doing so, children confront many novel and challenging experiences (e.g., social, academic, etc.) that provide opportunities to learn how to manage and cope with periods of anxiety. Those learning opportunities will continue through adolescence and adulthood as the life span presents challenging and anxiety-provoking experiences.

## Manifestations of Anxiety

Although the experience of anxiety takes on different forms and for different reasons among individuals, it typically is described as an unsettled and unpleasant sense of apprehension that cannot be readily assigned to a specific source. Not just a feeling, anxiety is usually accompanied by a variable range of somatic symptoms (Table 16.1),

*Table 16.1*　Physical Manifestations of Anxiety

| Symptom |
| --- |
| Chest tightness |
| Diaphoresis |
| Diarrhea |
| Headache or dizziness |
| Hyperventilation |
| Muscle tension or spasm |
| Nausea or upset stomach |
| Sighing respiration |
| Tachycardia or palpitations |
| Urinary frequency, hesitancy, urgency |

including muscle tension, upset stomach, and sighing respiration. In addition, behavioral or psychological symptoms (Table 16.2) such as nervousness, poor focus, and restlessness often interact with somatic symptoms to create a sustained cycle of distress for anxious people.

Anxiety disorders usually do not appear in isolation among adolescents and are often accompanied by a range of maladaptive symptoms and behaviors, including shyness, social withdrawal, poor self-confidence, dysphoria, and hypersensitivity (Quay and LaGreca, 1986). These comorbid features may be the result of common etiological conditions (physiological or psychosocial) or may

*Table 16.2*　Behavioral Manifestations of Anxiety

| Symptom |
| --- |
| Avoidance |
| Instability |
| Irritability |
| Negativity |
| Nervousness |
| Poor focus |
| Restlessness |
| Unrealistic or excessive worry |

reflect the negative impact that anxiety asserts developmentally. In either case, the variability and comorbidity of adolescent disordered anxiety requires special attention.

## Disordered Anxiety

Unfortunately, anxiety can sometimes grow beyond a normal, manageable level as it permeates thoughts, overwhelms coping resources, and disrupts healthy functioning. Anxiety disorders are one of the most prevalent categories of childhood and adolescent psychopathology (Anderson, Williams, McGee, & Silva, 1987; Costello, 1989; Kashani and Orvaschel, 1990; McGee et al., 1990), with approximately 9% of adolescents meeting the clinical criteria for at least one of several subtypes of disordered anxiety. About 25% of Americans between the ages of 15 and 54 years struggle with anxiety disorders during their lifetimes (Kessler et al. 1994), driving an estimated societal cost in excess of $42 billion per year in job disruption, mortality, and treatment expenditures (Greenberg et al., 1999). Whether specifically diagnosed as a formal disorder (e.g., panic disorder) or more generally as anxiousness or stress, anxiety can present some individuals with challenges that are not easily traversed.

Determining whether or not anxiety is normal or clinically disordered is not an easy task because individuals experience anxiety in a variety of ways. For most, an anxious state is a temporary and relatively mild experience that subsides within minutes, hours, or days. For others, anxiety can be short but terrifyingly intense (e.g., panic disorder) or chronic and debilitating (e.g., generalized anxiety disorder).

Unlike other psychiatric disorders, disordered anxiety shows great variability of expression and normality across individual and sociocultural contexts. For instance, in some social contexts or cultures, anxiety is expressed most often via somatic sensations, whereas in others the experience of anxiety is a prominent cascade of negativistic or catastrophic thoughts. An important implication is that clinicians consider the individual's sociocultural context when attempting to determine whether the expression of signs and symptoms is excessive.

Although chronic or recurrent bouts of anxiety are typically diagnosed as one of several subtypes of anxiety disorder (Table 16.3), inconsistent occurrences of anxiety are more difficult to clinically diagnose. It is important to note that, because anxiety varies in duration and intensity, the physical (Table 16.1) and behavioral (Table 16.2) symptoms may also vary greatly between individuals. Overall, if anxiety serves to distress or disrupt any important aspect of an individual's functioning (i.e., physical, social, or vocational) then intervention is appropriate. Thus, in considering patient care, anxiety should be viewed as an individualistic and complex combination of factors and varying and subjective degrees of distress or debilitation.

For the purposes of this chapter two exemplars of disordered anxiety, generalized anxiety disorder (GAD) and panic disorder (PD), will be described briefly along with the DSM-IV-TR (*Diagnostic and Statistical Manual of Mental Disorders,* 4th edition, text revision, APA.) criteria for each. GAD and PD were selected to illustrate the differences and range of symptoms and dysfunction that can result within the broad and variable clinical category of anxiety disorders.

---

*Table 16.3*   Anxiety Disorder Subtypes

Acute Stress Disorder
Generalized Anxiety Disorder
Obsessive-Compulsive Disorder
Panic Disorder
Panic Disorder with Agoraphobia
Posttraumatic Stress Disorder
Social Phobia
Specific Phobia

---

## Generalized Anxiety Disorder

The features of GAD include persistent and excessive anxiety or worry and significant symptoms of muscle tension, restlessness, fatigue, difficulty concentrating, irritability, and sleep disturbances (see Figure 16.1.)

Clinically, adolescents with chronic or pervasive anxiety are often diagnosed as struggling with what is known as GAD. GAD is characterized by generalized, excessive, and unrealistic anxiety or worry within a variety of contexts. Adolescents with this disorder often are perfectionists. They may spend hours doing and redoing homework or other tasks that most of their peers would dash off in a short period. Restlessness, tiredness, difficulty concentrating, irritability, muscle tension, sleep disturbance and feeling on edge all characterize the disorder. In severe cases, young people may refuse to go to school. Excessive worry accompanied by one of these physical symptoms occurring for many days over a 6-month period is a signal that the youngster may be suffering from generalized anxiety disorder.

Individuals with GAD are commonly hypervigilant with regard to their internal state and poor overall functioning, creating a vicious cycle of negativity and exacerbating their distress.

### Panic Disorder

Panic-disordered individuals experience recurrent, unexpected episodes of extreme anxiety that rapidly escalates to a point at which the individual feels a complete loss of self-control and panics. The symptoms of panic attacks are more severe in nature than generalized anxiety disorder and include heart palpitations, sweating, feeling of choking, fear of dying or losing control, chills or hot flushes, and chest pain (see Figure 16.2).

Having experienced at least one attack, panic disordered individuals associate certain internal cues and/or situations with the past terrifying episode and persistently concern themselves with

---

*Figure 16.1*    Diagnostic Criteria for Generalized Anxiety Disorder

A. Excessive anxiety and worry (apprehensive expectation), occurring more days than not for at least 6 months, about a number of events or activities (such as work or school performance).

B. The person finds it difficult to control the worry.

C. The anxiety and worry are associated with three (or more) of the following six symptoms (with at least some symptoms present for more days than not for the past 6 months). Note: Only one item is required in children.
   (1) Restlessness or feeling keyed up or on edge
   (2) Being easily fatigued
   (3) Difficulty concentrating or mind going blank
   (4) Irritability
   (5) Muscle tension
   (6) Sleep disturbance/difficulty

D. The focus of the anxiety and worry is not confined to features of an Axis I disorder, such that the anxiety or worry is not about having a panic attack (as in Panic Disorder), being embarrassed in public (as in Social Phobia), being contaminated (as in Obsessive-Compulsive Disorder), being away from home or close relatives (as in Separation Anxiety Disorder), gaining weight (as in Anorexia Nervosa), having multiple physical complaints (as in Somatization Disorder), or having a serious illness (as in Hypochondriasis), and the anxiety and worry do not occur exclusively during Posttraumatic Stress Disorder.

E. The anxiety, worry, or physical symptoms cause clinically significant distress or impairment in social, occupational, or other important areas of functioning.

F. The disturbance is not due to the direct physiological effects of a substance (e.g., drugs of abuse, medication) or a general medical condition (e.g., hyperthyroidism) and does not occur exclusively during a mood disorder, a psychotic disorder, or a pervasive developmental disorder.

---

*Source: DSM-IV-TR, APA, 2000*

the prospect of additional attacks. In addition, they worry about implications of having another attack (e.g., losing control, having a heart attack), or an inappropriate change in behavior related to the attack often leads to agoraphobia (see Figure 16.3).

## Cognitive–Behavioral Approach to Anxiety

Sensitivity to the context of adolescent anxiety is of fundamental importance during the evaluation stage of intervention. However, after accounting for the contextual challenges, resources, and capacities of an individual patient, a mode of intervention must be applied. Adolescent anxiety is an amalgam of many internal and external contextual

factors that interact in complex ways. Nevertheless, interventions that address the behavioral and cognitive aspects of anxiety seem to yield the most effective and robust results. Thus, after accounting for the patient's context and experience of anxiety, standard cognitive–behavioral interventions may be customized to best fit that individual.

### BEHAVIORAL PERSPECTIVES

Behavioral and learning theorists assert that formally neutral events acquire anxiety-provoking properties by association with painful or otherwise distressing stimuli. According to this perspective, when a neutral event is paired with one that is painful, the formally neutral one is said to become aversive. This theory essentially externalizes the cause in the stimulus so that it is the

---

*Figure 16.2*    Diagnostic Criteria for Panic Attack

A discrete period of intense fear or discomfort, in which four (or more) of the following symptoms develop abruptly and reach a peak within 10 minutes:

1. Palpitations, pounding heart, or accelerated heart rate
2. Sweating
3. Trembling or shaking
4. Sensations of shortness of breath or smothering
5. Feeling of choking
6. Chest pain or discomfort
7. Nausea or abdominal distress
8. Feeling dizzy, unsteady, lightheaded, or faint
9. Derealization (feelings of unreality) or depersonalization (being detached from oneself)
10. Fear of losing control or going crazy
11. Fear of dying
12. Paresthesias (numbness or tingling sensations)
13. Chills or hot flushes

---

*Source: DSM-IV-TR, APA, 2000*

stimulus that acquires anxiety-provoking properties. This orientation may explain why a patient who had particularly painful or distressing experience at a past medical office visit may have recurrent anxiety relating to future visits even though they may not involve the same or even similar procedures as were originally aversive.

The behaviorist perspective may also explain why anxiety can be inappropriately maintained once it has been established: Behavior will continue if it is reinforced or rewarded. For example, the patient described above who experiences anxiety relating to medical appointments might avoid scheduling them or going to them. This avoidance of anxiety-provoking situations is reinforcing because it alleviates the patient's anxiety and avoidance becomes a learned response.

Social learning theorist Albert Bandura (1997) asserts that the threat attended to by anxious people is a relational matter concerning the match between perceived coping capabilities and potentially hurtful aspects of the environment. Therefore, to understand people's appraisals of ex-

ternal threats and their affective reactions to them, it is necessary to analyze their judgments of their coping capabilities. According to Bandura (1997), efficacy beliefs subjectively determine how threatening a situation is. As a consequence, disordered anxiety is not the product of one's perceived inability to control environmental threats but rather is associated with a perceived inefficacy to control oneself.

### COGNITIVE PERSPECTIVES

The influence of cognitive or perceptive labeling of anxiety levels was recognized by Stanley Schachter (1964). His Two-Factor Theory of emotion considered physiological arousal and cognitive interpretation as necessary elements of emotion, but that neither is independently sufficient to explain it. As shown in Figure 16.4, Schachter suggested that different emotions often have similar physiological features and that the actual emotion experienced (e.g., nervousness, worry, etc.) depends on the individual's appraisal of the situation.

*Figure 16.3*    Diagnostic Criteria for Panic Attack with Agoraphobia

A.  Both (1) and (2):
    (1)  Recurrent unexpected Panic Attacks
    (2)  At least one of the attacks has been followed by 1 month (or more) of one (or more) of the following:
         (a) persistent concern about having additional attacks, (b) worry about the implications of the attack or
         its consequences (e.g., losing control, having a heart attack, "going crazy"), (c) a significant change in
         behavior related to the attacks
B.  The presence of Agoraphobia broadly defined as severe anxiety relating to being in places from which es-
    cape might be difficult (or embarrassing) or in which help may not be available in the event of having an
    unexpected or situationally triggered Panic Attack or panic-like symptoms.
C.  The Panic Attacks are not due to the direct physiological effects of a substance (e.g., a drug of abuse, a
    medication) or a general medical condition (e.g., hyperthyroidism).
D.  The Panic Attacks are not better accounted for by another mental disorder, such as Social Phobia (e.g., oc-
    curring on exposure to feared social situations), Specific Phobia (e.g., on exposure to a specific phobic situa-
    tion), Obsessive-Compulsive Disorder (e.g., on exposure to dirt in someone with an obsession about
    contamination), Posttraumatic Stress Disorder (e.g., in response to stimuli associated with a severe stressor),
    or Separation Anxiety Disorder (e.g., in response to being away from home or close relatives).

*Source: DSM-IV-TR, APA, 2000*

When people experience arousal for which they have no plausible explanation, their cognitive appraisal of situational factors will determine what emotion they feel (or focus on). For some individuals, physiological arousal may be labeled and experienced as "anxiety" in distressing contexts such as a public-speaking engagement and as "nervousness" in a competitive golf tournament. In addition, research suggests that individuals who make negative attributions by default when presented with unexplained arousal are more likely to experience anxiety (Marshall & Zimbardo, 1979; Maslach, 1979; Schachter & Singer, 1962).

Physiological arousal itself is often generated cognitively by arousing trains of thought. Schwartz (1971) and later Beck (1976) looked at the connection between arousing trains of thought and physiological arousal. This cognitive model of arousal provides an explanation for anxiety, panic attacks, and phobias which are said to result from a malfunction of the body's physiolog-ical alarm system induced by dysfunctional schemas (integrated patterns of thought in memory) that make it respond to unreal threats.

## COGNITIVE COPING STRATEGIES

Coping may be broadly defined as an individual's attempt to gain a sense of control over an environmental or internal challenge to the extent that a personally valued outcome is achieved. It is a dynamic process guided by internal and external appraisals of a challenge (threat), assessments of one's ability to respond, and the behaviors (strategies) directed toward that challenge (Lazarus, 1993; Lazarus & Folkman 1984).

Essentially, a sense of control facilitates one's empowerment to engage a challenge and apply strategies to cope with it. Adolescents are only just beginning to build their sense of control over themselves and their contexts. They may feel or act confident, but their sense of control is not as sturdy as that of an experienced adult. When an adolescent finds herself within an unfamiliar or

*Figure 16.4*    Stanley Schachter's Two-Factor Theory of Emotion

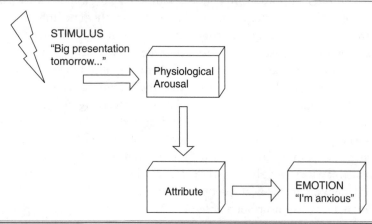

intimidating situation, she may struggle to maintain a sense of control and become unable to cope effectively with challenges therein.

**Lack of Personal Control.**    Anxiety is derived less from a perceived inability to control environmental threats and more from a perceived inefficacy to control oneself or one's level of functioning. Inefficacy sometimes involves perceived vulnerability to total loss of personal control rather than momentary lapses in functioning. Through inefficacious trains of thought, anxious patients distress themselves and constrain and impair their level of functioning (Lazarus & Folkman, 1984; Meichenbaum, 1977). The anxious individual focuses on irrational contingencies that maintain a psychological (and physiological) cycle of negativity that builds and eventually overwhelms.

During a panic attack, for example, the thought of dying during a cardiac stress test may evoke an image of suffocation that causes chest tension and a pounding heart. Interpreted as signs of impending physical or mental collapse, these symptoms exacerbate the patient's anxiety, which increases physical tension, and so on. As a consequence of this cycle of negativity and growing tension, potentially reassuring information has no access to the patient's cognitive focus and thus reasoning is disturbed. Eventually the patient may suffer mainly from anticipatory anxiety. For chronically anxious patients, stress and worry may saturate their lives, leaving only small "islands" of anxiety-free functioning.

One study found that cancer patients who believed that they had control over the course of their cancer or that others (i.e., health professionals) could control the outcome of their illness were generally less distressed (Taylor, Helgeson, Reed, & Skokan, 1991; Thompson, Sobolew-Shubin, Galbraith, Schwankovsky, & Cruzen, 1993). In contrast, patients with disordered levels of anxiety may be overestimating the likelihood of a threat and underestimating their ability to cope with it. As a result, they pay selective attention to the negative aspects of a circumstance or dwell on the worst possible outcomes. Thoughts, feelings, and physical sensations then reinforce one another in an escalating cycle of myopic negativity. Whether maintaining or releasing control, the individual must have confidence in her own ability to cope (coping efficacy).

**A Perception of Helplessness.** Lack of control transforms over time and degree into a growing perception of helplessness. For example, when severe pain is not treated appropriately, patients may develop pain symptom complexes leading to anxiety, depression, and hostility that in turn may exacerbate a patient's perceptions of pain and discomfort (Wolman & Lutterman, 1988). Chronic pain can also give rise to a pervasive sense of helplessness in patients who perceive that the experience and management of pain is out of their control. These patients may increasingly view the relatively normal challenges of medical procedures or rehabilitative tasks as insurmountable obstacles provoking distress and fear that accumulate to greater levels of personal negativity.

Similarly, a study of breast cancer patients found that those who perceived a lack of control had poorer global adjustment (Lowery, Jacobsen, & DuCette, 1993). In contrast, one study of cancer patients found that subjects with a perceived control over the symptoms of their illness were more positively adjusted (Taylor et al., 1991). Another study found that cancer patients who felt in control of their emotions and of their physical symptoms had lower scores on an anxiety–depression scale (Thompson et al., 1993). High perceived control and the use of problem-focused coping have been associated with lower psychological distress among all age cohorts throughout a variety of environmental challenges (Compas, Malcarne, & Fondacaro, 1988; Conway & Terry, 1992; Forsythe & Compas, 1987).

As an example, an interesting line of research was designed to take advantage of the phenomenon that, among patients with panic attack disorder (an anxiety disorder), panic attacks can be provoked when patients with the disorder breathe air that is enriched with carbon dioxide ($CO_2$) over a period of time. Researchers (Sanderson, Rapee, & Barlow, 1989) found that perceived control could transform threatening situations into safe ones even when physiological factors that provoke elevated anxiety are present.

Research procedures called for the formation of a sample of 20 patients with panic disorder and arranged for them to inhale a mixture of $CO_2$-enriched air for 15 minutes. All 20 patients were informed that when a light bulb directly in front of them was illuminated, this would be a signal that they could decrease the amount of $CO_2$ that they were receiving, if they felt they needed to, by turning a dial. The patients were divided into 2 groups of 10. Each of the patients in the first group were presented with an illuminated light signal during the entire time that they were breathing the $CO_2$.

Patients in the second group were never presented with the illuminated signal. What both groups of patients did not know is that all inhaled the same amount of enriched $CO_2$ mixture regardless of their use of the dial because the dial itself was ineffective. Thus, although patients in the first group were led to believe they could regulate the amount of $CO_2$ they received by manipulating a dial, this perceived control was illusionary. However, those patients who believed they were exercising control remained calm and rarely experienced panic attacks or catastrophic thoughts, but those who knew they could not exercise any control experienced mounting anxiety and a greater likelihood of panic attacks. In this instance, it was not the moderation of the event itself that reduced anxiety; it was the ability to positively frame one's perspective of the event that moderated anxiety.

## COPING EFFICACY

Anxiety is generally the result of one's inability or perceived inability to cope with a salient challenge that has breached a personal threshold of coping efficacy. Studies have shown that the implementation and effectiveness of different coping strategies is related to the objective characteristics of the challenge and the patient's appraisals of the challenge, with the individual's appraisals of his control over the challenging environment commanding the most influence (Folkman, 1984; Thompson et al., 1993).

Coping efficacy is the extent to which an individual believes his repertoire of coping skills can be effectively applied to produce a desired outcome. We each have a threshold of personal coping efficacy that can change depending on the context in which we are situated. For example, an adolescent may feel confident in her ability to manage a complex challenge within academic studies but feel very vulnerable and distressed when confronted with an illness that forces her to re-evaluate herself outside of her familiar and mastered personal context.

Chronically ill patients who measure highly on mastery (control) and self-efficacy (appraisal of effectiveness) are less likely to struggle with psychological distress (Brown, Andrews, Harris, Adler, & Bridge, 1986; Holahan & Holahan, 1987). Although coping efficacy is influenced by social norms and experience, it is guided by an individual's direct or indirect decision process. Indeed, converging lines of evidence corroborate the influential role of coping efficacy as a buffer against anxiety and stress within medical and other challenging contexts (Connell, Davis, Gallant, & Sharpe, 1994; Krause, 1987; Pearlin, Lieberman, Menaghan, & Mullen, 1981; Roberts, Dunkle, & Haug, 1994; Smith, Dobbins, & Wallston, 1991).

## C.O.P.E

In the early 1990s, Dr. John Dacey of Boston College began to investigate the relationship of self-control, coping-skills inventories, and self-efficacy among children and adolescents with various behavioral challenges. He viewed negative social-emotive behaviors as being the product of deficient internal control. This self-control model of behavior was based on the premise that individuals learn (formally and informally) a repertoire of cognitive skills and strategies for coping with complicated contexts involving self and behavior (Dacey, Amara, & Seavey, 1993). To Dacey and his associates, the negative behaviors and conceptions of self were not as much a function of emotional or social states but of deficiencies in or misdirected applications of cognitive-based coping skills. Because these coping skills and strategies are learned, the prospect of re-teaching these cognitive abilities provided the possible treatment of a wide range of child and adolescent problems (Dacey, et al., 1993; Dacey & Fiore, 2000).

Dacey et al. (1993) found that most adolescents experience the same four challenges when they operate within anxiety-provoking contexts. These challenges are as follows.

1. *Inability to effectively calm (C) themselves.* Anxious people enter a vicious cycle of increasing distress as they focus on their distress in the face of an anxiety-provoking context. The ability to regulate one's physiological and psychological arousal is a crucial first step in addressing and effectively alleviating one's level of anxiety. The inability to maintain a manageable level of arousal will only serve to distract the individual from rational and organized thinking.

2. *Deficient ability to originate (O) options and plans for dealing with the anxious moments or context in which one finds oneself.* The powerful negativity that accompanies the realization that one is trapped within a dreadful circumstance without an alternative or exit serves to feed the physiological and psychological arousal of the anxious person. However, when one is enabled to derive rational inventories of personal and contextual capacities the individual is then more likely to effectively deal with the anxiety-provoking context in a productive way.

3. *Inability to persevere (P) in efforts to maintain control when operating within anxiety-provoking contexts.* Even when attempting to use strategies to help gain control over their anxiety, anxious individuals often have difficulty maintaining focus and

rational attention. Often, even the best-laid plan for dealing with an anxious context is broken as physiological distress interacts with irrational thinking, thus serving to distract and undermine the anxiety-alleviating efforts.

4. *Inability to make an accurate and functional evaluation of one's condition (E).* The distress exerted on anxious individuals is often perceived as a consistent state of distress saturating one's life. This is an inaccurate evaluation of one's condition; however, it is a powerfully negative perception that is difficult for the anxious person to disconfirm. It is crucial for an anxious person using anxiety-alleviating strategies to have the ability to accurately evaluate his level of anxiety and thus the functionality of his efforts. Without an effective understanding of how to accurately evaluate one's condition, any skill or strategy designed to alleviate anxiety will be inaccurately assessed by the anxious person and thus soon dispersed amongst overpowering anxiety.

Dacey and colleagues organized a cognitive training program called "COPE" to address the four above-described challenges as they occur among anxious adolescents. The core components included strategies for calming of the nervous system (C), originating several plans for dealing with the problem (O), persevering when the temptation to quit trying becomes strong (P), and evaluating the progress of the initiative and making changes to improve it (E) (Dacey et al., 1993; Connelly, 1996; DeSalvatore, 1998).

# References

American Psychiatric Association. (2000). *Diagnostic and statistical manual of mental disorders* (4th ed., text revision). Washington, DC: Author.

Anderson, J. C., Williams, S., McGee, R., & Silva, P. A. (1987). DSM-III disorders in preadolescent children: Prevalence in a large sample from the general population. *Archives of General Psychiatry, 44,* 69–76.

Bandura, A. (1997). *Self-efficacy: The exercise of control.* New York: W.H. Freeman.

Beck, A. (1976). *Cognitive therapy and emotional disorders.* New York: International Universities Press.

Brown, G. W., Andrews, B., Harris, T. O., Adler, Z., & Bridge, L. (1986). Social support, self-esteem and depression. *Psychological Medicine, 16,* 813–831.

Bronfenbrenner, U. (1979). *The ecology of human development.* Cambridge, MA: Harvard University Press.

Compas, B. E., Malcarne, V., & Fondacaro, K. (1988). Coping with stress in older children and young adolescents. *Journal of Consulting and Clinical Psychology, 56,* 405–411.

Connell, C. M., Davis, W. K., Gallant, M. P., & Sharpe, P. A. (1994). Impact of social support, social cognitive variables, and perceived threat on depression in elderly adults with diabetes. *Health Psychology, 13,* 263–273.

Connelly, M. (1996). What types of classroom instruction in self-control significantly effect the locus of control of inner-city seventh grade students? Unpublished doctoral dissertation, Boston College.

Conway, V. J., & Terry, D. J. (1992). Appraised controllability as a moderator of the effectiveness of different coping strategies: A test of the goodness of fit hypothesis. *Australian Journal of Psychology, 44,* 1–7.

Costello, E. J. (1989). Child psychiatric disorders and their correlates: a primary care pediatric sample. *Journal of American Academy of Child and Adolescent Psychiatry, 28,* 851–855.

Dacey, J., Amara, D., & Seavey, G. (1993). Reducing dropout rate in inner city middle school children through instruction in self control. *Research on Middle Level Education Quarterly, 17,* 109–116.

Dacey, J. S., & Fiore, L. B. (2000). *Your anxious child: How parents and teachers can relieve anxiety in children.* San Francisco: Jossey Bass.

DeSalvatore, L. E. (1998). An examination of the effectiveness of classroom teacher implementation of the Boston College conflict prevention program in reducing conflict behaviors in sixth and seventh grade Boston Public School students. Unpublished dissertation, Boston College.

Elder, G. H., Jr. (1980). Adolescence in historical perspective. In J. Adelson (Ed.), *Handbook of adolescent psychology* (pp. 3–46). New York: Wiley.

Elder, G. H., Jr., Modell, J., & Parke, R. D. (1993). Studying children in a changing world. In G. H. J. Elder, J. Modell, & R. D. Parke (Eds.), *Children in time and place: Developmental and historical insights* (pp. 3–21). New York: Cambridge University Press.

Folkman, S. (1982). An approach to the measurement of coping. *Journal of Occupational Therapy, 3,* 95–107.

Folkman, S. (1984). Personal control and stress and coping processes: A theoretical analysis. *Journal of Personality and Social Psychology, 46,* 839–852.

Ford, D. L., & Lerner, R. M. (1992). *Developmental systems theory: An integrative approach.* Newbury Park, CA: Sage.

Forsythe, C. J., & Compas, B. (1987). Interaction and cognitive appraisals of stressful events and coping: Testing the goodness of fit hypothesis. *Cognitive Behavior Therapy, 11,* 473–485.

Gottlieb, G. (1992). *Individual development and evolution: The genesis of novel behavior.* New York: Oxford.

Greenberg, P. E., Sisitsky, T., Kessler, R. C., Finkelstein, S. N., Berndt, E. R., Davidson, J. R., et al. (1999). The economic burden of anxiety disorders in the 1990s. *Journal of Clinical Psychiatry. 60,* 427–435.

Hetherington, E. M., Lerner, R. M., & Perlmutter, M. (Eds.). (1988). *Child development in life-span perspective.* Hillsdale, NJ: Erlbaum.

Holahan, C. K., & Holahan, C. J. (1987). Self-efficacy, social support, and depression in aging: A longitudinal analysis. *Journal of Gerontology: Psychology Sciences, 42,* 65–68.

Kashani, J. H., & Orvaschel, H. (1990). A community study of anxiety in children and adolescents. *American Journal of Psychiatry, 147,* 313–318.

Kessler, R. C., McGonagle, K. A., Zhao, S., Nelson, C. B., Hughes, M., Eshleman, S., et al. (1994). Lifetime and 12-month prevalence of DSM-III-R psychiatric disorders in the United States. Results from the National Comorbidity Survey. *Archives of General Psychiatry, 51,* 8–19.

Kendall, P., Chansky, T., & Kane, M. (1992). *Anxiety disorders in youth: Cognitive-behavioral interventions.* New York: Plenum.

Kendall, P., & MacDonald, J. (1993). Cognition in the psychopathology of youth, and implications for treatment. In K. S. Dobson & P. C. Kendall, Eds., *Psychopathology and Cognition,* San Diego, CA: Academic Press.

Krause, N. (1987). Life Stress, social support, and self-esteem in an elderly population. *Psychology and Aging, 2,* 349–356.

Lazarus, R. S., & Folkman, S. (1984). *Stress, appraisal, and coping.* New York, Springer.

Lazarus, R. S. (1993). Coping theory and research: Past, present, and future. *Psychosomatic Medicine, 55,* 234–247.

Lerner, R. M. (1986). *Concepts and theories of human development* (2nd ed.). New York: Random House.

Lerner, R. M., & Spanier, G. B. (Eds.). (1978). Child influences on marital and family interaction: A life-span perspective. New York: Academic.

Lowery, B. J., Jacobsen, B. S., & Ducette, J. (1993). Causal attribution, control, and adjustment to breast cancer. *Journal of Psychosocial Oncology, 10,* 37–53.

Maccoby, E. E. (1980). *Social development: Psychological growth and the parent–child relationship.* New York: Harcourt Brace Jovanovich.

Marshall, G., & Zimbardo, P. (1979). Affective processes of inadequately explained physiological arousal. *Journal of Personality and Social Psychology, 37,* 970–988.

Maslach, C. (1979). Negative emotional biasing of unexplained arousal. *Journal of Personality and Social Psychology, 37,* 953–969.

McGee, R., Feehan, M., Williams, S., Partridge, F., Silva, P. A., & Kelly, J. (1990). DSM-III disorders in a large sample of adolescents. *Journal of American Academy of Child and Adolescent Psychiatry, 29,* 611–619.

Meichenbaum, D. (1977). *Cognitive behavioral modification: An integrative approach.* New York: Plenum Press.

Ollendick, T., & Cerney, J. (1989). *Clinical behavior therapy with children.* New York: Plenum.

Pearlin, L. I., Lieberman, M. A., Menaghan, E. G., & Mullen, J. T. (1981). The stress process. *Journal of Health and Social Behavior, 22,* 337–356.

Quay, H. C., & LaGreca, A. M. (1986). Disorders of anxiety, withdrawal, and dysphoria. In H. C. Quay, & J. S. Werry (Eds.), *Psychopathological Disorders of Childhood,* 3rd ed. (pp. 111–155). New York: Wiley.

Roberts, B. L., Dunkle, R., & Haug, M. (1994). Physical, psychological, and social resources as moderators of the relationship of stress to mental health of the very old. *Journal of Gerontology: Social Sciences, 49,* 535–543.

Saarni, C. (1999). *The Development of Emotional Competence.* New York: Guilford Press.

Sanderson, W. C., Rapee, R. M., & Barlow, D. H. (1989). The influence of an illusion of control on panic attacks induced via inhalation of 5.5% carbon dioxide-enriched air. *Archives of General Psychiatry, 46,* 157–162.

Schachter, S. (1964). The interaction of cognitive and physiological determinants of emotional state. In L. Berkowitz (Ed.), *Advances in Experimental Social Psychology* (Volume 1, pp. 49–80). New York: Academic.

Schachter, S., & Singer, J. (1962). Cognitive, social and physiological determinants of emotional state. *Psychological Review, 69,* 379–399.

Schwartz, G. (1971). Cardiac responses to self-induced thoughts. *Psychophysiology, 8,* 462–467.

Smith, C. A., Dobbins, C. J., & Wallston, K. A. (1991). The mediational role of perceived competence in psychological adjustment to rheumatoid arthritis. *Journal of Applied Social Psychology, 21,* 1218–1247.

Taylor, S. E., Helgeson, V. S., Reed, G. M., & Skokan, L. A. (1991). Self-generated feelings of control and adjustment to physical illness. *Journal of Social Issues, 47,* 91–109.

Thompson, R. A. (1998). Early sociopersonality development. In N. Eisenburg (Ed.), *Handbook of Child Psychology* (5th ed.), *Volume 3: Social emotional, and personality development* (pp. 25–104). New York: Wiley.

Thompson, S. C., Sobolew-Shubin, A., Galbraith, M. E., Schwankovsky, L., & Cruzen, D. (1993). Maintaining perceptions of control: Finding perceived control in low-control circumstances. *Journal of Personality and Social Psychology, 64,* 293–304.

Wolman, R. L., & Lutterman, A. (1988). Management of pain from burn injury. *Contemporary Surgery, 3* (Supplement 20-5) 33.

# Chapter 17

# The Roots of Violence and Aggression

Mary Walsh

Jamie Barrett

## Case Example

John was sent to see the school nurse, Mrs. Price, because he had just been in a fight in the hallway. He had a swollen hand and cuts and bruises on his face. John is a 13-year-old, eighth-grade student whom the nurse remembered had been in her office about two months ago. On that occasion John had been sent to her by the principal who suspected that John may have been "high." A small amount of marijuana had been found in his schoolbag. However, Mrs. Price was unable to determine if John had been "using" that day in school. Mrs. Price recalled that John had been very reluctant to talk when she asked him if he was using drugs. John had replied that maybe he did use and maybe he did not, but the drugs that the principal found were not his. When Mrs. Price asked whose drugs they were, he replied that he was not going to tell anyone because he could get in a lot of trouble if he told.

Mrs. Price again found that John was very reluctant to talk with her or to provide an explanation of the fight in the hallway. John would only reveal that he had a "problem" with another student and they settled it. When the nurse informed him that students can be suspended for fighting, John replied, "I don't give a damn."

Mrs. Price accessed John's school file and found that he lives in a housing project about a 15-minute walk from the school. The records indicated that John lives with his mother and his three younger brothers and that John's father is not in contact with the family. There was a report from Social Services on record charging abuse and neglect by John's mother's boyfriend. The report had been substantiated and John was placed in foster care for two months. John's mother has not attended many school meetings and is rarely in contact with the school. John's record also indicates that he missed two months of school last year as a result of having been placed in a juvenile detention facility. He had been charged with assault and battery stemming from a fight with a peer in a park near the school.

After consulting the record, Mrs. Price went to speak with Mr. Lawrence, John's guidance counselor. He reported that John has been associating with a group of peers who are known for being disruptive in class and fighting after school. Mr. Lawrence also reported that other students are afraid of John and state that he has a very short temper. According to Mr. Lawrence there are many people in the school, including teachers and staff, who fear John is going to really hurt someone during one of his violent outbursts.

John's case is a difficult one for any school's student support staff. They must address multiple questions such as: "How much of a threat to himself or others is John?" "How can John be reached?" "Should intervention take place in the school or in the home?" It is clear that John is at a critical point in his development; the adults in his world worry that if he does not receive the proper care and services now, he could well be on the road to physical injury, juvenile detention, or worse. To intervene effectively with youth such as John, it is important to have an understanding of violence and aggression and the related behaviors as well as appropriate and effective interventions.

# The Need for Action

National tragedies such as the Columbine school shootings have focused attention on the need for health care providers to understand how to prevent acts of violence and aggression by youth (Gance-Cleveland, 2001). Violence in school, family, and community settings is now recognized as a public health crisis (Prothrow-Stith, 1995). Health care providers play a critical role in violence prevention and intervention because they are often the primary contact with both children and adults and are the "frontlines" of service delivery. Their encounters are not limited to traditional inpatient and outpatient health care settings; health care providers now play a key role in a range of community agencies and programs as well as in schools.

Research in the areas of psychology, public health, and health science has yielded a number of effective strategies for optimizing intervention and preventive efforts with violent children, ado-

lescents, and adults (Gance-Cleveland, 2001). However, it is often not clear which interventions will have the most benefit for specific clients. For example, should we send an aggressive child to individual therapy, family treatment, or an anger management group?

Although knowledge of effective intervention strategies is clearly necessary, it is insufficient without an understanding of how, when, or where to intervene. The problem of violence and aggression is complex and multifaceted. It spans biological, psychological, social, and cultural domains. Thus, there is no way that we can limit interventions to any single domain across a wide range of clients. The Surgeon General's report on youth violence points out that a critical aspect of the intervention and prevention of any deleterious behavior lies in understanding how the behavior developed in the first place (U.S. Department of Health and Human Services, 2001). Explaining the development of psychopathology requires a theoretical framework that allows us to understand the impact and interaction of the various and complex factors that contribute to the development and manifestation of the problem behaviors (Lerner, 1995). Such a theoretical framework serves as a guide for the articulation and application of various prevention and intervention strategies for aggressive and violent behavior. An understanding of how aggression and violence develop is critical to providing effective care.

This chapter first explores traditional definitions and understandings of violence and aggression. We then describe a more recent conceptualization of the development of aggression—a perspective that expands and enriches our previous understandings and leads to new ways of thinking about intervention. Against the backdrop of this new conceptualization of development, we examine the manifestation and course of pathological violence in both children and adults. Further, we describe optimal, comprehensive, and collaborative interventions for aggressive behaviors. Finally, we conclude by applying our knowledge and understanding of violence and aggression to the case of John.

# Definitions of Violence and Aggression

*Aggression* can best be defined as an act or any form of behavior that is carried out with the immediate intention to harm or injure another being who is motivated to avoid such harm (Coie & Dodge, 1998; Anderson & Bushman, 2002). *Violence* is considered an aggressive act that has extreme harm as its goal. Thus all violence is aggressive, but not all aggression is violent. Aggressive acts that do not inflict extreme harm would not be considered violent (Anderson & Bushman, 2002). For example, a child pushing another child would be considered aggressive, whereas a man stabbing another man would be considered violent.

It is also important to distinguish between hostile and instrumental aggression. Hostile aggression is considered to be impulsive, unplanned, and driven by anger with the goal of harming the victim. Instrumental aggression is a premeditated way of using aggression to obtain a goal other than harming the victim, and it is often considered proactive rather than reactive (Coie & Dodge, 1998)

For instance, pushing another man out of frustration after being bumped at a crowded sporting event would be considered hostile aggression, whereas boxers trying to knock each other out in a match to obtain prize money would be considered instrumental aggression. In the developmental literature, aggression tends to describe a broad category of human behavior, whereas violence tends to refer to specific aggressive actions (e.g., acts of domestic violence, community violence, school violence).

# Traditional Understandings of the Development of Violence and Aggression

It is important to review how violence and aggression have traditionally been understood from the perspective of the behavioral sciences.

Aggressive and violent behavior in humans is hardly a new problem. Traditional explanations for this behavior vary in the degree to which they rely upon psychology, sociology, biology, medicine, anthropology, and public health to explain aggression and violence. We will now review some of the primary ways in which violence and aggression have been conceptualized.

## Ethological Theories of Aggression

Ethology is the study of the biological bases of human and animal behavior and the comparison between the two. It is fundamentally based on the assumption that adaptations and maturation drive the developmental process for animals and humans (Parke & Slaby, 1983; Lester & Goldney, 1997). Humans and animals develop fixed action patterns, which are innate responses to certain stimuli. If those responses produce desirable results, they are repeated as efficient ways to achieve a goal (Lorentz, 1966). Thus, aggression and violence in humans has arisen as an adaptive mechanism to perpetuate one's own genes by warding off potential threats.

Ethologists also argue that aggressive and violent behaviors are adaptive in the competition for limited resources. In particular, these theorists argue that differential patterns of aggression in males and females can be attributed to reproductive strategies (Archer, 1995). The crux of this understanding is the assumption that men are more likely than women to be aggressive and kill because men are competing for the opportunity to advance their genes through repeated procreation. Ethologists argue that men heighten their own chances to procreate repeatedly if they eliminate the competition. In contrast, women are thought to be more selective in their choice of partners because of their greater time investment in pregnancy and child-rearing. In short, ethological theorists posit that aggression in males has arisen as a mechanism to compete for the advancement of their genes.

## Biological Mechanisms

Other research has moved beyond the evolutionary or adaptive functioning of aggression and focused on the biological mechanisms that promote aggressive behavior. Temperament is a construct frequently proposed to account for the development of aggression in children. Temperament is comprised of relatively stable, biologically based, individual characteristics of behavior. These characteristics are assumed to arise as a result of a combination of genetic predispositions, developmental maturation, and early experiences (Rothbart & Bates, 1998). Difficult temperaments have been shown to influence parental caregiving, which can in turn affect the emergence of aggressive patterns of behavior. Children who are fussy or difficult to soothe often do not elicit as much warmth from adults as children who are peaceful and engaging. As a result, children with difficult temperaments often develop poor attachments and negative early relationships, which have been shown to influence the development of aggressive or antisocial behaviors (Rothbart & Danberry, 1981).

The hormonal system constitutes another biological mechanism that has been shown to have an impact on the development of aggression. Earlier studies on hormones and aggression attempted to examine a link between testosterone, aggression, and criminal behavior (Kreuz & Rose, 1972; Persky, Smith, & Basu, 1971). Although these studies could not find conclusive support for a link between aggression and criminal behavior, there was evidence of a link between testosterone and some types of aggression (Parke & Slaby, 1983).

Recent research, however, has moved away from looking at testosterone and other biological agents as the primary factor in the development of aggression and has focused instead on the inhibitory neurotransmitter serotonin. Suomi (2000) writes that testosterone has limited utility in distinguishing between highly aggressive and non-highly aggressive individuals. He points to research by Kruesi and colleagues (1990) that has linked low concentrations of a serotonin metabolite with overly aggressive behavior by children toward their mothers and peers. As our understanding of hormonal influences on behavior continues to develop, the relationship between hormones and aggression will become clearer. Despite our incomplete understanding of these biological influences, one cannot deny the impact they have on human beings and the expression on aggression and violence.

## Social Learning Theory

Social learning theory accounts for violence and aggression by examining the ways in which these acts are modeled or learned. Albert Bandura (1965, 1973) conducted one of the most notable studies on learned aggression by exposing children to models of aggressive and nonaggressive behaviors. In the study, children watched adults play with an inflatable doll. Some adults hit the doll, while others played in a nonaggressive manner with the doll. The children were then given an opportunity to play with the doll and their behaviors were observed. The children who witnessed the aggressive modeling were found to be more aggressive with the doll than the children who were not.

Social learning theory posits that aggressive and violent behaviors are learned and shaped not only by witnessing the behaviors but also by feedback about those behaviors through rewards and punishment (Parke & Slaby, 1983). The person may then internalize those behaviors, and if he or she feels that these aggressive behaviors will be rewarding or will help to achieve a goal, they are more likely to be rehearsed and practiced. Thus, social learning theories, along with social cognitive theories, build on ethnographic and biological theories of aggression by recognizing that humans are not influenced solely by biological instincts or adaptive mechanisms. Rather, humans are also profoundly influenced by our ability to learn and process social cues and information.

## Frustration Hypothesis

The "frustration-aggression" hypothesis posits that aggression arises from the experience of frustration (Geen, 2001). Certainly, anyone who has stubbed his or her toe while doing chores or waited in a long line at a store understands how frustration can lead to feelings of aggression. Dollard and colleagues (1939) are credited with first proposing that in order for aggression to occur it must first be preceded by a state of frustration. However, other studies have modified this hypothesis by positing that although frustration can lead to aggression, it is not a necessary condition, and indeed, people can learn to modify their responses to frustration in order to avoid aggressive responses (Davitz, 1952).

Indeed, a person's attributions or beliefs about the intent of the person who caused the frustration often have an effect on whether the person responds aggressively (Berkowitz, 1989). Dill and Anderson (1995) evidenced this reformulation of the frustration-aggression hypothesis with a study of responses to frustration with college students. The results revealed that when the research participants perceived that the frustration was justified, they were likely to respond in a less aggressive manner than if they perceived the frustration to be unjustified. Participants who experienced no frustration displayed fewer aggressive responses than either of the frustrated groups. This study lends further validity to the notion that frustration will not unequivocally and inevitably lead to aggression; there are moderating variables that have a profound outcome on how the experience of frustration impacts aggression.

# Critique of Traditional Theories of Aggression

As this brief overview suggests, traditional theories have provided us very different accounts of how aggression develops. Over the years, these various views have been the subject of considerable debate and critical examination. Although each of the traditional approaches has yielded a significant amount of knowledge, the formulations are often seen as competing with one another and lead to efforts that explain aggression in terms of one or a few causal factors. This rather narrow approach often leads providers who work with violent children and adults to ask "black and white" questions such as

> "Is aggression explained by genes or the family environment?"
>
> "Are video games and popular music primarily to blame for the rise of violence in our schools?"
>
> "Do children who are aggressive have any hope of changing this behavior by the time they reach adulthood?"
>
> "What risk factor needs to be removed to help these children become nonaggressive?"

In many ways, these questions were shaped by earlier notions of human development in which the development of any behavior was understood as a universal phenomenon that occurred in the same way regardless of a person's race, ethnicity, gender, class, family, or community. Piaget's (1970) stages of cognitive development provide one of the clearest examples of this type of understanding of human development. The various stages of cognitive development are assumed to occur in the same form and sequence for all children regardless of their particular circumstances.

These traditional developmental theories also tended to focus on a single domain of development (e.g., psychological) with little acknowledgement of the explicit contribution of other domains (e.g., the biological or social) on behavioral outcomes. The biological, psychological, and social realms were considered as separate and discrete domains with no account of their mutual influence on one another.

This traditional view of development was also evidenced in the lack of focus on adult development and the related assumption that development effectively stopped at age 18. Thus, a person was considered to have developed consistent and stable patterns of behavior prior to reaching adulthood. With no clear understanding of adult development, these theories did not consider how adults at different developmental levels impact the development of children in both positive and negative ways. We now know that development continues into adulthood, and we are continuously becoming aware of how earlier development impacts the expression of behavior in adulthood (Lerner, 1986).

Finally, the traditional theories of development were preoccupied with risk factors. They were focused on deficits and negative developmental outcomes. With such a heavy emphasis on risk, they paid scant attention to sources of strength and resilience. The critique of these theories of aggression, and indeed, developmental theory more generally, have led in the past two decades to newer and more complex theories of human development and the specific behaviors that it encompasses.

# A Comprehensive Framework for Conceptualizing Aggression and Violence

Over the past two decades, contemporary theorists in the fields of psychology and human development have begun to view human development in a comprehensive and holistic way. These modern theorists view development as a complex phenomenon and suggest that it involves a reciprocal relationship between the person and his or her context. Therefore, an issue such as violence in the family will impact the development of aggression differentially as a function of a person's context (e.g., ethnicity, gender, community, social supports). Further, the status of a person's development will, in turn, impact his or her context. For example, a child who behaves aggressively may contribute to furthering violence in the family.

Additionally, contemporary theorists believe that development does not occur solely at one level (e.g., psychological) but occurs simultaneously at the bio-psycho-social levels. These various organizational levels not only develop at the same time but continually interact with and change one another. Consequently, we cannot reduce the etiology of aggression to one of these developmental factors. Indeed, psychological, biological, and social factors have a profound and interactive effect on the development of any behavior.

These recent formulations of developmental theory recognize that not only are there multiple levels of development but also that these levels continue to develop over the life span. However, the development of any behavior over the life span does not occur in a uniform manner because development can follow a variety of pathways. These pathways reflect the complexity of development. That is, the same pathway can lead to different outcomes, while the same outcome can result from different pathways. Consequently, two children may look as if they are on the same path toward the development of aggression, yet because of the presence of different moderating and mediating factors (e.g., the family, community, school climate), one child may move away from violence while the other may engage in violent behavior.

In considering these myriad outcomes, contemporary developmental theories do not focus solely on risk factors that contribute to negative outcomes but also on protective factors that promote positive outcomes and foster resiliency throughout the life span. They propose that the prevention of violence and aggression is not achieved by merely reducing the risk factors that contribute to the development of the behavior. Rather, it requires the presence and development of protective factors in a young person's life. Protective factors are now recognized as powerful contributors to the prevention of violence and aggression.

If we view the questions that were asked at the beginning of this section (e.g., "Is it genes or the family environment that explains aggression?") through the lens of modern developmental theory we quickly see that there are no simple or easy answers. In fact, the questions themselves oversimplify the issues. There is no simple intervention that can completely address aggression and violence. The development of violence or aggression is too complex to be understood or addressed at a simple level, that is, by addressing one factor in isolation (e.g., video games, or the family, or biology). To truly understand aggression and violence we need a framework that can encompass this complexity. It must also account for the manifestation of aggression over the life span as well as the risk and protective factors that contribute to its development, prevention, and intervention.

Contemporary developmental theory provides a conceptual framework for understanding the development of aggression in a comprehensive manner. This holistic conceptualization of aggression can lead to developmental interventions that are realistic and meaningful. Let us now consider how the fundamental assumptions of this view of human development can assist us to better understand violence and aggression. We illustrate each of these assumptions with a salient example from the research literature on violence and aggression. In short, we illuminate how the often wide-ranging and even conflicting research outcomes in the field of aggression can be synthesized to form a more comprehensive understanding of this behavior.

## Context

Human development is involved in a reciprocal relationship with context. In other words, development is affected by context, while at the same time a person's development affects that context. Therefore, a comprehensive, developmental conceptualization of aggression will account for the mutual impact of both the context and the person on the development of violent or aggressive behavior. *Context* includes both the context of the individual (e.g., family, neighborhood, school, social connections) as well as the larger context in which the person develops (e.g., culture, economics, technological advances, and social problems such as poverty and racism).

As the individual develops, the way in which he or she interacts with contextual influences shapes the impact of the context on the behavior. For example, a child who begins to bully others in school may influence other children to react violently, and slowly a culture of violence begins to develop in the school. Similarly, one or two children may start to share a very violent video game with their friends. Soon, there are many children in the school playing the game, and then that violent video game is part of the popular culture in the school. Indeed, one of the areas where the impact of context on aggressive behavior has been examined in detail is in the research on the effect of media on aggression.

### EFFECT OF MEDIA

Video games and other aspects of the electronic media (e.g., television, movies, music, DVDs) are some of the most powerful and pervasive contextual factors that have been linked to violence and aggression in young people (Bushman & Anderson, 2001). One of the most contentious recent debates has revolved around the impact of television, popular music, and video games on young children, specifically in relation to the development of aggressive and violent behaviors. As the proliferation of technology in the home continues to increase, so too does our attention to the influence this technology has on children and adolescents. Longitudinal studies with boys have demonstrated that watching violent television programs at a young age is correlated with the expression of aggressive behaviors up to 10 years later (Eron, Huesmann, Lefkowitz, & Walder, 1972; Huesmann, Eron, Lefkowitz, & Walder, 1973).

Just as television has become more and more prominent in homes across the country, video games are gaining popularity as technological advances afford video game manufacturers the ability to produce increasingly better graphics and more realistic game-play (Vessey & Lee, 2000). Meta-analyses on the research conducted on video games reveal that studies have supported a link between children playing violent video games and then displaying increased levels of aggression shortly thereafter (Bensley & Van Eenwyk, 2001; Griffiths, 1999). Another meta-analysis found that violent video game play was linked to increased aggression in children but that this effect was less significant than that of watching violent television programs (Sherry, 2001).

To further explore this relationship and to determine if these effects are replicated with older children and adolescents, there clearly is a need for further research on violent video games and their effects on children (Anderson & Bushman, 2002; Dill & Dill, 1998). In the meantime, parents and adults are encouraged to monitor children to determine if they are spending an excessive amount of time playing video games and limit video game use. Vessey and Lee (2000) suggested that if a child is playing a video game almost everyday and for many hours a day, plays the game for excitement or tries to beat a personal best, gets restless when unable to play, tries unsuccessfully to limit playing, and chooses video games over social activities, he or she may be playing video games excessively.

Similar to video games, popular music, particularly heavy metal and hip-hop music, has been traditionally linked to violence and aggression in children and adolescents. Today, CDs have parental warnings on the labels that are intended to alert consumers and parents to violent or graphic content in the lyrics of the songs. Even though the public is receiving warnings, there is still debate over the extent of music's impact on behavior.

Research has yielded mixed results on whether or not music with violent lyrical content actually influences aggressive behavior in the listener. Rubin and colleagues (2001) examined dispositions and attitudes in relation to musical preferences and found that heavy metal listeners exhibited more aggression and a decreased regard for women, and that rap listeners exhibited more aggression and distrust. This is not to say that a type of music causes aggression because someone with an aggressive personality may choose a type of music that matches his or her mood or disposition. However, other research has found that adolescents who are exposed to violent rock and rap videos tend to be more accepting of violent behavior immediately after viewing the videos than were control groups (Huesmann, Moise, & Podolski, 1997).

## Bio-Psycho-Social Levels

It is critical to account for the multiple organizational levels of development (bio-psycho-social) that are impacting the expression of aggressive or violent behavior. For example, a person may have a biological predisposition to act aggressively, often attribute the motivations of others as being hostile, and live in a neighborhood where physical violence is the norm for settling disputes. One would be remiss to attempt to reduce this person's violent behavior to one of these factors alone. It is the dynamic interaction of these biological, social, and psychological variables within the context of the person's development that provides a comprehensive understanding of the behavior. One of the constructs that spans the bio-psycho-social domains and has received a great deal of attention in aggression research is gender.

### GENDER

Gender has a complex influence on development in that it has biological determinants but is also subject to powerful socialization forces as well as internalized, psychological beliefs about what it means to be a man, woman, or transgendered. Gender's pronounced effect on the bio-psycho-social levels of development has led researchers to examine the links between gender and the expression of violent and aggressive behaviors.

It has been commonly accepted that males tend to be more aggressive and violent than females. Indeed, this belief has been supported by research that shows boys display more aggressive behaviors and are more likely to threaten physical harm to peers than are girls (Coie & Dodge, 1998; Maccoby & Jacklin, 1980). However, this difference between genders is not as clearly delineated as some past studies would lead us to believe.

Whereas boys are socialized to use physical aggression as a means to preserve the social order, achieve goals, and express their frustration, girls are socialized to use nonconfrontational aggression for many of the same reasons. Consequently, boys typically are described as expressing direct aggression, whereas girls are described as expressing indirect aggression. As boys and girls develop into adolescents, these differences in the expression of aggression become more marked (Cairns & Cairns, 2000). This is often seen in middle school where boys will physically hurt one another, whereas girls will often gossip and tease one another behind each other's backs (Simmons, 2002).

Both forms of aggression, indirect and direct, may have profound and painful effects on young girls and boys. Boys who are physically weaker and nonaggressive are taught not to cry or show feelings of fear or embarrassment when they are hurt or threatened. The socialization of boys instructs them that the proper way to respond is to take the abuse "like a man" or to fight back with physical violence (Pollack & Shuster, 2000). There is no outlet or recourse for those boys who do not want to fight or who are scared to engage in a physical fight.

Although girls do not have to fear physical confrontation to the degree that boys do, the indirect and social aggression that girls experience can be just as punishing. At a time when children are establishing themselves socially, there are few things as painful as being shunned by former friends or being mercilessly teased by peers. Those girls who are not as socially adept as their peers suffer the most from this indirect aggression (Simmons, 2002).

## Risk and Resilience

Traditional approaches to understanding violence and aggression have tended to focus on deficits in the individual that have led to pathological aggression. However, human development in any domain involves both deficits *and* strengths—risk as well as resilience. Risk and protective factors are the dynamic and interactive agents that influence our development.

Factors that place someone at risk for developing aggressive or violent behaviors include family conflict, a difficult child temperament, neurological problems, cognitive deficits, past physical or emotional abuse, rigid or harsh discipline practices, past substance use, past school experience, birth complications, maternal substance abuse, eating poorly or not having enough to eat, faulty attributions of other's behaviors, associating with deviant peers, membership in a gang, social forces such as racism, and prior life experience in impoverished or dangerous environments (Dodge, 2001). Factors that would act as protective agents that would keep a person from being prone to violence or aggression include coming from a stable home, having supportive and caring relationships as a child with adults, associating with peers with prosocial attitudes, belonging to clubs that promote prosocial values, participating in healthy recreational activities, maintaining a proper diet, having cognitive strengths, and having social strengths (Dodge, 2001). Following is an examination of how one risk factor—in particular, family violence—can influence the development of aggressive behavior in children and what can help to mitigate this risk.

### FAMILY VIOLENCE

Family relationships can serve as either a powerful risk or protective factor for aggression, depending on the quality and intensity of the relationships within the family. A caring and supportive family can serve to insulate and protect an individual from the development of aggression, whereas a family whose relationships are marked by violence can foster aggression in an individual (Dodge, 2001; Geen, 2001). Family violence and domestic violence in particular have been the cause of increasing concern among psychologists, researchers, educators, and law enforcement officials. A staggering amount of the violence in this country takes place in the home. An estimated 3.2 million children were reported as suspected victims of child abuse or neglect in 1999. Of these reported cases, over 1 million cases were confirmed; indicating a victimization rate of 15 per 1,000 (Stop Family Violence, 1999). In addition, those children who witness violence in the home must cope with living in a volatile environment and often have to adjust to frequent disruptions in the family structure and living situation (Ericksen & Henderson, 1992). This exposure to violence in the home can leave a profound impact on the future expression of aggression and violence by the victims. Children who learn violence as a way to communicate, discipline, or maintain control within the family may be more prone to exhibiting violent or aggressive behavior themselves (Parke & Slaby, 1983).

Widom (1989) compared children who had been physically abused or neglected in the home during childhood to a group that had not suffered abuse or neglect to see if abuse had an impact on future violence as an adult. He found that both physical abuse and neglect predicted adult criminal violence, with physical abuse in childhood being a stronger predictor than neglect. Family relationships that are characterized by violence often perpetuate a cycle of violence in which children replicate these patterns of violence in their own relationships (Geen, 2001; Parke & Slaby, 1983). Recent research indicates that a woman today is more likely to be attacked, raped, or killed by a male partner than any other type of assailant (Koss et al., 1994). It is critical that we can inter-

vene with these children before the pattern of violence spills over into adult relationships.

Currently, educators and policy makers are focusing on the importance of fostering resilience in protecting children from the pernicious impact that family violence can have on the development of aggressive behavior (McLaughlin, Irby, & Langman, 1994). Just as risk factors, such as community violence and a disadvantaged school environment, exacerbate the risk for violence, the presence of protective factors, such as membership to the local YMCA or after-school program, mitigate the risk for future violence (Dodge, 2001; Rutter, 2001).

Indeed, the nurturance and support that is provided in community and neighborhood youth organizations can supercede the effects of the violence that many children experience in the home and community. For example, a child who benefits from the protective factors of an after-school program (e.g., supportive relationships with adults, a safe haven from community violence, supervised interaction with peers) is at less risk for violence than a child who is without these supports and is susceptible to negative peer influences during out-of-school time (McLaughlin et al., 1994). Therefore, violence prevention and intervention efforts should be just as focused on fostering resiliency as they are on reducing risk.

## Life Span Development

Aggression and violent behaviors develop over the life span. Often, early experiences with aggression impact the way one expresses aggression and violence later in life. Anyone who has taken some time to observe young children interact with one another has surely witnessed aggressive acts among children. Aggressive behavior in children often first occurs when a child tries forcefully to take an object, such as a toy, away from another child (Tremblay et al., 1998). Preschool children display this instrumental aggression as a way to achieve their goal of gaining or retaining possession of a valued object. There are also certain periods in development, however, where young children manifest aggressive behaviors with no apparent goal as a motivation for the behavior.

For example, Tremblay and colleagues (1998) found that 2-year-olds display more physical aggression, much of which is unprovoked, than any other age group. These findings indicate that there may not be certain conditions (e.g., negligent parenting, the use of corporal punishment) that lead to or cause the origins of aggressive behavior; rather, it may be that factors such as harsh discipline reinforce or maintain the expression of aggressive behaviors in young children (Cairns & Cairns, 2000).

As children become older there is a sharp decline in physical aggression. This decline is followed by a marked increase in verbal aggression, such as teasing (Hartup, 1974; Parke & Slaby, 1983). Aggressive behavior evolves into teasing when the child is able to formulate a mental representation of another child and understand what words will hurt that child.

As the child moves into middle childhood, he or she also develops the awareness of when someone intends to do harm. At this point children are able to engage in retaliatory aggression and also are able to make judgments about when this aggression is appropriate (Herzberger & Hall, 1993). Aggressive behavior then moves from acting as a tool to maintain possession of an object or being manifested at random to an action with socially constructed meaning, such as when a boy strikes another child who has teased him so as not to look weak in front of his peers. In our society boys are often socialized to believe that only "wimps" allow others to taunt or humiliate them (Pollack & Shuster, 2000). In this example, the boy is using a physically aggressive act to conform to a social norm around boys retaliating when they have been insulted.

As children make the transition toward understanding the meaning of aggression, adults play a powerful role in shaping their experiences with aggression. The way in which adults respond to aggressive behavior can have a profound impact on later aggressive behavior. For example, overly authoritarian and overly permissive parenting styles have been associated with contributing to hostile and aggressive behavior in children (Baumrind, 1996). Parents who are harsh and too strict with their children do not allow them to develop a sense of self-efficacy in their own socialization and in the development of prosocial behaviors. Parents who are too "hands-off" do not provide sufficient support and guidance to help lead the child away from deviant or aggressive behavior (Baumrind, 1991). Although overly authoritarian and permissive parenting styles can contribute to antisocial and aggressive behavior in children, an authoritative yet caring parenting style can play a critical role in fostering more socially appropriate behaviors in children (Rutter, 2001).

Parents and adults can provide civilizing influences that help children to manage or control aggressive impulses or feelings and in turn develop prosocial behaviors. Indeed, the structure and rules inherent in society help children to understand that violent behavior is not an acceptable way to resolve conflicts and that hurting other people results in consequences to the aggressor. Just as children at a young age begin to understand the social meaning and consequences associated with violence, they also begin to understand the social implications of prosocial behavior.

Research in the area of prosocial competencies has provided support for the notion that adult modeling is very important in promoting development along positive pathways and avoiding negative pathways. Teachers and parents who have undergone training in promoting prosocial behavior have demonstrated success in influencing children to develop social competencies (Elksnin & Elksnin, 2000; Hune & Nelson, 2002). In addition, a recent study has shown that children who believe that their parents will react positively to prosocial behavior displayed lower levels of delinquency and aggression and higher levels of prosocial behavior (Wyatt & Carlo, 2002). Thus, although there is strong research evidence supporting the detrimental effects that adults and forces in the media can have concerning children and aggression, it is equally important to recognize and attend to the powerful positive effects that adults can have on helping children develop prosocial competencies and skills.

## PROXIMAL AND DISTAL FACTORS

One way to understand the development of aggressive behaviors over the life span is through proximal and distal factors. Proximal and distal factors provide for us a way to conceptualize the experiences and factors that place someone at risk for future violent or deviant behavior (Dodge, 2000). Distal risk factors include all of the influences in the development of a pattern of behavior that have occurred in the past and are not subject to intervention. These distal risk factors have set the stage for the current externalizing problems that the conduct-disordered child is manifesting. Unfortunately, we are not able to travel back in time and prevent the child from abusing substances, nor can we erase the memories of an abusive childhood. We can, however, intervene with the proximal risk factors that the child is manifesting in the present.

Proximal factors can be characterized as the cognitive and emotional processes that perpetuate aggressive or violent behaviors (Dodge, 2000; Kazdin, 2000). Dodge (2000) provided an example of the way a youth could react to being laughed at and teased by a group of peers. The youth could respond by laughing with them, ignoring them, teasing them back, or by striking them. The youth with conduct disorder will likely perceive the teasing as a threat and lash out in violence at a group of peers. Violent youth often view the world through a lens of hostility, which leads them to act aggressively and perpetuates the violation of norms and rules (Pettit, Polaha, & Mize, 2001).

Delineating the distal and proximal processes involved in violence and aggression allows for an understanding of what has happened in a person's past to influence or promote aggressive behavior as well as what is happening in the present to perpetuate these behaviors. Thus, optimal interventions for aggressive behavior are ones that recognize and attend to the distal processes and also work to alleviate the proximal risk factors that are propagating the violent behaviors.

In short, we have demonstrated how the research on aggression reflects the complexity of the developmental process, which influences the origins and expression of aggressive behavior. The role of context, bio-psycho-social domains, a life span perspective, and resilience all illuminate and complicate our understanding of aggression. Although the development of aggression can often be avoided or diverted through effective interventions and preventive measures, there are still many children and adults for whom aggressive behavior is serious and problematic.

# Pathological Aggression

It is important that we first make a distinction between normative and pathological aggression before we describe the characteristics of pathological aggression. It is a truism that every human being is capable of aggressive or violent behavior. Indeed, this behavior can serve an adaptive purpose at times. If one were ever cornered alone by an attacker, one would hope that he or she would have mechanisms available to direct energy into aggressive behavior for the purposes of self-preservation. Similarly, we all can recall instances where mild forms of aggression may have helped us in an athletic pursuit, to get to work on time, or to get on a crowded subway train. Yet, how do we separate "normal" aggressive behavior or instincts from pathological aggression? How do we distinguish between a child who gets into a fight at school due to situational factors and one who is at a serious risk for developing life-course persistent violent behavior?

To answer these questions it is necessary to consider the intent, the context, and the outcome of the behavior. For example, accidentally harming another motorist in a minor traffic incident is a completely different situation than using his or her vehicle to try to run another off of the road. Likewise, the context of the violent action also has a profound impact on how society views the behavior. For instance, two professional hockey players can physically beat one another and receive 5 minutes in the penalty box. But if that same behavior occurred on the street, it would likely result in a criminal charge of assault and battery. Finally, the outcome of the aggressive act is another powerful factor in how we view acts of aggression. The child who stabs another child will do far greater damage and receive much more severe consequences than the child who pushes his peer on the playground.

Following are examples of disorders or conditions that can be considered pathological violence. In these instances the course of development has resulted in the individual developing behaviors that are dangerous to him or herself or to others. The following examples of pathological violence demand our full attention as health care providers if we are to make our children healthier and our communities safer places in which to live.

## Bullying

Teachers, parents, school staff, and mental health professionals are growing increasingly concerned about the prominence of bullying in schools and communities (Olweus, 1994). Bullying can be defined as physical or verbal aggression that is intended to harm or threaten intimidated individuals (Olweus, 1993). For a long time, bullies and bully victims were considered to be part of normal child development. However, recent research has pointed to the deleterious impact that bullying can have on healthy child development. Bullying has been associated with depression, low self-esteem, anxiety, and overall maladjustment up to 10 years after the bullying has occurred (Olweus, 1994). Bullying is now viewed as a public health problem related to school violence, and researchers are working to better understand what fosters bullying in the school environment (Spivak & Prothrow-Stith, 2001).

Olweus (1994) identified typical characteristics associated with bullies and bully-victims. In particular, he found that bullies tend to be more aggressive and physically stronger than their peers. Bullies express a need to dominate and lacked empathy for their victims. In contrast, bully-victims tend to be more anxious, passive, withdrawn, sensitive, cautious, and insecure than their peers. Bully-victims are also more likely to be physically weaker than their peers and to experience greater feelings of isolation and loneliness.

Recent research on bullying has focused on the domain of social competence and how it impacts bullying behavior. Crick and Dodge (1999) proposed that children who are proactively aggressive, such as bullies, are likely to experience verbal and physical aggression as more rewarding than are nonaggressive children. The authors also contended that proactively aggressive children are deficient in terms of encoding social cues and responding to social situations in prosocial ways.

In contrast, Sutton and colleagues (1999a, 1999b) argue that bullies are actually quite competent at processing and encoding social cues as evidenced by the way they can manipulate others to acquiesce to them and the way in which they can deflect teasing and criticism from others. Bullies are often considered the leaders of their peer group, which would require them to be quite proficient at processing social cues. Thus, it is possible that bullies may not attend to the cues that help other children to act in a prosocial manner, while at the same time they may excel at manipulating social situations so that they are in a position of power over their peers. Even though we do not have a clear empirical understanding of the precise role of social cognition in bullying behavior, we must address the significant impact of aggressive and bullying behavior in schools and peer groups.

Recent focus on aggression and peer groups has shifted to include the role that peers can play in mediating conflict as well as what parents can do to protect their children from the harmful effects of bullying. Vessey (1999) believes that adults can help "bully-proof" children by instilling in them a sense of pride and teach them to be assertive but not aggressive. If children have a positive self-image and know how to defend themselves in a nonaggressive manner, they are less likely to suffer at the hands of bullies. Adults can also help by modeling proper conflict resolution skills and by noticing behavioral changes in children (e.g, withdrawing from activities, being late to school) that may indicate that the child is being bullied.

More research is needed to examine how peers, teachers, parents, and school staff can intervene to prevent bullying and to help minimize the negative consequences this behavior can have on both bullies and bully-victims, including depression and feelings of isolation (Salmon, James, & Cassidy, 2000). It is crucial that the perception of bullying shifts from being part of growing up to a serious problem that deserves our full attention. Indeed, if bullying is not curbed there is the possibility that the behavior could develop into a more pervasive pattern of aggressive behavior that is characteristic of conduct disorder.

## Conduct Disorder

When children consistently behave in ways that transgress the rules and norms of our society and violate the safety and physical well-being of others, they are traditionally diagnosed with conduct disorder (CD). Inclusive in the description of CD is the expression of violent and aggressive behaviors. The extensive research base that has been de-veloped on understanding and intervening with CD can serve to inform a conceptualization of the risk factors that influence the development of deviant patterns of behavior, such as violence and aggression.

The essential feature of CD is a pattern of behavior in which the child or youth ignores the rights of others or violates age-appropriate norms (American Psychiatric Association, 1994). Children who have been diagnosed with this disorder typically are aggressive with people and animals (e.g., bullies, initiates fights, physically cruel to either people or animals), destructive with property (e.g., deliberate fire setting), deceitful or engage in thefts (e.g., breaking into another's house, car, or building), or other serious violations of rules (e.g., running away, truancy). CD has two subtypes: childhood-onset type (where at least one conduct problem was present prior to age 10) and adolescent-onset type (where no conduct problems were present prior to age 10) (American Psychiatric Association, 1994).

The aggressive and violent symptoms associated with CD are not going to be manifested in the same way across the life span and across individuals. In fact, one of the most crucial determinations to make when assessing an individual with CD is the age of onset for the symptoms of CD. The trajectory of CD, the severity of violent behaviors, and the prognosis for treatment are all related to the age of onset of the symptoms (Moffitt & Caspi, 2001; Moffitt, Caspi, Harrington, & Milne, 2002; Patterson, Forgatch, Yoerger, & Stoolmiller, 1998). There is a much greater risk for CD to develop into pathology in adult life if risk factors are present in childhood (Kazdin, 1997). This delineation is crucial to distinguishing between *adolescent limited* (AL) CD and *life-course persistent* (LCP) CD. Youth with AL CD tend not to display aggressive or antisocial behaviors until adolescence, when they gravitate toward negative peers. Youth with LCP CD, in contrast, tend to display a constellation of risk factors during childhood that place them at risk for persistent conduct problems—factors that will now be discussed.

Moffitt and colleagues (2002) followed LCP and AL offenders to the age of 26. Their results showed that LCP offenders rated higher than AL offenders on measures of psychotic personality traits, mental health problems, substance dependence, financial problems, problems in the workplace, and drug-related and violent crime. Patterson and colleagues (1998) studied chronic offenders and also discovered a trajectory or pathway for chronic offending that began with risk factors in childhood, continued through early age of first arrest, then to chronic arrest, and finally to a pattern of adult recidivism. Both studies provide compelling evidence for the profound impact of age of onset on the severity of prognosis of CD and violent and deviant behavior.

Childhood factors that place someone at risk for early-onset CD have been delineated by Kazdin (1997), who separated them into child factors, parent and family factors, and school-related factors. As we will see, the identified factors encompass biological, psychological, and social influences.

The "child factors" defined by Kazdin (1997) include a difficult child temperament, neuropsychological deficits, attention difficulties, poor social skills, and poor academic and intellectual performance. "Parent and family factors" include prenatal and perinatal complications, a family history of psychopathology, harsh parent–child punishment, poor supervision or monitoring of the child, family relationships characterized by a lack of warmth and affection, marital discord, large family size, siblings with antisocial behavior, and socioeconomic disadvantage. Finally "school-related factors" include the child attending a school where there is little emphasis on academic work, little teacher time spent on lessons, infrequent teacher use of praise and appreciation for schoolwork, little emphasis placed on individual responsibility of the students, and poor working conditions for students.

While the above risk factors characterize LCP youth with CD, there are also risk factors in adolescence that predict AL youth. As can be inferred from the above list, the risk factors for LCP youth are often characterized by biological influences such as temperament or a neurological disorder, or the psychological effects of negligent parenting. AL youth, however, often enter into adolescence with few of the problems present in LCP youth and typically do not display overly aggressive or violent behaviors during childhood (Moffit & Caspi, 2001). The primary risk factors for AL youth are usually located in the social influences they encounter when they enter into adolescence.

For example, a young boy who comes from a supportive family is still at significant risk to join a gang or to associate with negative or deviant peers if that is the norm in his neighborhood. This is especially true during the adolescent years when it is normative for youth to seek independence and to align themselves more with peers than with their families (Prothrow-Stith, 1993). Delinquent gangs, in particular, have become an especially violent and deadly form for socializing youth to commit violent acts (Bing, 1992). If juveniles do not receive services and supports, the chronic violence that is associated with both gang involvement and CD can persist into adulthood.

# Pathological Aggression in Adults

## Antisocial Personality Disorder

When chronic and pathological aggressive and violent behavior persists from childhood into adulthood, the diagnosis of antisocial personality disorder must be considered. To be diagnosed with antisocial personality disorder the individual must have been previously diagnosed with CD. The other diagnostic criteria include a pervasive pattern of disregard and violation of the rights of others, since age 15, as indicated by three or more of the following: 1) failure to conform to social norms with respect to lawful behaviors; 2) deceitfulness; 3) impulsivity or failure to plan ahead; 4) irritability and aggressiveness; 5) reckless disregard for the safety of others or self; 6) consistent irresponsibility; and 7) lack of remorse (American Psychiatric Association, 1994). Approximately 40% of boys and 25% of girls who are diagnosed with CD are later diagnosed with antisocial personality disorder (Black, 1999).

Those who develop antisocial personality disorder are considered very dangerous to themselves and others. Antisocial individuals are characterized by a lack of remorse and a complete disregard for the established rules of society (Black, 1999). Ted Bundy, Charles Manson, and other "cold-blooded" killers portrayed in the media are all popular examples of people whose violent behavior can be deemed antisocial. This propensity for unchecked violence has researchers and practitioners studying how and why antisocial personality disorder develops and what can be done to treat these individuals.

There has been substantial research evidence to support that there is a biological or molecular component involved in the development of antisocial personality disorder (Black, 1999; McGuffin & Thapur, 1998). Twin studies, as well as longitudinal studies, have shown that there are genetic factors involved with antisocial behavior and traits, including aggressive and violent behavior. Difficulty in defining the disorder along the continuum of antisocial behavior has limited some of these studies.

For example, as antisocial behavior continues from adolescence into adulthood, at what point does the individual officially become antisocial? More complete definitions of the disorder and further research is needed to try to locate and determine the specific genes that may influence the development of antisocial personality disorder (McGuffin & Thapur, 1998). Nevertheless, antisocial personality disorder cannot be reduced solely to genetic factors. The family environment, social environment, substance abuse, and past neglect

and abuse have all also been correlated with the disorder (Black, 1999; Ridenour et al., 2002).

## Alcohol Abuse and Aggression

Alcohol consumption can have a variety of effects on human behavior, including increased aggression. Excessive consumption of alcohol is associated with increased physical aggression in the general population (Bushman & Cooper, 1990; Wells, Graham, & West, 2000). It has been theorized that the aggression results from an impaired ability of an intoxicated person to process social cues (Steele & Josephs, 1990). An intoxicated person is more likely to attend to aggression-related cues and less likely to attend to the social cues that prevent a sober person from acting aggressively (Geen, 2001). The perceptual scope becomes narrowed to the point where not all available information and cues are considered, thus making conflict and aggressive responses more likely (Gibbs, 1986).

The social climate of barrooms and norms of drinking behavior may also impact the increased likelihood of alcohol-related aggression. The bar is a setting where social norms are relaxed and people can blame deviant behavior on having too much to drink (Goldstein, 1994). Graham and Wells (2001) conducted a naturalistic study of alcohol-related aggression in bars. The authors found that four general themes were likely to be at the center of aggressive incidents: conflict with staff; bar activities; troublemaking and offensive behavior; and interpersonal and relationship issues. Thus, in the context of the barroom certain forms of violence and aggression are going to be more likely than others.

# Violence Prevention and Intervention

In summary, we have described violent and aggressive behavior as a complex phenomenon that is rooted in the multiple levels of the individual (bio-psycho-social) and contextual domains (e.g., family, school, culture, environment,). Therefore, it follows that successful intervention with violent and aggressive children and adults requires programs and techniques that can attend to the complexity of the problem. Moreover, the prevention of future acts of violence and aggression requires programs, measures, and policies that impact on these multiple contexts and levels (e.g., the school, community, family). Two approaches in particular that have been recognized nationally for their effectiveness in the prevention of youth violence include Second Step, a program consisting of activity-based lessons designed to identify feelings, solve problems, and get along with others, and PATHS (Promoting Alternative Thinking Strategies), a classroom-based program designed to build social competencies and reduce aggression and behavior problems in elementary school children (Frey, Hirschstein, & Guzzo, 2000; Greenberg, Kusche, & Mihalic, 1998; Walsh & Murphy, 2003).

For a complete listing of empirically supported approaches to the prevention of youth violence, the Surgeon General's *2001 Report on Youth Violence* delineates programs that are evidence based and consistent with contemporary developmental theory (U.S. Department of Health and Human Services, 2001). These programs met rigorous standards for inclusion to be among the best approaches we have in addressing youth violence and aggression. Following are brief descriptions of two programs that have been recognized by the Surgeon General for their effectiveness in addressing youth violence (U.S. Department of Health and Human Services, 2001).

tems that encompass the individual (e.g., peer group, family, community supports) (Henggeler & Hoyt, 2001). MST therapists are available 24 hours a day, 7 days a week, and the treatment is delivered in the natural environments of the children and families (i.e., home, school). Therapists have small, manageable caseloads so they can focus on client needs and truly engage with client and family. MST is an ecological approach, therefore therapists work closely with the schools, courts, social service agencies, and other health care providers. MST therapists are held accountable for treatment outcomes, and in some cases their rate of compensation is based upon demonstrating desired outcomes (Henggler, 2001; Henggeler & Hoyt, 2001).

Multisystemic therapy has been shown to be efficacious with very difficult-to-treat populations of children and adolescents who struggle with significant conduct and emotional problems (Kazdin, 2000). MST was found to effectively improve family functioning and family cohesion as well as to reduce delinquent peer affiliation and delinquent behavior with serious juvenile offenders (Huey, Henggeler, Brondino, & Pickrel, 2000). There is also recent research evidence that home-based MST may be more effective at decreasing externalized symptoms and improving family functioning and school attendance for children and adolescence with psychiatric emergencies than inpatient hospitalization (Henggeler et al. 1999). Finally, the theoretical underpinnings of MST are very much aligned with the developmental framework presented earlier in this chapter.

## Multisystemic Therapy

Multisystemic therapy (MST) is an intensive family- and community-based treatment that is designed to address the multiple factors associated with youth violence and delinquency (e.g., problems in school, trouble with peers and family, violent neighborhood). MST is designed to work with the individual and the interconnected sys-

## FAST Track

FAST Track is a comprehensive prevention program that targets severe conduct problems by using a multi-modal, early intervention approach. FAST Track is grounded in the notion that antisocial behaviors, such as violence and aggression, have multiple, interactive causes and therefore require multiple, cooperative interventions. FAST

Track intervenes at the level of the school, the home, and the individual and seeks to improve communication among these domains, as well as to increase problem-solving skills and coping mechanisms for the individual. The expected result is that disruptive and antisocial behavior will decrease in the home and at school (Conduct Problems Prevention Research Group, 1992).

The FAST Track Program focuses on the transition points in school (e.g., first grade, middle school) but spans grades 1 through 6. It includes a parent training component (e.g., effective discipline techniques, communication skills, techniques to foster academic achievement), which is followed by biweekly home visits to reinforce these parenting skills. In addition, the children receive individual social skills, peer relations, and anger management training that is augmented by classroom interventions (McMahon, Greenberg, & The Conduct Problems Prevention Research Group, 1995).

The FAST Track program is in the early stages of evaluation, but to date there is strong evidence that the program has contributed to improved social skills and peer relationships in the participating students. Additionally, parents who participated in the intervention evidenced more positive involvement in their children's academic progress and increased communication with the schools as well as more effective discipline strategies at home. The hope is that these intermediate outcomes will contribute to the long-term developmental outcome of decreased conduct problems (Conduct Problems Prevention Research Group, 1999a, 1999b).

## The Role of School Nurses and Health Professionals in Treatment and Intervention

The field of nursing has also developed programs that fit into the "best practices" model for violence prevention and intervention. For example, the Nurse-Family Partnership (NFP) has been recognized by the University of Colorado's Center for the Study and Prevention of Violence (1996) as a "Model Program" in violence prevention. The Nurse-Family Partnership is designed to improve prenatal health and the outcomes of pregnancy by having home visitors work with families from pregnancy through the first 2 years of the child's life. Through parent education and family care, the NFP has been linked to decreased instances of child abuse and neglect, decreased maternal substance abuse, and decreased child behavioral problems (Olds, Hill, Mlhalic & O'Brien, 1998).

Nursing's emphasis on both preventive care and intervention makes it particularly well suited to engage in violence prevention on both the individual and community domains (Beauchesne, Kelly, Lawrence, & Faquharson, 1997). For example, the school is in particular need of nurses and health professionals to aid in the struggle to stop violence (Strawhacker, 2002). Effective violence prevention in the schools requires the collaborative and cooperative efforts of principals, teachers, student support staff, families, and community agencies. School nurses and school health professionals play an important role in this prevention process because they are often the first people to see students after a violent encounter. School nurses and school health professionals are also in contact with primary care physicians, who are often a parent's first resource when a child is in trouble. It is critical that school health professionals be knowledgeable about how to detect abuse and violence as well as how to link students to proper resources for intervention and prevention (Gioiella, 1994; Ross et al., 1998).

Gance-Cleveland (2001) pointed to the Columbine shootings to reinforce how important it is for school nurses and health professionals to be aware of the climate in their schools and the risk factors for violence. In addition to recognizing the warning signs for violence (e.g., sense of powerlessness, feelings of rage, ostracization by peers) and attending to the presence of risk and protective factors outlined earlier in this chapter, school health professionals are positioned to design and evaluate violence prevention programs in the schools, engage in community outreach around violence prevention initiatives, and to advocate for legislation that supports violence prevention (Gance-Cleveland, 2001).

## Applied Prevention and Intervention

In applying a framework that accounts for the complex nature of aggression to the case of "John" that was introduced at the beginning of this chapter, we can see that there will not be a "one-shot cure" for his violent behavior. John's violent behavior seems to be the product of multiple risk factors that have been present over the course of his development. There is little evidence of interventions and scant evidence of any supports that are available to him.

John has grown up in a context where he witnesses violence in his family and his neighborhood. He has a history of violence that started when he was young and was incarcerated at a young age. Both of these factors place him at elevated risk for developing long-term conduct problems. His current peer group seems to endorse violence as a means of intimidation. In addition, John's substance use may be an attempt to self-medicate some of the internal disturbances that are contributing to his aggressive behavior. Finally, it is also crucial to note that John has been described as having a short temper, which could be indicative of biological factors that predispose him to aggression.

Mrs. Price is now faced with the daunting task of integrating all of the above information and formulating treatment recommendations. However, she cannot be expected to do this on her own. Clearly, one trip to the nurse's office is not going to permanently alter behavior that is complex and longstanding. Mrs. Price should seek out the school team that is charged with addressing the nonacademic barriers to learning. Stemming

the tide of aggressive and violent behavior will require nurses, physicians, psychologists, social workers, and school counselors to work together to assess the student's needs and design an intervention plan. These plans should take into account multiple contexts, bio-psycho-social domains, development over the life span, and potential sources of risk and resilience (Lerner, 1986)

Thus, a comprehensive treatment for John would address the biological (e.g., medication evaluation, substance abuse treatment), social (e.g., locating and accessing resources during out-of-school time), and psychological (e.g., individual counseling, family therapy) factors that contribute to his violent and aggressive behavior. It is critical that the treatment providers and adults in John's life recognize the full context in which these behaviors have developed and work in conjunction with one another so that the interventions and services are coordinated and effective. There is no one-shot intervention that will provide immediate relief for John, but through a concentrated effort, health practitioners and services providers can support and help John.

The goal of this unified support system will be to alter John's developmental path away from a consistent and stable pattern of antisocial and violent behavior. The adults in John's life can help him follow this positive path by working to decrease the risk factors for violence (e.g., exposure to family violence, association with a delinquent peer group, lack of adult supervision) and to introduce protective factors (e.g., increasing John's connectedness with the school, finding him a mentor, engaging him in prosocial after-school activities). It is critical to link John to these resources and supports as soon as possible before he seriously hurts himself or someone else.

# Conclusion

Earlier theories of aggression and violence helped us with our emergent understandings of the problem, but they often led to dichotomous thinking (e.g., explaining aggression as either learned or innate). As a result, aggression was conceptualized in a narrow and circumscribed manner, which in turn led to interventions that were simplistic. Professionals who work with violent and aggressive clients know from experience that attempting to reduce aggressive behavior to one or two root causes is unrealistic. In addition, these professionals may have been frustrated with interventions that did not take into account the complexity that they were seeing in their client's problems. For example, a health care professional may become very disheartened to find interventions that focus solely on anger management skills or medication treatment, when it is clear that there is much more contributing to the client's difficulty.

A more recent understanding of human development has helped us to recognize that the development of aggression and violence can be traced not only to individual traits but also to influences in the family, school, community, and society. Further, aggression does not develop in a universal manner across all people, but varies as a result of both the risk factors and supports that are in place as well as the developmental status of the person (e.g., child, adolescent, adult). This newer understanding of human development has lead to a much richer and deeper understanding of the roots and treatment of aggression and violence. It also reflects the significant complexity that practicing professionals experience in their day-to-day work with clients.

Finally, this more complex understanding of aggression has helped to provide a stronger base for prevention and intervention. Researchers now know that intervention and prevention efforts that impact multiple areas (e.g., the person, classroom, home, neighborhood) in a coordinated manner are more likely to be effective. Interventions must reflect the multifaceted nature of violence and aggression that characterizes clients in hospitals, clinics, mental health centers, and schools. As a result, health care professionals can feel better prepared to work together to pro-vide comprehensive treatment for both children and adults who manifest aggressive and violent behavior.

# References

American Psychiatric Association. (1994). *Diagnostic and statistical manual of mental disorders* (4th ed.). Washington, DC: Author.

Anderson, C. A., & Bushman, B. J. (2002). Effects of violent video games on aggressive behavior, aggressive cognition, aggressive affect, physiological arousal, and prosocial behavior: A meta-analytic review of the scientific literature. *Psychological Science, 12,* 353–359.

Archer, J. (1995). What can ethology offer the study of human aggression? *Aggressive Behavior, 21,* 243–255.

Bandura, A. (1965). Influence of models' reinforcement contingencies on the acquisition of imitative responses. *Journal of Personality and Social Psychology, 1,* 585–595.

Bandura, A. (1973). *Aggression: A social learning analysis.* New York: Holt.

Buamrind, D. (1991). Parenting styles and adolescent development. In R. M. Lerner, A. C. Petersen, & J. Brooks-Gunn (Eds.), *Encyclopedia of adolescence* (Volume 2, pp. 746–758). New York: Garland Publishing.

Baumrind, D. (1996). The discipline controversy revisited. *Family Relations, 45,* 405–414.

Beauchesne, M. A., Kelly, B. R., Lawrence, P. R., & Faquharson, P. E. (1997). Violence prevention: A community approach. *Journal of Pediatric Health Care, 11,* 155–164.

Bensley, L., & Van Eenwyk, J. (2001). Video games and real-life aggression: Review of the literature. *Journal of Adolescent Health, 29,* 244–257.

Berkowitz, L. (1989). Frustration-aggression hypothesis: Examination and reformulation. *Psychological Bulletin, 106,* 59–73.

Bing, L. (1992). *Do or die.* New York, NY: Harper Perennial.

Black, D. W. (with Larson, C. L.). (1999). *Bad boys, bad men: Confronting antisocial personality disorder.* New York: Oxford University Press.

Bushman, B. J., & Anderson, C. A. (2001). Media violence and the American public: Scientific facts versus media misinformation. *American Psychologist, 56,* 477–489.

Bushman, B. J., & Cooper, H. M. (1990). Effects of alcohol on human aggression: An integrative research review. *Psychological Bulletin, 107,* 341–354.

Cairns, R. B., & Cairns, B. D. (2000). The natural history and developmental functions of aggression. In A. J.

Sameroff, M. Lewis, & S. M. Miller (Eds.), *Handbook of Developmental Psychopathology* (2nd ed. pp. 403–429). Dordrecht, Netherlands: Kluwer Academic Publishers.

Center for the Study and Prevention of Violence. (1996). Blueprints for violence prevention. Retrieved February 20, 2003, from University of Colorado website *http://www.colorado.edu/cspv/blueprints/index.html*.

Coie, J. D., & Dodge, K. A. (1998). Aggression and antisocial behavior. In W. Damon and N. Eisenberg (Eds.), *Handbook of child psychology: Volume 3. Social, emotional and personality development* (5th ed., pp. 779–862). New York: Wiley.

Conduct Problems Prevention Research Group. (1992). A developmental and clinical model for the prevention of conduct disorders: The FAST Track Program. *Development and Psychopathology, 4,* 509–527.

Conduct Problems Prevention Research Group. (1999a). Initial impact of the Fast Track Prevention Trial for conduct problems: I. The high-risk sample. *Journal of Consulting and Clinical Psychology, 67,* 631–647.

Conduct Problems Prevention Research Group. (1999b). Initial impact of the Fast Track Prevention Trial for conduct problems: II. Classroom effects. *Journal of Consulting and Clinical Psychology, 67,* 648–657

Crick, N. R., & Dodge, K. A. (1999). 'Superiority' is in the eye of the beholder: A comment of Sutton, Smith, and Swettenham. *Social Development, 8,* 128–131.

Davitz, J. R. (1952). The effects of previous training on postfrustration behavior. *Journal of Abnormal & Social Psychology, 47,* 309–315.

Dill, J. C., & Anderson, C. A. (1995). Effects of frustration justification on hostile aggression. *Aggressive Behavior, 21,* 359–369.

Dill, K. E., & Dill, J. C. (1998). Video game violence: A review of the empirical literature. *Aggression and Violent Behavior, 3,* 407–428.

Dodge, K. A. (2000). Conduct Disorder. In A. J. Sameroff, M. Lewis, & S. M. Miller (Eds.), *Handbook of Developmental Psychopathology* (2nd ed. pp. 447–463). Dordrecht, Netherlands: Kluwer Academic Publishers.

Dodge, K. A. (2001). The science of youth violence prevention: Progressing from developmental epidemiology to efficacy to effectiveness to public policy. *American Journal of Preventive Medicine, 20*(1S), 63–70.

Dollard, J., Doob, L. W., Miller, N. E., Mowrer, O. H., Sears, R. R., Ford, C. S., et al. (1939). *Frustration and aggression.* Oxford, England: Yale University Press.

Elksnin, L. K., & Elksnin, N. (2000). Teaching parents to teach children to be prosocial. *Intervention in School and Clinic, 36,* 27–35.

Ericksen, J. R., & Henderson, A. D. (1992). Witnessing family violence: The children's experience. *Journal of Advanced Nursing, 17,* 1200–1209.

Eron, L. D., Huesmann, L. R., Lefkowitz, M. M., & Walder, L. O. (1972). Does television violence cause aggression? *American Psychologist, 27,* 253–263.

Frey, K. S., Hirschstein, M. K., & Guzzo, B. A. (2000). Second Step: Preventing aggression by promoting social competence. *Journal of Emotional and Behavioral Disorders, 8,* 102–122.

Gance-Cleveland, B. (2001). Pediatric nurses: Advocates against youth violence. *Journal of the Society of Pediatric Nurses, 6,* 133–142.

Geen, R. G. (2001). *Human aggression* (2nd ed.). Philadelphia, PA: Open University Press.

Gibbs, J. J. (1986). Alcohol consumption, cognition and context: Examining tavern violence. In A. Campbell & J. J. Gibbs (Eds.), *Violent transactions: The limits of personality.* Oxford: Basil Blackwell.

Gioiella, E. C. (1994). Reducing violence—The next curriculum imperative. *Journal of Professional Nursing, 10,* 130.

Goldstein, A. P. (1994). *The ecology of aggression.* New York: Plenum Publishers.

Graham, K., & Wells, S. (2001). Aggression among young adults in the social context of the bar. *Addiction Research and Theory, 9,* 193–219.

Greenberg, M. T., Kusche, C., & Mihalic, S. (1998). Promoting alternative thinking strategies (PATHS). In D. S. Elliott (Series Ed.), *Blueprints for violence prevention.* Boulder, CO: Center for the Study and Prevention of Violence, Institute of Behavioral Science, University of Colorado at Boulder.

Griffiths, M. (1999). Violent video games and aggression: A review of the literature. *Aggression and Violent Behavior, 4,* 203–212.

Hartup, W. W. (1974). Aggression in childhood: Developmental perspectives. *American Psychologist, 29,* 336–341.

Henggeler, S. D. (2001). Multisystemic therapy. *Residential Treatment for Children and Youth. Special Issue: Innovative Mental Health Interventions for Children: Programs that Work, 18*(3), 75–85.

Henggeler, S. W., & Hoyt, S. W. (2001). Multisystemic therapy with juvenile offenders and their families. In J. M. Richman & M. W. Fraser (Eds.), *The context of youth violence: Resilience, risk and protection.* Westport, CT: Praeger.

Henggeler, S. W., Rowland, M. D., Randall, J., Ward, D. M., Pickrel, S. G., Cunningham et al. (1999). Home-based multisystemic therapy as an alternative to the hospitalization of youths in psychiatric crisis: Clinical outcomes. *Journal of the American Academy of Child and Adolescent Psychiatry, 38,* 1331–1339.

Herzberger, S. D., & Hall, J. A. (1993). Consequences of retaliatory aggression against siblings and peers: Urban minority children's expectations. *Child Development, 64,* 1773–1785.

Huesmann, L. R., Eron, L. D., Lefkowitz, M. M., & Walder, L. O. (1973). Television violence and aggression: The causal effect remains. *American Psychologist, 28,* 617–620.

Huesmann, L. R., Moise, J. F., & Podolski, C. L. (1997). The effects of media violence on the development of antisocial behavior. In D. M. Stoff, J. Breiling, & J. D. Maser (Eds.), *Handbook of antisocial behavior* (pp. 181–193). New York: John Wiley & Sons.

Huey, S. J., Henggeler, S. W., Brondino, M. J., & Pickrel, S. G. (2000). Mechanisms of change in multisystemic therapy: Reducing delinquent behavior through therapist adherence and improved family and peer functioning. *Journal of Consulting and Clinical Psychology, 68,* 451–467.

Hune, J. B., & Nelson, C. M. (2002). Effects of teaching a problem-solving strategy on preschool children with problem behavior. *Behavioral Disorders, 27,* 185–207.

Kazdin, A. E. (1997). Conduct disorder across the lifespan. In S. S. Luthar, J. A. Burack, D. Cicchetti, & J. R. Weisz (Eds.), *Developmental psychopathology: Perspectives on adjustment, risk, and disorder* (pp. 248–272). New York: Cambridge University Press.

Kazdin, A. E. (2000). Treatments for aggressive and antisocial children. *Child and Adolescent Psychiatric Clinics of North America, 9,* 841–858.

Koss, M. P., Goodman, L. A., Browne, A., Fitzgerald, L. F., Keita, G. P., & Russo, N. F. (1994). *No safe haven: Male violence against women at home, at work, and in the community.* Washington, DC: American Psychological Association.

Kreuz, I. E., & Rose, R. M. (1972). Assessment of aggressive behavior and plasma testosterone in a young criminal population. *Psychosomatic Medicine, 34,* 321–322.

Kruesi, M. J., Rapoport, J. L., Hamburder, S., Hibbs, E., Potter, W. Z., Leanne, M., et al. (1990). Cerebrospinal fluid monoamine metabolites, aggression, and impulsivity in disruptive behavior disorders of children and adolescents. *Archives of General Psychiatry, 47,* 419–426.

Lerner, R. M. (1986). *Concepts and theories of human development* (2nd ed.). New York: Random House.

Lerner, R. M. (1995). *America's youth in crisis: challenges and options for programs and policies.* Thousand Oaks, CA: Sage.

Lester, D., & Goldney, R. D. (1997). An ethological perspective on suicidal behavior. *New Ideas in Psychology, 15,* 97–103.

Lorentz, K. (1966). *On aggression.* New York: Harcourt, Brace & World.

Maccoby, E. E., & Jacklin, C. N. (1980). Sex differences in aggression: A rejoinder and reprise. *Child Development, 51,* 964–980.

McGuffin, P., & Thapur, A. (1998). Genetics and antisocial personality disorder. In T. Millon, E. Simonsen, M. Birket-Smith, & R. D. Davis (Eds.), *Psychopathy:*

*Antisocial, criminal, and violent behavior.* New York: The Guilford Press.

McLaughlin, M. W., Irby, M. A., & Langman, J. (1994). *Urban sanctuaries: Neighborhood organizations in the lives and futures of inner city youth.* San Francisco, CA: Jossey-Bass.

McMahon, R. J., Greenberg, M. T., & the Conduct Problems Prevention Research Group. (1995). The FAST Track Program: A developmentally focused intervention for children with conduct problems. *Clinician's Research Digest, 13,* 1–2.

Moffit, T. E., & Caspi, A. (2001). Childhood predictors differentiate life-course persistent and adolescence-limited antisocial pathways among males and females. *Development and Psychopathology, 13,* 355–375.

Moffit, T. E., Caspi, A., Harrington, H., & Milne, B. J. (2002). Males on the life-course persistent and adolescence-limited antisocial pathways: Follow-up at age 26 years. *Development and Psychopathology, 14,* 179–207.

Olds, D., Hill, P., Mlhalic, S., & O'Brien, R. (1998). *Blueprints for violence prevention, book seven: Prenatal and infancy home visitation by nurses.* Boulder, CO: Center for the Study and Prevention of Violence.

Olweus, D. (1993). Bullies on the playground: The role of victimization. In C. H. Hart (Ed.), *Children on playgrounds: Research perspectives and applications* (pp. 85–128). Albany: State University of New York Press.

Olweus, D. (1994). Bullying at school: Long-term outcomes for the victims and an effective school-based intervention program. In L. R. Huesmann (Ed.), *Aggressive behavior: Current perspectives* (pp. 97–130). New York: Plenum Press.

Parke, R. D., & Slaby, R. G. (1983). The development of aggression. In P. H. Mussen (Ed.), *Handbook of child psychology* (Volume 4, pp. 548–641). New York, NY: John Wiley & Sons.

Patterson, G. R., Forgatch, M. S., Yoerger, K. L., & Stoolmiller, M. (1998). Variables that initiate and maintain an early onset trajectory for juvenile offending. *Development and Psychopathology, 10,* 531–547.

Perskey, H., Smith, K. D., & Basu, G. K. (1971). Relation of psychological measures of aggression and hostility to testosterone production in man. *Psychosomatic Medicine, 33,* 265–277.

Pettit, G. S., Polaha, J. A., & Mize, J. (2001). Perceptual and attributional processes in aggression and conduct problems. In J. Hill & B. Maughan, (Eds.), *Conduct disorders in childhood and adolescence* (pp. 292–319). New York, NY: Cambridge University Press.

Piaget, J. (1970). Piaget's theory. In P. H. Mussen (Ed.), *Carmichael's manual of child psychology* (Volume 1, pp. 703–732). New York, NY: John Wiley & Sons.

Pollack, W. S., & Shuster, T. (2000). *Real boys' voices*. New York, NY: Penguin Books.

Prothrow-Stith, D. (1993). *Deadly consequences*. New York: Harper Collins.

Prothrow-Stith, D. (1995). The epidemic of youth violence in America: Using public health prevention strategies to prevent violence. *Journal of Health Care for the Poor and Underserved, 6,* 95–101.

Ridenour, T. A., Cottler, L. B., Robins, L. N., Campton, W. M., Spitznagel, E. L., & Cunningham-Williams, R. M. (2002). Test of the plausibility of adolescent substance use playing a causal role in developing adulthood antisocial behavior. *Journal of Abnormal Psychology, 111,* 144–155.

Ross, M. M., Hoff, L. A., McComas, J., Carswell, A., Bunn, H., & Coutu-Wakulczyk, G. (1998). Strengthening the interdisciplinary education of nurses in violence prevention, detection and intervention. *Nurse Educator, 23*(3), 17–18.

Rothbart, M. K., & Bates, J. E. (1998). Temperament. In N. Eisenberg (Vol. Ed.) & W. Damon (Ed.), *Handbook of child psychology: Volume 3. Social, emotional and personality development* (5th ed., pp. 105–176). New York: Wiley.

Rothbart, M. K., & Danberry, D. (1981). Development of individual differences in temperament. In M. E. Lamb & A. L. Brown (Eds.), *Advances in child developmental psychology*. Hillsdale, NJ: Erlbaum.

Rubin, A. M., West, D. V., & Mitchell, W. S. (2001). Differences in aggression, attitudes towards women, and distrust as reflected in popular music preferences. *Media Psychology, 3,* 25–42.

Rutter, M. (2001). Psychosocial adversity: Risk, resilience, and recovery. In J. M. Richman & M. W. Fraser (Eds.), *The context of youth violence: Resilience, risk and protection*. Westport, CT: Praeger.

Salmon, G., James, A., & Cassidy, E. L. (2000). Bullying a review: Presentations to an adolescent psychiatric service and within a school for emotionally and behaviourally disturbed children. *Clinical Child Psychology & Psychiatry, 5,* 563–579.

Simmons, R. (2002). *Odd girl out: The hidden culture of aggression in girls*. New York, NY: Harcourt Trade Publishers.

Spivak, H., & Prothrow-Stith, D. (2001). The need to address bullying—An important component of violence prevention. *Journal of the American Medical Association. Special Issue, 285*(16), 2131–2132.

Steele, C. M., & Josephs, R. A. (1990). Alcohol myopia: Its prized and dangerous effects. *American Psychologist, 45,* 921–933.

Stop Family Violence (1999) Family violence statistics. Retrieved February 27, 2003, from *http://www.stopfamilyviolence.org/sfvo/stats_ca.html.*

Strawhacker, M. T. (2002). School violence: An overview. *Journal of School Nursing, 18*(2), 68–72.

Suomi, S. J. (2000). A biobehavioral perspective on developmental psychopathology: Excessive aggression and serotonergic dysfunction in monkeys. In A. J. Sameroff, M. Lewis, & S. M. Miller (Eds.), *Handbook of Developmental Psychopathology* (2nd ed., pp. 237–256). Dordrecht, Netherlands: Kluwer Academic Publishers.

Sutton, J., Smith, P. K., & Swettenham, J. (1999a). Social cognition and bullying: Social inadequacy or skilled manipulation? *British Journal of Developmental Psychology, 17*(3), 435–450.

Sutton, J., Smith, P. K., & Swettenham, J. (1999b). Bullying and 'theory of mind': A critique of the 'social skills deficit' view of anti-social behaviour. *Social Development, 8,* 117–127.

Tremblay, R. E., Japel, C., Perusse, D., Boivin, M., Zoccolillo, M., Montplaisir, J., et al. (1998). The search for the age of onset for physical aggression: Rousseau and Bandura revisited. *Criminal Behavior and Mental Health, 9*(1), 8–23.

U.S. Department of Health and Human Services (2001). Youth violence: *A report of the Surgeon General*. Washington, DC: U.S. Public Health Service. Available from *http://www.surgeongeneral.gov/library/youthviolence/chapter1/sec1.html.*

Vessey, J. A. (March, 1999). Bully-proof your child. *The Johns Hopkins Health Insider, 2*(4), 8.

Vessey, J. A., & Lee, J. E. (2000). Violent video games affecting our children. *Pediatric Nursing, 26,* 607–612.

Walsh, M. E., & Murphy, J. A. (2003). *Children, health and learning: A guide to the issues*. Westport, CT: Greenwood Publishing Group.

Wells, S., Graham, K., & West, P. (2000). Alcohol-related aggression in the general population. *Journal of Studies on Alcohol, 61,* 626–632.

Widom, C. S. (1989). Child abuse, neglect, and adult behavior: Research design and findings on criminality, violence, and child abuse. *American Journal of Orthopsychiatry, 59,* 355–367.

Wyatt, J. M., & Carlo, G. (2002). What will my parents think? Relations among adolescents' expected parental reactions, prosocial moral reasoning and prosocial and antisocial behaviors. *Journal of Adolescent Research, 17,* 646–666.

# Part Four

## TOWARD DEVELOPMENTALLY APPROPRIATE CARE

# Chapter 18

# Development of Children with Chronic Illness

Kathleen Thies

Three-year-old Deon is admitted to the hospital to rule out pneumonia—again. Born prematurely, he has bronchopulmonary dysplasia (BPD) and cerebral palsy. He also has delays in language acquisition. Irritable and difficult, he alternately clings to and rejects his mother while in the hospital, leading staff to question the quality of his parenting.

Nine-year-old Deanna and her mother are meeting with the assistant principal and nurse of Deanna's new school. The mother explains that her daughter was diagnosed with cystic fibrosis as an infant and that her health regimen at school includes taking dietary enzymes before meals and using inhalers as needed. The school nurse explains that she is in the building only two days each week. Deanna proudly announces that she can take her pills and use her inhalers by herself. The assistant principal asks Deanna's mother to sign a permission slip so that she can do so.

Twelve-year-old Nicole is at a restaurant with her traveling soccer team. When she takes her time in the bathroom, the coach checks on her and finds that she had been checking her blood glucose—which was fine. She feels like everyone is staring at her when she returns to her seat. Later, Nicole complains to the nurse in the clinic that

everyone is always watching her and she hates being different. Given Nicole's distress, the nurse wonders if a support group would help.

Sixteen-year-old John is on chemotherapy for the second time in 4 years. He has been difficult to deal with at home. His schoolwork has deteriorated. The morning of his sister's high school graduation, John goes dirt biking with friends and dislodges the catheter that was inserted into a large vein in his chest to accommodate administration of chemotherapy. It needs to be removed surgically immediately, and his doctor is clearly annoyed about it. His sister is furious with him and his friends for not being more careful. John tells her it's his life, so butt out.

Eighteen-year-old Ryan needs to have his wisdom teeth removed. His health insurance will not cover the costs of having the procedure in a same-day surgical center with general anesthesia, as recommended by his oral surgeon and requested by his parents. Ryan has Down syndrome. Dental visits have always been a challenge with Ryan, and no one is listening to their concerns that he will become frightened and thus uncooperative.

These are examples of children and adolescents with chronic health conditions. According to the

Social Securities Act of 1985, "children with special health care needs" include those with 1) developmental disabilities, mental retardation, and learning disabilities; 2) chronic medical illness, such as diabetes and asthma; and 3) emotional/behavioral difficulties, including attention deficit disorder (ADD) (Ireys, 1994). Health professionals typically use the term *chronic health condition* when referring to the first two of these groups, conditions that involve pathophysiology of and treatments for major body systems. About 6% to 15% of American children have a chronic condition that affects their physical health (Hoffman, Rice, & Sung, 1996) and potentially their developmental trajectory as well.

This group of children and adolescents constitute one of the "special" groups of patients cared for by health professionals in inpatient and community-based settings. Accreditation standards from the Joint Commission on Accreditation of Healthcare Organizations (JCAHO) stipulate that staff who care for "special" groups—for example, the young and old—must meet age-specific competencies. This has generated a surge of programs to train staff across disciplines to meet the JCAHO standards. Given the increased attention to evidenced-based practice, the JCAHO standard has created a two-pronged challenge. The first is to clarify the content of the "age-specific" knowledge base underlying competent practice. The second is to identify practice criteria by which staff competence can be assessed. That is, we lack the evidence that informs what *age-appropriate care* means, in theory and in practice.

The purpose of this chapter is to address the first challenge of age-appropriate care: that is, identifying some of the developmental knowledge necessary to provide care to children and adolescents. In the first part of the chapter, we examine the meaning of *age-appropriate care* from a developmental life span perspective and present the rationale for why *developmentally appropriate care* is the more suitable term. In the second part of the chapter, we apply developmental theory and research to the care of children and adolescents with chronic illness and disability.

# Age-Appropriate Versus Developmentally Appropriate Care

The lack of evidence for age-appropriate care reveals an interesting conundrum for several reasons. First, although there are theories of aging—for example, stochastic and nonstochastic explanations for how the body changes after it has reached maturity (Ebersole, Hess, & Luggen, 2004)—there is no theory of age per se. Age is a construct based on linear time. By itself, age does not guarantee development and, as a marker for predictable changes over time, is moderately associated with physical and psychosocial development at best (Rutter, 2002; Zigler & Glick, 1986). Age lacks a theoretical framework within which to build the research for evidence-based practice across the life span.

We propose that *age-appropriate care* can be revised as *developmentally appropriate care,* which by definition would be person and family centered, as well as culturally sensitive. It also would provide a theoretical framework for explaining the organization of physical and psychosocial change from the prenatal through the post maturity period.

Second, a great deal of research in the health professions has focused on adaptation to illness and disability, with an eye to developing models of care. Unfortunately, such models by their very nature are deficit driven. That is, illness and disability are the phenomena around which the model is developed. Because poor health is considered counter to normal experience, it is viewed as a stressor or threat to development. Although illness is indeed stressful, models of adaptation to illness that do not account for adaptation to life in general presume that the processes underlying normal development and response to stress are different, an assumption nullified by research on resilence in the face of chronic stress (Chapter 4 by Thies). For people with chronic illness and disability, especially children, adaptation to illness and to life is in fact the same thing.

Third, health professionals tend to separate adaptation to illness from normal development because we are woefully uninformed about the adaptive processes that contribute to development, normal or otherwise, in the first place. When we create models of adaptation to illness and disability without regard for theories of human development, we squander a valuable trove of research on which to base evidence for developmentally appropriate care, evidence that can help providers to support optimal growth and development in patients and families. A growing body of literature has begun to integrate models of normal development with clinical-developmental approaches to psychotherapy (Noam, 1998) and with developmental psychopathology (Cicchetti & Hinshaw, 2002; Rutter et al., 1997). This literature recognizes that the underlying processes are potentially the same, albeit organized differently and with different outcomes. To be effective clinicians, health care professionals more "at-home" with the exception need to become more familiar with the norm.

Fourth, developing standards for the appropriate care of the "special" group of children and adolescents with chronic conditions is complicated by the lack of a consistent definition of this group. Health care providers, educators, and state and federally funded programs use different formal and informal definitions, and for different purposes, including demographic research and eligibility for services (Thies, 1999). Using a developmental framework for the "appropriate care" for this "special" population would bypass the problem of illness, disability, or age as the defining criterion.

## A Developmental Perspective

Although several chapters in this book have addressed the meaning of a developmental life span perspective (see Chapter 3 by Lerner and Ashman and Chapter 4 by Thies), the basic concepts are worth repeating here. We review the developmental perspective, explain why *age* is not the same thing as *development,* and evaluate several existing conceptualizations of age-appropriate care in light of the developmental perspective. Key concepts of the developmental perspective are the relationship between the person and environment, organization, and change over time.

### THE RELATIONSHIP BETWEEN PERSON AND ENVIRONMENT

Bronfenbrenner's ecology of human development is familiar to most health care providers (Bronfenbrenner, 1979), sometimes referred to as a biopsychosocial approach to human development. As noted in earlier chapters, it is represented by expanding concentric rings of social influence, centered around the individual: immediate family (microsystem); immediate community of peers, school, and work (mesosystem); the larger social structures of society (exosystem); and finally culture and history (macrosystem). The "bio" aspect of the model has traditionally focused on what unique characteristics the individual brings to his/her relationship with the ecosystem, such as gender, temperament, or health status. However, we also have come to appreciate that biophysical aspects of the environment, such as air and water, as well as constructed aspects of the environment, such as shelter and transportation, contribute to development of the individual and family as well.

**Development Occurs Through Transactions Between Person and Environment.** Although the biopsychosocial model is familiar to health care professionals, most do not appreciate its implications for the complex relationship between the individual and the ecosystem. That relationship is characterized by reciprocal transactions; that is, people shape their environments and vice versa (Lerner, 1982, 1986; Sameroff, 1975). The relationship is dynamic. Both the person and the environment are constantly changing; they develop together and because of each other (Lerner, 1986).

On a micro level, the reciprocal shaping between child and environment occurs through multiple small transactions; through what is said and not said, and how; and through gestures, touching, attitudes, actions, and so on. For example, the second child is not born into the same family or to the same parents as the first child. The parents as individuals and the family structure as a whole have been changed by the presence of the first child. The characteristics of the first child—gender, temperament, health status, and so on—contribute to the parents' own development and expectations about the second child, all of which shape the first child in turn and so on over time, leading to the observation that persons create their own environments by being part of them (Scarr & McCartney, 1983).

As we move further out in the concentric rings of the biopsychosocial framework, transactions occur between individuals and groups of people and/or institutions, between groups and between institutions, and so on. The term *transaction* implies that each party is changed in some way by the relationship, whereas the term *interaction* does not have the same implication. For example, one child with a serious disability can have a profound affect on a local school budget. Conflicting policies between institutions (e.g., an insurance company and a hospital) may complicate access to care, which affects the child and the family. The emergence of special populations, such as those with developmental disabilities, affects public policy for everyone. Even macrosystems can change in response to individual development.

**Human Development and Biological Readiness.** Biological readiness to interact with the environment is key to development, in both typical and atypical developmental trajectories. Observation of healthy children leaves the impression that certain milestones are universal among human beings and thus appear to be genetically programmed in a way that is referred to as *canalization* (Waddington, 1966). Reflexes, when an infant rolls over, sits, stands, cuts first teeth, says first words, and so on, are so remarkably similar among healthy infants that all children seem to be moving down the same "canal" at the same pace in the first 3 years of life, regardless of environmental input.

Canalization makes clear that we cannot teach a newborn to crawl, a 6-month-old to walk, or a toddler to ride a bicycle. The key neurosensory and neuromuscular pathways have not yet developed, so the behavior cannot be learned until the child is ready. However, these physical abilities are the product of more than physical development; they represent the organization of multiple developmental systems at a point in time. For example, it is no accident of nature that infants develop depth perception at about the same time they learn to crawl.

Canalization leads to the common notion that development naturally unfolds in predetermined sequential stages, which is a misreading of developmental theory. This false belief is often referred to as the *ontogenetic fallacy*, the belief that individual development unfolds along its own unique course untouched by environmental events. The evidence does not support this understanding of development. The biologically ready organism develops because it can take advantage of the environment.

Example by exception illustrates the evidence for development as a product of the transaction between person and environment. An infant with physical and cognitive disabilities will not develop emotionally, socially, or intellectually in the expected way because the child is biologically not able to take advantage of her relationship with the environment in a manner that shapes typical development. Thus, on the one hand, we can see that the milestones that are the measure of typical development are based on observations of healthy children who bring their full developmental potential to their relationship with the environment. Their development did not "just happen." On the other hand, children with disabilities have a developmental trajectory that reflects the extent of their ability to make use of the environment, resulting in a developmental picture that is both similar to and yet different from the norm.

## DEVELOPMENT AS AN ORGANIZED PROCESS

Development is a process, that is, it is always happening across and within all levels of the ecosystem at the same time. Most clinicians are familiar with domains of development (physical, cognitive, emotional, etc.). A developmental perspective emphasizes the processes by which so-called domains of development work together, rather than discrete stages in each domain. A life span developmental perspective recognizes that we cannot explain human development by examining a person in cross-section at a point in time. The course of human development is actively embedded within an ecosystem of multiple levels of influence and dynamic transactions that occur concurrently within and between individuals and systems and in the context of history and over time (Lerner, Walsh, & Howard, 1998).

For example, we are familiar with biological processes that integrate perception with motor activity (see Chapter 9 by Eckrich and Strohmeyer on motor development). The attachment system organizes all domains into observable behaviors (see Chapter 6 by McCartney and O'Connor). In developmental psychology, we also refer to the self-system (Harter, 1999), the parenting system (Baumrind, 1978; Belsky, 1984), systems of peer relationships and social cognition (Fiske & Taylor, 1991; Hartup, 1983; Rubin, Bukowski, & Parker, 1998; Selman & Schultz, 1990), self-regulation as a system (Bronson, 2000), and so on. All of these systems involve multiple domains of development in organized and sometimes predictable patterns.

**The Hierarchical Integration of Development.** Although no one theory explains development, Werner (1957) has postulated that development proceeds from global diffusion through increasing differentiation to hierarchical integration. To interpret this principle as meaning that development proceeds from simple to complex would be an oversimplification. Mature development is hierarchically integrated, characterized by complexity, flexibility, and internalization. Mature behavior is mediated by thought. In this model, earlier, less mature levels of development continue to be accessible to mature individuals because early development provides the building material for and becomes integrated into later development, a phenomenon sometimes referred to as a *nested hierarchy.*

For example, it is not enough to say that a 9-year-old child is a concrete thinker. The child can still subscribe to more magical preoperational ways of thinking typical of preschool-aged children, and may do so, especially under duress (Thies, 1996; Thies & Walsh, 1999). It is unlikely that the 9-year-old can think abstractly, which tends to emerge in early adolescence and is associated with physical, social, and neurological changes. However, we cannot support development toward abstract thinking if we do not appreciate how a child became a concrete thinker beforehand.

Furthermore, we cannot appreciate the process of thinking if we are not clear what the child is thinking about; that is, the content of thought and the process of making sense are intricately related. Novel or anxiety-laden information and experiences may initially be processed at less mature levels of development regardless of age. We do not "regress" in such circumstances, a construct found in psychoanalytic theory (Freud, 1924/1952). In developmental theory, we would say that all of the domains of development are not organized at the same level of maturity, and that under duress we rely on patterns of organization that are familiar albeit less well organized or effective than we can manage under more optimal circumstances.

**Development as an Uneven Process.** The process of hierarchical integration is uneven because there is so much variation in the environment and the person's readiness to make sense of it. As a result, the mix and match among the domains of development at any one point in time yield a dynamic mosaic. A single person may have very mature and very immature levels of development coexisting within her understanding of herself and the world at the same time. For example, a child with health problems may be fairly sophisticated interacting with doctors and nurses and woefully inadequate interacting with peers. Similarly, two persons of the same age may be of very different developmental levels either because their experiences have been very different and/or their readiness to make sense of experience has been different.

**Cognition: The Primary Processor of Experience.** Human beings are active organisms who construct their understanding of the world through their ability to take in and make sense of environmental information (Piaget, 1950; White, 1976). The developmental perspective maintains that cognition is the primary processor of human experience, through the development of cognitive structures that become increasingly complex with maturity (Piaget, 1950) and which serve to organize experience, including emotion (Block, 1982; Sroufe, 1979). This premise is known as a cognitive-developmental approach to human development. Although Piaget did not refer specifically to brain structures, research in neuroscience recognizes the relationship between brain development and cognition (see Chapter 7 on cognitive development by Travers). The cognitive-developmental framework has implications for children whose neurodevelopment has been adversely affected by illness, disability, injury, or treatment (Brown, 1999), which is addressed later in this chapter.

### SENSITIVE PERIODS IN DEVELOPMENT

As noted in Chapter 4 by Thies on resilience, there appear to be sensitive periods for optimal development in any one individual in selected areas, such as attachment to caregivers (Chapter 6 by McCartney and O'Connor) and language

(Chapter 7 by Travers). Time is critical in the historical sense, within and between cohorts and cultures. Americans born in the 1920s versus the 1950s grew up with different resources and expectations (Elder, 1995). Similarly, children born in the 1980s may share the same historical time period, but American and Eastern European members of this cohort have experienced the time very differently. Important transitions and events occur at points in time in a person's life, reshaping that person's developmental trajectory and potentially the trajectory of generations to follow (Bronfenbrenner & Ceci, 1994; Rutter, 1996).

## Toward Developmentally Appropriate Care

Although health care has used developmental theories—especially those of Erikson and Piaget—to *describe* life stages, we have not applied a developmental framework to *explain* how development and human response to illness are integrated. Using ages and stages to describe human development is a convenient heuristic, but it is one that an appreciation for the principles of human development reveals as unnecessarily simplistic and possibly misleading.

### EXAMPLE BY EXCEPTION: CHILDREN WITH DEVELOPMENTAL DISABILITIES

Exceptions often help to illustrate the rule. Children with developmental disabilities provide an excellent test case for why age-appropriate care falls short of its intention for children with and without disabilities. For example, children with Down syndrome have a wide range of intellectual, social, and physical potential. Despite delays in reaching normative developmental milestones, these children display coherence in the organization of their development that reflects developmental trends while at the same time is uniquely their own.

Attachment to caregivers, play behavior, and sense of humor in children with Down syndrome emerge in more or less the same sequence as in children who are not mentally retarded and tend to be organized similarly (Beeghly & Cicchetti, 1987; Beeghly, Perry, & Cicchetti, 1989; Cicchetti & Beeghly, 1990; Cicchetti & Sroufe, 1976). For example, for both infants with Down syndrome and those who develop typically, physical humor emerges first. Appreciating physical humor is based on the tension associated with anticipating an expected result from an action and the release of tension when something different and pleasantly surprising happens instead.

The later timing of the emergence of a sense of humor in children with Down syndrome reflects delays in their development but also that the cognitive, affective, and social systems that make up humor are organized in a way similar to cognitively comparable children who are not retarded when humor does emerge. Similarly, these systems work together to support the development of the symbols required for attachment behavior, communication, and play much as they do in normal development. For example, a block can be a car and "drive" across the floor.

Other examples by exception involve the physical development of children with Down syndrome. When sitting unsupported in a room that tilts visually but not actually, normal infants reach out to steady themselves, the visual feedback telling them they are off balance even though postural feedback says they are not. By comparison, those with Down syndrome are older when they sit alone, but do not perceive the discrepancy between visual and postural feedback in the "tilting" room and so do not reach out (Butterworth & Cicchetti, 1978). In other words, the perceptual-sensory-motor system of children with neurodevelopmental disabilities is organized differently than is typical, so that physical milestones not only emerge later but present a different neuromotor clinical picture (Capute & Accardo, 1996), especially regarding balance—a potential safety issue in their care.

Persons with Down syndrome also tend to have soft neurological signs, consistent with hypotonia.

A small oral cavity and soft jaw and mouth musculature contribute to drooling but also increase the risks associated with choking and suctioning. Developmentally appropriate mouth care, feeding, and assisted ventilation need to consider not only these physical differences, but the health care professional also needs to take cognitive differences into account when explaining medical procedures to a person with Down syndrome. In the case of Ryan, the teenager with Down syndrome who was introduced at the beginning of this chapter and who needs his wisdom teeth removed, his physical and cognitive-behavioral development require modifications in his care while treating him like the teenager he is (Chapter 13 by Singer).

We can see that using age as the criterion for appropriateness of care represents an atheoretical approach to care that ultimately undermines its effectiveness. Similarly, assuming that a 9-year-old with Down syndrome is at the same developmental stage as a typical 4-year-old is neither accurate nor effective for either child. Example by exception tells us a great deal about the organization of development in both typical and atypical trajectories.

## AGE, STAGE, AND DEVELOPMENT

The example of individuals with Down syndrome helps make the case for why age-appropriate care is a misnomer:

- Age does not equal stage.
- Age does not equal development.
- Age does not equal maturity (Rutter, 2002).

Age, stage, and development may be related, but they are not the same thing. Age, stage, and development are most closely related during the highly canalized period of the first 3 years of normal growth and development. However, the relationship among age, stage, and development becomes more variable over time in healthy populations and is different in those with developmental disabilities from the outset. There can be predictable developmental trends in a relatively homogenous cohort exposed to similar life experiences and culture, for example, healthy middle-class white American children born during the 1950s. However, there is sufficient variation in individual makeup and experience such that developmental trends can paint only the broadest strokes of a complex picture. As Eckrich and Strohmeyer point out in Chapter 9, the concept of *average* motor ability becomes less appropriate as people grow older.

The developmental perspective may momentarily confound the health care provider who is comfortable with the stage heuristic. Also, the addition of *developmentally appropriate* to the lexicon of philosophies of care may seem taxing. We have care that is *person-centered, family-centered* (Institute for Family-Centered Care, 2003; Shelton & Stepanek, 1994), *community-based* (Hunt, 1998), and *culturally sensitive* (Bonder, Martin, & Miracle, 2002). On closer inspection, we see that the person, family, community, and culture are all part of the ecology of human development (Bronfenbrenner, 1979; Bronfenbrenner & Ceci, 1994).

Care that is developmentally appropriate must also be appropriate for individual persons and families in their communities and cultures. Individual human development is embedded within these spheres and cannot be considered apart from them. The case can be made that a life span developmental perspective can provide the overarching theoretical framework to establish "appropriate" standards of care for all persons regardless of age, ability, health status, and culture.

## LESSONS LEARNED FROM OTHER FIELDS

Early childhood educators are ahead of most health professionals in appreciating the concept of developmental appropriateness. Developmentally appropriate educational practices are those that are both age appropriate and individually appropriate (Bredekamp, 1987/1993). Age is used as a criterion because of the canalization of early growth and development in healthy children in

the first 3 to 5 years. Knowledge of the typical developmental trajectory enables teachers to provide an environment that will promote its development. Individual appropriateness recognizes that individual differences exist within even a homogenous cohort and that all children do not march in step along one developmental path.

Those who work with special populations, such as those with developmental and learning disabilities, also appreciate that a developmental approach to individual and family interventions is superior to one based on age (Shelton & Stepanek, 1994) (Chapter 13 by Singer, Chapter 14 by Hauser-Cram). A careful assessment of current and previous functioning in all of the domains of development coupled with close observation of the organization of behavior is the foundation for interventions that are appropriate for the individual and his/her needs and potential. Although these fields have their challenges, they have attempted to use a theoretical framework to develop their standards for care and education, rather than rely on age.

By comparison, age-appropriate care for both children and elders has focused on accommodating presenting physical characteristics. For example, equipment and supplies such as catheters and medications must be appropriate for small and aging bodies, respectively. Similarly, an appreciation for physical differences in oxygen exchange and the liver's ability to metabolize medications has led to modifications in therapeutic interventions. To this end, age-appropriate approaches to care for pediatric patients have included improving team organization to maximize the use of discipline-specific specialty knowledge in complex situations, such as trauma and subacute care (Grebin & Kaplan, 1995; Long, Katz, & Pokorni, 1989; Schweer & Ose, 1995).

Appropriate care of elders has also focused on "concerns" and areas of "need" common among clients requiring nursing care. Areas of concern include the psychosocial, physical, and educational; communication; the involvement of family and/or significant others; as well as special factors and stressors that might be predicted within each age group. These factors were based on "general information about developmental stages and other age-dependent factors" (Hall, 1999, p. 243). Areas of need address the "normal changes that occur as individuals age and the effects those changes have on individuals' responses to the disease process" (Travis & Duer, 1999, p. 105).

## Conclusion

The case can be made that a developmental perspective can provide the overarching theoretical framework to establish "appropriate" standards of care for all persons regardless of age, ability, health status, and culture. It is especially fitting for children and adolescents who have chronic health conditions that affect how their physical, cognitive, and social development is organized. In the next section, we review a large body of research that has identified predictable normative trends in cognitive, emotional, and social development, and identify implications for how children with chronic conditions adapt not just to illness but to life with illness.

# Developmental Trends in Children and Adolescents: Toward Developmentally Appropriate Care

This section focuses on the development of the individual child and adolescent, rather than on family development. In particular, we focus on normative developmental trends in emotional development (Saarni, Mumme, & Campos, 1998), concepts of self (Harter, 1999) and other (Selman & Schultz, 1991), perceptions of control (Connell, 1985; Rothbaum, Weisz, & Snyder, 1982), and coping (Donaldson, Prinstein, Danovsky, & Spirito, 2000; Knapp, Stark, Kurkjian, & Spirito, 1991). These domains of development have been shown to have implications for children and adolescents with chronic illness in the following areas: understanding illness (Bibace & Walsh, 1981), appraising and coping with illness-related stress (Spirito, Stark, Gil, & Tyc, 1995; Spirito, Stark, & Williams, 1988; Thies, 1994; Thies & Walsh, 1999), psychosocial adjustment (Thompson & Gustafson, 1996; Wallander, Thompson, & Alriksson-Schmidt, 2003), adherence to medical regimens (see Chapter 19 on adherence by Nansel), and resilience (see Chapter 4 on resilience by Thies). Implications for developmentally appropriate care for children and adolescents with chronic conditions are integrated into the review.

It is important to note that most of the research involved presumably healthy middle-class American children, unless otherwise noted. Furthermore, given that most of the research used a cognitive-developmental framework, the subjects can be considered to be cognitively normal. In addition, as much of the research involved either interviews with children or the use of self-reports by children, the findings are necessarily influenced by children's use of language. That is, children's ability to discuss a phenomenon may not do justice to their ability to understand it. This is a well-recognized weakness of research with child subjects.

## Cognition: Knowledge of Illness

Travers has reviewed the major theories and characteristics of cognitive development in Chapter 7. Cognition incorporates development of the neurological structures that support biological readiness for hand-eye coordination, visual and auditory scanning, memory, and language, as well as how information is processed and in what context. Theories of how children learn include Vygotsky's (1978) zone of proximal development, which is the area between what children are able to accomplish on their own and what they are able to do with maximum support. A corollary is teaching through scaffolding, in which the environment provides the supports for learning (Bruner & Haste, 1987).

For the purposes of this chapter, we address cognition as an organizer of experience in the neo-Piagetian sense, particularly regarding how children report their understanding of illness (Bibace & Walsh, 1981). Nevertheless, a neo-Piagetian construction of illness should not be confused with models of information processing that have implications for the learning styles of children, especially those with learning differences in auditory processing, attention, and memory.

Children's conceptual development of illness follows the predictable Piagetian developmental trend: preoperational, concrete logical, and early and abstract logical. This trend reflects qualitative, not quantitative, differences in complexity, causality, and reference (external vs. internal cues). However, the relationship between a child's age and Piagetian stage is not absolute and may be domain specific. Remember that development is uneven. For example, children's conceptualization of illness tends to lag behind their more basic knowledge of physical causality (Bearison, 1998; Thompson & Gustafson, 1996). That is, it would not be unusual for a young person who is capable of abstract thinking in science to conceptualize illness in a way more typical for a concrete thinker. Indeed, many adolescents and adults have a very concrete understanding of the human body and thus of its pathophysiology.

It is easy to assume that children with chronic illness mature faster in their knowledge of illness than peers. However, this assumption confuses quantitative and qualitative differences in knowing. For example, 9-year-old concrete thinkers can reel off reams of facts about baseball players, rock collections, soccer, diabetes, and so on—whatever is salient to them. Similarly, children's script knowledge of recurring events, including medical events, is highly schematic, detailed, and more accurate with age and time (Bearison, 1998), leav-

ing the impression that children with chronic illness are more mature in their understanding of illness than would be expected for their age.

It is important for the clinician to realize that knowing *more* is not the same thing as *how* knowing is organized, or what one does with the knowledge. The evidence suggests that children's conceptualization of health and illness does not outpace their developmental level (Bearison, 1998). That is, a 9-year-old concrete thinker may know more, but does not have the cognitive flexibility and complexity of an early abstract thinker of age 13.

## PRESCHOOL: AGES 3 TO 6

Preoperational thinkers describe illness in terms of phenomena and contagion (Bibace & Walsh, 1981). An illness is its associated activities or symptoms. For example, Deon, the young child with broncopulmonary dysplasia and mild cerebral palsy introduced at the beginning of this chapter, might describe his illness as when "I breathe with the tube [oxygen] at night." He appreciates the scripted ritual involved in his care, for example, putting his leg braces on, but could not explain it or reproduce it on his own.

The outward appearance of illness and disability are especially salient to very young children. If they cannot observe a phenomenon, such as the inside of the body, it is not meaningful to them. Therefore, they do not perceive a person with an invisible illness as different. Illness has a negative physical and moral valence; not only does it hurt, but people who get it are perceived as bad. Because young children cannot anticipate that something good will come from something bad, medical interventions that hurt cannot be helpful. For preoperational thinkers, illness just happens by chance, like magic, and so all illness is contagious (Bibace & Walsh, 1981). Indeed, many adults during the early days of the AIDS crisis were all too willing to subscribe to primitive beliefs about how the virus is spread, due in part to illogical fear.

## EARLY TO MIDDLE CHILDHOOD: AGES 6 TO 10

The concrete thinker describes illness as a sequence of causal events, with external origins, which can be reversed (Bibace & Walsh, 1981). The body is a machine: it malfunctions; you fix it. Nine-year-old Deanna might tell you that "sometimes the tubes in my lungs get clogged up and I can't breathe and the inhaler unclogs them." She knows that something may hurt before she can feel better, such as her chest physical therapy.

Concrete thinkers love rules because rules make life predictable and manageable. Deanna can have the scripted routine and language of a medical regimen down pat—"I always take my enzymes at 11:30 because I have lunch at noon." She can tell you all about cystic fibrosis. However, it is easy to read too much into her self-confidence. Difficulties with problem solving in the face of irregularities in either the illness or routine reveal a lack of cognitive flexibility and depth of understanding. What if she takes her enzymes at 11:30 but there is a fire drill at 11:45, and she doesn't get lunch until 12:30? Deanna may have learned a rule to fit this situation, but applying it when needed, under duress, or in novel circumstances, is another story. Indeed, variation in routine may confuse and upset the concrete thinker, and she will tell you that you are doing "it" all wrong.

The school wants to know when Deanna can manage her illness by herself. The lesson of a developmental approach to adherence is that independence is a false goal at any age. The question is not when she can manage alone but how she can manage which aspects of her illness with what support at which point in time. Factors that need to be considered include how she understands her illness and the health regimen (propositional and procedural knowledge), how she learns, her interpretation of symptoms, her motivation to manage the illness, her psychomotor ability, variations in the illness itself, environmental supports (parents, school personnel, peers), and so on (Chapter 19 by Nansel) (Iannotti & Bush, 1993). In other words, knowing about cystic fibrosis and being able to take pills at a certain time are necessary but not sufficient for illness self-management.

## EARLY TO LATE ADOLESCENCE: AGES 11 TO 17

The young adolescent/older child can demonstrate early abstract thinking in selected areas of knowledge, whereas abstract thinking across multiple domains is more typical later in the teen years and into young adulthood. For the early abstract thinker, the body is still a machine but now has multiple interacting parts. Illness is an internal process involving multiple causes and effects (Bibace & Walsh, 1981). Twelve-year-old Nicole might explain her diabetes this way: "you need insulin to make energy out of food, otherwise it stays in your bloodstream as sugar and that's why my readings are high sometimes."

With maturity, conceptions of illness become more complex, with a greater appreciation for internal versus external cues, multiple interacting causes and effects, and less vulnerability to chance occurrence (Bearison, 1998). The more mature abstract thinker explains how multiple causes and effects interact by describing transformations at the cellular level (Bibace & Walsh, 1981): "Insulin lets glucose into the cell where it is made into energy. My pancreas doesn't make enough insulin so I take it as a shot, but I still have to check to make sure my blood sugar isn't too high or too low because sometimes it's hard to balance how much I eat with how much insulin I use." High versus low blood glucose levels have different causes and effects, so interventions can be tailored to the specific circumstances.

Nicole may provide an early abstract explanation of her illness—perhaps she has learned it well by rote—but still be relatively rule-bound in how she manages it. Again, development is uneven. By her mid-teen years, she may be more flexible cognitively and could troubleshoot high and low blood glucose readings on her own under optimal and predictable circumstances, for example, during a soccer game when a coach, family, or friends who know about her illness are present.

As a person capable of abstract thinking, John, the 16-year-old on chemotherapy, should be able to appreciate the relatively concrete mechanics of having a catheter in his chest and the implications for physical activity, such as falling off of a dirt bike. In his case, his risk-taking behavior may have more to do with his sense of self than with his ability to understand his illness and its management. Again, development is uneven, and adherence is complicated.

Although Ryan is 18 years old, it is difficult to assess his concept of illness or of a medical procedure, in part because of language difficulties common among some people with Down syndrome. Thus, there is insufficient evidence regarding his cognitive-developmental level in the neo-Piagetian sense. Although many persons with mental retardation are capable of some concrete reasoning, functional assessments are often more effective with individuals with neurodevelopmental disabilities (Msall, 1996).

## Implications of Knowledge for Adherence and Management

As was the case with Deanna, knowledge about an illness and a health regimen are necessary but not sufficient for adherence and self-management. As Nansel points out in Chapter 19, adherence integrates physical, cognitive, and psychosocial aspects of development. As some illnesses and their treatments have known cognitive implications for memory, attention, and concentration, allowances for individual differences in intellectual ability need to be incorporated into standards for developmentally appropriate care as well (Brown, 1999; Brown & Sawyer, 1998; Thies, 1999).

## Emotion, Control, and Coping

Emotional development incorporates physiological arousal (Lazarus, 1984; Piaget, [1950] 1981), self-regulation and control (Bronson, 2000;

Selman & Schultz, 1991), and the social-cognitive ability to interpret the emotional meaning in situations (Saarni et al. 1998). Emotional valence—whether something feels "good" or "bad"—is the cornerstone of emotional development beginning in infancy. Intense negative valence is especially salient as well as highly adaptive because it is often experienced as a sympathetic "fight or flight" response to actual or perceived threat (Darwin, 1859; Izard, 1977). Together, psychological meaning of events, negative emotion states, and sympathetic arousal are a powerful and sophisticated integrated system that can either serve us well or wear us down (McEwen, 2002).

Reasons for behavior, especially in response to a situation with a negative valence, follow a developmental trend from external to internal sources of motivation and control (Ryan & Connell, 1989). A person is externally motivated when he or she acts to follow the rules and avoid punishment: "Because I'm supposed to. Because I'll get in trouble." Introjected reasons for behavior include taking on the values of someone else, especially to please or avoid displeasing the other or self: "Because I want people to like me. Because I'll feel badly if I don't."

Mature individuals act based on standards and values that they have identified as their own: "Because I think it's important. Because I want to learn it." Interestingly, regardless of age and maturity, we need no reason for doing something with a positive valence other than intrinsic pleasure (White, 1959), which also may be accompanied by a parasympathetic response (McEwen, 2002): "It's fun." "I like it."

The developmental trend in control also moves from the external to the internal. It begins by attributing control to some unknown factors ("I don't know"), moves toward the external ("powerful others are in control"), and then to the more mature internal ("I am in control") (Connell, 1985; Harter & Connell, 1984). A truly mature control is neither external nor internal; rather, the mature person has sufficient self-control and flexibility to assume or relinquish control as the situation warrants (Deci & Ryan, 1985, 1987).

Not surprisingly, coping and control are related. Coping using primary control involves externally oriented efforts to shape events through some type of activity. Doing something about it, thinking about something else, and telling other people what to do are examples. Coping using secondary control is an internally directed effort to modify one's own subjective psychological state. Secondary control can include external activities, but the goal is internal (e.g., doing something so that you feel good about yourself or talking a situation out with a trusted friend). Other examples include developing introspective insight, changing how you think about something so that you can change how you feel about it, and telling yourself you're OK (Rothbaum et al., 1982).

The development of problem- and emotion-focused coping also demonstrates externalizing and internalizing trends. Like primary control, problem-focused coping is more action oriented, such as doing something. Emotion-focused coping is similar to secondary control. Efforts to manage feelings include the generally less mature (and less effective) wishful thinking and avoidance as well as the more mature changing how one feels. Effective emotion-focused coping, like secondary control, develops later because of its internal focus. With maturity and experience, children develop a broader variety of both emotion- and problem-focused coping mechanisms and are more effective at selecting one appropriate for the situation (Donaldson et al., 2000; Knapp et al., 1991; Spirito et al., 1988).

## PRESCHOOL: AGES 3 TO 6

Preschool-aged children name their feelings and recognize them in others, with variations on happy, mad, sad, and scared. They realize that a feeling is associated with an external event ("he was mean"), but their appraisal of a stressful situation focuses on the experience of being upset rather than its cause (Harter, 1988; Selman &

Schultz, 1991; Thies & Walsh, 1999). Intense negative feelings are physiological and psychological intrusions into a sense of self, so that "being mad" and "being bad" become the same. Very young children may experience shame and guilt, as Erikson (1950) suggested, but they lack the linguistic and introspective maturity to identify these emotions. Shame is feeling "bad."

They aren't always sure who or what is control of a situation or why they behave as they do (Connell, 1985; Thies, 1994): "I don't know." Their coping repertoire may complement the physical and emotional experience of intrusion (e.g., a meltdown, striking out)—unless the environment supports self-regulation (Bronson, 2000; Selman & Schultz, 1991), for example, holding the child or redirecting the child's attention using calm but firm words. Becoming a civilized human being is a key developmental task for this age group.

For young Deon, who has cerebral palsy, and other children with neurodevelopmental disabilities, emotional self-regulation and attachment behaviors to caregivers may be organized differently than in typically developing children, due to the dissociation of development in cognitive, motor, and behavioral systems (Capute & Accardo, 1996; Carlson, Samson, & Sroufe, 2003; Shapiro, 1996). For Deon, physiological self-regulation may be further compromised by the side effects of medical treatments. For example, beta-agonist bronchodilators and prednisone, used in BPD, contribute to irritability and poor sleep. Medical and nursing staff who have concerns about the quality of parenting need to assess the attachment relationship between Deon and his mother using standards developed for special populations (Shapiro, 1996; Szymanski & King, 1999).

## EARLY TO MIDDLE CHILDHOOD: AGES 6 TO 10

By the time they enter school, children appreciate that the link between external situations and internal emotions is causal rather than associative (Saarni et al., 1998). They prefer to identify distress as caused by events and other people, whereas good feelings are part of the self (Harter, 1985). Indeed, they see their own behaviors as the primary cause of good outcomes in most situations and are less likely to find themselves at fault when things do not go well (Connell, 1985; Harter, 1999). This tendency helps to explain the overconfidence of school-aged children in their ability to manage their illness, such as 9-year-old Deanna, who has cystic fibrosis. She does not appreciate that supportive adults, such as her mother and the nurse at her former school, have contributed to her history of good health outcomes.

Concrete school-age thinkers classify emotions along two dimensions—intensity (level of arousal) and valence—a classification system that continues to serve young adults reasonably well (Russell & Ridgeway, 1983; Smith & Ellsworth, 1985). That is, one can be very happy or a little sad. However, the child is less likely to differentiate among internal feelings, such as feeling angry and guilty at the same time. Interestingly, children ages 8 to 9 with chronic illness report being moderately sad equally and moderately angry in comparison to older children and adolescents when asked about illness-related feelings (Thies & Walsh, 1999).

**Social-Emotional Expression.** By ages 8 to 10, children know the social rules governing emotional expression (Saarni et al., 1998). They display socially appropriate feelings even if they don't feel them, or will hide feelings as a way of avoiding trouble or embarrassment. For example, Deanna might insist that she is fine when she is not so that her teacher leaves her alone. This can lead to emotional displays inappropriate for the situation, such as smiling when upset. Older and emotionally more mature school-aged children begin to develop a second-person perspective: they can put themselves in another's shoes. They can empathize with another, but they also know they can hurt someone else's feelings by breaking

the social rules that discourage acting on mean intentions—and will do so (Selman & Schultz, 1991). Deanna's friends know they can hurt her feelings by teasing her, even though they know they shouldn't.

**Control, Coping, and Appraisal.** In general, strategies to regulate distress focus on primary control that is externally oriented (Band & Weisz, 1990; Bearison, 1998; Deci & Ryan, 1987) For example, Deanna may try to change an illness-related stressor, such as being teased, by telling a peer what to do ("Leave me alone!"), or she might just try to get away (Selman & Schultz, 1991). Another example includes substituting pleasant thoughts for unpleasant ones (Carroll & Steward, 1984) ("I thought about how I was going to play with my friends after school.").

As concrete thinkers, school-aged children are not terribly introspective. Thinking about something pleasant is a kind of primary control coping and centers on thinking about different events as a distraction rather than on developing insight about the relationship between current events and feelings. The latter strategy, which is both more secondary and emotion focused, develops with experience and support (Band & Weisz, 1990; Bearison, 1998).

Compliance with rules to avoid trouble is a strong source of motivation also linked to primary control that emerges during this period: "I have to or else" (Ryan & Connell, 1989). For example, 9-year-old Deanna when asked what is "hard" about having cystic fibrosis might say, "I sometimes have to leave the playground during recess because I need to use the inhaler." When asked why she did this, she would reply, "If I don't use the inhaler, my breathing will get worse and then the nurse calls my mother." Primary forms of control that involve avoiding consequences are often given by this age group as the reason for acting as they do to manage distress (Band & Weisz, 1990; Thies, 1994; Thies & Walsh, 1999). This form of primary control is operative across the life span.

## LATE CHILDHOOD TO EARLY ADOLESCENCE: AGES 10 TO 13

Ages 10 to 13 mark a transitional period between childhood and adolescence, characterized by emerging self-awareness, fickle emotions, and conflict (Elkind, 1984). Internal emotional experience becomes better differentiated (e.g., feeling two emotions such as sad and relieved at the same time, or liking and not liking the same person at the same time) so that emotional conflict and ambivalence begin to churn (Harter, 1986; Whitesell & Harter, 1989). Nicole, the 12-year-old with diabetes, may be both annoyed that her coach checked up on her and somewhat relieved at the same time (emotions she prefers to not display, which by itself causes conflict).

The second-person perspective becomes well established as transitional children realize that players on both sides of a relationship have their own thoughts and feelings (Selman & Schultz, 1991). Nicole is aware that she might stare at a friend returning from the bathroom just as her friends are staring at her. She is also aware that positive and negative feelings can arise from both external events and from her own inner thoughts (Harris, 1985), perhaps feeling guilty that she would be annoyed with friends for the very behavior she herself would display if the situation were reversed.

**Control, Coping, and Appraisal.** There begins a subtle integration of the interpretation of arousal, the management of affective disequilibrium, and the rules for the expression of emotion. By age 13, young adolescents realize that parents have both emotional and behavioral expectations for them, and their internal distress is related to perceptions of competence in fulfilling these expectations (Phares & Compas, 1990). Nicole realizes that others expect her to be increasingly competent in managing not only her diabetes but also emotional distress.

When inner experience becomes open to evaluation, and negative feelings arise from inner states, there follows the expectation that affective disequilibrium should be managed internally as well. Increasingly, both appraising illness-related stress and the response to it revolves around meeting the expectations of other people and avoiding their disapproval (Thies, 1996; Thies & Walsh, 1999). For Nicole, being liked by her friends and being competent in managing her diabetes are both at stake in the incident at the restaurant. She hoped to avoid embarrassment and scrutiny by leaving the table to check blood glucose, while at the same appearing to be self-sufficient. Effective emotion-focused coping can develop more fully now, but then again, it may not if the support is not in place.

## ADOLESCENCE: AGES 13 TO 17

With the onset of abstract complex thinking, adolescents begin to distinguish how situations, their own feelings and behavior, and the feelings and behavior of others work together (Harris, 1985). Emotions are understood to have several layers of causes (Nannis, 1988). The link between situations and emotions is mediated by a conscious inner dialogue, which by itself can be a source of distress. Adolescents can live in their heads (Elkind, 1984), so John, the 16-year-old on chemotherapy, reports that just thinking about his cancer can be stressful (Thies & Walsh, 1999). Perhaps because of this, adolescents with chronic illness also report being more frustrated and upset than younger peers during illness-related stress, although they are equally angry. Indeed, adolescents report more overall negative emotions in general (Thies & Walsh, 1999).

**Social-Emotional Awareness.** Adolescents can take a third-person perspective (Selman, 1980). That is, John can stand outside of himself and observe himself interacting with his friends and sister (Selman & Schultz, 1991). He is aware of being aware of himself. For John, like other adolescents with and without illness, evaluating the self he observes is a source of distress because he measures himself against standards for behavior that he has begun to internalize but not may meet (Harter, 1985, 1988; Thies, 1996; Thies & Walsh, 1999). At the same time, understanding the emotional needs of others, such as his sister (Selman & Schultz, 1991), and managing distress through introspection is becoming important to him (Nannis, 1988), even if he is not effective at doing so.

**Control, Coping, and Appraisal.**   Strategies to manage distress expand during adolescence to include secondary forms of control (Band & Weisz, 1990; Bearison, 1998; Deci & Ryan, 1987), such as developing insight and talking through distress with a trusted friend. The motivation to deal with illness-related stress can come from within, based on internalized standards (Thies, 1996; Thies & Walsh, 1999). Ideally, we would hope that John would avoid risky behavior based on his own desire to be healthy or to not ruin his sister's graduation.

However, as he seems more motivated to win approval from friends—a strategy more common among younger than older adolescents—he resorts to more primary forms of control as a reliable method of dealing with emotional disequilibrium. He distracts himself with physical activities and tells his sister what to do: Butt out. John may be trying to make his own rules for managing his illness, not because he is being irresponsible or rebelling, but because he wants the illness to fit his life rather than the other way around (Thies, 1996). Unfortunately, how he makes it fit doesn't work.

Being capable of complex abstract thinking does not mean that adolescents are able to effectively cope with the associated emotions. They are flooded with states of physiological arousal that are new, different, and difficult to control and interpret at the same time that conflicting social expectations about how to do so are presented. On the one hand, adolescents can conceive of multifocal strategies to manage distress (Selman & Schultz, 1991), that is, efforts directed at the three parts of any situation: other people, the situation itself, and self. On the other hand, the emotional and behavioral skill to manage layers of meaning in a situation cannot develop without considerable support. Consequently, adolescents can think, feel, and behave at very different developmental levels at the same time—and, like John, often do.

Ryan, who has Down syndrome, is also flooded with physiological arousal and new demands for appropriate behavior. Less able to keep up with the social life of typically developing childhood friends, but capable of the desire to do so, he also feels conflict and confusion. However, differences in his understanding of the social situations that lead to emotional arousal complicate his ability to manage the associated feelings.

## Development of Understanding Self and Other

A sense of self incorporates self-as-agent ("I am, I do, I can"), self-as-object ("about me"), as well as self in relation to others, especially peers (Harter, 1999; James, 1890; Rubin et al., 1998; Selman & Schultz, 1991). As a developmental system, self is the process by which "the individual evaluates his or her status within particular contexts with respect to three fundamental psychological needs: competence, autonomy, and relatedness" (Connell & Wellborn, 1991, p. 51). Competence is perceptions about one's ability in four domains and is related to control: physical, active, social, and psychological (Damon & Hart, 1986). Autonomy refers to self-regulation and relatedness to management of interpersonal relationships. Competent children and adolescents are psychologically healthier than their less competent peers. Indeed, competence is the foundation for self-esteem (James, 1890; Masten & Coatsworth, 1995).

The literature on children and adolescents with chronic illness makes the case that relationships with peers is a major source of stress (Reiter-Purtill & Noll, 2003; Stewart, 2003). Of course, the same could be said for all children to some extent (Rubin et al., 1998). A developmental perspective asks not just *what* is stressful but *how* the stressor is organized; that is, what is the meaning of the peer relationship at any given point that makes it vulnerable to the disconfirmation we know as stress (Block, 1982), especially for children with illness?

The research suggests that relationships with self and other are what is most at stake during illness-related stress. In interviews, children and adolescents with chronic illness reported that it was not the illness regimen per se that is stressful for them, it is people. They may not like insulin injections, for example, but that is not what is "hard." Stress is dealing with other people, especially peers, during illness episodes (Thies, 1996). Furthermore, their appraisal of how dealing with other people, especially peers, was "hard" changes with maturity (Thies & Walsh, 1999). Because the self is an actor in the same events that have emotional meaning, the development of emotional self-regulation in response to stress is part of the self-system. Consequently, strategies for managing stressful feelings, events, and other people are related, albeit unevenly.

## PRESCHOOL: AGES 3 TO 6

For preschoolers, the key domain of *self* is physical (Damon & Hart, 1986). Three-year-old Deon would say, "I have brown eyes. I like music." He would unlikely refer to his disability in his self-description because it is not salient to him and he does not appreciate that other people might see him as different. He might refer to something he has, such as a wheelchair or a dog. *Liking, having, wanting,* and *doing something* go together.

Among young children, competence has an all-or-none quality to it without regard for comparative ability (Harter, 1985). Everyone in kindergarten is the fastest runner. Relationships with others are egocentric, which means the "my" perspective is the only perspective of which they are aware. Preschoolers do not appreciate mali-cious aforethought, their own or another's (Harter, 1985). They can identify another person as the transgressor, but do not concern themselves with intent: it is the experience of being transgressed upon that matters (Selman & Schultz, 1991).

**Self, Other, and Appraisal.** It was noted earlier that negative events are experienced as emotionally intrusive on the self. At this developmental level, emotion and self are not separate, so that "being upset" is at stake. When feeling intruded upon, literally or psychologically, a person may strike out at the offender or run away, in true fight-or-flight fashion, unless that person is capable of internal mental manipulations to control their response or change the meaning of events (Selman & Schultz, 1991). Young children do not engage in self-generated internal dialogue. You may overhear them talking to themselves or a pet—"It's OK"—but they are using the words from trusted others to calm themselves. They need guidance from attachment and parenting figures to shape such self-regulatory behaviors (Bronson, 2000).

Although intrusive behaviors are common among typically developing young children, most develop the self-regulatory capacity and learn the social cues required to play with peers, to cooperate with adults, and to manage distress. Because children with developmental disabilities have more difficulty with self-regulation, and because their cognitive and language differences may cause them to misread social cues, they tend to be more intrusive in their play behavior (Wilson, 1999), which may be mistakenly interpreted as aggression. Helping young children with disabilities develop social competence is an important strategy not only for mainstreaming (Odom, McConnell, & McEvoy, 1992) but also for managing stress when relationships are at stake.

## EARLY TO MIDDLE CHILDHOOD: AGES 6 TO 10

For concrete thinkers, inner and outer experience become differentiated. They have a sense that mind, body, and volition are separate but related parts of a whole self (Harter, 1999). "My" thoughts, feelings, and intentions are private, and I know yours are as well. Doing things is a key domain of self-definition (Damon & Hart, 1986) and contributes to a sense of competence (Harter, 1985, 1999). Peer comparisons are an important standard for measuring competence (Rubin et al., 1998): Everyone knows who the fastest runner is. As long as children like Deanna are developing other areas of competence, such as swim team and Brownies, not being the fastest doesn't have to matter.

Being competent is a pleasant experience (White, 1959), and pleasant experiences fit within a self-structure that has rules for incorporating "good" within the self and leaving the "not-so-good" outside of the self (Harter, 1985). Here again, we see the integration of emotional development and the self-system: Deanna may take credit for successful illness management (pleasant) and blame failure (unpleasant) on external factors, such as other people or events, like a fire drill at lunch time or an uncooperative teacher.

**Unilateral Perspective: Self and Appraisal.** Younger school-aged children have unilateral, or one-way, relationships with the social environment (Selman & Schultz, 1991). There's "me" and there's "you." Peer relationships are based on liking the same things, doing stuff together—and on dominance. At the unilateral level of development, interpersonal strategies are aimed at putting one's self first: doing what I like to do, and getting the other person to do what I want to do. They include enlisting the assistance of powerful others, such as telling the teacher, being directive ("do this"), and making threats ("or else") or teasing. Teasing is classic dominance behavior, that is, putting the other down. It first appears in the rough-and-tumble play of the preschool years and morphs into verbal sparring in childhood and potentially into bullying and harassment later (see

Chapter 17 by Walsh and Barrett). Sometimes surrendering to the dominating child or situation is an effective short-term strategy when other strategies are not part of the child's repertoire.

Stress is appraised as a one-way external press: something (illness) or someone is imposing unwanted restrictions on preferred activities, making the child do something she doesn't want to do, or keeping the child from doing something she wants to do. Because "doing things" is a key part of self-definition, it is not surprising that "doing what I want to do" is at stake during illness-related stress at this level. When asked what is "hard" (that is, stressful) about having cystic fibrosis, Deanna would report, "I had to stop playing because I couldn't breathe." For her, playing with friends, a normal childhood activity, was at stake during illness-related stress. Teasing is a related example. In interviews, when children were asked what they wanted to have happen instead of being teased (that is, what is at stake), most reported, "I wanted them to play with me" (Thies, 1996; Thies & Walsh, 1999).

At the same time, children at this level are motivated to comply with the rules, less there be consequences from powerful others, including the illness. Deanna might say, "I went into the nurse's office to use my inhaler so that I wouldn't get more sick." Or "I told them to stop teasing me." When she says, "It's not fair that I couldn't play, " she is not making a moral statement but expressing disgruntlement at not getting what she wants.

**Second-Person Perspective: Self and Appraisal.** Older school aged-children, or about ages 9 to 11, develop a second-person perspective; that is, they can put themselves in someone else's shoes, which is fundamental for reciprocal, or two-way, relationships (Selman & Schultz, 1991). Emotional and self-development become integrated with social rules, and concrete thinkers love rules. Because this development overlaps with the developmental level of transitional children, the implications of the second-person perspective are discussed in the next section.

## LATE CHILDHOOD TO EARLY ADOLESCENCE: AGES 10 TO 13

As noted earlier, this is a transitional period in which inner experiences become differentiated. Self-concept also revolves around more abstract traits (Damon & Hart, 1986; Harter, 1999). Twelve-year-old Nicole might report, "I'm a caring person. I'm smart." The ability to see one's self as others might, and to measure one's self against one's own expectations, enables children to be self-reflective and to evaluate their own competence (Harter, 1985). Increasingly, there is a move toward internalizing standards from family and respected others (Harter, 1999; Selman & Schultz, 1991): "I like being smart because then I might get scholarships for college."

**Second-Person Perspective: Self and Appraisal.** The second-person perspective, discussed earlier, is a hallmark of older school-aged and transitional children, beginning as early as 9 in more mature children and evolving into the third-person perspective among some young adolescents. There is considerable variability among 10- to 12-year-olds in their social and emotional maturity, with girls typically maturing a bit earlier than boys. Thus, the developmental implications for girls like Deanna and Nicole, ages 9 and 12, respectively, overlap.

In a two-way reciprocal relationship, the agreement—sometimes spoken, sometimes implied—is that friends are supposed to like and help each other. "Being nice" means not teasing, liking me, being chums. Charges of "that's not fair" and "he was mean to me" signify that a trust has been broken and is a key ingredient of conflict. Conflict signifies potential loss and a threat to the self-system: friendship, trust, being liked (Rubin et al., 1998; Selman & Schultz, 1991).

For children with chronic illness, "being liked" and "being competent" are at stake, and illness-related stress is a violation of agreement (Thies &

Walsh, 1999). Approval from others and self, as well as avoiding disapproval of same, is a potential source of motivation for action during stress, but the fallback strategy of complying with rules to avoid punishing consequences is often more reliable.

For example, Deanna can put herself in her friends' shoes and realizes they can do the same; thus, she now realizes that teasing is intended to hurt her feelings. As hurting people is against the rules—indeed, the Golden Rule is based on reciprocity in relationships—she may invoke rules to keep that from happening again: "The rules at school are that friends are supposed to be nice to each other." Concrete thinkers who favor primary forms of control know there are consequences to breaking rules, such as experiencing the wrath of the same powerful others that children will enlist to support their cause. In other words, Deanna will tell the teacher (Thies, 1996).

Although Deanna may feel singled out for teasing because of her illness, many of her peers feel the same. In other words, cystic fibrosis is not the reason for being teased per se. Peer comparisons are an important source of competence information among school-aged children. Any perceived violations of the norm are fair game for teasing (Keltner, Capps, Kring, Young, & Heerey, 2001). But, because children on both sides know it is intended to be harmful, tolerance for this behavior suggests that harm is an accepted part of interpersonal relationships.

Nicole's age group is particularly concerned with being treated like "normal," which means like everyone else (Thies, 1996). Because they can see themselves from another's point of view, they might not like what they see. As inner experience becomes open to inspection, emotions become more fickle, and psychological safety lies in conformity. That is, Nicole may say she feels different because she has diabetes, but, in fact, every 12- to 13-year-old feels different. It's not about being different as much as it is about being the same as everyone else.

A common strategy for regulating two-way relationships, especially among older school-aged children and transitional children, is persuasion. If Nicole can see things from her friends' perspective, then she expects they should be able to see things from hers. Other strategies include guilt-tripping, showing off, or postponing one's own goals in order to gain favor with others (Selman & Schultz, 1991). Self-conscious about thinking she is being stared at, she might entreat them with, "C'mon you guys, you wouldn't like it if I stared at you." Often, transitional children like Nicole can appraise an illness-related stressor at a reciprocal level but manage it at the less mature unilateral level with primary control, for example, by invoking rules, making threats, or telling other people what to do. "OK, just cut it out and leave me alone."

Interestingly, the illness may be one party in a two-way reciprocal relationship. In interviews, transitional children like Nicole and many adolescents reported that they did everything they were supposed to do but got sick anyway. Nicole may say that she followed the agreed-upon rules of diabetes management, like eating right, but still had difficulty with high blood glucose levels. The implication is that the illness did not keep up its end of the agreement, that is, blood glucose levels did not do what they were supposed to do (Thies, 1996).

## ADOLESCENCE: AGES 13 TO 17

With the onset of abstract thinking, the self is appreciated as more complex (Harter, 1999). Adolescents think of themselves in psychological terms, which include thoughts, intentions, desires, hopes and fears, and how they are seen by others (Damon & Hart, 1986; Nannis, 1988; Selman & Schultz, 1991). As noted by Elkind (1984), he summarizes the social, cognitive, and emotional changes in adolescence as "thinking in a new key."

Around age 14, there is a peak in both self-consciousness (i.e., the imaginary audience,

"Everyone is watching me.") and internal conflict ("Who am I?") (Harter, 1988). In other words, it is normal to feel different. Again, the reason Nicole believes that everyone is staring at her in the restaurant is that she is a 12-year-old young adolescent, not because she has diabetes. (Girls may experience the imaginary audience earlier than boys.) She may be convinced they stare because they think she is different due to her diabetes, but her peers have their own reasons for feeling different as well, which she may not yet appreciate. Given this heightened self-consciousness, information control about the illness is paramount (Thies, 1996). Parents and health care professionals need to be especially careful about mentioning a child's illness in front of peers without involving the child in how or whether to do so.

Because adolescents live in their heads, egocentric thinking—"It's about me."—is common. Given their moody nature, egocentric thinking is validated by parents' increased attention and concern. Egocentric thinking also lends itself to a romantic sense of destiny known as the personal fable. For John, a belief in his physical prowess may be particularly important.

## Third-Person Perspective: Self and Appraisal

The egocentric thinking of adolescents should not be confused with the egocentric thinking of preschoolers. Young children do not step outside of their reality, whereas adolescents can take a third-person perspective of themselves (Selman & Schultz, 1991). This is Freud's phenomenon of the observing ego: "I am aware of being aware of myself." Monitoring one's own behavior and self-criticism (Harter, 1985, 1988) are hallmarks of this period. John is distressed that he can be a different person in different situations: Which is the real John?

John should be able to see himself and others as part of a larger, interconnected system: they all have a part to play. His includes not risking his health while riding dirt bikes because the consequences affect everyone: his sister, his parents, and even his friends and physician. His relationships should begin to move toward mutuality, where there is collaborative sharing and a sense of commitment to the relationship itself (Selman & Schultz, 1991). His sister is already at this point. She wants to feel that she, John, and his friends are on the same psychological wavelength, in which there is a shared mutual interest in John's health and in her graduation. She can anticipate and integrate his needs with her own and expects him to do the same in order to strike a balance in the relationship.

There is a down side to thinking in a new key. With more sophisticated social cognition regarding motivation and intent, adolescents who are trying to strike a balance of mutuality in friendships are also vulnerable to disillusionment and betrayal. John's sister feels betrayed by him, and he may feel disillusioned about friends who encouraged him to behave recklessly. Teasing can be perceived as playful and affectionate when there is implied mutual agreement about the motivation and intent (Keltner et al., 2001).

Adolescents appraise illness-related stress as upsetting the balance of a relationship. For adolescents with chronic health conditions, "being myself" and "maintaining the relationship" are at stake, with boys favoring the former and girls the latter. When John says "It's my life," he sees his very self at stake. Increasingly, adolescent's reasons for their behavior are internalized standards of their own, which they talk out with other people: "I know I need to take care of myself" (Thies & Walsh, 1999). The desire to set the standards, to strike a balance, and to make their own rules can extend to their relationship with their illness. As noted earlier, John wants the illness to adapt to his life, which includes dirt biking (Thies, 1996). Unfortunately, his choice doesn't balance the relationship because he failed to consider "who" the illness is—its demands, its limits, and so on—in the relationship.

Once again, John's understanding of a situation may be developmentally more mature than his ability to manage it. Under duress, he experiences his sister's anger with him as an external pressure and attempts to remove the stressor by telling her to leave him alone. Although this pattern of appraisal and coping is well established among 8- to 9-year-olds, in the integrated hierarchy of development it is still available to John when more mature strategies are not yet reliable. Clinicians who understand the clinical-developmental implications of John's behavior can help him to reorganize at more age-appropriate levels of maturity (Noam, 1998). If being himself is at stake, he needs to identify a more mature part of himself to fight for, rather than risking himself through identification with an activity that could be harmful.

There is another important area of development for adolescents—time. Although even young children can talk in the past and future tense, it is not until the onset of abstract thinking that adolescents appreciate that the future is *their* future (Harner, 1982). A future orientation adds complexity to the relationship with the environment. Worries about their future prospects and about the impact of current events on their future are verbalized.

## Conclusion and Recommendations

Tables 18.1, 18.2, and 18.3 summarize the developmental trends reviewed above. There are a number of lessons that health care providers can take from this brief review of the developmental literature.

First, development proceeds in predictable trends from early childhood through adolescence (and into adulthood as well), but this observation is made from only the broadest population-based perspective. Furthermore, broad trends in development do not account for individual differences among people, or the unevenness of development within any one person at a given point in time.

*Table 18.1*  Developmental Trends in Emotion, Self and Other, and Motivation

| | Emotions[1,2,3,4] | Self and Friendships with Peers[5,6,7] |
|---|---|---|
| Pre-K 3–6 years old | Negative feelings are global and intrusive, without reference to cause.<br><br>Feelings and situation blend. | Focus is on the physical self, such as liking, wanting, having things, and being all good or all bad.<br><br>Can be empathetic to others' feelings but cannot step outside of own reality. Experience and self blend so that negative experiences are intrusive. |
| School-age 5–9 years old | Negative feelings have external cause that child blames on others or tries to change ("unfair!"), thinks of pleasant things as distraction. | Differentiation of self and other, so that each has their own feelings and intentions, but what "I" want takes precedence.<br><br>A real friend does what "I" want to do because "we" like the same things. The focus is on doing things, on being active, and being capable.<br><br>Competence is based on rule compliance. |
| Transition overlap 8–12 years old | Feelings caused by external and internal factors.<br><br>Feels conflict; can have two feelings at once.<br><br>Internal self-talk, distracts self. | Inner self becomes differentiated, develop self-reflection, self-evaluation, and second-person perspective. Intentions are deliberate.<br><br>Focus on social self and traits (e.g. "nice").<br><br>Relationships are a two-way pact. "If I can understand you, you can understand me, so I will persuade you to understand me." |
| Adolescent >12 years old | Feelings have multiple causes and layers; feels off balance; conscious inner dialogue to set things right. | Integration of self and other into a larger system of multiple perspectives and connections/commitments; develop third-person perspective.<br><br>Balance within the system is important.<br><br>Self is introspective, monitors behavior and conscious inner dialogue. |

## Reasons for Acting/Motivation[8,9,10]

| Any age Preschool age | Absolute preference: Does something because it's inherently pleasurable or avoids it because it's inherently unpleasant and intrusive; fundamental to human experience "I like to eat candy . . . just cuz it's yummy." Or, doesn't know why he/she did something. "Just did. I don't know." |
|---|---|
| Younger school-aged children | External orientation: Complies with rules to avoid bad consequences. External authority are agents who maintain rules and mete out punishment. "Teacher says" or "I'll get you in trouble." An external orientation provides a source for standards for behavior as well as someone to blame. The illness is an external other with its own set of "comply or get sick" rules. |
| Older school-aged children into young adolescence | Internal orientation/introject: Reasons are framed internally but are esteem-based pressures to act, such as getting approval of others or one's self or by avoiding the disapproval of others or own guilty/embarrassing feelings. External standards are becoming internalized. May want to blame others but recognizes that one is responsible. Feels betrayed when others intentionally preempt self's authority. Feels inner conflict about making decisions. Wants to appear competent to others re: illness compliance. |
| Older adolescence | Integrated/identifications: Has own standards for acting, based on wanting to do the right or important thing, or based on self-understanding. Says "should" to refer to own rules. Takes context into account; shares control with the environment. Failure to live up to own standards meets with self-criticism. Wants illness to fit own life rather than the other way around. |

[1] Harris, 1985.
[2] Harter, 1986.
[3] Nannis, 1988.
[4] Whitesell & Harter, 1989.
[5] Damon & Hart, 1986.

[6] Harter, 1999.
[7] Selman & Schultz, 1991.
[8] Connell, 1985.
[9] Deci & Ryan, 1985, 1987.
[10] Ryan & Connell, 1989.

*Table 18.2*   Developmental Trends in Appraisal of Illness-Related Stress[1,2]

| Developmental Level | Experience of Stress |
| --- | --- |
| **Intrusive: preschool**<br>"Being upset" is at stake. | Stressors are perceived as global, diffuse, without boundaries and as emotionally intrusive and overwhelming. |
| **External press: young to middle school-age**<br>"Doing what I want" is at stake. | Stressors are perceived as a one-way external pressure, as rigid, uncompromising.<br>The illness is a pressure; it has "comply or else get sick" rules.<br>Competence is rule compliance. |
| **Violation of contract: older school-age and young adolescent**<br>"Being competent and being liked" are at stake. | Stressors perceived as a violation of a two-party contract, in which friends are nice to each other.<br>Illness can be the other party. "I did what I was supposed to do, and I got sick anyway."<br>Concerned about competence in decision making, resetting the pact. |
| **Out of balance: adolescent**<br>"Being myself" and "maintaining the relationship" are at stake. | Stressors are perceived as upsetting the balance in an integrated system, in a relationship.<br>Illness throws it off balance.<br>Competence based on setting standards for how illness fits into system of self and other. |

[1]*Thies, 1994, 1996.*
[2]*Thies & Walsh, 1999.*

For example, trends tell us that 9-year-old Deanna is not yet able to think abstractly, regardless of how much she seems to know about her cystic fibrosis at this point in time. We know that she likely will be able to think abstractly by the time she is a teenager, but developmental trends alone do not tell us exactly when that will happen or if it will apply equally to all areas of thought, especially under duress. In fact, there is no guarantee that it will happen at all, especially if the environment does support this development.

Second, adaptation to illness and disability is adaptation to life. As Chapter 4 by Thies on resilience suggests, resilience in the face of chronic stress is not a matter of invulnerability but of staying the normative course of development as much as possible. The factors that contribute to resilience in children in the studies cited in Chapter 4—positive personality, intelligent, good social skills, supportive parenting—are found in children with chronic illness as well.

That does not mean that illness is not stressful; rather, the nature of the stress associated with chronic illness is related to normative life events, such as peers, school, and a sense of self. For example, it is normal for a 12-year-old girl to think everyone is looking at her; the girl with diabetes organizes that self-consciousness around her illness, just as another girl may organize it around being overweight. The adaptive effort is the process by which meaning is made of this phenomenon in her own life and how it shapes her sense of self and her relationship with the environment.

Third, the age/stage heuristic that most clinicians have learned in their lectures on growth and development is necessary but insufficient evidence for providing care that is developmentally appropriate for a given individual in the context of his/her family, community, culture, and historical time. Better assessment tools and intervention strategies need to be developed to ensure that each

*Table 18.3*  Developmental Trends in Coping with Illness-Related Stress

| Type of Coping | Explanation | Examples |
|---|---|---|
| **Primary Control**<br>First shows up at about 5–6 years, predominates among pre-formal/ concrete thinkers (school-age), but found throughout life. | Primary coping behavior involves efforts to modify or otherwise influence events, circumstances, or other people so as to enhance rewards by bringing objective conditions into line with what the child wants; externally directed. | "I did my blood test and took my insulin. I had to."<br>"I was out of breath so I played four square instead." |
| | **Instrumental type: based on activity**<br>Complying with rules<br>Try to do something different instead | "I can't have any of the cake. It would make my sugar too high."<br>"I thought about how we were going to go to the fair after the game."<br>"I watched TV." |
| | **Cognitive type: thoughts**<br>Telling yourself what you should or shouldn't do<br>Forget about it, distract mind with activity<br>Think about good things instead | |
| | **Social type: self/other**<br>Directing/influencing the behavior of other people | "I told her to stop teasing me."<br>"I told the nurse to be really careful with my shot."<br>"I said 'why can't you eat what I eat so we're the same?'" |
| **Secondary control**<br>Doesn't show up consistently until child is a formal thinker (adolescent); uses both primary and secondary coping. | Secondary coping behavior involves efforts to modify or otherwise influence the child's own subjective psychological state (mood, attributions, expectations, wishes, interpretations) so as to enhance rewards by achieving comfortable accommodation or goodness-of-fit with respect to conditions as they are; internally directed | |
| | **Instrumental type**<br>Doing something so that you feel good about yourself | "I stick to my diet because I want to be healthy." |
| | **Cognitive type**<br>Talking to yourself, relaxing your mind<br>Telling yourself you're doing the right thing, that it will be all right | "I tell myself that I am probably healthier than most people because I take care of myself."<br>"I just remember that they are not really my friends anyway." |
| | **Social type**<br>Sharing thoughts and concerns with someone else | "I talk to my mother."<br>"I told my friends how I felt so we could work it out." |

[1] *Band & Weiss, 1990.*
[2] *Bearison, 1998.*
[3] *Donaldson, Prinstein, Danovsky, & Spirito, 2000.*
[4] *Spirito, Stark, Gil, & Tye, 1995.*
[5] *Spirito, Stark, & Williams, 1988.*

person receives care that not only meets his/her current developmental needs and abilities but that also promotes optimal development through the provision of environmental support for the person and at the system levels of family, community, and culture. Health care providers need to develop theoretically sound evidence for appropriate and effective care delivery.

Fourth, the emphasis on the relationship between person and environment is consistent with emerging models of community-based care. For nurses in particular, the role of the environment in health care should be very familiar: Florence Nightingale noted that nurses must manipulate the environment (physical and social) in order to optimize the body's nature healing processes (Nightingale, 1859).

We suggest the following principles for developmentally appropriate care:

1. Developmentally appropriate care recognizes that adaptation to illness is also adaptation to life for persons with chronic illness and disability.

2. Developmentally appropriate care recognizes that development at any point in the life span is a product of the transactional relationship between person and environment over time. This applies to physical/biological, psychosocial/behavioral, and intellectual domains of development, as well as to developmental systems, such as peer relationships.

3. Developmentally appropriate care recognizes that there are broad normative trends in development across the life span often associated with the passage of time, but that time alone does not guarantee development.

4. Developmentally appropriate care recognizes that there are significant individual differences in development and that development is uneven.

5. Developmentally appropriate care is age appropriate, in that persons are treated with respect for their life's experience and expectations. For example, an adolescent with a developmental disability is an adolescent first regardless of differences in ability.

6. Developmentally appropriate care is person centered, in that it fits an individual's presented developmental capacities while supporting reestablishment of reported optimal capacities. That is, begin at the level the person presents clinically, but design care to support the person's usual or expected level outside of a clinical situation, as reported by the person, family, or other caregivers.

7. Developmentally appropriate care promotes optimal competence in physical/biological, psychosocial/behavioral, and intellectual domains, as well as in self-management of care, by providing the environmental supports across family and community systems to do so. For example, Deanna will continue to need guidance and support as she manages her illness in new situations and at different levels of her own development.

8. Developmentally appropriate care is designed in partnership with the individual, family, and community. For example, ask Deon's and Ryan's family what works best when their sons are distressed.

9. Developmentally appropriate care incorporates the meaning of an illness or disability for the individual, family, community, and culture at that point in historical and personal time.

Health care providers take care of people who live with illness and disability. Unfortunately, we know more about the illnesses and disabilities than we do about the people. It is time that we apply the lessons from the field of human development to health care.

# References

Band, E., & Weisz, J. (1990). Developmental differences in primary and secondary control coping and adjustment to juvenile diabetes. *Journal of Personality and Social Psychology, 39,* 968–976.

Baumrind, D. (1978). Parental disciplinary patterns and social competence in children. *Youth and Society, 9,* 229–276.

Bearison, D. J. (1998). Pediatric psychology and children's medical problems. In K. A. Renninger (Ed.), *Child Psychology in Practice* (5th ed., Vol. 4, pp. 635–709). New York: John Wiley & Sons.

Beeghly, M., & Cicchetti, D. (1987). An organizational approach to symbolic development in children with Down syndrome. *New Directions in Child Development, 36,* 5–29.

Beeghly, M., Perry, B., & Cicchetti, D. (1989). Structural and affective dimensions of play development in young children with Down syndrome. *International Journal of Behavioral Development, 12,* 257–277.

Belsky, J. (1984). The determinants of parenting: A process model. *Child Development, 55,* 83–96.

Bibace, R., & Walsh, M. E. (1981). Development of children's concepts of illness. In M. E. Walsh (Ed.), *Children's concepts of health, illness, and bodily functions.* San Francisco: Jossey-Bass.

Block, J. (1982). Assimilation, accommodation and the dynamics of personality development. *Child Development, 53,* 281–295.

Bonder, B., Martin, L., & Miracle, A. (2002). *Culture in clinical care.* Northoboro, NJ: SLACK.

Bredekamp, S. (Ed.). (1987/1993). *Developmentally appropriate practice in early childhood programs serving children birth through age 8.* Washington, DC: National Association for the Education of Young Children.

Bronfenbrenner, U. (1979). *The ecology of human development.* Cambridge, MA: Harvard University Press.

Bronfenbrenner, U., & Ceci, S. (1994). Nature-nurture reconceptualized in developmental perspective: A bioecological model. *Psychological review, 101,* 568–586.

Bronson, M. B. (2000). *Self-regulation in early childhood: Nature and nurture.* New York: Guilford.

Brown, R. T. (Ed.). (1999). *Cognitive aspects of chronic illness in children.* New York: Guilford.

Brown, R. T., & Sawyer, M. G. (Eds.). (1998). *Medications for school-age children: effects on learning and behavior.* New York: Guilford.

Bruner, J., & Haste, J. (Eds.). (1987). *Making sense: the child's construction of the world.* London: Methuen.

Butterworth, G., & Cicchetti, D. (1978). Visual calibration of posture in normal and motor retarded Down's syndrome infants. *Perception, 7,* 513–525.

Capute, A. J., & Accardo, P. J. (1996). A neurodevelopmental perspective on the continuum of developmental disabilities. In P. J. Accardo (Ed.), *Developmental disabilities in infancy and childhood* (2nd ed., Vol. I: Neurodevelopmental diagnosis and treatment, pp. 1–24). Baltimore: Paul H. Brookes Publishing.

Carlson, E. A., Samson, M. C., & Sroufe, A. (2003). Implications of attachment theory and research for developmental-behavioral pediatrics. *Developmental and Behavioral Pediatrics, 24,* 364–379.

Carroll, J., & Steward, M. (1984). The role of cognitive development in children's understanding of their own feelings. *Child Development, 55*(4), 1486–1492.

Cicchetti, D., & Beeghly, M. (1990). An organizational approach to the study of Down syndrome: contributions to an integrative theory of development. In M. Beeghly (Ed.), *Children with Down syndrome: a developmental perspective* (pp. 29–62). New York: Cambridge University Press.

Cicchetti, D., & Hinshaw, S. (2002). Development and psychopathology: prevention and intervention science: contributions to developmental theory. *Development & Psychopathology, 14,* 667–671.

Cicchetti, D., & Sroufe, A. (1976). The relationship between affective and cognitive development in Down's syndrome infants. *Child Development, 47,* 920–929.

Connell, J. P. (1985). A new multidimensional measure of children's perceptions of control. *Child Development, 56,* 1018–1041.

Connell, J., & Wellborn, J. Competence, autonomy, and relatedness. In Megan, G. & Sroufe, L. (Eds.), *Self-processes and Development.* Minnesota Symposia on Child Psychology. Hillsdale, NJ: Erlbaum.

Damon, W., & Hart, D. (1986). Stability and change in children's self-understanding. *Social Cognition, 4*(2), 102–118.

Darwin, C. (1859). *The origin of the species by means of natural selection.* London: John Murray.

Deci, E. L., & Ryan, R. M. (1985). *Intrinsic motivation and self-determination in human behavior.* New York: Plenum.

Deci, E. L., & Ryan, R. M. (1987). The support of autonomy and the control of behavior. *Journal of Personality and Social Psychology, 53,* 1024–1037.

Donaldson, D., Prinstein, M. J., Danovsky, M., & Spirito, A. (2000). Patterns of children's coping with life stress: Implications for clinicians. *American Journal of Orthopsychiatry, 70,* 351–359.

Ebersole, P., Hess, P., & Luggen, A. (2004). *Toward healthy aging* (6th ed.). St. Louis, MO: Mosby.

Elder, G. H. (1995). The life course paradigm: social change and individual development. In P. Moen, G. H. Elder, & K. Luscher (Eds.), *Examining lives in context: Perspectives on the ecology of human development* (pp. 101–140). Washington, DC: American Psychological Association.

Elkind, C. (1984). *All dressed up and no place to go: Teenagers in crisis.* Reading, MA: Addison-Wesley.

Erikson, E. H. (1950). *Childhod and society.* New York: W. W. Norton & Company.

Fiske, S. T., & Taylor, S. E. (1991). *Social cognition.* New York: McGraw-Hill.

Freud, S. (1924/1952). *A general introduction to psychoanalysis* (J. Riviere, Trans.). New York: Washington Square Press.

Grebin, B., & Kaplan, S. C. (1995). Toward a pediatric subacute care model: Clinical and administrative features. *Archives of Physical Medicine and Rehabilitation, 76*(12-S), SC16-20.

Hall, J. (1999). Developing meaningful age-appropriate competencies for clinical services. *Journal for Nurses in Staff Development, 15,* 241.

Harner, L. (1982). Talking about the past and future. In W. Friedman (Ed.), *The developmental psychology of time.* New York: Academic.

Harris, P. (1985). What children know about the situations that provoke emotion. In C. Saarni (Ed.), *The socialization of emotions* (pp. 161–185). New York: Plenum.

Harter, S. (1985). Competence as a dimension of self-evaluation: Toward a comprehensive model of self-worth. In R. Leahy (Ed.), *The development of the self.* New York: Academic Press.

Harter, S. (1986). Cognitive developmental processes in the integration of concepts about emotions and the self. *Social Cognition, 4,* 119–151.

Harter, S. (1988). Developmental and dynamic changes in the nature of self-concept: Implications for child psychotherapy. In S. Shirk (Ed.), *Cognitive development and child psychotherapy.* New York: Plenum.

Harter, S. (1999). *The construction of the self: A developmental perspective.* New York: Guilford.

Harter, S., & Connell, J. P. (1984). A model of the relationship among children's academic achievement and their self-perceptions of competence, control and motivational orientation. In J. Nicholls (Ed.), *The development of achievement motivation* (pp. 219–250). Greenwich, CT: JAI.

Hartup, W. W. (1983). Peer relations. In E. M. Hetherington (Ed.), *Socialization, personality and social development* (Vol. 4, pp. 103–196). New York: Wiley.

Hoffman, C., Rice, D., & Sung, H. Y. (1996.). Persons with chronic conditions: Their prevalence and costs. *Journal of the American Medical Association, 276,* 1473–1479.

Hunt, R. (1998). Community-based nursing: Philosophy or setting? *American Journal of Nursing, 98*(10), 45–48.

Iannotti, R. J., & Bush, P. J. (1993). Toward a developmental theory of compliance. In S. J. Yaffe (Ed.), *Developmental aspects of health compliance behavior* (pp. 59–76). Hillsdale, NJ: Lawrence Earlbaum Associates.

Institute for Family-Centered Care. (2003). *Family-centered care: Questions and Answers.* Retrieved December 30, 2003, from www.familycenteredcare.org.

Ireys, H. T. (1994). *Children with special health care needs: Evaluating their needs and relevant service structures* [unpublished paper]. Baltimore, MD: Institute of Medicine, Johns Hopkins University.

Izard, C. (1977). *Human emotions.* New York: Plenum.

James, W. (1890). *The principles of psychology.* New York: Holt, Rinehart and Winston.

Keltner, D., Capps, L., Kring, A. M., Young, R. C., & Heerey, E. A. (2001). Just teasing: A conceptual analysis and empirical review. *Psychological Bulletin, 127,* 229–248.

Knapp, L. G., Stark, L. J., Kurkjian, J. A., & Spirito, A. (1991). Assessing coping in children and adolescents: Research and practice. *Educational Psychology Review, 3,* 309–334.

Lazarus, R. (1984). On the primacy of cognition. *American Psychologist, 39*(2), 124–129.

Lerner, R. M. (1982). Children and adolescents as producers of their own development. *Developmental Review, 2,* 342–370.

Lerner, R. M. (1986). *Concepts and theories of human development.* New York: Cambridge University Press.

Lerner, R. M., Walsh, M. E., & Howard, K. A. (1998). Developmental-contextual considerations: Person-context relations as the bases for risk and resiliency in child and adolescent development. In T. Ollendick (Ed.), *Children and adolescents: Clinical formulation and treatment* (Vol. 5, pp. 1–24). New York: Elsevier Science Publishers.

Long, T., Katz, K., & Pokorni, J. (1989). Developmental intervention with the chronically ill infant. *Infants and Young Children, 1*(4), 78–88.

Masten, A. S., & Coatsworth, D. J. (1995). Competence, resilience and psychopathology. In D. Cicchetti & D. Cohen (Eds.), *Risk, disorder and adaptation* (Vol. 2, pp. 715–752). New York: Wiley.

McEwen, B. (2002). *The end of stress as we know it.* Washington, DC: Joseph Henry.

Msall, M. E. (1996). Functional assessment in neurodevelopmental disabilities. In P. J. Accardo (Ed.), *Developmental disabilities in infancy and childhood* (2nd ed., Vol. I: Neurodevelopmental diagnosis and treatment, pp. 371–392). Baltimore: Paul H. Brookes.

Nannis, E. (1988). Cognitive-developmental differences in emotional understanding. In P. Cowan (Ed.), *New directions for child development: Developmental psychopathology and its treatment* (pp. 31–49). San Francisco: Jossey-Bass.

Noam, G. (1998). Clinical-developmental psychology: Toward developmentally differentiated interventions. In K. A. Renninger (Ed.), *Child psychology in practice* (Vol. 4, pp. 585–634). New York: John Wiley & Sons.

Odom, S. L., McConnell, S. R., & McEvoy, M. A. (Eds.). (1992). *Social competence of young children with disabilities.* Baltimore: Paul H. Brookes.

Phares, V., & Compas, B. (1990). Adolescent's subjective distress over their emotional/behavioral problems. *Journal of Consulting and Clinical Psychology, 58,* 596–603.

Piaget, J. (1950). *The psychology of intelligence.* London: Kegan Paul, Trench & Trubner.

Reiter-Purtill, J., & Noll, R. B. (2003). Peer relationships with chronic illness. In M. C. Roberts (Ed.), *Handbook of Pediatric Psychology* (pp. 176–197). New York: Guilford Press.

Rothbaum, F., Weisz, J., & Snyder, S. (1982). Changing the world and the self: a two-process model of perceived control. *Journal of Personality and Social Psychology, 42,* 5–37.

Rubin, K. H., Bukowski, W., & Parker, J. G. (1998). Peer interactions, relationships and groups. In N. Eisenberg (Ed.), *Social, emotional and personality development* (5th ed., Vol. 3, pp. 619–700). New York: John Wiley & Sons.

Russell, J., & Ridgeway, D. (1983). Dimensions underlying children's emotion concepts. *Developmental Psychology, 19,* 795–804.

Rutter, M. (1996). Transitions and turning points in developmental psychopathology. *International Journal of Behavioral Development, 19,* 603–626.

Rutter, M. (2002). Nature, nurture and development: From evangelism through science toward policy and practice. *Child Development, 73*(1), 1–21.

Rutter, M., Dunn, J., Plomin, R., Simonoff, E. et al. (1997). Integrating nature and nurture: Implications of person-environment correlations and interactions for developmental psychopathology. *Development & Psychopathology, 9,* 335–364.

Ryan, R. M., & Connell, J. P. (1989). Perceived locus of causality and internalization: Examining reasons for acting in two domains. *Journal of Personality and Social Psychology, 57,* 749–761.

Saarni, C., Mumme, D. L., & Campos, J. J. (1998). Emotional development: Action, communication, and understanding. In N. Eisenberg (Ed.), *Social, Emotional, and Personality Development* (5th ed., Vol. 3, pp. 237–309). New York: John Wiley & Sons.

Sameroff, A. (1975). Transactional models in early social relations. *Human Development, 18,* 65–79.

Scarr, S., & McCartney, K. (1983). How people make their own environments: A theory of genotype-environment effects. *Child Development, 54,* 425–435.

Schweer, L., & Ose, M. B. (1995). Implementation of a regional pediatric trauma center: Transformation from a pediatric institution to a regional pediatric trauma center. *AORN Journal, 61,* 558.

Selman, R. (1988). *The growth of interpersonal understanding.* New York: Academic Press.

Selman, R., & Schultz, L. (1990). *Making a friend in youth.* Chicago: University of Chicago Press.

Shapiro, B. K. (1996). Neurodevelopmental assessment of infants and young children. In P. J. Accardo (Ed.), *Developmental disabilities in infancy and childhood.* (Vol. I: Neurodevelopmental diagnosis and treatment, pp. 311–322). Baltimore: Paul H. Brookes.

Shelton, R., & Stepanek, J. (1994). *Family-centered care for children needing specialized health and developmental services.* Bethesda, MD: Association for the Care of Children's Health.

Smith, C., & Ellsworth, P. (1985). Patterns of cognitive appraisal in emotion. *Journal of Personality and Social Psychology, 48,* 813–838.

Spirito, A., Stark, L. J., Gil, K. M., & Tyc, V. L. (1995). Coping with everyday and disease-related stressors by chronically ill children and adolescents. *Journal of the American Academy of Child and Adolescent Psychiatry, 34,* 283–290.

Spirito, A., Stark, L. J., & Williams, C. (1988). Development of a brief coping checklist for use with pediatric populations. *Journal of Pediatric Psychology, 13,* 555–574.

Sroufe, A. (1979). The coherence of individual development. *American Psychologist, 34,* 834–841.

Stewart, J. L. (2003). Children living with chronic illness: An examination of their stressors, coping resources and health outcomes. In D. Holditch-Davis (Ed.), *Research on child health and pediatric issues* (Vol. 21, pp. 203–243). New York: Springer.

Szymanski, L., & King, B. H. (1999). Practice parameters for the assessment and reatment of children, adolescents, and adults with mental retardation and comorbid mental disorders. *Journal of the American Academy of Child and Adolescent Psychiatry, 38* (suppl), 5S–31S.

Thies, K. M. (1994). *A developmental analysis of cognitive appraisal of stress in chronically ill children.* Unpublished dissertation, Boston College, Chestnut Hill, MA.

Thies, K. M. (1996). A developmental perspective on stress appraisal: How children understand the everyday challenges of living with a chronic health condition. In J. Sowers (Ed.), *Making our way: Building self-competence among youth with disabilities* (pp. 97–114). Baltimore, MD: Paul Brookes.

Thies, K. M. (1999). Identifying the educational implications of chronic illness in children and adolescents. *Journal of School Health, 69,* 392–397.

Thies, K. M., & Walsh, M. E. (1999). A developmental analysis of cognitive appraisal of stress in children and adolescents with chronic health conditions. *Children's Health Care, 28,* 15–32.

Thompson, R., & Gustafson, K. (1996). *Adaptation to chronic childhood illness.* Washington, DC: American Psychological Association.

Travis, S. S., & Duer, B. (1999). Preparing staff to deliver age-appropriate nursing care to elderly patients. *Journal of Continuing Education in Nursing, 30*(3), 105.

Vygotsky, L. (1978). *Mind in society: The development of higher psychological processes.* Cambridge, MA: Harvard University Press.

Waddington, C. H. (1966). *Principles of development and differentiation.* New York: Macmillan.

Wallander, J. L., Thompson, R., & Alriksson-Schmidt, A. (2003). Psychosocial adjustment of children with chronic physical conditions. In M. C. Roberts (Ed.), *Handbook of Pediatric Psychology* (3rd ed., pp. 141–158). New York: Guilford.

Werner, E. E. (1989). High risk children in young adulthood. *American Journal of Orthopsychiatriy, 59,* 72–81.

Werner, H. (1957). The concept of development from a comparative and organismic point of view. In D. B. Harris (Ed.), *The concept of development* (pp. 125–148). Minneapolis: University of Minnesota Press.

White, R. (1959). Motivation reconsidered: The concept of competence. *Psychological Review, 66,* 297–333.

White, S. H. (1976). The active organism in theoretical behaviorism. *Human Development, 19,* 99–107.

Whitesell, N., & Harter, S. (1989). Children's report of conflict between simultaneous opposite-valence emotions. *Child Development, 60,* 673–682.

Wilson, B. J. (1999). Entry behavior and emotion regulation abilities of developmentally delayed boys. *Developmental Psychology, 35,* 214–222.

Zigler, E., & Glick, M. (1986). *A developmental approach to adult psychopathology.* New York: John Wiley.

# Chapter 19

# Adherence to Health Care Regimens

Tonja Nansel

Nonadherence to treatment regimens is one of the most common and frustrating issues dealt with by health professionals. Almost two decades ago, nonadherence was described as "the best documented, but least understood, health-related behavior" (Becker & Maiman, 1975, p. 11). Although much progress has been made since then in understanding the problem, nonadherence will likely remain an ongoing challenge for health care providers. Adherence to medication and treatment regimens is problematic across diagnoses. This chapter reviews the problem of adherence and traditional views of its definition and intent. A developmental perspective on adherence based on a self-regulation model of human behavior is presented, with examples from children and elders. Finally, strategies to promote adherence are discussed.

## The Problem of Nonadherence

A review of literature on medication adherence published from 1975 to 1996 yielded an average rate of 76% adherence to medication for physical disorders (Cramer & Rosenheck, 1998). Adherence to antidepressant and antipsychotic medications was somewhat lower, averaging 65% and 58%, respectively. Adherence to lifestyle changes such as diet or exercise is typically even poorer than adherence to medication regimens (Carmody, Matarazzo, & Istvan, 1987; Glanz, 1979; Marcus et al., 2000; Sluijs & Knibbe, 1991). Even for conditions in which nonadherence carries severe medical consequences, adherence remains problematic. Studies of transplant patients have found that approximately 20% of patients are nonadherent with immunosuppressive therapy (Laederach-Hofmann & Bunzel, 2000), and a study of renal transplant patients found that 34% missed three or more laboratory report calls in a row during the first 12 months after transplant (Rudman, Gonzales, & Borgida, 1999).

Nonadherence to medication and other treatment regimens results in significant adverse health outcomes, including antibiotic-resistant organisms (Gibbons, 1992; Schwarzmann, 1998), hospitalizations (Maronde et al., 1989), disease progression and complications (Dunbar-Jacob & Schlenk, 1996), and even transplant failure (Rovelli et al., 1989). Overall, costs associated

411

with medication nonadherence are estimated to be over $100 billion per year (National Pharmaceutical Council, 1992). An examination of Medicaid drug and hospital claims data found that irregular medication use was one of the strongest predictors of hospital use and costs in persons with severe and persistent mental illnesses even after controlling for diagnosis, baseline functioning, previous hospitalizations, and demographic characteristics (Svarstad, Shireman, & Sweeney, 2001). Irregular users had twice as many hospitalizations, four times as many hospital days, and 3.8 times greater hospital costs.

## Authoritarian Versus Patient-Centered Approaches

To understand the problem of nonadherence, we must first examine the way in which adherence is conceptualized. Traditionally, adherence has been addressed from an authoritarian perspective. The health care provider (i.e., authority) provides instructions, and the patient is expected to follow them. Lack of adherence, then, indicates a deficit in the patient. However, an attempt to understand nonadherence from this perspective has shown little utility. Nonadherence is not associated with a disregard for one's health, and there are no identifiable patient characteristics that distinguish those who adhere from those who do not. This may in part explain why provider estimates of patient adherence are typically inaccurate.

A more useful conceptualization is that of a patient-centered approach to adherence (Bauman, 2000). From the patient's point of view, the provider is an important source of information about health, illness, and treatment. However, the instructions given may be complex, anxiety provoking, and challenging to implement. They may be incompatible with personal and cultural beliefs, and may contradict the advice of family, friends, or even other providers. Rather than assuming adherence, then, the provider should proceed under the assumption that adherence is

difficult to achieve and, as such, needs to be negotiated, planned, evaluated, and reassessed over time. Such an approach changes the way in which we conceptualize adherence. Rather than reflecting "obedience" to the provider's instructions, adherence refers to a person's ability to incorporate new goals, information, and behaviors into established routines (Ewart, 1993).

Failure to achieve the provider's desired or expected level of adherence may be either intentional or unintentional on the part of the patient. Although nonadherence is often treated as a single concept, intentional and unintentional nonadherence in fact represent very different behaviors. In intentional, or volitional, nonadherence the patient makes a reasoned choice not to comply. Patients may disagree with the provider's instructions, or they may decide that they are unable to follow them. In inadvertent nonadherence, however, the patient accepts the instructions and intends to comply but is unable to do so adequately. Patients may believe they are adhering but have misunderstood instructions, or they may have difficulty adhering to the degree needed for optimal outcomes. In such inadvertent nonadherence, patients may not be aware that they are not adhering sufficiently. For example, patients may forget a medication dose occasionally but believe that they are adhering well enough, or may believe that they have decreased dietary fat intake but in reality have not done so.

Risk factors for volitional and inadvertent nonadherence may be quite different. Important risk factors for volitional nonadherence are those that result in the patient believing that not adhering represents a better choice than adhering. These include factors such as denial of the diagnosis, divergent beliefs from the physician regarding the condition and how it should be treated, skepticism about the effectiveness of the prescribed treatment, fears about the treatment, cost of the treatment, adverse effects of the treatment, or receiving differing advice from multiple providers. Important risk factors for inadvertent nonadherence, on the other hand, are those that create barriers to patients carrying out their intentions. These include patient characteristics such as poor mental, physical, or emotional functioning; lack of social support; competing demands; presence of multiple caregivers; low literacy; or language barriers. In addition, developmental characteristics such as parent–child conflict, cognitive maturity, social/emotional maturity, or autonomy-seeking may be responsible. Other factors increase the risk of either type of nonadherence. Poor patient–provider communication or lack of a strong patient–provider therapeutic alliance may lead to the patient not sufficiently understanding or not trusting the provider's advice. Greater difficulty, complexity, or disruptiveness of the regimen may result in the patient deciding that it is not worth the effort and is also likely to interfere with patients' ability to carry out the regimen even if they intend to do so.

## Relationship Between Adherence and Health Outcomes

The problem of adherence is compounded by the reality that the relationship between adherence and health outcomes is far from perfect (Figure 19.1). Although greater adherence typically re-

sults in better health outcomes, individual patients who are highly adherent may nonetheless experience poor outcomes, and patients who are poorly adherent may experience good outcomes. Treatments are not always effective, and disease courses and responses to treatment are not uniform. Thus, while undertaking efforts to promote patient adherence, we must recognize that some patients will receive greater benefit from these efforts than will others. Although health care providers may imply that perfect adherence will always result in an optimal outcome in order to attempt to motivate the patient, doing so can result in discrediting the provider's advice if the treatment is not effective.

# Developmental Framework: A Self-Regulation Perspective on Adherence

A self-regulation perspective provides a useful framework for conceptualizing adherence. This perspective conceptualizes adherence as the patient's attempt to integrate and act on medical information. Self-regulation models view persons as self-regulating systems—as active problem solvers (Leventhal, Leventhal, & Cameron, 2001;

***Figure 19.1***    Relationship Between Adherence and Health Outcomes

| | | ADHERENCE | |
| | | *Good* | *Poor* |
|---|---|---|---|
| **OUTCOME** | *Good* | Ideal situation<br>Reflects adequate match of treatment to illness. | Illness may be self-limiting.<br>Patient may be sufficiently resilient to recover without treatment. |
| | *Poor* | Treatment may not be optimal or adequate for patient.<br>Illness may be resistant to treatment. | Patient may be unconvinced of need or may quit due to side effects.<br>Patient may wish to adhere but have difficulty doing so. |

*(Adapted from Sackett & Haynes, 1976)*

Leventhal, Leventhal, & Contrada, 1998) who respond to health threats through a problem-solving process. This problem-solving process is represented in the upper portion of Figure 19.2. People observe and interpret health-related situations, forming an appraisal of that situation. They select and implement actions to manage the situation and evaluate their initial perceptions and the response to their actions based on the feedback they receive. Adherence or nonadherence to health-related behaviors, then, is based on a person's appraisal of the condition, the availability and relevance of particular actions for management of the health threat, and an evaluation of the outcomes (both costs and benefits) of those actions.

For example, a patient's decision about taking antihypertensive medication will be influenced by factors such as beliefs about the nature and meaning of "high blood pressure" (e.g., whether it is transient or persistent, whether it is symptomatic, how serious it is), beliefs about the effectiveness of the medication for improving health, alternative methods for managing blood pressure, side effects of taking the medication, and financial cost of the medication. If the patient decides to take the medication, he or she will then attend to any changes in symptoms, side effects, or other feedback believed to be relevant in order to determine whether the medication is beneficial.

As depicted in the lower portion of Figure 19.2, the problem-solving process itself is a prod-

*Figure 19.2* Self-Regulation Processes

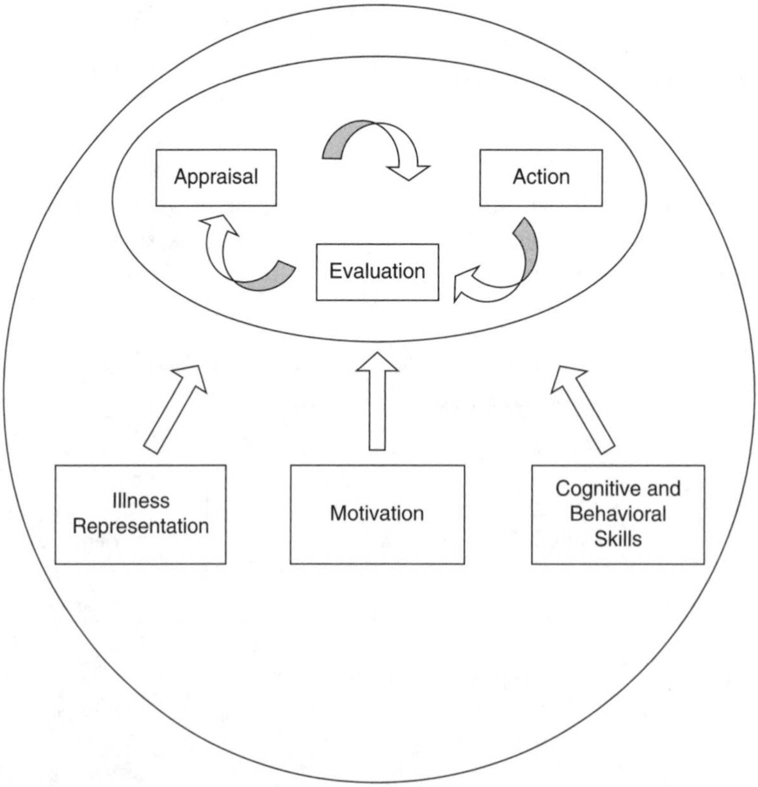


*(Adapted from Leventhal, Leventhal, & Cameron, 2001)*

uct of multiple factors: 1) the person's understanding of the health threat, or *illness representation,* 2) level of motivation, 3) cognitive and behavioral skills, and 4) the socio-cultural environment (Leventhal, Diefenbach, & Leventhal, 1992; Leventhal et al., 2001). A person's illness representation includes beliefs about the label and symptoms of the illness; the timeline for the development, duration, and treatment of the illness; the cause of the illness; the consequences of the illness; and the expected responsiveness of the condition to treatment (Schober & Lacroix, 1991). One's illness representation may or may not be based on its biomedical nature or the medical procedures optimal for its management. However, it is this representation that shapes the generation of actions for management and the evaluation of the outcomes of these actions.

The problem-solving process is further affected by the individual's level of motivation, as well as his or her cognitive and behavioral skills. The greater the person's level of motivation, the more he or she is likely to engage in active problem solving. The greater the person's level of cognitive and behavioral skills, the more successful those problem-solving processes will be. Individuals are more likely to select responses that they believe they are capable of carrying out, especially those that they have used successfully in the past. Finally, the problem-solving process is shaped by the sociocultural environment. An individual's perceptions of the attitudes and beliefs of those in his or her social and cultural environment can influence that person's appraisal of a health condition and evaluation of outcomes, as well as motivation for engaging in specific behaviors. Further, one's environment affects the development of cognitive and behavioral skills as well as the behavioral choices available.

## Comparison with Other Models

A self-regulation perspective offers greater utility for understanding and promoting adherence than models based primarily on cognitions such as the health belief model (Rosenstock, 1974). First, this perspective takes into account not only beliefs but also individual capabilities. A person may hold beliefs that favor adoption of a health behavior, but lack the skills to maintain that behavior. Second, a self-regulation perspective is ecological, taking into account environmental influences on behavior. Finally, self-regulation provides a framework by which one can understand relevant developmental factors (Leventhal, Leventhal, Robitaille, Brownlee, 1999). Developmental processes, including cognitive, emotional, and social development, directly affect one's ability to problem-solve. Life experiences also shape a person's development of perceptions, skills, and expectations, thereby influencing the problem-solving process. Social environments change throughout the life span, further affecting self-regulation.

## Developmental Changes

Developmental models of adherence differ from other models because a developmental model accounts for how adherence can and does change. The development of self-regulation, and thus adherence, reflects changes in cognitive, physiological, behavioral, and social domains of development, as well environmental influences, for example, those that shape illness representation. Although typical changes can be anticipated across the life span, individual differences in the development of adherence should be expected.

Developmental changes in the individual affecting adherence include changes in both cognitive and physiological processes. In youth, the progression in cognitive development influences one's understanding of health and illness, understanding of causality and consequences, and ability to problem-solve. Thus, self-regulation capability develops alongside cognitive maturity. Emotional development further influences self-regulation via the emergence of more advanced and adaptive coping skills. In the elderly, cognitive decline may occur, resulting in cognitive processing and memory difficulties affecting adherence. Elderly persons must also deal with age-related biological changes, increasing the difficulty of health-related problem-solving. For example, as individuals age, they typically experience increased symptoms overall, yet these symptoms are often more vague. Thus, they must determine the significance of and appropriate action for gradually appearing, blunted symptoms in the presence of already-existing age-related somatic changes. For example, a person with mild arthritis may be uncertain as to whether a new but somewhat vague pain is simply a part of her arthritis or a sign of a different problem.

Developmental changes affecting adherence also occur in the social environment. Among young children, adherence is primarily an issue of parental adherence; thus, the family environment exerts the greatest influence in adherence. As children mature, they gradually take more responsibility for health care, and adherence is influenced by both family and peer environments. Peer influences become increasingly important as the youth matures and may be a key source of social support. Parents continue to have a significant influence, especially for providing assistance with problem-solving and ongoing supervision. Throughout adulthood, key social environments include family, friends, and workplace. These settings may provide environmental stability and support for health behaviors, but they may also impose stressors and competing demands. Throughout the life span, developmental changes in the information available to people may occur, exposing them to discussion about symptoms, beliefs regarding health promotion and illness management, and other relevant information. With increasing age, individuals also experience greater morbidity and mortality in their social networks, which may result in a sense of nonspecific vulnerability.

## EXAMPLE OF A SELF-REGULATION PERSPECTIVE

The utility of a self-regulation perspective for understanding adherence was demonstrated in a study of HIV-infected late middle-age and older adults (Siegel, Schrimshaw, & Dean, 1999). Researchers found that participants relied heavily on their symptoms and a subjective sense of well-being to assess the effectiveness of their prescribed medications. An increase in symptoms was typically perceived as a sign of the medication being ineffective or doing more harm than good. Even in the presence of clinical indicators of improvement, such as increased T-cell count, patients questioned the effectiveness of medication if they perceived greater symptoms or side effects. Moreover, patients did not usually talk to their physicians before discontinuing or decreasing medication dose. These findings support the proposition that patients engage in a decision-making, hypothesis-testing process regarding adherence to medications. They formulate hypotheses about the cause of symptoms, alter their medical regimen, and evaluate the effect. Thus, when nonadherence has a perceived positive effect, patients believe that their nonadherence is the appropriate course of action.

A self-regulation framework helps delineate the multiple factors that must be addressed to promote adherence to recommended health-related behavior changes (Leventhal, 1993). An accurate understanding of the health condition is needed to form an accurate appraisal and evaluation of outcomes. Motivational factors create the desire to adopt healthy behaviors and stop health-damaging ones. Skill factors are needed for the selection and execution of appropriate actions and for the maintenance of these actions in the face of obstacles. For example, a person attempting to make dietary changes to promote weight loss must have a sufficient understanding of nutrition to determine what food choices are wisest, sufficient motivation to persevere in the face of obstacles, and sufficient problem-solving skills to manage difficult situations such as eating out and weight plateaus. Finally, effective management of negative affective states, such as anxiety and distress, is needed so that these emotions do not block effective action. An individual's social and cultural environment may influence any of these factors; as such, it represents yet another important factor in efforts to promote adherence.

## Promoting Adherence

Early efforts at enhancing adherence often focused only on addressing knowledge or motivational factors. Traditional patient education methods attempted to increase adherence through increasing understanding of the health condition, while early interventions addressing health risks typically attempted to enhance motivation with persuasive messages. Research on such efforts has shown that both methods are generally insufficient for promoting and sustaining behavior change. An accurate understanding of the health condition or issue is necessary but not sufficient for change, and messages about health threats have not been found to influence behavior unless they were combined with concrete information defining a plan of action (e.g., Leventhal, Singer, & Jones, 1965; Leventhal, Watts, & Pagano, 1967). This is because health behavior change requires not only adequate motivation but also the problem-solving skills to carry out the intended behaviors (Ewart, 1991, 1993; Leventhal et al., 2001). Problem-solving activities thus form the link from motivation to actual behavior change. The importance of problem-solving activities in connecting motivation to behavior is supported by several studies finding that greater problem-solving ability is associated with greater adherence among both children (Hanna, Ewart, & Kwiterovich, 1990) and adults (Fehrenbach & Peterson, 1989).

# Adherence at Each End of the Developmental Spectrum

A developmental perspective on adherence is best articulated by comparing the two ends of the developmental spectrum: children and elders. Among children and adolescents, the role of the family in promoting adherence is paramount. Among elders, the picture changes as the complexity of the medication regimen increases as cognitive flexibility declines.

## Children and Adolescents

Among children and adolescents, the majority of illnesses are acute. In such cases, nonadherence is often not associated with adverse health outcomes for the individual patient, but it contributes to the development of resistant strains of bacteria and associated costs (Gibbons, 1992; Schwarzmann, 1998). Overall, about one-third of pediatric patients do not adhere adequately to regimens for acute illness (Rapoff & Barnard, 1991). In treatment for acute illness, adherence tends to decrease over time, as symptoms decrease. While typical courses of antibiotics run 10 days, children often begin to feel better by the third or fourth day. With symptom relief no longer functioning as a motivator, parents and youth may believe that they no longer need the medication. Studies of adherence to 10-day antibiotic regimens for otitis media have shown that 19% to 59% of children do not get at least 50% of the prescribed medication, and 84% to 95% do not get 80% of the prescribed course (Charney et al., 1967; Dickey, Mattar, & Chudziker, 1975; Feldman, Momy, & Dulberg, 1988; Mattar, Marklein, & Yaffee, 1975; Mclinn, McCarty, Perrotta, Pichichero, & Reindenberg, 1995).

Levels of nonadherence to chronic disease regimens vary widely according to the disease and particular behavior studied, but it is estimated that 50% to 55% of pediatric patients with a chronic illness are insufficiently adherent (Rapoff & Barnard, 1991; Rapoff, 1999). Nonadherence increases with the complexity and intrusiveness of the regimen and often increases with duration of the disease. Adherence to medical regimens for chronic illness is associated with both short- and long-term negative health outcomes, including school absence, hospitalizations, complications, and decreased life span.

## PARENT–CHILD RELATIONSHIPS

Understanding adherence among children and adolescents requires attention to both child development and parent–child dynamics. Children's concepts of physical illness appear to develop in a manner consistent with cognitive development (Bibace & Walsh, 1980; Burbach & Peterson, 1986). As children mature, they progress from a more nonspecific understanding of illness, typically unable to differentiate symptoms of illness from causes of illness, to an understanding of specific symptoms, diseases, and physiological processes. Perceived control over illness also typically increases with cognitive maturity. Thus, patient education and efforts to promote adherence need to be appropriate to the child's level of cognitive development. As predicted by self-regulation models, adherence among youth with chronic illness has been found to be related to illness perceptions, including belief in the importance and/or necessity of the regimen and controllability of the illness (Buston & Wood, 2000; Byer & Myers, 2000; Griva, Myers, & Newman, 2000).

Adherence to a chronic illness regimen involves changing roles and responsibilities between parent and child. As children mature, they take on increasing responsibility for day-to-day management. However, the complexity of chronic illness management often requires greater problem-solving skills than the youth has developed, and developmental issues of adolescence may result in inconsistent adherence. As such, an effective and flexible parent–child partnership is needed for optimal adherence. When the child's degree of responsibility is too high for his/her level of cognitive maturity, poor adherence and health outcomes result (Wysocki et al., 1996). Both family conflict (Christiaanse, Lavigne, & Lerner, 1989; Friedman et al., 1986; Hauser et al., 1990; Miller-Johnson et al., 1994) and parental involvement (Anderson, Ho, Brackett, Finkelstein, & Laffel, 1997; Beck et al., 1980; Ingersoll, Orr, Herrold, & Golden, 1986; Tebbi, Richards,

Cummings, Zevon, & Mallon, 1988) have consistently been found to be important determinants of adherence to health care regimens for chronic illness. Programs that promote active parent involvement with appropriate negotiation of responsibility (Anderson, Brackett, Ho, & Laffel, 2000) and improved overall family functioning (Wysocki, Greco, Harris, & White, 2000) have been shown to result in greater adherence to treatment regimens.

## ADOLESCENCE

Adherence to medical regimens during adolescence can be especially challenging. During adolescence, rapid changes in both the self and the social context occur. The peer group becomes increasingly important for providing a sense of identity and belonging, and adolescents experience a strong desire to avoid being different from their peers (Harter, 1990). Cognitive development, particularly the development of formal reasoning skills, occurs throughout the adolescent years. Early adolescents may still use concrete operations in making decision about health care, and they are less likely to use formal reasoning in emotionally charged decisions. In difficult situations, they may perceive a narrow range of solutions, ignore long-term consequences, and make premature decisions. Adolescents also tend to feel a sense of invulnerability and attention to the present (Elkind, 1967; Keating, 1990); as such, the long-term consequences of poor adherence are not particularly salient.

Negotiating independence within the context of the parent–child relationship is an important task of adolescence (Montemayor & Flannery, 1991). However, the desire to assert independence may result in the youth choosing to neglect illness management tasks that are dictated by parents or health care providers in order to assert autonomy. For example, if parents of a youth with diabetes use authoritarian means to enforce prescribed blood glucose monitoring, the youth may begin to skip blood sugar checks to demonstrate independence. Therefore, it is important for parents and health care providers to avoid placing adolescents in a situation where they have to choose between the conflicting goals of autonomy and self-care (Anderson & Coyne, 1991). Instead, a shared-responsibility, partnership approach will allow the youth to gradually take on greater amounts of responsibility while continuing to receive the assistance and supervision needed for effective self-management.

From childhood through adolescence, health care providers may shape their interactions with youth to promote healthful behaviors (Ewart, 1993). During early childhood, it is important to build favorable outcome expectations for healthful behaviors and expose children to healthy social models. As children progress through middle childhood, they can understand behavior-outcome relationships and benefit from explicit self-standards for desired health behaviors. Providers may promote the selection of healthful behavioral goals and provide supportive feedback for goal attainment. During adolescence, it is important to also teach and encourage the use of problem-solving skills for avoiding or managing difficult social situations. Through an understanding of both the factors influencing adherence and developmental processes in youth, health care can be provided in a way that maximizes adherence and health-promoting behavior.

## Elders

Inadequate adherence to medication regimens among elderly adults appears to occur with considerable frequency, with estimates ranging from one-fifth to over one-half among various samples of older adults (Botelho & Dudrak, 1992; Col, Fanale, & Kronholm, 1990; Coons et al., 1994; Cooper, Love, & Raffoul, 1982). Both intentional and unintentional nonadherence have been found to be prevalent. In an in-home survey of adults age 60 to 90 (Cooper et al., 1982), 73% of nonadherence (primarily underuse of prescribed medications) was intentional. The most common

reasons for intentional nonadherence were believing that one did not need the medication in the dose prescribed and experiencing side effects. Those who were unintentionally nonadherent cited forgetting and not being able to afford or obtain the medication as the primary reasons for nonadherence. In a study of hospital admissions among the elderly, somewhat differing results were obtained, with unintentional nonadherence being the most prevalent (Col et al., 1990). Among this hospitalized population, the most common cause of noncompliance was forgetfulness, followed by side effects, and then the medication being perceived as unnecessary.

Among the elderly, unintentional nonadherence appears to be particularly influenced by changes in cognitive skills. Adherence to a medication regimen involves four processing components: 1) comprehension of the instructions, 2) integration of medication schedules with each other into a daily plan, 3) remembering the medication schedule once it is integrated, and 4) remembering to take the medication at the appointed time. There is evidence that the elderly are disadvantaged at each of these steps, with age-related declines in inference, working memory, long-term memory, and prospective memory (Park, 1999).

As such, it is not surprising that adherence declines with age in older adults (Morrel, Park, Kidder, & Martin, 1997; Park, Morrell, Frieske, & Kincaid, 1992) and that nonadherence is associated with greater numbers of prescribed medications and more complex medication schedules (Col et al., 1990; Coons et al., 1994; Hulka, Cassel, Kupper, & Burdette, 1976). In one study, adherence to prescriptions taken once or twice daily was 72%, versus 54% for medications taken three or four times daily (Botelho & Dudrak, 1992). However, in another study, the oldest adults demonstrated adherence equal to that of the young-old adults when provided with cognitive aids, including a detailed hour-by-hour medication schedule and a weekly medication organizer with four daily slots (Park et al., 1992). Thus, the decline in adherence observed with aging may be accounted for by cognitive changes associated with aging and may be compensated for by the use of cognitive aids.

Nonadherence in the elderly is associated with significant adverse health outcomes. In a study of hospital admissions among the elderly, 11.4% of admissions were due to noncompliance (Col et al., 1990). Moreover, a Medicaid three-drug limit on drug reimbursement implemented in New Hampshire was associated with a decrease in prescription drug use among those who had taken three or more medications before implementation of the limit and more than double the rates of admission to nursing homes (Soumerai, Ross-Degan, Avorn, McLaughlin, & Choodnovskiv, 1991). After the three-drug limit was discontinued, the rates of prescription drug use and nursing home admissions returned to baseline (prelimit) levels. These findings demonstrate both the importance of adherence for health outcomes as well as the effect of health care policy on adherence behaviors.

# Promoting Improved Adherence

Reviews of interventions designed to increase adherence have shown that systematic efforts designed to improve understanding and problem solving, decrease barriers, and facilitate memory can in fact improve adherence (Newell, Bowman, & Cockburn, 1999; Newell, Bowman, & Cockburn, 2000; Posavac, Sinacore, Brotherton, Helford, & Turpin, 1985; Yabroff, Kerner, & Mandelblatt, 2000). Typically, greater effort is required to increase adherence to lifestyle changes or preventive care than to specific treatments such as medications. Especially effective are programs that assist patients to incorporate the treatment regimen into their daily routine, as well as those that target modifying the provision of care. Interventions need to be designed to address both

intentional and unintentional nonadherence and may need to address provider, practice, and patient factors.

## Provider–Patient Interaction

The development of an effective provider–patient partnership, or treatment alliance, builds the foundation for the provision of health care and the promotion of patient adherence. Components of a strong treatment alliance include mutual positive regard, shared problem solving and decision making, shared goals, and high motivation for attaining goals. Although the concept of treatment alliance has been studied primarily within the field of psychotherapy (Hovarth & Luborsky, 1993; Hovarth & Symonds, 1991), findings demonstrating more positive outcomes with greater treatment alliance have important implications for medical treatment as well. By involving the patient in decision making about the treatment regimen, the regimen is more likely to be appropriate for the patient's particular needs and limitations, and the patient is more likely to be vested in carrying out the regimen. Indeed, a study of adolescents with severe asthma demonstrated that a more positive treatment alliance was associated with greater adherence and more optimal medical outcomes (Gavin, Wamboldt, Sorokin, Levy, & Wamboldt, 1999).

Effective provider–patient communication is important both for creating an effective provider–patient alliance and for promoting improved understanding of the provider's recommendations and reasons for them. Communication about a medical treatment or regimen should include insuring that the patient thoroughly understands what she or he is being asked to do and why, and then respectfully determining whether the patient in fact intends to follow through with the provider's recommendations. If there is discrepancy, the provider can then determine the reasons for the patient's reluctance, attending to relevant beliefs, social norms, and barriers.

Communication should address the patient's beliefs about the costs, benefits, and likely effectiveness of a treatment as well as the degree of practical difficulties. In addition, the provider should assist the patient to anticipate and problem-solve potential barriers to adherence. For example, if a patient is being instructed in dietary changes, the provider may ask about situations in which it will likely be difficult to follow these changes and problem-solve ways to handle these situations. When prescribing medications, it is important for providers to discuss expected side effects, encourage the patient to report any new symptoms, take patients' concerns seriously, work with the patient to reduce side effects, and enhance patients' abilities to determine the cause of symptoms they experience. A system of provider–patient communication termed "PREPARED" (DiMatteo, Reiter, & Gambone, 1994; Gambone & Reiter, 1991) assists providers in addressing these components (Figure 19.3).

For addressing adherence to difficult behavior or lifestyle changes, such as smoking cessation, exercise, or dietary changes, an approach that has been shown to be particularly useful is that of motivational interviewing (Figure 19.4). Motivational interviewing was originally developed and used within the field of addictions (Emmons & Rollnick, 2001; Miller & Rollnick, 1991;

Rollnick,& Miller, 1995), but its use has expanded to many areas of health behavior change (Rollnick, Heather, & Bell, 1992; Rollnick, Mason, & Butler, 1999). This approach arose out of observations that, rather than trying to convince clients to change, counselors were more effective when they elicited arguments for change from the clients themselves. A motivational interviewing approach is based on the recognition that direct persuasion can push the patient into a position of defensiveness. Patients typically feel ambivalence regarding behavior change. They may recognize a given behavior as healthful but also have negative feelings toward the behavior. For example, patients may acknowledge that an exercise program would benefit their cardiac status but find exercise to be unpleasant or time consuming. Therefore, advice-giving or overt persuasion will typically lead to resistance and counter-arguments ("yes, but . . .").

Motivational interviewing instead provides a greater degree of personal autonomy by encouraging patients to explore their ambivalence, express their own reasons for concern and arguments for change, and thereby move toward behavior change. The practitioner uses reflective listening, empathy, and objective feedback to facilitate the patient's delineation of discrepancy between personal goals and current behavior, assisting the

---

*Figure 19.3*    "PREPARED" System of Provider–Patient Communication

**P**—The recommended **procedure** or **prescription**

**R**—The **reason** for the recommendation in terms of the observed or potential harm that is or could be threatening the patient's health status

**E**—The patients' and providers' outcome **expectations** in terms of preventing or reversing any harm

**P**—The **probability** of achieving those expectations

**A**—Reasonable **alternatives** to what has been recommended, including expectant management or watchful waiting

**R**—All significant **risks** associated with what has been recommended

**E**—**Expenses,** including direct and indirect costs

**D**—The **decision**

*(DiMatteo, Reiter, & Gambone, 1994; Gambone & Reiter, 1991)*

---

*Figure 19.4*    Key Motivational Interviewing Concepts

1. Motivation to change is elicited from the client and not imposed from without.
2. It is the client's task, not the counselor's, to articulate and resolve his or her ambivalence.
3. Direct persuasion is not an effective method for resolving ambivalence.
4. The counseling style is generally a quiet and eliciting one.
5. The counselor is directive in helping the client to examine and resolve ambivalence.
6. Readiness to change is not a client trait, but a fluctuating product of interpersonal interaction.
7. The therapeutic relationship is more like a partnership or companionship than expert/recipient roles.

---

*(Rollnick & Miller, 1995)*

patient in resolving ambivalence and enhancing self-efficacy and optimism for change. The patient maintains responsibility for the decision to change, with motivation to change elicited from the patient rather than being imposed by the practitioner. Recent research supports the usefulness of motivational interviewing as a promising approach for promoting adherence to smoking cessation, HIV risk reduction, diet, exercise, medication use, and outpatient follow-up (Dunn, Deroo, & Rivara, 2001; Kemp, Kirov, Everitt, Hayward, & David, 1998; Safren et al., 2001; Swanson, Pantalon, & Cohen, 1999).

## Practice Characteristics

Characteristics of the medical practice and treatment regimen may also be designed to improve adherence. Practice characteristics may affect the development of a treatment alliance, the patient's understanding of illness and treatment, and the degree of barriers to adherence. For example, providing a consumer-friendly clinical setting (e.g., ease of making appointments, reduced waiting time) and facilitating ease of contact with the provider between office visits will promote positive treatment alliance and also increase the likelihood that a patient will contact the provider if difficulties with the treatment occur. Providing patient-centered counseling as a standard part of practice will improve patients' understanding of the treatment regimen and increase motivation

for adherence, and a proactive approach to reducing and managing adverse effects will reduce barriers to adherence. Prescribing practices that minimize regimen complexity and cost will also reduce barriers to adherence, as will the provision of reminders between visits. Tailoring the treatment regimen to the patient's particular needs and lifestyle will further reduce barriers and promote a positive treatment alliance.

In understanding adherence as an outcome that is difficult to achieve and therefore must be actively negotiated, the provider will create an environment in which difficulties with adherence can be openly discussed and problem solving may occur. Regular medical care should include an assessment of the degree of adherence achieved, problems encountered, and the patient's appraisal of treatment effectiveness. Assessment tools, such as the Brief Medication Questionnaire (Svarstad, Chewning, Sleath, & Claesson, 1999), may be useful for identifying patients who are having difficulty with adherence so that appropriate actions may be taken (e.g., modification of the regimen, assistance from family members, use of memory aids, etc.).

For patients who have difficulty remembering to take medications, providers may facilitate adherence by providing cognitive aids or even modifying the prescription itself. Cognitive aids found to facilitate adherence include the use of medication schedules and organizers (Park et al., 1992), as well as other strategies such as pairing the medication-taking with routine activities and using visual memory reminders (Wallsten et al., 1995). In addition to the use of such tactics, adherence may also be increased through modifications in prescribing. In assessments of patients seen for geriatric medical consultations, it was found that dosage intervals could be reduced in one out of three patients, and one in eight patients could be switched from a multiple-dose regimen to a once-daily regimen (Sweetman, Howard, & O'Neill, 1999). Considering that the use of once-daily regimens may increase adherence by as much as 25% (Eisen, Miller, Woodward, Spitznagel, & Przybeck, 1990), changes in prescribing practices could have a substantial impact on improving adherence.

## Patient Education

A self-regulation perspective on adherence is useful for guiding patient education practices to facilitate adherence (Leventhal, 1993). Because symptoms are seen as an indicator of disease, patients expect treatment to ameliorate both symptoms and the underlying disease. Thus, patient education should include preparing people to accurately interpret symptoms and to understand treatment effects and their timeline. The patient's representation of a health problem may be markedly different from the health professional's view, and it is this representation that guides behavior. If the patient's expectations regarding symptoms, treatment effects, and timeline are not congruent with the reality of the disease process and treatment, nonadherence is likely to occur. Moreover, patients make appraisals based on their experience as to the nature of the health problem, the adequacy of the treatment used, and their ability to perform the treatment regimen. These appraisals affect the maintenance of motivation for behavior. As such, educational interventions designed to improve adherence should address patient appraisals, goals, and self-evaluated capabilities. Various interventions utilizing a patient-centered counseling or coaching approach, supplemented with appropriate behavioral and practice support (such as special medication containers, self-monitoring procedures, mailed reminders, and tailoring of regimens), have demonstrated the effectiveness of this approach for promoting medication adherence and even changing lifestyle behaviors (Bailey et al., 1990; Haynes et al., 1976; Logan, Milne, Achber, Campbell, & Haynes, 1979; Ockene et al., 1991; Ockene et al., 1999; Peterson, McLean, & Millingen, 1984; Vale, Jelinek, Best, & Santamaria, 2002).

For difficult or complex adherence behaviors, education focusing on perceptions and appraisals may not be sufficient. Patients often fail to adhere adequately to behaviors even when they fully intend or desire to do so. Adherence to lifestyle changes or other treatment regimens may involve daily behaviors that are difficult, time consuming, and unpleasant. For example, a person may desire to stop smoking but have difficulty doing so because of uncomfortable withdrawal symptoms. Someone with diabetes may intend to perform a blood sugar check before every meal but falter when socializing with friends. As such, behavioral approaches may be especially useful for enhancing adherence to more difficult behaviors and regimens.

Behavioral approaches are designed to increase a person's skills, bridging the gap between motivation and performance. Behavioral programs that involve modeling and behavioral rehearsal (Hammond, Lincoln, & Sutcliffe, 1999), self-monitoring (Sperduto, Thompson, & O'Brien, 1986), goal setting and contracting (Hammond et al., 1999; Heinssen, Levendusky, & Hunter, 1995; Wysocki, Green, & Huxtable, 1989), and training in problem solving (Delamater et al., 1991; DeVellis, Blalock, Hahn, DeVellis, & Hochbaum, 1988) have been shown to promote improved adherence to lifestyle changes and treatment regimens. For example, in a program developed for patients with arthritis (DeVellis et al., 1988), patients were assisted to identify problems associated with adherence, identify and evaluate strategies to deal with the problem, and develop an action plan. Follow-up telephone calls were then used to evaluate progress and revise the plan as needed. The program was found to be successful in helping patients resolve problems with adherence.

# Summary

Although much progress has been made in understanding the factors that promote and inhibit adherence, this understanding has yet to be systematically applied to routine health care practice. A collaborative model of practice, in which the provider serves as an expert consultant and the patient as the person responsible for day-to-day health care management, creates the foundation for efforts to promote adherence. Adherence to a treatment regimen is a problem-solving process, influenced by one's understanding, motivation, skills, and sociocultural environment, and nested in a developmental context. Thus, the facilitation of adherence requires attention to the patient's perception of the illness and treatment regimen, motivation for adherence to the regimen, problem-solving skills for overcoming obstacles, and sociocultural environment. Providers have the ability to assist patients' self-care efforts by enhancing their understanding, motivation, and skills, as well as by addressing environmental supports and barriers. Efforts to promote adherence through improving patient–provider interaction, creating patient-centered health care practices, providing quality patient education, and facilitating the development of behavioral skills have been shown to be effective in improving patient adherence across various diagnoses and treatment regimens.

# References

Anderson, B. J., Brackett, J., Ho, J., & Laffel, L. M. (2000). An intervention to promote family teamwork in dia-

betes management tasks: Relationships among parental involvement, adherence to blood glucose monitoring, and glycemic control in young adolescents with type 1 diabetes. In D. Drotar (Ed.), *Promoting adherence to medical treatment in chronic childhood illness: Concepts, methods, and interventions* (pp. 347–366). Mahwah, NJ: Lawrence Erlbaum Associates.

Anderson, B., Ho, J., Brackett, J., Finkelstein, D., & Laffel, L. (1997). Parental involvement in diabetes management tasks: Relationships to blood glucose monitoring adherence and metabolic control in young adolescents with insulin-dependent diabetes mellitus. *Journal of Pediatrics, 130,* 257–265.

Anderson, B. J., & Coyne, J. C. (1991). "Miscarried helping" in the families of children and adolescents with chronic diseases. In. J. H. Johnson & S. B. Johnson (Eds.), *Advances in child health psychology* (pp. 167–177). Gainesville, FL: University of Florida Press.

Bailey, W. C., Richards, J. M. Jr., Brooks, C. M., Soong, S., Windsor, R. A., & Manzella, B. A. (1990). A randomized trial to improve self-management practices of adults with asthma. *Archives of Internal Medicine, 150,* 1664–1668.

Bauman, L. J. (2000). A patient-centered approach to adherence: Risks for nonadherence. In D. Drotar (Ed.), *Promoting adherence to medical treatment in chronic childhood illness: Concepts, methods, and interventions* (pp. 71–94). Mahwah, NJ: Lawrence Erlbaum Associates.

Beck, D. E., Fennell, R. S., Yost, R. L., Roginson, J. D., Geary, D., & Richards, G. A. (1980). Evaluation of an educational program on compliance with medication regimens in pediatric patients with renal transplants. *Journal of Pediatrics, 96,* 1094–1097.

Becker, M. H., & Maiman, L. A. (1975). Sociobehavioral determinants of compliance with health and medical care recommendations. *Medical Care, 13,* 10–24.

Bibace, R., & Walsh, M. E. (1980). Development of children's concepts of illness. *Pediatrics, 66,* 913–917.

Botelho, R. J., & Dudrak, R. (1992). Home assessment of adherence to long-term medication in the elderly. *The Journal of Family Practice, 35,* 61–65.

Burbach, D. J., & Peterson, L. (1986). Children's concepts of physical illness: A review and critique of the cognitive developmental literature. *Health Psychology, 5,* 307–325.

Buston, K. M., & Wood, S. F. (2000). Non-compliance amongst adolescents with asthma: listening to what they tell us about self-management. *Family Practice, 17,* 134–138.

Byer, B., & Myers, L. B. (2000). Psychological correlates of adherence to medication in asthma. *Psychology, Health and Medicine, 5,* 389–393.

Carmody, T. P., Matarazzo, J. D., & Istvan, J. A. (1987). Promoting adherence to heart-health diets: A review of the literature. *Journal of Compliance in Health Care, 2,* 105–124.

Charney, E., Bynum, R., Eldreye, D., Frank, D., MacWhinney, J. B., McNabb, N., et al. (1967). How well do patients take oral penicillin? A collaborative study in private practice. *Pediatrics, 40,* 188–195.

Christiaanse, M. E., Lavigne, J. V., & Lerner, C. V. (1989). Psychosocial aspects of compliance in children and adolescents with asthma. *Developmental and Behavioral Pediatrics, 10*(2), 75–80.

Col, N., Fanale, J. E., & Kronholm, P. (1990). The role of medication noncompliance and adverse drug reactions in hospitalizations of the elderly. *Archives of Internal Medicine, 150,* 841–845.

Coons, S. J., Sheahan, S. L., Martin, S. S., Hendricks, J., Robbins, C. A., & Johnson, J. A. (1994). Predictors of medication noncompliance in a sample of older adults. *Clinical Therapeutics, 16,* 110–117.

Cooper, J. K., Love, D. W., & Raffoul, P. R. (1982). Intentional prescription nonadherence (noncompliance) by the elderly. *Journal of the American Geriatrics Society, 30,* 329–331.

Cramer, J. A., & Rosenheck, R. (1998). Compliance with medication regimens for mental and physical disorders. *Psychiatric Services, 49,* 196–201.

Delamater, A. M., Smith, J. A., Bubb, J., Davis, S. G., Gamble, T., White, N. H., et al. (1991). Family-based behavior therapy for diabetic adolescents. In J. H. Johnson & S. B. Johnson (Eds.), *Advances in child health psychology* (pp. 293–306). Gainesville, FL: University of Florida Press.

DeVellis, B. M., Blalock, S. J., Hahn, P. M., DeVellis, R. F., & Hochbaum, G. M. (1988). Evaluation of a problem-solving intervention for patients with arthritis. *Patient Education and Counseling, 11,* 29–42.

Dickey, F. F., Mattar, M. E., & Chudziker, G. M. (1975). Pharmacist counseling increases drug regimen compliance. *Hospitals, 49,* 85–89.

DiMatteo, M. R., Reiter, R. C., & Gambone, J. C. (1994). Enhancing medication adherence through communication and informed collaborative choice. *Health Communication, 6,* 253–265.

Dunbar-Jacob, J., & Schlenk, E. A. (1996). Treatment adherence and clinical outcome: Can we make a difference? In R. J. Resnick & R. H. Rozensky (Eds.), *Health psychology through the life span: Practice and research opportunities* (pp. 323–343). Washington, DC: American Psychological Association.

Dunn, C., Deroo, L., & Rivara, F. P. (2001). The use of brief interventions adapted from motivational interviewing across behavioral domains: A systematic review. *Addiction, 96,* 1725–1742.

Eisen, S. A., Miller, D. K., Woodward, R. S., Spitznagel, E., & Przybeck, T. R. (1990). The effect of prescribed daily dose frequency on patient medical compliance. *Archives of Internal Medicine, 150,* 1881–1884.

Elkind, D. (1967). Egocentrism in adolescence. *Child Development, 38,* 1025–1034.

Emmons, K. M., & Rollnick, S. (2001). Motivational interviewing in health care settings: Opportunities and limitations. *American Journal of Preventive Medicine, 20,* 68–74.

Ewart, C. K. (1991). A social problem-solving approach to behavior change in coronary heart disease. In S. A. Shumaker, E. B. Schron, & J. K. Okene (Eds.), *The handbook of health behavior change* (pp. 153–190). New York: Springer Publishing Company.

Ewart, C. K. (1993). Health promotion and disease prevention: A social action conception of compliance behavior. In N. A. Krasnegor, L. Epstein, S. Bennet Johnson, & S. J. Yaffe, *Developmental aspects of health compliance behavior* (pp. 251–280). Hillsdale, NJ: Lawrence Erlbaum Associates.

Feldman, W., Momy, J., & Dulberg, C. (1988). Trimethoprim-sulfamethoxazole vs. amoxicillin in the treatment of acute otitis media. *Canadian Medical Association Journal, 139,* 961–964.

Fehrenbach, A. M., & Peterson, L. (1989). Parental problem-solving skills, stress, and dietary compliance in phenylketonuria. *Journal of Consulting and Clinical Psychology, 57,* 237–241.

Friedman, I. M., Litt, I. F., King, D. R., Henson, R., Holtzman, D., Halverson, D., et al. (1986). Compliance with anticonvulsant therapy by epileptic youth. *Journal of Adolescent Health Care, 7,* 12–17.

Gambone, J. C. & Reiter, R. C. (1991). Quality improvement in health care. *Current Problems in Obstetrics, Gynecology, and Fertility, 14,* 151–175.

Gavin, L. A., Wamboldt, M. Z., Sorokin, N., Levy, S. Y., & Wamboldt, F. S. (1999). Treatment alliance and its association with family functioning, adherence, and medical outcome in adolescents with severe, chronic asthma. *Journal of Pediatric Psychology, 24,* 355–365.

Gibbons, A. (1992). Exploring new strategies to fight drug-resistant microbes. *Science, 257,* 1036–1038.

Glanz, K. (1979). Dieticians' effectiveness and patient compliance with dietary regimens: A pilot study. *Journal of the American Dietetic Association, 75,* 631–636.

Griva, K., Myers, L. B., & Newman, S. (2000). Illness perceptions and self efficacy beliefs in adolescents and young adults with insulin dependent diabetes mellitus. *Psychology and Health, 15,* 733–750.

Hammond, A., Lincoln, N., & Sutcliffe, L. (1999). A crossover trial evaluating an educational-behavioural joint protection programme for people with rheumatoid arthritis. *Patient Education and Counseling, 37,* 19–32.

Hanna, K. J., Ewart, C. K., & Kwiterovich, P. O. (1990). Child problem solving competence, behavioral adjustment and adherence to lipid-lowering diet. *Patient Education and Counseling, 16,* 119–131.

Harter, S. (1990). Self and identity development. In S. S. Feldman & G. R. Elliott (Eds.), *At the threshold: The developing adolescent* (pp. 352–387). Cambridge, MA: Harvard University Press.

Hauser, S. T., Jacobson, A. M., Lavori, P., Wolfsdor, J. I., Herskowitz, R. D., Milley, J. E., et al. (1990). Adherence among children and adolescents with insulin-dependent diabetes mellitus over a four-year longitudinal follow-up: II. Immediate and long-term linkages with the family milieu. *Journal of Pediatric Psychology, 15,* 527–542.

Haynes, R. B., Sackett, D. L., Gibson, E. S., Taylor, D. W., Hackett, B. C., Roberts, R. S., et al. (1976). Improvement of medication compliance in uncontrolled hypertension. *Lancet, 1*(7972), 1265–1268.

Heinssen, R. K., Levendusky, P. G., & Hunter, R. H. (1995). Client as colleague: Therapeutic contracting with the seriously mentally ill. *American Psychologist, 50,* 522–532.

Horvath, A. O., & Luborsky, L. (1993). The role of the therapeutic alliance in psychotherapy. *Journal of Clinical and Consulting Psychology, 61,* 561–573.

Horvath, A. O., & Symonds, B. D. (1991). Relation between working alliance and outcome in psychotherapy: A meta-analysis. *Journal of Counseling Psychology, 38,* 139–149.

Hulka, B. S., Cassel, J. C., Kupper, L. L., & Burdette, J. A. (1976). Communication, compliance, and concordance between physicians and patients with prescribed medications. *American Journal of Public Health, 66,* 847–853.

Ingersoll, G. M., Orr, D. P., Herrold, A. J., & Golden, M. P. (1986). Cognitive maturity and self-management among adolescents with insulin-dependent diabetes mellitus. *Journal of Pediatrics, 108,* 620–623.

Keating, D. P. (1990). Adolescent thinking. In S. S. Feldman & G. R. Elliott (Eds.), *At the threshold: The developing adolescent* (pp. 54–89). Cambridge, MA: Harvard University Press.

Kemp, R., Kirov, G., Everitt, B., Hayward, P., & David, A. (1998). Randomised controlled trial of compliance therapy. *British Journal of Psychiatry, 172,* 413–419.

Laederach-Hofmann, K., & Bunzel, B. (2000). Noncompliance in organ transplant recipients: A literature review. *General Hospital Psychiatry, 22,* 412–424.

Leventhal, H. (1993). Theories of compliance, and turning necessities into preferences: Application to adolescent health action. In N. A. Krasnegor, L. Epstein, S. Bennet Johnson, & S. J. Yaffe, *Developmental aspects of health compliance behavior* (pp. 91–124). Hillsdale, NJ: Lawrence Erlbaum Associates.

Leventhal, H., Diefenbach, M., & Leventhal, E. A. (1992). Illness cognition: Using common sense to understand treatment adherence and affect cognition interactions. *Cognitive Therapy and Research, 16,* 143–163.

Leventhal, H., Leventhal, E. A., & Cameron, L. (2001). Representations, procedures, and affect in illness self-regulations: A perceptual-cognitive model. In A. Baum, T. A. Revenson, & J. E. Singer (Eds.), *Handbook of Health Psychology* (pp. 19–47). Mahwah, NJ: Lawrence Erlbaum Associates.

Leventhal, H., Leventhal, E. A., & Contrada, R. J. (1998). Self-regulation, health, and behavior: A perceptual-cognitive approach. *Psychology and Health, 13,* 717–733.

Leventhal, E. A., Leventhal, H., Robitaille, C., & Brownlee, S. (1999). Psychosocial factors in medication adherence: A model of the modeler. In D. C. Park, R. W. Morell, & K. Shifren (Eds.), *Processing of medical information in aging patients: Cognitive and human factors perspectives* (pp. 19–47). Mahwah, NJ: Lawrence Erlbaum Associates.

Leventhal, H., Singer, R., & Jones, S. (1965). Effects of fear and specificity of recommendations upon attitudes and behavior. *Journal of Personality and Social Psychology, 2,* 20–29.

Leventhal, H., Watts, J. C., & Pagano, R. (1967). Effects of fear and instructions on how to cope with danger. *Journal of Personality and Social Psychology, 6,* 313–321.

Logan, A. G., Milne, B. J., Achber, C., Campbell, W. P., & Haynes, R. B. (1979). Work-site treatment of hypertension by specially trained nurses: A controlled trial. *Lancet, 2*(8153), 1175–1178.

Marcus, B. H., Dubbert, P. M., Forsyth, L. H., McKenzie, T. L., Stone, E. J., Dunn, A. L., et al. (2000). Physical activity behavior change: Issues in adoption and maintenance. *Health Psychology, 19*(1 Suppl.), 32–41.

Maronde, R. F., Chan, L. S., Larsen, F. J., Strandberg, L. R., Laventurier, M. F., & Sullivan, S. R. (1989). Underutilization of antihypertensive drugs and associated hospitalization. *Medical Care, 27,* 1159–1166.

Mattar, M. F., Marklein, J., & Yaffe, S. J. (1975). Pharmaceutic factors affecting pediatric compliance. *Pediatrics, 55,* 101–108.

McLinn, S. E., McCarty, J. M., Perrotta, R., Pichichero, M. E., & Reindenberg, B. E. (1995). Multicenter controlled trial comparing ceftibuten with amoxicillin/clavulantae in the empiric treatment of acute otitis media. *Pediatric Infectious Disease Journal, 14,* 5108–5114.

Miller, W., & Rollnick, S. (1991). *Motivational interviewing: Preparing people to change addictive behaviors.* New York: Guilford Press.

Miller-Johnson, S., Emery, R. E., Marvin, R. S., Clarke, W., Lovinger, R., & Martin, M. (1994). Parent-child relationships and the management of insulin-dependent diabetes mellitus. *Journal of Consulting and Clinical Psychology, 62,* 603–610.

Montemayor, R., & Flannery, D. J. (1991). Parent-adolescent relations in middle and late adolescence. In R. M. Lerner, A. C. Petersen, & J. Brooks-Gunn (Eds.), *Encyclopedia of adolescence* (Vol. 2) (pp. 729–734). New York: Garland Publishing.

Morrell, R. W., Park, D. C., Kidder, D. P., & Martin, M. (1997). Anderence to antihypertensive medications across the life span. *The Gerontologist, 37,* 609–619.

National Pharmaceutical Council. (1992). Noncompliance with medication regimens: An economic tragedy. *Emerging Issues in Pharmaceutical Cost Containment, 2*(2), 1–13.

Newell, S. A., Bowman, J. A., & Cockburn, J. D. (1999). A critical review of interventions to increase compliance with medication-taking, obtaining medication refills, and appointment-keeping in the treatment of cardiovascular disease. *Preventive Medicine, 29,* 535–548.

Newell, S. A., Bowman, J. A., & Cockburn, J. D. (2000). Can compliance with nonpharmacologic treatments for cardiovascular disease be improved? *American Journal of Preventive Medicine, 18,* 253–261.

Ockene, I. S., Hebert, J. R., Ockene, J. K., Saperia, G. M., Stanek, E., Nicolosi, R., et al. (1999). Effect of physician-delivered nutrition counseling training and an office-support program on saturated fat intake, weight, and serum lipid measurements in a hyperlipidemic population. *Archives of Internal Medicine, 159,* 725–731.

Ockene, J. K., Kristeller, J., Goldberg, R., Amick, T. L., Pikow, P. S., Hosmer, D., et al. (1991). Increasing the efficacy of physician-delivered smoking intervention: A randomized clinical trial. *Journal of General Internal Medicine, 6,* 1–8.

Park, D. C. (1999). Aging and the controlled and automatic processing of medical information and medical intentions. In D. C. Park, R. W. Morell, & K. Shifren (Eds.), *Processing of medical information in aging patients: Cognitive and human factors perspectives* (pp. 3–22). Mahwah, NJ: Lawrence Erlbaum Associates.

Park, D. C., Morrell, R. W., Frieske, D., & Kincaid, D. (1992). Medication adherence behaviors in older adults: Effects of external cognitive supports. *Psychology and Aging, 7,* 252–256.

Peterson, B. M., McLean, S., & Millingen, K. S. (1984). A randomized trial of strategies to improve patient compliance with anticonvulsant therapy. *Epilepsia, 25,* 412–417.

Posavac, E. J., Sinacore, J. M., Brotherton, S., Helford, M. C., & Turpin, R. S. (1985). Increasing compliance to medical treatment regimens: A meta-analysis of program evaluation. *Evaluation & The Health Professions, 8,* 7–22.

Rapoff, M. A. (1999). *Adherence to pediatric medical regimens.* New York: Kluwer Academic/Plenum.

Rapoff, M. A., & Barnard, M. U. (1991). Compliance with pediatric medical regimens. In J. A. Cramer & B. Spilker (Eds.), *Patient compliance in medical practice and clinical trials* (pp. 73–98). New York: Raven Press.

Rollnick, S., Heather, N., & Bell, A. (1992). Negotiating behaviour change in medical settings: The development of brief motivational interviewing. *Journal of Mental Health, 1,* 25–37.

Rollnick, S., Mason, P., & Butler, C. (1999). *Health behavior change: A guide for practitioners.* Edinburgh: Churchill Livingstone.

Rollnick, S., & Miller, W. (1995). What is motivational interviewing? *Behavioural and Cognitive Psychotherapy, 23,* 325–324.

Rosenstock, I. M. (1974). The health belief model and preventive health behavior. *Health Education Monographs, 2,* 354–386.

Rovelli, M., Palmeri, D., Vossler, E., Bartus, S., Hull, D., & Schweizer, R. (1989). Noncompliance in organ transplant recipients. *Transplantation Proceedings, 21,* 833–834.

Rudman, L. A., Gonzales, M. H., & Borgida, E. (1999). Mishandling the gift of life: Noncomplaince in renal transplant patients. *Journal of Applied Social Psychology, 29,* 834–851.

Sackett, D. L., & Haynes, R. B. (1976). *Compliance with therapeutic regimens.* Baltimore: Johns Hopkins University Press.

Safren, S. A., Otto, M. W., Worth, J. L., Salomon, E., Johnson, W., Mayer, K., et al. (2001). Two strategies to increase adherence to HIV antiretroviral medication: Life-Steps and medication monitoring. *Behaviour Research and Therapy, 39,* 1151–1162.

Schober, R., & Lacroix, J. M. (1991). Lay illness models in the enlightenment and the 20th century: Some historical lessons. In J. A. Skelton & R. T. Croyle (Eds.), *Mental representation in health and illness* (pp. 10–31). New York: Springer-Verlag.

Schwarzmann, S.W. (1998). Novel cost-effective approaches to the treatment of community-acquired infections. *Annals of Pharmacotherapy, 32*(1), S27–S30.

Siegel, K., Schrimshaw, E. W., & Dean, L. (1999). Symptom interpretation and medication adherence among late middle-age and older HIV-infected adults. *Journal of Health Psychology, 4,* 247–257.

Sluijs, E. M., & Knibbe, J. J. (1991). Patient compliance with exercise: Different theoretical approaches to short-term and long-term compliance. *Patient Education & Counseling, 17,* 191–204.

Soumerai, S. B., Ross-Degnan, D., Avorn, J., McLaughlin, T. J., & Choodnovskiv, I. (1991). Effects of Medicaid drug-payment limits on admission to hospitals and nursing homes. *New England Journal of Medicine, 325,* 1072–1077.

Sperduto, W. A., Thompson, H. S., & O'Brien, R. M. (1986). The effect of target behavior monitoring on weight loss and completion rate in a behavior modification program for weight reduction. *Addictive Behaviors, 11,* 337–340.

Svarstad, B. L., Chewning, B. A., Sleath, B. L., & Claesson, C. (1999). The Brief Medication Questionnaire: A tool for screening patient adherence and barriers to adherence. *Patient Education and Counseling, 37,* 113–124.

Svarstad, B. L., Shireman, T. I., & Sweeney, J. K. (2001). Using drug claims data to assess the relationship of medication adherence with hospitalization and costs. *Psychiatric Services, 52,* 805–811.

Swanson, A. J., Pantalon, M. V., & Cohen, K. (1999). Motivational interviewing and treatment adherence among psychiatric and dually diagnosed patients. *Journal of Nervous and Mental Disease, 187,* 630–635.

Sweetman, L., Howard, D., & O'Neill, D. (1999). Once-daily medications for older patients in the general hospital. *Journal of the American Geriatrics Society, 47,* 629.

Tebbi, C. K., Richards, M. E., Cummings, K. M., Zevon, M. A., & Mallon, J. C. (1988). The role of parent-adolescent concordance in compliance with cancer chemotherapy. *Adolescence, 28,* 599–611.

Vale, M. J., Jelinek, M. V., Best, J. D., & Santamaria, J. D. (2002). Coaching patients with coronary heart disease to achieve the target cholesterol: A method to bridge the gap between evidence-based medicine and the "real world"–randomized controlled trial. *Journal of Clinical Epidemiology, 55,* 245–252.

Wallensten, S. M., Sullivan, R. J., Hanlon, J. T., Blazer, D. G., Tyrey, M. J., & Westlund, R. (1995). Medication taking behaviors in the high- and low-functioning elderly: MacArthur field studies of successful aging. *The Annals of Pharmacotherapy, 29,* 359–364.

Wysocki, T., Greco, P., Harris, M. A., & White, N. H. (2000). Behavioral family systems therapy for adolescents with diabetes. In D. Drotar (Ed.), *Promoting adherence to medical treatment in chronic childhood illness: Concepts, methods, and interventions* (pp. 367–382). Mahwah, NJ: Lawrence Erlbaum Associates.

Wysocki, T., Green, L., & Huxtable, K. (1989). Blood glucose monitoring by diabetic adolescents: Compliance and metabolic control. *Health Psychology, 8,* 267–284.

Wysocki, T., Taylor, A., Hough, B. S., Linscheid, T. R., Yeates, K. O., & Naglieri, J. A. (1996). Deviation from developmentally appropriate self-care autonomy: Association with diabetes outcomes. *Diabetes Care, 19,* 119–125.

Yabroff, K. R., Kerner, J. R., & Mandelblatt, J. S. (2000). Effectiveness of interventions to improve follow-up after abnormal cervical cancer screening. *Preventive Medicine, 31,* 429–439.

# Chapter 20

# EagleEyes: Technologies for Nonverbal Persons

Philip DiMattia

James Gips

The inclusion of a chapter in a book on human development on teaching and learning how to use assistive technology may help to demonstrate and deepen understanding of how similar the work is for all professional in the delivery of service to people in need. The following vignette may help to clarify the similarity of roles among professional human service providers: "There is no way to the end of the journey but to travel the road that leads to it." An ALS patient wrote this after one session using a technology called EagleEyes that was developed at Boston College. The patient had a successful career in business and was a respected and active member of his community until ALS began to gradually diminish his capacity to effectively communicate. Such drastic change in his ability to act upon his environment shut him out of the world that he had known, that he had worked in and lived in throughout his life—a world with which he was familiar and comfortable and where he enjoyed a level of prestige and authority, but also a world that gradually became more and more difficult to access.

Technology has the potential to become a great equalizer when both designers and service providers come together to develop models of collaboration that combine talents and interests in ways that attempt to improve the quality of life for persons whose access to their natural environment has been rendered difficult as a result of disease and/or other forms of disability. Technology can help to supplement an individual's innate ability to meet his or her biological needs and also to help an individual with severe communication disorders mediate a relationship with the environment. The aforementioned tasks are often the same for other human service providers when attempting to meet the health care needs of those they serve.

This chapter describes the use of assistive technology with children and youth with severe physical and communication disabilities to discover themselves as persons among persons and to experience events among events that promote a lifelong journey. The use of technology to mediate the relationship between the individual and the environment within an educational context is similar to the one attempted within the various fields of human service providers.

EagleEyes is a technology developed at Boston College that allows a person to operate a computer by simply moving his or her eyes or head. The first generation of EagleEyes that was developed in 1993 uses surface electrodes attached to the head (Gips, Olivieri, & Tecce, 1994). A second generation of EagleEyes, called the Camera Mouse, developed in 1999, uses a camera to track head movement (Betke, Gips, & Fleming, 2002). The two technologies work as mouse substitutes, allowing individuals to control the mouse pointer on the screen by moving their eyes or head.

In 1994, shortly after the first EagleEyes development, one of the principal developers, Dr. James Gips, a faculty member in the Computer Science Department of the Boston College Carroll School of Management, and Dr. Philip DiMattia, Director of the Boston College Campus School of the Lynch School of Education,[1] entered into agreement to form a research and service collaboration. This joint effort, which became known as the Boston College Campus School EagleEyes Program, was developed to assist individuals with severe disabilities and major health care needs. Special attention has been given to children with severe physical disabilities and severe communication disorders who may benefit by the use of EagleEyes as a means for furthering their ability to communicate and to access and enhance more formal educational opportunities.

# The Boston College Campus School

The Boston College Campus School serves learners with multiple challenges, including complex health care needs. The program provides learner-centered educational and therapeutic services in a school-based setting. Using a transdisciplinary team approach that includes major special education and clinical/medical disciplines, student growth and development is believed to be best achieved through the provision of a stimulating environment and challenging instruction tailored to the needs of the individual. Many of the students served in the school have little to no expressive language as a result of their physical disabilities. The curriculum of the school is driven by the Massachusetts Curriculum Frameworks with adjustments made consistent with the identified special learning needs of each student. Emerging assistive technologies are allowing assessments of previously unknown capabilities for many of the students.

## Extent of the Problem

In the United States, there are more than 140,000 children suffering from cerebral palsy. Each year, an additional 5,000 to 10,000 children join their ranks (McCormick, Gortmaker, & Sobol, 1990). Perhaps the greatest tragedy is that more than 70% of the children afflicted by this debilitating motor dysfunction are estimated to have normal to near normal intelligence. Cerebral palsy is a potentially devastating condition that results from injury to the immature brain. Cerebral palsy is not a disease but a lifelong condition; its essential features are impairment of muscle function, with significant numbers having severe communication disorders as well. The vast majority of these children, despite their normal intelligence, are limited in their educational development by their inability to communicate verbally. Neonatology, the specialization of newborn medicine, has developed significantly over the past two decades. During this time there has been a substantial increase in premature infant survival rates at ever lower mean birth weights. The medical profession has become increasingly more aware of various disabilities and has also become better able to diagnose at an earlier age.

In 1980 the birth trauma survival rates for infants was approximately 21%. Currently, as a result of extraordinary medical advances, the survival rate for such incidents is approximating 80% (Roth, Resnick, & Ariet, 1995). Thus, children are alive today who just a few years ago would not have survived premature birth. This remarkable attainment is not without the unintended consequence of a significant increase in the number of children surviving with lifelong developmental and neurological issues of a substantial magnitude (McCormick et al., 1990) Unfortunately, the advances made in the medical field have far surpassed the accomplishments of technology and education. Because the number of children with cerebral palsy is growing so rapidly, technology and education must anticipate this growth and develop appropriate supports and accommodations to serve this population.

## The Impact of Severe Disabilities

The National Institutes of Health has estimated that cerebral palsy costs the United States $5 billion each year. A substantial part of this cost emanates from the loss of meaningful employment. This is in part the result of inadequate education of children assumed to be severely retarded because of their inability to communicate and their often-disfiguring motor symptoms. By helping them to communicate through the use of state-of-the-art assistive technology such as EagleEyes, individuals would be better prepared to access appropriate educational curriculum that would assist in reducing the problem of unemployment.

Another important issue to address deals with raising the learning standards of children with severe disabilities. Traditionally, functional literacy has been the curriculum of choice for individuals with multiple disabilities, giving no notice to their potential for higher-order thinking and learning that would help them. The EagleEyes program has sought to raise expectations so that students will have increased opportunity to access the general education content found in schools. This latter effort presents a formidable challenge to special and regular educators, to those involved in the preparation of teachers, and to educational policy makers who call for the inclusion of all students in spite of any limitations into our schools. One of the most recent of such efforts has been the passage of PL 107-110, Leave No Child Behind Act of 2001 (LNCB).

One of the highest priorities of the LNCB is to prepare all students to score at a proficient level and show continuous progress attaining, for example, state standards as measured by the Massachusetts Comprehensive Assessment System (MCAS) tests, by 2014.

The profound impact on the way society functions, resulting from the technology revolution, provides a strong rationale for encouraging the development of assistive technologies that can help to promote the independence of intelligent individuals whose inherent capacities are trapped in unresponsive bodies. School districts under the Individual with Disabilities Education Act (IDEA) of 1990 (Public Law 101-476) are required to provide the emerging technologies so students with severe physical disabilities and severe communication disorders can access appropriate educational experiences that ensure Free and Appropriate Public Education (FAPE). However, a major limitation exists in that the effectiveness of using assistive technologies by schools has not received adequate attention. The development of state-of-the-art research-based programs and studies that systematically examine results is lacking.

# A Rationale for EagleEyes

The conceptual framework underlying the EagleEyes program has been described in an earlier report by the authors entitled *An Eye Control Device for Students Without Language Expressive Capacity: EagleEyes* (DiMattia, Curran, & Gips, 2001). In this work the authors argue that all children possess a common human nature and inherent intellectual capacities. While there can be and there are disabled senses, there can be no disabled intellects because the intellect is an immaterial faculty. As a result of starvation through a lack of stimulation, the intellect may become stagnant and impotent. Each child is a human being and is equal in this commonality with every other. The essence and nature of being human best illustrates the age-old philosophical question of the "one and the many." All children are members of the same common species and possess the very same inherent powers and capabilities that are given a visible manifestation in a multitude of physical, intellectual, and psychological expression.

Individual differences are always only differences in degree, never differences in kind. The fact that individuals possess common traits to different degrees is itself proof that they share a common nature.

Mortimer J. Adler, writing in the trilogy called *The Paidiea Proposal,* states a similar position as that expressed above by stating that all children learn and argues for the same K–12 schooling for all of them. For Adler, those who do not experience success in school were not properly taught, reaffirming that all children have specifically unique personalities, each with his or her own physical, intellectual, and psychological characteristics.

## The Need for Stimulation

As noted earlier, young children with severe physical disabilities and severe communication disorders who survive catastrophic birth trauma are estimated to have normal to near normal intelligence. Without ongoing special attention and specialized aids that assist in creating access to the regular educational curriculum, such children become at serious risk for experiencing educational developmental closure. The difference between formal schooling and all other forms is that knowledge has been organized both in scope and sequence for the learner to experience. Thoughtful and creative teachers who welcome the challenge of designing innovative strategies that result in increased learning help to ensure that each child is able to use his/her natural capacity to become his/her own agent and instrument for learning. It is the rescue of this "lost" stratum of society using advanced technologies that has been the central goal of the Boston College Campus School EagleEyes Program.

In her work on what teacher preparation needs to include, Blackwell (2003) identifies several benchmarks regarding student learning and teacher need. The first benchmark is that knowledge and understanding based on prior experience informs an individual's preconceptions. A second benchmark refers to the notion of usable content knowledge and how teachers come to understand how children learn content knowledge.

## Identifying Learner Potential

These benchmarks form the basis for initial meetings that take place between students enrolled in the Campus School and volunteers. As part of orientation, observers are asked to think about and respond to the following three questions.

1. From your observation(s), can you identify **something** that the student demonstrates that he/she knows?

2. How do you think the student learned that **something?**

3. How do you know that the student knows that **something?**

The observer affirms the existence of preconceptions on the part of the child (pupil) as well as the process used by the pupil in learning a useable content knowledge. An observer, after several meetings with a child, reported the experience in the following way:

*When I first met B there was no response or indication of any human interaction. I had a brief one-way conversation telling her how pleased I was to meet her and to be able to visit with her. B was hooked up to what was described as the electrode EagleEyes system and was attempting to do an eye painting. This was described as analogous to finger painting. Wherever B looked, bright colors appeared on the screen, forming a burst of colorful shapes and lines. She worked very deliberately filling in spaces as her eyes moved across the computer screen. After about 30 minutes of sustained effort, B finished covering the entire computer screen surface. Throughout the task, B did not show any observable affect. However, when the teacher asked if she wanted to use this painting as a Mother's Day card, B responded with a big smile and facial gesture that without question conveyed a definitive yes response.*

From this sample observation, one could conclude that **B** was not only able to demonstrate specific knowledge about what she thought made a quality art product but also useable knowledge in that she would use her product to make a Mother's Day greeting card. What might be yet another conclusion is that **B** demonstrated the capacity to be a participant in her environment rather than merely a spectator. The impact upon observers is often sufficiently powerful that they become persuaded as to the potential of EagleEyes to help individuals without voice.

This brief example of how we are using EagleEyes, the electrode system, and the Camera Mouse system offers some insight regarding the learning potential that children with severe disabilities and severe communication disorders present. The remaining sections of this chapter present a literature review of assistive technology, selected literature reviews of eye gaze systems, three cases of students of various ages (two electrode users and one Camera Mouse user), a discussion of findings to date, and finally, some predictions for the future.

# Literature Review

The Technology-Related Assistance for Individuals with Disabilities Act of 1988 (Public Law 100-407, August 19, 1988) defines an assistive technology device as "any piece of equipment, or product system, whether acquired commercially or off the shelf, modified or customized, that increases, maintains, or improves functional capabilities of individuals with disabilities." The term *assistive technology service* means any service that directly assists a student with a disability in the selection, acquisition, or use of an assistive technology device. IDEA further defined assistive

technology service to include a number of specific supports, the first of which demands that the student have access to an evaluation of technology needs. The school district is also responsible for providing training and technical assistance to the student and his or her family and "for professionals, employers, or other individuals who provide services to, employ, or otherwise are substantially involved in the major life functions of the individual with disabilities" (20 USC 1401 [26]).

Assistive technology advances over the past 20 years have changed the lives of individuals with disabilities in profound ways. People with impaired vision, profound hearing loss, orthopedic disabilities, and others with multiple disabilities are functioning more independently as a direct result of developments in the field of assistive technology. Input and output devices that include switches, pointing devices, voice recognition, video screens, voice synthesizers, telecommunications, and language boards are some of the assistive devices that are contributing not only to learning and education, but providing independence and opportunity for the fullest possible development to various groups of individuals with disabilities (DiMattia et al., 2001).

## The Importance of Assistive Technology

Assistive technology actually dates back farther than 20 years. Hearing aids, for example, were first patented in the 1890s, and the essential mechanism for amplifying sound has not changed over the years. The first suction attachment for lower limb prosthesis was a socket developed in 1863. This type of socket is still used in modern prosthesis. However, what has changed dramatically is the structure of the technology and the materials used in creating these devices.

The most effective state-of-the-art technology has become available only during the past 15 years due to the recent advances in electronics. The single most important change in computer design and construction was the reduction in complexity brought about by the development of the microprocessor electronic circuit "chip." Computers are built into virtually every piece of electronic assistive technology. This innovation, the microprocessor, resulted in reduced size and cost of assistive devices and greatly increased functional capabilities (Cook & Hussey, 2002).

Although people with disabilities have used assistive devices for decades, assistive technology to help students in their classroom setting is a relatively new phenomenon that is constantly changing the ways students with disabilities are treated. Assistive technology has ultimately grown up in the field of medicine and has only recently begun to be truly utilized in the domain of education. Gray (1997), an assistive technology specialist speculates,

> As awareness and acceptance of the field of augmentative and alternative communication (AAC) has increased, the need for public schools to provide AAC for students with severe communication disabilities has become more evident. Speech-language pathologists, educators, parents, and other professionals are becoming more informed regarding the legislation that ensures the right to a free, appropriate public education for students with disabilities.

Because federal law now mandates that assistive technology be incorporated into educational programs through the Technology-Related Assistance for Individuals with Disabilities Act (PL 100-407), it becomes necessary to carefully examine ways to incorporate these technologies into best-practice approaches of special education (Judge & Parette, 1998).

With the emerging trend to include assistive technology in all classrooms, Bruder (1996) suggests that the field of special education must be prepared to use any technology necessary to enhance a student's learning. For this to occur, educators must be skillful in assessing a student's current use of, or need for, assistive technology for survival or enhanced learning and, subsequently,

must be able to use the most appropriate technology for each student's need. Cook and Hussey (2002) suggest using the Technology Integration Plan developed by Church and Glennen (1992) as a way for educators to form strategies about using assistive technology in the classroom. Church and Glennen propose that activities using assistive devices should

1. occur frequently,

2. be motivating and enjoyable,

3. present opportunities for independence in one of several areas, and

4. be activities that the student could not effectively complete utilizing current modes and methods.

Cook and Hussey (2002) affirm that in all functional areas there are educational technologies that aid in the acquisition of the necessary skills.

## The Need For Communication

A crucial skill that a school-aged child learns is how to communicate. Olsen and DeRuyter (2002) describe for teachers the importance of establishing communication and integrating development in opportunities to learn to communicate early on in life. Goossens and colleagues (1994) outlined several techniques to incorporate best-practice strategies to promote communication. The first strategy is that any training should be conducted within the natural environment of the classroom. This is important because the child must become comfortable with using his or her device with the teacher and students in the class. Secondly, students should be provided with frequent examples of assistive technology use. For them to become skilled enough to use the devices, they must observe other individuals modeling interactive use of their systems. Finally, assistive technology training should foster communication interaction between peers. Merbler and colleagues (1999) recommend that, whenever possible, devices that can be customized be used. This allows changes to be made to the device as needs of the learner and his or her academic program change.

Beukelman and Mirenda (1998) conceptualize academic participation as occurring at four levels.

1. The first is *competitive,* in which the learner who has a disability has the same expectations as his or her nondisabled peers. The workload is adjusted, but the student's academic progress is evaluated in the same way as peers.

2. The second level is *active* participation, in which the workload is also adjusted and the evaluations are based on individualized standards. The expectations are less than for nondisabled peers.

3. The third level is *involved,* in which academic expectations are minimal and inclusion occurs via alternative activities.

4. At the fourth level, *passive,* there are no academic expectations and the student passively observes learning activities in the regular classroom.

One of the major goals of the Boston College EagleEyes program is to utilize the technology in a way that every student functions at the competitive level.

This review of the assistive technology literature has identified some of the benefits to individuals with disabilities and as well as several standards that promote best practice

## Review of Eye-Controlled Systems

Duchowski (2003) reports on four types of eye-tracking systems, two of which have been used in assistive technology systems.

In one type of device, the eye is tracked by shining an infrared light toward the head and tracking the reflections of the light from the eye using an infrared camera attached to a computer. The software processes the camera image to determine where the user is looking (gaze point), and the mouse pointer is then placed at the gaze point.

Mouse clicks can be done with a slow eye blink or a hardware switch or by using dwell time (holding the mouse pointer in a small area for a certain period of time). These systems can either be external systems, mounted near the monitor, or they can be head-mounted systems.

The Quick Glance Eye Tracking System, produced by Eye Tech Digital Systems, is one example of an eye-controlled system of this type. Requirements for using this system are the ability to keep the head steady and good eye control. The system costs about $4,000. Another example of this type of system is the Eye Gaze System by LC Technologies. To use this system, the user needs good control of one eye, the ability to keep the head still, and some reading or word recognition skill. There are portable and stationary versions of the system. An example of a head-mounted system is Vision Key by H.K. EyeCan Ltd.

The second type of eye tracking reported by Duchowski (2003) that has been used in eye-controlled assistive technology is based on the EOG, or electro-oculographic potential. The EOG results from the corneal-retina potential, the cornea of the eye being electrically positive and the retina being electrically negative. As the person moves the eyes, the EOG changes by about 10 microvolts for each degree of rotation. The EOG is measured using five surface electrodes placed around the eyes. Two electrodes are used to measure the vertical EOG, two the horizontal EOG, and one is used as a reference ground. The EagleEyes electrode system is an example of an eye-control assistive technology of this type.

## Review of Head-Controlled Systems

Head movement to control a mouse is another means of communication for persons without speech. The movement can be tracked with infrared, ultrasound, or video technology.

One example is the HeadMouse, which translates the movements of a user's head into directly proportional movements of the computer mouse pointer. The HeadMouse is a wireless optical sensor that tracks a tiny and disposable target that is placed on the user's forehead or glasses.

The Head Tracking Mouse by NaturalPoint is a similar device in that it sits on top of a computer monitor and tracks a reflector placed on the person's head or eyeglasses. Once calibrated, the movement of the user's head relates exactly to the direction the onscreen cursor will travel. This program can be used with Dwell Select software, which allows the user to perform a mouse click by dwelling on an area target for a certain number of seconds. The HeadMouse is available for approximately $300.

The Camera Mouse, the second-generation EagleEyes system also developed at Boston College, uses a video camera located above or below the monitor as a mouse replacement.[2] An image from the camera is displayed on the screen. The camera can be focused on the user's nose, chin, thumb, or foot, any body part over which the individual has control. The Camera Mouse has been showcased in Paraplegia News and TechCommunications publications in 2002 as an up-and-coming hands-free computer control system. The product is available now from CM Solutions, Inc. (www.cameramouse.com).

# EagleEyes Program Methodology

The EagleEyes program has developed a methodology to examine the effects of the use of the EagleEyes system on the learning development of each individual. The work with each student is evolving and continues in hopes that the program will be able to report additional developments as they occur and as individuals reach various milestones. Because EagleEyes is a work in progress, responses to each of the study questions are expected to evolve over time as well. However, the information reported gives some indication of where each student is in his or her learning supported by their teachers and parents.

## The Research Questions

The following research question guides the activities of the program: To what extent does the use of EagleEyes, either the electrode system or the Camera Mouse system, affect the learning and teaching behavior when provided with regular education tasks and measured by evaluating the student's ability to follow directions, examining evidence of new learning, and understanding the relationship between cause and effect? Other questions include:

1. What happens to the student's intellectual development?

2. What happens to the student's communication skills?

3. What happens to the student's emotional development?

4. What happens to the student's social development?

5. What happens to the student's educational progress?

6. What happens to the student's interpersonal relationships?

7. What happens to the student's home life?

The following are academic questions for evaluation of the students:

1. What evidence is there that the student is aware of self and of others?

2. How long can the student remain on task? Follow directions?

3. Does on-task behavior change by academic task?

4. What evidence is there that the student is able to initiate interaction?

5. What evidence exists that the student comprehends the spoken word? The written word?

The following are social questions for evaluation of the students:

1. To what extent does the student demonstrate social skills with age-appropriate peers? With adult helpers? With others?

2. To what extent does the student demonstrate the ability to take turns? Engage peers in play? Listen to others? Make requests to others?

The following are emotional questions for evaluation of the students:

1. What evidence is there that the student can express joy? Empathy? Anger? Fear? Humor?

Data are collected from various sources, such as multiple field notes, direct observations made by classroom teachers and assistants, interviews with parents and other professional and ancillary providers with direct access to the student, and classroom work products produced by students themselves.

## Personal Stories

Earlier in this chapter it was noted that one goal of the EagleEyes is to raise awareness of the potential for higher-order learning among children with severe physical disabilities and severe communication disorders. The authors believe that one of the best ways to achieve this is to empower individuals to become self-advocates by telling personal stories that describe some of the effects experienced by the use of EagleEyes as an assistive device for communication and learning. Personal stories provide an additional means of evaluating the effectiveness of the EagleEyes program.

The following vignette might be best viewed within a **"prove that he belongs"** framework, an attitudinal disposition often communicated to parents by others.

*On opening day a mother escorts her 7-year-old daughter **D** to her second-grade classroom, where **D** is greeted by her new teacher in a warm and friendly manner, with excitement about the year ahead and anticipation of new friendships and the new academic learning that is expected to take place. **D** is excited, comfortable, and eager to take up the teacher's invitation to explore her new classroom, the colorful books, the spots on "Timothy the Turtle's tummy," the aquarium, and the colorful posters positioned neatly around the classroom. Mother is pleased and happy that **D** is off to such a good beginning as she walks to her vehicle to retrieve her second child, **E**, and escort him to his classroom. **E** is 12 years old, with cerebral palsy that severely limits his physical mobility, and he also has a severe communication disorder. He cannot speak, requires a wheelchair, and wears a body jacket that is difficult to tolerate and affects his comfort and morale as a result. As Mother wheels **E** into his classroom, he is greeted by his teacher in a friendly but also rather stern manner. **E** is told by his teacher that she hopes this year will be better than last, that he becomes more serious about his work and shows greater enthusiasm and cooperation with the staff. As mother leaves the building and reflects about what she has just experienced, she finds herself asking, "Why is my daughter made to feel that she clearly belongs, while my son made to feel that he needs to prove that he does? Why is it so difficult for people to see the other person in a more human way? How can distorted perceptions be changed into more positive ones? How can people be helped to be more sensitive to other human beings? While it is so frustrating to me, I can only imagine how my son must feel. After all, he experiences such insensitivity."*

The cases that follow in the next section attempt to show that the richness of individual personalities are only different in degree and not in kind, and that all children possess a common human nature and inherent intellectual capacities that through encouragement, nurturance, support, and wisdom of adult helpers are allowed to grow and to flourish into fruition.

# Case Studies

Three cases are included in this section. The ages of the subjects range from 10 to 21 years of age. Two are male and one is female. Two of the subjects reside in Massachusetts; one attended a regular public school, graduating with a certificate of completion in June 2002, and a second is enrolled in a Collaborative Public School Program. A third subject resides in another state and is enrolled in a regular public school third-grade classroom. The primary diagnosis of the three subjects is cerebral palsy with related health care conditions and severe physical and communication disorders. The first two cases describe electrode EagleEyes users, whereas the third case reports on a Camera Mouse user.

## Case 1: G

### BACKGROUND

G is a 17-year-old male who has a diagnosis of quadriparesis, agenesis of corpus collosum, hydrocephalus ex vacuuo, and a seizure disorder that is currently well under control and for which he takes medication. G has decreased visual acuity, status post gastroesophageal reflux, and a hypoplastic left kidney. G uses a manual wheelchair for mobility, wears a body jacket that he tolerates, and double upright metal braces with orthopedic high-top shoes during the daytime. Before G became an electrode EagleEyes user, a primary method for him to communicate was through the use of an augmentative language board and a chin switch to answer multiple-choice questions.

### SCHOOL HISTORY

G has been a special education student for all of his school-age years. He has been enrolled in collaborative special education programs with other students with disabilities from a very early age. In such programs, academic expectations have been minimal. The major goals of these programs have attempted to strike a strong balance between G's severe health care needs and the need for functional literacy and understanding. There have been periods when G's health care needs have taken priority over other developmental needs. G has benefited from having a stay-at-home mother who has also acted as a home teacher, reinforcing lessons learned at school. Other family members have also been very supportive and have contributed to the creation of an active learning environment that has provided G with extraordinary experiences, especially in math and history, two areas of special interest. G used his augmentative language board and eye gaze to communicate with family members.

G has been an EagleEyes user for approximately 6 years. During the first 3 years with EagleEyes, G's participation was inconsistent and sporadic. G's time in the EagleEyes classroom at Boston College was increased during his 4th and 5th year because of his increased motivation and expanded curriculum opportunities. This past year he has been coming to the Boston College EagleEyes classroom for 3 hours weekly.

G has an electrode EagleEyes system at home that he uses regularly. He comes to the Boston College EagleEyes classroom 3 days per week for 1 hour each day where he works on academic tasks, further development of eye control, and on prosocial skills. The latter is structured around a network of five to six undergraduate students who engage in a variety of social experiences with G that include games, conversation, and attending athletic events on and off campus. G has responded to these experiences in several interesting ways. He is more outgoing and receptive of others. He enjoys competing in games (e.g., Tic Tac Toe) using his EagleEyes technology with other males, but shows both sensitivity and restraint when competing with the females in his group.

Finding appropriate software for students such as **G** can be rather challenging. For the past 2 years **G** has completed distance learning courses over the Internet using the electrode EagleEyes technology. **G** has completed free history courses offered over the internet through Barnes and Noble (www.barnesandnobleuniversity.com.), including "Pearl Harbor" and "The Railroad in American History." **G** completed each required lesson and all of the assignments, and took quizzes as part of the requirements of each course using EagleEyes. In addition to learning the material, **G** was able to make contact with other people who were taking the courses who do not have physical disabilities. During one such experience, **G** was able to have a long-distance correspondence with a woman in Brazil. He posted that he was taking the course using only his eyes. The woman was amazed and wrote to him, asking many questions about him and the access technology he uses, telling him that he was an inspiration. Through these experiences **G** continues to discover more about himself as a person among persons. In this way, he experiences acceptance with his peers as a full-fledge member, affirming more and more that he is just like them.

classes, Michael was enrolled in a collaborative special educational program where there was little attention to academics.

Michael turned 22 in October 2003. As part of the aging-out transitioning requirements, a neuropsychological reevaluation was conducted that revealed sufficient evidence that Michael was of at least average intelligence, which resulted in his being decertified as eligible for Mental Retardation services. Consequently, the Massachusetts Rehabilitation Commission has become the state agency of responsibility for providing a long-term educational and vocational program. The educational component will include further academic preparation with a long-term goal of attending college to prepare for work in public relations. He is planning to continue using the EagleEyes technology to which he was introduced at age 13 and has used ever since as a major strategy for communication and academic work. A film documentary was recently completed where Michael tells a compelling story of self-discovery and attempts to overcome his limitations through learning about himself and the world. Michael coauthored the script by using the EagleEyes technology.

## Case 2: Michael

Michael N. recently graduated from Marshfield Massachusetts High School with a Certificate of Completion. He began attending a regular school when he was 13 years old. A special education teacher attended all classes with Michael and was responsible for modifying and transferring academic content into a format that Michael could access using the EagleEyes system and a language board assistive device. This approach allowed Michael to be an active and competitive participant in all academic work in each classroom. Workloads were adjusted, but academic progress was evaluated in the same way as the other students in the classroom. Before he attended regular

*Figure 20.1* Michael with EagleEyes Electrodes

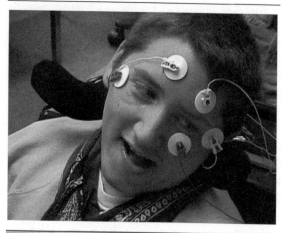

## Early History and Education

Michael was born with a diagnosis of spastic quadriplegic cerebral palsy. On three separate evaluations, because Michael was not able to be responsive to his examiners, he was diagnosed as having the mental age of an 18-month-old infant. For the first 10 years of schooling he was enrolled in various collaborative educational programs where maintenance effort was the dominant practice and where academic learning was not an option. When Michael was 6 years old and attending one of these programs, he met his current personal teacher who at that time was a program aide, and they have been together ever since. During the early years of attendance at the collaborative programs, very little was expected of Michael by way of effort, and during this time he was a spectator of life rather than a participant. While the program settings provided good quality personal attention, care, and service, they offered little structured education.

A good deal of the following data is taken from a number of oral history interviews with Maureen Gates, Michael's personal teacher who has been with him since he was 6 years old; his mother, Kathy, who has been Michael's major advocate; and from the personal experiences of the authors.

Michael's personal aide, Maureen, began to take notice that when she brought Michael home he would be greeted by his mother who would ask him questions about his day and would watch his eye movements for his responses. His mother would often validate a response by repeating a question in a slightly different manner. Maureen began to notice other characteristics and behavior about Michael. For instance, she observed that during the program day Michael would smile and show facial signs reacting to humorous situations. She found herself talking more often directly to Michael and learned to read his response behaviors. These consisted of two paired eye movements—up versus down for yes or no responses, and left versus right for this or that choice-making responses. Thus Michael had been able to

show his mother, his father, sisters Kristen and Melissa, and now Maureen that he had a definitive yes or no response. There was no acknowledgement of this ability in his school record.

Thus, from age 3 to age 13 Michael's educational experiences did not include any formal learning and relied on observational learning on his part. At the same time, his mother and Maureen strongly sensed that Michael understood a great deal more than what he was able to express. They were two very supportive advocates who felt that there was a lot inside Michael ready to be released.

## Michael's Introduction to EagleEyes

While channel surfing one evening in early 1995, Michael's mother happened across a commentary regarding EagleEyes and the next day contacted us to ask if Michael could try the system. When he first used the EagleEyes system, it became obvious to several observers, the authors being among them, that he understood cause and effect probably much more than previously thought, and as time would eventually reveal. Pursuant to the requirements of special education regulations, his mother asked their school community to reconvene the special education team to take up the question of Michael's communication potential using the new cutting-edge EagleEyes technology. As a result, a referral was made to the EagleEyes program requesting that EagleEyes services be provided to address language arts development as expressed by the following two specific goals: first, teach Michael to say yes by raising his eyes and second, to say no by lowering his eyes. The plan was for Michael to come to the Boston College EagleEyes classroom twice weekly for 1-hour sessions, accompanied by his personal teacher, Maureen.

The following data is derived from field note observation recordings, oral history, and an examination of sample work products produced by Michael using the EagleEyes system. Since 1995, Michael has been a regular EagleEyes user with a system at home and one at the Boston College Campus School. Whether it was because of the presence of a number of faculty members, an undergraduate student providing technical supports, the young female EagleEyes teacher, or just the new opportunities that were now being presented, Michael, in a single activity, demonstrated to all present that not only did he indeed have a sense of humor but that he was also a very capable human being waiting to blossom. The following happened during an academic session to determine to what extent Michael recognized colors and understood shapes:

With Michael hooked up to the EagleEyes system, the teacher put several colorful shapes on the computer monitor and began by asking Michael to point to select ones. She asked Michael to locate and point to the yellow shape, then to the green shape, then to the blue shape. When she asked Michael to locate the red shape, he appeared to wander off and to lose interest. Up until then he was enthusiastic and motivated. His eyes became fixed on Eric, the undergraduate student who was providing technical support to the teacher. A few seconds passed before any of the individuals present realized that Michael was indeed on task finding the color red—he was looking at Eric who had red hair. As laughter began to fill the room, Michael was laughing with gusto for having been able to playfully trick a room made up of academics and researchers of some repute. That incident established a standard of expectation for Michael and for those who would be working with him: use humor and challenge Michael by expecting a lot from him. Shortly thereafter, an EagleEyes system was purchased for Michael to have at home where his mother and Maureen would be able to use it with him. When Michael was not at Boston College he was attending the collaborative program.

## TRANSITION AND BEGINNING OF FORMAL SCHOOLING

The superintendent of schools from Michael's hometown came to see one of the authors for academic advisement on a day when Michael was on the EagleEyes system. He was introduced to Michael and observed Michael working deliberately, following directions, and cooperating with the teacher. He commented that Michael demonstrates three basic characteristics of the successful student: compliancy, motivation, and cooperation with others. He raised the question of why Michael had to travel every day to a collaborative program at some distance from home while driving past the local middle school in the community where he lived. Shortly after the visit Michael was invited to enroll in the middle school in his home community, and Maureen was appointed his personal teacher with responsibility for shadowing him in classes to take subject-matter notes and note class assignments that Michael would complete at home using his EagleEyes system. Michael would also continue to attend the EagleEyes program at Boston College to continue working on eye control and to build confidence and endurance. He still came two times per week, but time was increased one additional hour each day.

In September 1996, 10 years after all of his contemporary peers, Michael commenced formal schooling where knowledge would be organized into scope and sequence. It was administratively decided that Michael would be introduced to academic classes incrementally based on how well he was able to assimilate information and complete work assignments. What a memorable beginning, as recalled by Maureen:

*On the first class day, when Michael and I showed up in Ms. A's English classroom, she questioned what he was doing being assigned to her academic class. She didn't know anything about children like him. "Why don't you see if there is another class that he could take?" I told her that Michael and I would not in any way be disruptive to her class, that I will take notes and modify all of the assignments in a format that Michael will be able to access to complete her assignments. I told her that we were just asking for a chance to show that Michael can do the work. She begrudgingly agreed to see how things would go.*

*Figure 20.2*    Michael Using the EagleEyes Electrodes System on a Large Screen

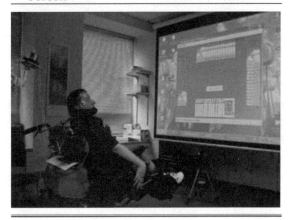

Note that the dynamic here clearly is the "prove that you belong" attitude identified earlier in this chapter.

The first couple of months went by without any major incident. Michael was highly motivated in undertaking all of the assignments, but there was little evidence that he belonged in the classroom. On one occasion, when the opportunity presented itself, it was suggested to Ms. A that she might wish to come to Boston College and meet EagleEyes faculty and see the EagleEyes system in action. Surprisingly, she seemed disposed to the suggestion and requested permission from the principal to accompany Michael and Maureen to Boston College. On the day of her visit Maureen had planned for Michael to work on a parts-of-speech exercise that was part of her class assignment for homework. She had arranged the academic material on a series of grids. With Ms. A observing and with a fairly rapid series of requests, Maureen asked Michael to locate different parts-of-speech in the text showing on the monitor. "Michael, can you locate a personal pronoun? A verb? An adjective? An adverb? Now locate a preposition." There were several other persons in the room at the time who were acknowledging

Michael's correct answers. Ms. A. was astonished and said: "Michael, this is terrific. We need to get others at school to hear about this work!"

At that moment Michael and Maureen just smiled at each other. They had just crossed over one bridge and somehow knew that others would be easier to build.

From that visit on, Ms. A became one of Michael's biggest cheerleaders at the Marshfield Middle School. The respect that other teachers held for her made her endorsement that much more meaningful. On another occasion Ms. A returned to the Boston College EagleEyes classroom and gave Michael a unit test that Maureen had organized into a multiple choice using a test format that had been customized for EagleEyes users. She gave Michael an 84% for a test grade and the next day sang his praises throughout the school community. From the middle school, Michael was promoted to Marshfield High School where his reputation as a highly motivated, cooperative, and enthusiastic student preceded his arrival.

That Michael was changing the perceptions of teachers about his disability was becoming fairly well established by the relative ease in enrolling in other courses of study. What was not expected was the unintended consequence of the impact on his peer group, as evidenced by another brief vignette that took place during a Friday afternoon Jeopardy activity. The social studies teacher created three-person teams of students who would then play a bonus round of Jeopardy. Michael's team members differed on an answer and Michael was asked to select what he thought would be the correct one. His selection turned out to be the correct one and his team won the round. Another student from a competing team raised her hand and stated that it wasn't fair because the team that won had Michael. The circle of belonging was completed with a bonus, namely that Michael, in addition to changing the perceptions of adults toward his abilities as a learner, was now changing his peers' perceptions.

## PREPARATION FOR ANOTHER TRANSITION

For the past school year Michael's time attending the EagleEyes classroom has been increased to 8 hours per week so that some attention can be given to help Michael develop age-appropriate social skills. This change in program is the result of Michael having graduated from high school in June 2002 with a certificate of completion and in preparation for transition from school to adult services through the Massachusetts Rehabilitation Commission. The achievement of being granted a certificate of high school completion at age 21 is extraordinary when one considers the fact that Michael did not begin any formal schooling until age 15, a full 10 years after his peers. There are two other important milestones that have taken place that are worth describing. The first is a change of official mental status, and the second is Michael's co-authoring of a script used to develop a documentary film.

## THE CHANGE IN OFFICIAL MENTAL STATUS

As part of transition preparation for transfer of program responsibility from the local public school district to a state human service agency, Michael was reevaluated. One of the major assessments involved a psychological appraisal to help determine if any changes in mental status had taken place since the earlier examinations. It is important to note that three other like assessments each confirmed a diagnosis that Michael had a mental age of an 18-month-old child. As a result of these findings Michael had been certified as mentally retarded and eligible for services of the Massachusetts Department of Mental Retardation for many years. As part of the reevaluation neuropsychological examination, Michael, his mother, and Maureen were interviewed by the examiner. They described for the examiner Michael's use of EagleEyes, what had been taken place educationally since the last assessment, and suggested that some part of the reevaluation include an alternative assessment component so that

Michael might be able to demonstrate more appropriately his newly discovered capabilities. As a result of this initial phase, the authors were asked to write their thoughts and suggestions about Michael with attention to his mental capabilities. In separate statements, the authors wrote to support the idea that Michael was at least of normal intelligence and in fact may have higher potential.

One author wrote, "One way to measure intelligence is to use a standardized instrument (i.e., a Stanford Binet); however, an alternative method would be to observe an individual in a new and unfamiliar situation that may reveal some index of his/her potential."

The second author wrote, "Michael was demonstrating on stage the electrode EagleEyes system to over 500 Boston College incoming freshman and their parents on a steamy August evening. Michael's grandmother was also in attendance in the audience. The electrode EagleEyes system works best when the surface electrodes are placed on dry facial skin. That evening the electrodes were not working well because of the perspiration on Michael's face. Michael discovered that by moving his tongue around he was able to compensate for the condition. He pointed to the word grandmother, which appeared on the screen twice, and to the picture of grandmother. This was not prearranged; no one in attendance had any idea that was what he was going to do. This feat, in my mind, was like an Olympic diver completing a 10-point dive with his hands tied behind his back. Michael showed everyone that evening the extraordinary ability under pressure to maintain composure and to problem-solve in spite of adverse circumstances."

A major finding of the reevaluation concluded that a diagnosis of mental retardation could not be supported and that there is demonstrative evidence to support that Michael falls within the normal range of intelligence. Shortly thereafter Michael received formal notification from the Massachusetts Department of Mental Retardation that he was no longer eligible for services. Michael and his family had a party to celebrate the welcomed news.

## MICHAEL'S EAGLEEYES DOCUMENTARY

Michael's EagleEyes documentary is the first in the "I'm In Here Series," a collaboration between the Boston College Campus School and the Boston College Fine Arts Department Graduate Film Studies program. Michael coauthored the script of a 23-minute documentary using his EagleEyes system that tells the story of his personal self-discovery and his continued journey to learn as much about the world as possible in spite of his physical limitations. One of the powerful messages contained in the film is the notion that there is no talent that cannot be cultivated.

## MICHAEL'S FUTURE

As indicated earlier, Michael is participating in planning for the next phase of his life with staff of the Massachusetts Rehabilitation Commission, his parents, special education staff of the Marshfield Public Schools, and members of the Boston College EagleEyes Program. Parameters have been identified for the new program to be developed for Michael that includes 1) work toward completion of the High School Equivalency (GED) requirements, 2) a social skills component, and 3) a vocational component with the use of EagleEyes technology as a center piece strategy. Michael's long-range hope is that he will someday be academically prepared to enroll in a college program that will lead to a career in public relations.

## Case 3: Amanda

Amanda is a 10-year-old female child who resides in Hopatcong, NJ. She has a severe neurological condition that leaves her with limited functional motor skills and no speech. As a result, she is not able to access a computer mouse in a traditional way. Amanda uses the EagleEyes Camera Mouse system that has been described earlier in this

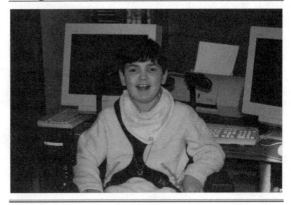

*Figure 20.3* Amanda

chapter. When individuals who are observing her using the Camera Mouse system are asked to describe the experience, they use words like *incredible, mind boggling, unbelievable, powerful,* and *emotionally moving.* Amanda began formal school in September 2002 when she was 9 years old and was assigned to a second-grade classroom as a result of informal assessment (Figure 20.3).

## EARLY HISTORY AND EDUCATION

Since preschool, Amanda has attended The Children's Center, a private, special education facility serving children with multiple disabilities located in Northern Central New Jersey. The referral information stated that, "Amanda has an undiagnosed disorder with an onset at 10 months of age that caused a period of acute deterioration of the white matter in her brain, resulting in her current motor impairments. She is wheelchair dependent with reflex influenced upper extremity movements. Her cognition appears to be intact. Her strongest mode of communication and most accurately controlled parts of her body are her eyes and head."

Amanda, while attending the Center's program, had been tried on several assistive technology devices with varying amounts of success. Amanda was able to use row-column visual scanning from the Dynavox 2c at a 2-second delay with a Spec switch placed to the side of her head.

Amanda most effectively used an encoding Etran, an eye-gaze communication board system, utilizing four colors with six fields of 4 to 24 symbols at a time. Center communication staff were not satisfied that Amanda's cognitive needs were being met through the use of these devices and wanted to explore other options that might be available for her.

## ACCESS TO CAMERA MOUSE

In the spring of 2000 after a staff member of the Center visited Boston College and tried out both the electrodes and the EagleEyes Camera Mouse system, Amanda traveled to Boston College with her parents to try EagleEyes. As a result of the initial trial, it was determined that Amanda would be a good candidate for the Camera Mouse system. In November 2000 three administrators from the Hopatcong Borough Schools visited the EagleEyes program and stated their desire to have a system at one of their schools for several children, including Amanda. In March 2001 the school district initiated the necessary paper work to purchase a Camera Mouse system. In October 2001, three EagleEyes staff members traveled to Hopatcong to test out the new system and to provide professional development training to staff of the district who would be working with the technology. During this time Amanda was still attending the Children's Center Program, and arrangements were made to have her attend the Hopatcong Elementary School for 1.5 hours weekly for social transitioning in preparation for full-time enrollment and use of Camera Mouse as a student in the regular classroom.

In late fall 2001, Amanda began using the Camera Mouse more regularly when a home system was donated by the father of a Camera Mouse user who had passed away. Her mother reported that Amanda was doing fine with the home system, loved using it, and that she was learning to recognize words. Her mother increased the negotiation tempo with Hopatcong school personnel to have Amanda transferred full time into an inte-grated classroom where she could regularly use the Camera Mouse technology.

## ENTRY INTO THE REGULAR CLASSROOM

In September 2002, Amanda was assigned to a regular second-grade classroom with a special education teacher and a personal aide assigned to provide in-class support throughout the school day. The placement in a second-grade classroom was based on available information from the Children's Center staff, parents, and observational impressions made by select members of the receiving school and what might constitute an appropriate peer group arrangement. In December 2002, three members of the EagleEyes program made a second trip to Hopatcong to meet with school personnel, Amanda, and her mother. The purpose of this visit was twofold. The first was to ensure that the technology was working properly, and the second purpose was to explore professional development needs of the classroom teacher and the in-class support staff.

## STUDY OF REGULAR CLASS PLACEMENT

The placement of Amanda in a regular classroom is an attempt to provide a more normalized school environment that is consistent with evidenced-based research that has been reported in the literature. As noted earlier, Beukelman and Mirenda (1998) reported the development of four levels of academic participation when students with disabilities are placed in a regular education classroom. The levels are Competitive, Active Participation, Involved, and Passive.

- The Competitive level of participation occurs when the student with disabilities has the same expectations as the nondisabled peers.

- At the Active level, participation takes place when the academic workload is adjusted and evaluated using individualized standards.

- At the Involved level, the academic expectations are minimal and inclusion occurs via alternative activities.

- At the Passive level, there are no academic expectations by the classroom teacher and the student passively observes learning activities as a spectator.

Although school staff and Amanda's mother stated that they wanted Amanda to be fully involved academically in the regular class placement at Competitive participation level, the reality, upon inspection, was that Amanda was operating at the Involved level, whereby current academic expectations were minimal and inclusion occurs via alternative activities with some spillover into Active participation level using individualized standards for evaluation of Amanda's work products.

The following question has been used to guide program activities and data collection: To what extent does the use of access technology that allows a student to control the mouse pointer by moving only the head affect learning and teaching behavior? Some other inquiry questions are

1. What happens to the student's communication skills?

2. What happens to the student's emotional development?

3. What happens to the student's social development?

4. What happens to the student's educational progress? Learning rate?

5. What happens to the student's home life?

### Impressions to Date

As a result of two on-site visits (the first in December 2002 and a second in March 2003), as well as a series of telephone and electronic mail communications, the information collected identified several issues that need to be addressed in order to have Amanda function at the Competitive level where expectations are the same as for her peers. Methods used to gather information included observations and conversations with the student; meetings with the teacher and aide; and conversations with the speech therapist, tech-

nology specialist, building administrators, central office leadership, and her mother. The information collected from group meetings and individual interviews covered five areas, including communication, social, emotional, academic, and quality-of-life aspects.

From the observational data and clinical impressions gathered from discussion with individuals directly involved with Amanda, a positive picture has begun to emerge concerning academic progress in the current placement. Amanda is communicating more using Camera Mouse with her special education teacher and her mother. She has a number of friends and engages peers easily. She laughs easily and shows happiness when others acknowledge her work. Her mother reports that at home she is always eager to use her Camera Mouse system and engage in challenging academic tasks. Creating a rich learning environment has been a priority at school and at home. Amanda has become very proficient in her eye control and has begun to build a sight vocabulary.

As shown in Figure 20.4, Amanda demonstrates her ability to communicate using her access technology by creating a message that she sent to a peer.

The message offers the reader some insight regarding Amanda's academic potential considering that she is still in her first formal school year, as well as some validation of her social development and status with a peer.

The spelling software used is custom-developed. It divides the alphabet into five groups. The student selects the group. Then a screen appears with the letters within the group. Each letter requires two clicks. There are also buttons to insert a space, delete, and for speaking the message aloud. The advantage of the program is that it allows the student to be less accurate with the access technology.

Teachers report that Amanda shows good social skills, not only in making friends but also in keeping them. Her peers are fond of her, want to be in her company, and show interest in the tech-

*Figure 20.4*   A Message Spelled Out by Amanda using Camera Mouse

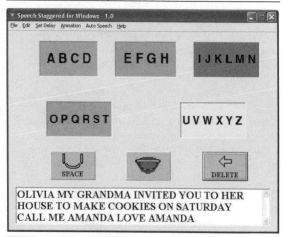

nology that she is using. Her teachers report that Amanda regularly demonstrates two learning behaviors that evidence-based research indicate are important: 1) compliancy and willingness to follow directions, and 2) the ability to demonstrate appropriate-time on-task behavior, both of which are valued by teachers. Teachers report that Amanda gives evidence of being able to remain on task for substantial periods of time and gets excited about her learning.

Amanda's home life is strong and vibrant. Her mother functions as an unofficial home teacher in specific areas of instruction and is an important part of Amanda's success. She helps Amanda to establish routines and personal structure, and to take increasingly more responsibility.

In summary, Amanda's first full year of enrollment in a regular classroom has been somewhat successful. She has shown through her motivation and enthusiasm that the placement decision was appropriate and has made some progress in adapting to the academic environment while still requiring related therapies that are now being provided more often after school. The school administration is currently determining next year's classroom placement for Amanda. There are several academic planning issues that have been identified that will be addressed during the summer and through contractual services by a unit of the Boston College Campus School, Project TEAM, during the next academic year. The goal for Amanda is to help her to function at the Competitive level academically and socially.

## ISSUES FOR THE 2005/2006 SCHOOL YEAR

There are several areas that the Hopatcong school staff, Amanda's mother, and the Boston College EagleEyes staff will be working on together during the summer before her class placement. Attention will be given to clarity of the regular teacher's responsibility regarding Amanda's academic program. The need to clarify ownership responsibility is vital to sustaining a focus on Amanda to participate at the Competitive level, so as to become a real part of her class. The scheduling and use of human resources in various ways will allow for planning time to be made available for the regular classroom teacher and the special education teacher so that parallel academic activities will dominate instruction during in-class and outside-of-class activities. Attention will also be given to the development of collaboration among the major constituencies that make up the support network. Standard third-grade curriculum materials will be adapted using software called Clicker 4 that allows information to be organized in various arrangements that will allow Amanda access using the Camera Mouse technology.

# What Has Been Accomplished to Date?

From the beginning, the Boston College Campus School EagleEyes Program has provided access to the EagleEyes technology to over 100 individuals in such locations as Massachusetts, Connecticut, New Hampshire, Arizona, New Jersey, New York, England, Northern Ireland, and Iceland. The collaborators have reported aspects of their work in a manuscript published in 2001, have made eight presentations at international assistive technology conferences, written six articles for inclusion in conference proceeding books, and have conducted numerous professional development workshops for educators and other professional noneducators. A most recent completed work by the collaborators is a coproduced 23-minute documentary on EagleEyes. It tells the story of one young person's (Michael) journey discovering himself, and offers testimony that when persons with severe physical disabilities and severe communication disorders are provided appropriate technology assistance, the possibility for them to communicate and become active learners arises. Such a development results in educational benefits to other members of society by altering misperceptions about individuals with severe physical disabilities and severe communication disorders.

## Notes

1. In addition to being the Director of the Boston College Campus School, Dr. Philip DiMattia is also a member of the faculty in the Lynch School of Education, Department of Teacher Education, Curriculum and Instruction and Special Education.

2. The Camera Mouse technology has been licensed by Boston College to CM Solutions, Inc. (www.cameramouse.com) of Austin, Texas. James Gips has a minor financial interest in the company.

## References

Adler, M. (1984). *The Paideia proposal, an educational manifesto.* New York: Macmillan.

Betke, M., Gips, J., & Fleming, P. (2002). The Camera Mouse: Visual tracking of body features to provide computer access for people with severe disabilities. *IEEE Transactions on Neural Systems and Rehabilitation Engineering, 10,* 1–10.

Beukelman, D. R., & Mirenda, P. (1998). *Augmentative and alternative communication, 2nd ed.* Baltimore: Brookes Publishing.

Blackwell, P. J. (2003). Student learning: Education's field of dreams. *Phi Delta Kappan,* January.

Bruder, M. B. (1996). An inservice model to build state personnel capacities on collaborations with families, staff, and agencies for early intervention. Final Report submitted to the U.S. Department of Education.

Church, G., & Glennen, S. (Eds.) (1992). *The handbook of assistive technology.* San Diego: Singular Publishing Group.

Cook, A., & Hussey, S. (2002). *Assistive technologies, principles and practice.* St. Louis: Mosby.

DiMattia, P., Curran, F. X., & Gips, J. (2001). *An eye control teaching device for students without language expressive capacity.* Lewiston: The Edwin Mellen Press.

Duchowski, A. (2003). *Eye tracking methodology: Theory and practice.* London: Springer-Verlag.

Gips, J., Olivieri, P., & Tecce, J. (1994). Direct control of the computer through electrodes placed around the eyes. In M. J. Smith, & G. Salvendy (Eds.), *Human-computer interaction: Applications and case studies,* Burlington, MA: Elsevier. (pp. 630–635).

Glennen, S., & Decoste, D. (1997). *Handbook of augmentative and alternative communication.* San Diego: Singular Publishing Group.

Goossens, C., Crain, S., & Elder, P. (1994). *Communication display books for engineered environments: Preschool environment, Books I and II.* Birmingham, AL: Southeast Augmentative Communication Publications.

Gray, D. High functioning autistic children and the construction of "normal family life." *Social Science & Medicine, 44*(8), 1099–1106.

Judge, S. L., & Parette, H. (Eds.). (1998). *Assistive technology for young children with disabilities.* Brookline, MA: Brookline Books.

McCormick, M. C., Gortmaker, S. L., & Sobol, A. M. (1990). Very low birthweight children: Behavior problems and school difficulties in a national sample. *Journal of Pediatrics, 117,* 687–693.

Olson, D., & DeRuyter, F. (Eds.). (2002). *Clinician's guide to assistive technology.* St. Louis: Mosby.

Roth, J., Resnick., M. B., & Ariet, M. (1995). Changes in survival patterns of very low birthweight infants from 1980–1993. *Archives of Pediatrics and Adolescent Medicine, 149,* 1311–1317.

Wolfe, P. (2001). *Brain matters: Translating research into classroom practice.* Alexandria, VA: Association for Supervision and Curriculum Development (ASCD).

# Chapter 21

# Living with Pain and Infirmity

Caryn Sheehan

Mary Kazanowski

Mr. G. is a 46-year-old male who is admitted to the hospital for pain control. He describes his pain as "unrelenting and excruciating." He has had multiple hospitalizations for a significant medical history including two myocardial infarctions, recent cardiac bypass surgery, amputations of three toes on his left foot, and a below-the-knee amputation of his right leg. For the past 2 years he has undergone dialysis three times a week for chronic renal failure related to his IDDM. Over the past 6 months repeated infections of his dialysis shunt have complicated his treatment. His current shunt is now painful to touch and erythematous.

Mr. G. is experiencing several types of pain: the chronic pain of peripheral neuropathy in his hands and legs, incisional pain from his sternal wound, and pain from his dialysis shunt, which increases during his dialysis treatments. Trials of medications and therapies have not provided him with substantial relief. Despite Mr. G.'s complicated medical history, until recently he was quite independent and even on admission to the hospital appears quite robust in his wheelchair. He interacts genuinely with his wife and teenage children until it is time for him to move into the bed. He asks his family to leave his room, saying that he does not want his family to see him in such pain.

During the past 2 years, the impact of Mr. G.'s physical pain has slowly become the focus of his life. Every movement, thought, and emotion is impeded by its presence. The pain has limited his ability to move even in bed, which has led to physical deconditioning. His arm and leg muscles have atrophied; he becomes short of breath simply by repositioning himself. He consciously tries to hide the severity of his pain from his family, which is easy to do during the day when his family is away at school and work. Mr. G. reports that the long sleepless nights are when his pain is at its worst. He fears that the pain will never be relieved and knows that it will intensify with each dialysis treatment and additional medical procedure. He has always had a healthy perception of himself and considered his life meaningful and fulfilling. His ability to reflect on his life and its meaning is now overshadowed by pain.

Pain is both a common and yet highly individualized experience. At its best, pain serves a vital function, signaling for attention to a dysfunction of a body part or system. At its worst, pain can become chronic, hovering relentlessly, despite having no apparent cause. The impact of pain on quality of life has been well documented (Lazarus & Neuman, 2001). The phenomenon of pain is multivariate, with physical, emotional, and social implications. Pain is often accompanied by an array of other distressing symptoms such as depression, isolation, insomnia, and cognitive and psychological impairment. The current treatment options for pain management are numerous, and identifying the particular option that effectively relieves a person's pain is often very difficult. Health care providers are responsible for making pain a priority and for identifying and implementing interventions that meet each individual's need until relief is obtained.

This chapter will describe the multifactorial nature of pain and its resulting infirmity, with discussion of its variation among different patient populations. The goal of this chapter is to assist health care providers in recognizing how different patient characteristics affect the pain experience, and how to best assess and manage pain in an individualized manner to ultimately maximize the quality of the person's life.

# The Problem of Pain

Pain is one of the most common reasons for seeking health care. According to a recent survey, 64% of American households report that they have one chronic pain sufferer, and 36% report at least two or more sufferers. Among these people with pain, 61% report that they have had pain for at least 5 years (Lazarus & Neuman, 2001). The economic impact that both short-term and long-term pain have on the health care system and on our society at large is immense (Waddell, 1996, as cited in Bennett & St. Marie, 2002). Pain that is poorly controlled leads to more visits with health care providers and prolonged hospital stays, as well as contributes to a variety of complications, including the development of chronic pain syndromes (AHCPR, 1992; Tasmouth, Estlanderb, & Kalso, 1996).

Time spent with health care providers and hospital stays take time away from work. Businesses assume the cost for lost employee work days, decreased productivity, and worker's compensation claims (Hemmila, 2002). Although health insurances pay for some treatments, surgeries, and medications, the burden of paying for pain management ultimately falls on the family of the person experiencing the symptom. Although the economic impact of pain can be staggering, most pain sufferers agree that the loss of functional capacity and quality of life is most costly.

## Quality of Life with Pain

There are many potential consequences of experiencing pain, including the following:

- Depression
- Insomnia
- Anxiety
- Impaired memory
- Physical deconditioning
- Impaired concentration
- Anger/frustration
- Social isolation
- Hopelessness

The combination of pain and its sequelae places people in pain among those with the lowest of quality of life. Quality of life is a measure that encompasses such indicators as physiological, psychological, sociological, and spiritual well-being. Research suggests that persons living with pain rate their quality of life lower than those living with progressive debilitating diseases such as coronary artery disease, chronic renal failure, or multiple sclerosis (Gerstle, All, & Wallace, 2001).

Over time, people with poorly managed pain often retreat from normal daily activities, such as exercise, hobbies, or even employment. This predisposes people with pain to significant physical deconditioning and social isolation. Furthermore, people with pain often have difficulty sleeping.

With insufficient sleep, and less activity offering distraction from their symptoms, they tend to become more preoccupied with the pain and experience additional suffering. Depression and/or anxiety exist in extremely high rates, ranging from 15% to 51%, depending on personal characteristics and the type of pain (Adams et al., 2001). A recent survey of chronic pain patients living at home revealed that almost one-third (31%) agreed with the statement, "some days the pain is so bad I just want to die" (Lazarus & Neuman, 2001).

The impact of pain and its potential consequences is so devastating that, as of January 1, 2001, the Joint Commission of Accreditation of Healthcare Organizations (JCAHO) established stringent new standards for pain assessment and management for all of its certified heath care facilities (http://www.JCAHO.com).

# About Pain

There are many different types of pain, which are important to distinguish because they respond differently to selected treatments. Types of pain can be classified based on the underlying mechanism of action and duration. These include cutaneous, visceral, somatic, and neuropathic pain, as well as acute and chronic pain.

*Cutaneous* pain occurs when superficial nerve fibers in cutaneous tissue are stimulated. It may result from mechanical injury, thermal injury, or chemical injury, such as a paper cut or a first-degree burn. Pain arising from stimulation of deeper nerve fibers (nocioceptors) may be visceral or somatic. *Visceral*, or organ, pain occurs in the gastrointestinal tract, pelvic, or cranial cavities. Common examples include menstrual pain or the pain associated with diverticulitis. It is diffuse, poorly localized, and frequently difficult to identify the source of pathology. *Somatic* pain, or structural pain arises in muscles, joints, bones, ligaments, tendons, or fascia. It is more easily localized by the client and is frequently associated with trauma or activity. Common examples of somatic pain are tendonitis or arthritis.

*Neuropathic* pain occurs as a result of damage to the peripheral or central nervous system, resulting in abnormal processing of sensory input by the peripheral or central nervous system. This differs from other types of pain mentioned above, which result from information transmitted through normal processing in the peripheral or central nervous system. With neuropathic pain, stimulation of nervous tissue is not necessary for perception of pain to occur. People often describe this type of pain as having a "shooting" or "electric" characteristic that can be particularly distressing.

The duration of pain may be either acute or chronic. Acute pain often develops as a result of a known physiologic cause. It is short lived, lasting less than 3 to 6 months, and typically resolves in response to treatment or time. Some examples of acute pain would be a headache, childbirth, or a fractured bone. In contrast, chronic pain lasts at least 3 to 6 months and is characterized by remissions and exacerbations. Chronic pain can be subdivided as either chronic malignant, that is, cancer pain, or chronic nonmalignant pain. Although a cause, usually the cancer, is commonly identified in chronic malignant pain, the source of the pain may not always be identified in chronic nonmalignant pain. Classic examples of chronic nonmalignant pain include low back pain lingering long after an initial injury, arthritis, or peripheral neuropathy.

## Pain Theory

An early theory of pain was specificity theory, which proposed that a specific pain system carried messages from pain receptors in the skin to a pain center in the brain (Melzack & Wall, 1983). During the 20th century, the elaborate anatomy and physiology of pain was described, which included sensory nerves that responded to external stimuli, carrying encoded messages to specific areas of the brain, and various types of sensory end organs with different receptors for touch, warmth, cold, and pain (Melzack & Wall, 1983). Other scientists identified thermal, mechanical, and chemical stimuli that activated sensory nerves when a threshold was reached, with transmission of information through specific peripheral and central pathways. Pain to free nerve endings was also found to stimulate A delta and C fibers with transmission of the pain message via the spinothalamic tract to pain centers in the thalamus (Melzack & Wall, 1983).

Although useful, specificity theory did not explain all types of pain sensations; why pain fibers could be cut, with persistence of pain; variation in pain tolerance among individuals and within the same individual; nor the absence of perceived pain when pain receptors were stimulated (Arnstein, 2002). Another theory, *pattern theory,* emphasized the importance of stimulus intensity and central summation in the pain experience, and acknowledged that there are variations within and among individuals in response to the same stimulus (Melzack & Wall, 1983).

In 1965, Melzack and Wall introduced the *gate control theory,* which proposed how thoughts and emotions might also play a role in pain (Figure 21.1). This theory retained elements of both specificity and pattern theories, and included components of psychosocial theories related to pain, proposing that affect, motivation, perception, and central control of the mind all contribute to the pain experience (Arnstein, 2002). The gate control theory proposed that small-diameter (A delta and C) fibers carry messages of pain to the dorsal horn of the spinal cord. A neural mechanism in this area (i.e., substantia gelatinosa) acts like a gate, which can increase or decrease nerve impulses from peripheral fibers to the central nervous system. Large-diameter (A beta) fibers can close the gate, reducing transmission of pain messages. The gating mechanism is influenced by the amount of input from the small and large fibers entering the spine and by central control processes of the brain (which evaluate pain in terms of past experience), and the system is modulated by motivational-affective, limbic, and reticular structures.

*Figure 21.1*    Gate Control Theory

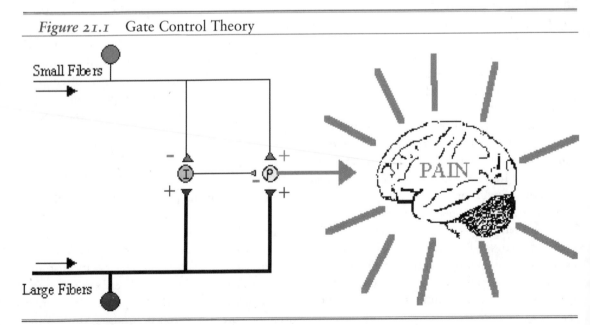

When noxious stimuli entering the spinal cord exceed a crucial level, T cells responsible for the subjective and objective experience are activated. These T cells are believed to be the link between the mind and the body (Arnstein, 2002).

Continuing research supports the gate control theory (Melzack & Wall, 1983, 1996) as the predominant pain theory. Examples of extensions to the theory include the following:

- With repeated moderate to severe pain, N-methyl-D-aspartate (NMDA) receptors are activated, which leads to an increase of amino acids, resulting in a greater-than-expected pain intensity, duration, and geographic distribution (Bennett & St. Marie, 2002; Coderre, Katz, Vaccarino, & Melzack, 1993);

- If moderate-to-severe pain persists for more than 24 hours, additional changes in the structures and function of the spinal segment of the nervous system occur (referred to as neuroplasticity); these changes lead to stimulation of pain fiber growth, resulting in more intense, widespread pain (Arnstein, 1997; Coderre et al., 1993);

- Multiple parallel nerve pathways, neurotransmitters, and inflammatory neuroactive substrates are involved in the generation, transmission, and modification of pain signals (Dubner & Gold, 1999; Urban & Gebhart, 1999).

The gate control theory helps explain why there are a variety of pain sensations perceived among clients, even with similar types of pain. The experience and response of a person to a pain stimulus is affected not only by the pain impulse but also by any factor that can open or close the gates within the central nervous system. The pain experience is individual and unique to each person. The client's physical and emotional response to the type and chronicity of the pain experience is also individual and unique. Research on the physiology of pain continues to accumulate,

which will likely extend gate control theory further.

Psychosocial theories also have been developed to describe the pain experience from a more holistic perspective. Cognitive-behavioral theory views pain as a complex multidimensional experience (Turk, Meichenbaum, & Genest, 1983). The theory assumes the patient, not the professional, is the expert in managing his or her own pain. The focus is on teaching individuals to monitor their thoughts, feelings, and actions while learning and using self-initiated skills.

# Managing Pain

Pain is a subjective experience; it is widely accepted that pain is "whatever the person experiencing it says it is" (McCaffrey & Pasero, 1999). The key to assessing pain is the ability to listen to the person's experience of the pain. The goals and strategies for assessing and managing acute versus chronic pain may differ.

## Acute Pain

The physical symptoms of acute pain are usually observable (Figure 21.2) and may or may not be congruent with clients' reports of pain. When acute pain is expected (e.g., after a surgical procedure), pain assessment is best accomplished with a pain scale. Scales come in different sizes and shapes, with a Likert scale as the most widely used

*Figure 21.2* Physical Manifestations of Pain

Crying
Wincing, grimacing
Guarding, bracing
Moaning, grunting
Agitation, irritability
Elevated heart rate or blood pressure
Tachypnea

*(McCaffery, 2002)*

*Figure 21.3* Faces Assess Scale and Linear Pain Scale

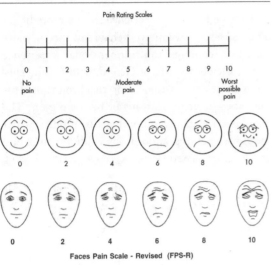

*(Reprinted by permission from Pediatric Pain Sourcebook, 2001; International Association for the Study of Pain.)*

the client's physical behaviors can assist the health care provider in assessing the likelihood of pain. Behavioral pain indicators consider behaviors such as crying, moaning, yelling, restlessness, or changes in vital signs such as an elevated respiratory rate, heart rate, or blood pressure; however, signs may be as subtle as a tensed brow or a generalized look of sadness (Figure 21.2). These types of scales should be used with caution: they attempt to ascertain whether a client is having pain, but are not intended to measure the intensity of pain. Furthermore, there is little research regarding the use of behavioral pain scales to substantiate their validity (McCaffery, 2002).

Often the most important assessment for clients who are unable to respond is to consider the recent pain history. Does the client have any chronic conditions that are known to cause pain? Has the client undergone any recent painful procedures? Is it likely that the client is in pain?

Pain scales are generally intended to measure the patient's reported intensity of pain. Other characteristics of the pain must also be assessed, such as the location, quality, and exacerbating and ameliorating factors, as well as the physical assessment of the site of pain. The health care provider needs to work collaboratively with the client to establish a mutually acceptable treatment plan and pain goal. Although it may seem that the pain goal should always be "0" (i.e., no pain), it may not be realistic to start with that goal. For example, immediately after major surgery, every client is going to experience some pain due to the temporary bodily insult. As the client awakens from surgery, there is often a period of transition in which the optimal amount and frequency of medication will be determined.

format. The client assigns a number from 0 to 10 to the level of pain at a given moment, with "0" being "no pain" and "10" being "the worst pain imaginable" (Figure 21.3). The number serves as a marker to initiate interventions and to evaluate progress in obtaining the client's pain management goals.

This type of scale is not appropriate for clients who may be unable to comprehend or correctly use a numerical scale to rate their pain (e.g., children less than 10 years old and older clients who are cognitively impaired due to dementia, delirium, psychosis, stroke, and/or coma). In some of these circumstances an effective alternative is the "Faces Pain Scale," which is valid for children ages 4 to 12 years and has been used successfully with cognitively impaired elders (McCaffrey, 2002). For non-English–speaking clients, versions of both the numeric and the faces scales have been translated into over eight different languages.

In the event that a client is severely cognitively impaired, minimally responsive, or comatose, the client should never be presumed to be pain free. In these cases, pain assessment scales that are based on

## Chronic Pain

For clients with chronic pain, a goal of "0" may never be possible. Therefore, negotiating a pain goal that is acceptable to the person in pain is paramount. A goal of "6" may allow one client to get out of bed in the morning, whereas a "4" means taking a ride in the car. A pain level of "2" may be necessary to partake in important activities, such as driving the car, working in the garden, or playing with grandchildren. Goals and activities, as well as pain management strategies, will vary depending on the client, his/her pain, and lifestyle. Doing a full pain assessment and working with clients to develop pain goals are not only essential for providing efficient pain management but are examples of the standards that are mandated by JCAHO.

Typically, health care providers have been better at assessing and managing acute pain than chronic pain. People in chronic pain often do not exhibit the physical features listed in Figure 21.3, which are manifestations of the sympathetic nervous system response to an acute stimulus, accompanied by an involuntary release of abnormally high levels of epinephrine and other stress hormones. This natural "fight-or-flight" response to a stressor cannot be maintained over an extended period of time. The stress response itself can potentially cause damage to the body if sustained, such as vessel wall damage with prolonged hypertension. Over time, the body recognizes that the stress response to chronic pain is futile and even potentially harmful, and even though the pain persists, the physical manifestations listed in Figure 21.2 subside.

### EXAMPLE

Consider Ms. F, a 41-year-old woman 1 day post-op after a right mastectomy and breast reconstruction. Despite requesting and taking 2 oxycodone (5 mg) with acetaminophen (325 mg) tablets every 4 hours, she rates her surgical pain around "7 or 8" on a 0 to 10 scale. The morning after surgery, as she is washing and moving more independently, she reports more pain and requests her oral medication more than 1 hour before it is due. The staff become concerned about her narcotic requests and use, especially since Ms. F. is resting quietly in bed most of the time. She is labeled by the health care providers as a "clock watcher" and "someone who likes her medication."

Her history reveals that she has suffered chronic neck, shoulder, and lower back pain since an automobile accident 6 years earlier. She has taken oxycodone at home on a regular basis for this pain. During the few weeks before her surgery, Ms. F. reported that her neck and back pain had been particularly painful, but her team of health care providers suggested treating her breast cancer before reevaluating her chronic pain management.

Ms. F.'s history offers insight into her postoperative pain management. First, it is likely that she has developed a tolerance to both her pain medication and the pain experience. That is, when the human body is chronically subjected to narcotics, over time gradual increases in dosage are needed to keep opiate receptors occupied. This would explain why she rates her pain very high while taking the maximum allotted doses of the narcotic postoperatively. Tolerance is not addiction, which denotes a compulsive craving for and use of medication to achieve some pleasure or euphoria. Whereas people with narcotic addiction may experience tolerance, people with drug tolerance are not drug addicts.

Second, having been exposed to pain for so long, her body no longer demonstrates the physiologic and psychological behaviors that many health care providers expect to see when someone is in acute pain. Ms. F. is not moaning; her vital signs are not elevated. Third, her pain is just as real as another postoperative patient's pain, if not more so, because she has both the chronic neck pain and the acute surgical pain concurrently.

### RELATIONSHIPS WITH HEALTH CARE PROVIDERS

When health care providers do not believe the patient's report of pain, a cycle of mistrust can be initiated. Peter and Watt-Watson (2002) describe unrelieved pain related to distrust as a matter of the clinician's own vulnerability. They propose that clinicians are reluctant to become too close to the patients or their pain, so they shield themselves with reluctance to prescribe potent pain medications, especially when the pain patients are minorities or belong to a lower socioeconomic class. There is a considerable degree of treatment variability and lack of confidence among physicians when making decisions about pain management (Green, Wheeler, LaPort, Marchant, & Guerrero, 2002).

Ultimately, health care providers continue to treat pain based on objective measures, despite the inherent subjectivity of the phenomena of pain. Patients seeking relief of pain are ever conscious of the aura of mistrust. When this type of relationship develops between provider and patient, the patient fears undertreatment of the pain and might "shop around" for a health care provider that will believe him. In the process of doing so, additional providers may deem this patient's behavior as suspicious.

Providers become skeptical when chronic pain patients request pain medication by specific name or dose, or at specific times. These behaviors do not necessarily indicate addiction. More often, these behaviors are a result of years of medication trial and error during which the patient has developed an awareness of what works best for his/her pain. The exaggerated fear of supplying an addict with pain medication is unfounded because the majority of people who report pain really do have pain (McCaffery, 2002).

In light of these special circumstances, the client with chronic pain requires an assessment tool that reflects the experience of pain over the long term, not just at the moment of assessment. Because chronic pain may be associated with psychosocial disturbances and physical deconditioning, most chronic pain questionnaires include assessment of physical capacity and emotional adjustment in addition to the detailed assessment of pain location, character, and intensity over a specified interval of time (Figure 21.4).

# Approaches to Pain Management

The importance of assessing pain cannot be underscored enough because the treatment plan is specific to the type and characteristics of the pain. For instance, lower back pain may respond well to physical therapy, whereas the acute renal colic pain from a kidney stone will likely require an opioid. Conventional Western medicine, also referred to as mainstream or allopathic medicine, has traditionally treated pain with medications. However, it is increasingly clear that a purely pharmacological approach to managing pain may be inadequate, especially for people with chronic pain.

Chronic pain patients are good candidates for a comprehensive, often multidisciplinary, approach to pain management, which utilizes a variety of interventions aimed at closing the gates and diminishing the pain experience. Pain management clinics are one means to obtaining a multidisciplinary plan of care. They will be discussed further at the end of this chapter. Because pain is such an individualized experience, each patient must have a pain management plan that is developed specifically for that particular person. The most successful approaches to pain management use a combination of therapies, including medications, physical measures, and some behavioral therapy, that are patient driven and provider supported.

## Analgesic Medications

Because the reader is familiar with common analgesic medications, and the focus of this chapter is not on the treatment of pain per se, this section will provide a very brief overview of the use of medications. The purpose is to put the individual client's needs and options into context, so that decisions about pain management can be patient centered and appropriate for the client's age and ability to manage. This section on managing pain will be followed by a discussion of the developmental implications for children, adults, and elders.

Medication for pain control is available in a variety of routes (oral, rectal, topical, subcutaneous, intramuscular, intravenous, intrathecal, and more) and in a variety of dosages. To further complicate the choice of treatment, categories of pain medications are not limited to analgesics and anesthetics; there are a variety of additional

*Figure 21.4* Chronic Pain Assessment Tool—Brief Pain Inventory

## BRIEF PAIN INVENTORY

Date_____/_____/_____ Time:_____

Name:_____
          Last          First          Middle Initial

1) Throughout our lives, most of us have had pain from time to time (such as minor headaches, sprains, and toothaches). Have you had pain other than these everyday kinds of pain today?

   1. Yes    2. No

2) On the diagram, shade in the areas where you feel pain. Put an X on the area that hurts the most.

Right    Left        Left    Right

3) Please rate your pain by circling the one number that best describes your pain at its WORST in the last 24 hours.

   | 0 | 1 | 2 | 3 | 4 | 5 | 6 | 7 | 8 | 9 | 10 |
   |---|---|---|---|---|---|---|---|---|---|----|

   No Pain                                Pain as bad as you can imagine

4) Please rate your pain by circling the one number that best describes your pain at its LEAST in the last 24 hours.

   | 0 | 1 | 2 | 3 | 4 | 5 | 6 | 7 | 8 | 9 | 10 |
   |---|---|---|---|---|---|---|---|---|---|----|

   No Pain                                Pain as bad as you can imagine

5) Please rate your pain by circling the one number that best describes your pain on the AVERAGE.

   | 0 | 1 | 2 | 3 | 4 | 5 | 6 | 7 | 8 | 9 | 10 |
   |---|---|---|---|---|---|---|---|---|---|----|

   No Pain                                Pain as bad as you can imagine

6) Please rate your pain by circling the one number that tells how much pain you have RIGHT NOW.

   | 0 | 1 | 2 | 3 | 4 | 5 | 6 | 7 | 8 | 9 | 10 |
   |---|---|---|---|---|---|---|---|---|---|----|

   No Pain                                Pain as bad as you can imagine

7) What treatments or medications are you receiving for your pain?

_____

_____

8) In the last 24 hours, how much relief have pain treatments or medications provided? Please circle the one percentage that shows how much RELIEF you have received.

   | 0% | 10 | 20 | 30 | 40 | 50 | 60 | 70 | 80 | 90 | 100% |
   |----|----|----|----|----|----|----|----|----|----|------|

   No relief                              Complete relief

9) Circle the one number that describes how, during the past 24 hours, pain has interfered with your:

A. General activity

   | 0 | 1 | 2 | 3 | 4 | 5 | 6 | 7 | 8 | 9 | 10 |
   |---|---|---|---|---|---|---|---|---|---|----|

   Does not interfere                     Completely interferes

B. Mood

   | 0 | 1 | 2 | 3 | 4 | 5 | 6 | 7 | 8 | 9 | 10 |
   |---|---|---|---|---|---|---|---|---|---|----|

   Does not interfere                     Completely interferes

C. Walking ability

   | 0 | 1 | 2 | 3 | 4 | 5 | 6 | 7 | 8 | 9 | 10 |
   |---|---|---|---|---|---|---|---|---|---|----|

   Does not interfere                     Completely interferes

D. Normal work (includes both work outside the home and housework)

   | 0 | 1 | 2 | 3 | 4 | 5 | 6 | 7 | 8 | 9 | 10 |
   |---|---|---|---|---|---|---|---|---|---|----|

   Does not interfere                     Completely interferes

E. Relations with other people

   | 0 | 1 | 2 | 3 | 4 | 5 | 6 | 7 | 8 | 9 | 10 |
   |---|---|---|---|---|---|---|---|---|---|----|

   Does not interfere                     Completely interferes

F. Sleep

   | 0 | 1 | 2 | 3 | 4 | 5 | 6 | 7 | 8 | 9 | 10 |
   |---|---|---|---|---|---|---|---|---|---|----|

   Does not interfere                     Completely interferes

G. Enjoyment of life

   | 0 | 1 | 2 | 3 | 4 | 5 | 6 | 7 | 8 | 9 | 10 |
   |---|---|---|---|---|---|---|---|---|---|----|

   Does not interfere                     Completely interferes classifications of drugs used to treat pain, including nonopioid analgesics, opioid analgesics, and analgesic adjuvants. The choice of medication is based on the type, location, and severity of pain.

One widely accepted treatment guide for pain management is the World Health Organization (WHO) Three Step Analgesic Ladder (WHO, 1990). Step One utilizes a nonopioid analgesic plus or minus an adjuvant medication. Step Two involves the addition of an opioid for mild-to-moderate pain with or without an adjuvant medication. Step Three involves use of opioids for moderate-to-severe pain such as morphine, with or without an adjuvant. Drug therapy has been the mainstay of treatment for the management of acute pain and chronic cancer pain in all age groups (American Pain Society, 1999).

For example, nonopioid analgesics (e.g., aspirin, acetaminophen, and nonsteroidal anti-inflammatory drugs [NSAIDS]) are useful for acute and chronic pain resulting from a variety of etiologies (American Pain Society, 1999). Low doses of opioids such as oxycodone (5 mg p.o.), codeine (30–60 mg p.o.), or hydrocodone (5–10 mg p.o.) are utilized for mild-to-moderate pain, sometimes in combination with a nonopioid analgesic for pain of greater severity. Severe pain requires opioids such as morphine, which do not have a ceiling; that is, there is no upper limit of tolerance, and the drugs can be titrated as needed to the patient's pain. For example, a narcotic-naïve person may start with a morphine dose of 5 mg to 15 mg by mouth, whereas individuals who have been taking opioids daily for chronic pain will tolerate oral doses as high as 30 mg to >300 mg. Severe pain that does not respond to oral opioids requires opioids via the parenteral (i.e., subcutaneous, intramuscular, or intravenous), epidural, or intrathecal routes, with the dose varying by route. Here again, persons who have developed a tolerance over time need and can tolerate surprisingly high doses of opioids without the adverse effects that an opioid-naïve person would surely experience. Equianalgesic charts assist health care providers in choosing appropriate doses (Acute Pain Management Guideline Panel, 1992).

Adjuvant analgesics are classified in categories other than analgesics but are also utilized for their analgesic properties. These include antidepressants, anticonvulsants, and corticosteroids. For example, benzodiazepines (e.g., Valium) is used for pain related to muscle spasm, sometimes in combination with nonopioids. Although pain management has traditionally focused on pharmacological approaches, there are also many nonpharmacologic means available. Sometimes the best pain management plans include both.

## Physical Measures

Nerve blocks may be beneficial in clients who do not obtain pain relief from standard analgesic therapy. They are particularly beneficial if pain is well localized or confined to a certain nerve distribution area. Nerve blocks may be temporary or permanent, dependent on the patient situation. Temporary nerve blocks commonly utilize local anesthetics, while permanent blocks (i.e., neuroablation) are accomplished with a chemical agent such as phenol or alcohol (Keane, McMenamin, & Polomano 2002). Permanent blocks and surgical procedures that involve cutting sensory nerves are necessary for only a small percent of individuals who do not respond to appropriate pharmacologic therapy.

Cutaneous stimulation either at the site of pain or at another site of the body can confound the gate control pain stimulus, reducing painful sensations. Examples of cutaneous stimulation include touch, pressure, massage, vibration, manipulation, and application of heat or cold. Massage is indicated for musculoskeletal pain (particularly related to immobility), circulation enhancement, relaxation, and stress reduction, each of which can impact an individual's pain (Vaughan, 2002). It directly affects soft muscle tissue, moves body fluids, and stimulates the nervous system, chemicals, and the endocrine system. It can help loosen contracted, shortened muscles and can stimulate weak, flaccid muscle, increasing the oxygen capacity of the blood between 10 and 15 percent (Goats, 1994). Most research on the effectiveness of massage for chronic pain has involved individuals with lower back pain (Rakel & Barr, 2003). A recent review of the literature by Furlan and colleagues (2002) concluded that massage may be beneficial for individuals with subacute or chronic lower back pain, especially when combined with exercise and education. Massage is also an effective treatment (in conjunction with analgesics) for cancer pain, particularly in males (Weinrich & Weinrich, 1990) and for neuropathic pain syndrome related to cancer (Martin, 1997).

Applications of heat increase blood flow to the skin and superficial organs, inducing vasodilatation, which increases oxygen and nutrient delivery to damaged tissues (Whitney, 1989). Heat also decreases joint stiffness by increasing the elastic properties of muscles (Vasudevan, Hegmann, Moore, & Cerletty, 1992). Cold therapy causes vasoconstriction and local hyperesthesia, which reduces inflammation, edema soon after an injury, burning perineal pain (Evans, Lloyd, & Jack, 1981), and muscle spasm (Vasudevan et al. 1992).

Physical therapy (PT) is another example of a physical measure utilized to decrease pain, increase function, and prevent further deconditioning. It utilizes a variety of approaches to decrease pain and increase function, including but not limited to massage, range of motion, stretching, exercise, heat or cold therapy, and transcutaneous electric nerve stimulation (TENS). TENS works by triggering a mild electric current across the skin to superficial nerves near the location of the pain. Whether the TENS is used externally or surgically implanted, it offers the patient some control over settings and duration of use. Physical therapy can increase the quality of life, especially for people with prolonged back pain (Hemmila, 2002).

## Behavioral Measures

Behavioral strategies that are cognitive, emotional, or psychosocial in nature can also be used to decrease pain. Behavioral strategies are commonly described as *complementary* or *integrative therapies*. In the past, they were also referred to as *alternative therapies*, but this term has lost favor because of the implication that it replaces conventional or mainstream medicine. Ideally, these therapies are utilized in conjunction with conventional medicine.

Mental and physical relaxation has been shown to reduce muscle tension, a contributing factor in pain (Ferrell-Torry & Glick, 1993). Although the relaxation response is a natural bodily response, it needs to be trained and practiced, particularly in people with pain, whose muscles are often tense as a response to pain. Relaxation can be achieved through controlled breathing exercises, visual or guided imagery, music therapy, distraction, humor, and biofeedback. Research has shown that meditation diminishes chronic pain (Kabat-Zinn, 1982; Kabat-Zinn et al., 1985; Kabat-Zinn et al., 1986). Individuals practicing mindfulness awareness have also reported that their relationship with the pain changes, and that they can choose to engage the pain or not.

Because Americans have recognized that these treatments are often effective as well as natural, the use and acceptance of complementary or integrative therapies has increased. Americans' utilization of nontraditional therapies was well documented in a landmark study by Eisenberg and colleagues (1998), who found that one-third of those responding to a survey had used at least one unconventional treatment in the previous year. Based on these findings, Eisenberg estimated that Americans made 425 million visits to providers of unconventional therapy in 1990. This figure exceeded the estimated number of visits to all primary health physicians for that year. In Eisenberg's sample, 36% used nonconventional treatments for back problems, 27% used it for headaches, and 26% for chronic pain.

In response to Americans' interest in these therapies, Congress established the National Center for Complementary and Alternative Medicine (NCCAM) at the National Institutes of Health in 1998 to develop and stimulate research on complementary therapies. The National Institutes of Health has classified complementary therapies into seven types of practice:

1. Herbal medicine

2. Diet, nutrition, and lifestyle changes

3. Mind/body or behavioral interventions (including several behavioral measures described previously)

4. Alternative systems of medical practice

5. Manual healing methods (including physical therapy and massage, described previously)

6. Bioelectromagnetics

7. Pharmacologic and biologic treatments, which include drugs and vaccines as yet unaccepted by mainstream medicine (National Center for Complementary and Alternative Medicine, 2000)

Many therapies considered complementary have been utilized in the treatment of pain. Research on the effect of these therapies on pain has been limited, but more research is being conducted, and support within and outside the medical community for the utilization of these techniques as adjuvants to traditional therapy has increased.

Multidisciplinary pain programs often utilize complementary or integrative therapies in their treatment of pain. Dr. Margaret Caudill's (1995) world-renowned program for individuals with chronic pain teaches individuals how to use a variety of mind–body behavioral strategies, including relaxation, imagery, visualization, self-hypnosis, and cognitive strategies to diminish the interference of pain in one's life. An inherent part of these therapies is the involvement of the client as an active participant in the treatment.

Participants are encouraged to individualize the program to their own needs by journaling and practicing personal thinking exercises.

Dr. Caudill's program has been shown to significantly lessen anxiety, depression, anger, and hostility, and, in many cases, the severity of pain. Individuals participating in these programs have also been shown to use fewer analgesics and have had fewer visits to physicians than those not involved in such programs (Caudill, 1995). Unfortunately, health insurance reimbursement for complementary therapies is often limited to chiropractic services and occasionally acupuncture. Most other services such as reflexology, massage, naturopathy, and nutritional counseling are not covered (Cleary-Guida, Okvat, Oz, & Ting, 2001).

## Barriers to Pain Management

The volume of choices available for treating pain is enough to daunt any uninformed health care provider. In some cases, poor pain management may be directly related to the health care provider. These barriers to pain management include the following (U.S. Dept of Health & Human Services, Management of Cancer Pain, 1994):

- Inadequate assessment or knowledge of pain management

- Not believing the client's report of pain

- Fear of regulatory repercussions for frequently prescribing controlled substances

- Fear of illegal diversion of opioids

- Fear of opioid-induced side effects, such as respiratory depression, sedation, and constipation

- Fear of contributing to a patient's addiction

- Short duration of office visits

In other cases, the person in pain may actually contribute to poor assessment or treatment of pain. Following are some examples of patient characteristics that create barriers to pain relief

(Davis, Hiemenz, & White, 2002; Lansbury, 2000):

- Failure to report pain when asked, so as not to "bother" the health care provider
- Viewing pain as a normal part of aging or expected as a consequence of a certain disease (arthritis) or diagnosis (cancer)
- Hesitancy to take medications that are strong enough
- Fear of addiction
- Fear of side effects
- Saving medication for when pain becomes severe
- Skeptical of trying new or complementary therapies
- Lack of transportation or finances to visit the health care provider or inability to pay for medical equipment (TENS unit) or pain medications
- Fear of diagnostic tests
- Comorbidities causing noncompliance with treatment plan (cannot participate in exercise because of emphysema)
- Not using support devices because of social stigma
- Fear of loss of independence

## Developmental Aspects of Pain

To manage pain well, it must be done in a manner that is developmentally sensitive. Although a broad overview of pain theories and management strategies have been included here, each must be applied within the context of the patient's developmental characteristics. Just as medication dosages must be modified for both the pediatric and elderly clients, the behavioral approaches to pain management should be modified to suit the particular needs of the developmental stage. However, age-specific biases and assumptions should be validated. For instance, it is widely understood that the injection of narcotics is not a preferred route for the delivery of pediatric pain medication, based on the assumption that children fear needles and that injections cause additional pain. Despite the obvious aversion that children have toward needles, one study revealed that a majority of pediatric clients who had tried acupuncture to treat their pain described it as both pleasant and effective (Kemper et al., 2000). In fact, many complementary therapies, such as imagery, relaxation, biofeedback, massage, and heat, have been used and recommended to treat children in pain (American Academy of Pediatrics, 2001). Complementary, cognitive and behavioral, and traditional pain therapies have been used to manage pain throughout the life span, each with slightly different emphasis depending on the developmental needs of the client.

Specifically, the pediatric pain experience poses a challenge to both the family and the health care community, primarily because of the relative lack of scientific study specific to this population. The American Academy of Pediatrics and the American Pain Society Taskforce on Pain in Infants, Children and Adolescents describes the care of this population as inadequate and often ineffective (American Academy of Pediatrics, 2001). This is particularly distressing because one of their recommendations is that most acute pediatric pain can and must be anticipated and managed with the correct resources. Furthermore, the task force recommends that health care providers should approach pediatric pain patients and their families with a developmentally sensitive, multimodal, and multidisciplinary approach.

### INFANTS

Children with pain are a particularly vulnerable population. Infants up to 1 year old are trying to establish trust with their primary caregivers, the parents (Wong, 1993). Thus, parent participation in the care of a child with pain is essential. Because infants have no voice, it is especially important that clinicians address pain in this population in order to cultivate trust with both parent and child. Infants have historically been considered the most innocent and resilient of any age group. However, the conventional assumption that infants do not "know" pain or will not "remember" pain has been dispelled. Furthermore, it is now widely accepted that pain management is a legitimate concern for this age group, as evidenced by the American Academy of Pediatrics' recent recommendation that all circumcisions be performed with some type of anesthetic (American Academy of Pediatrics, 1999).

## PRESCHOOL CHILDREN

Preschool children have all experienced some type of pain, but our appreciation for their understanding of the phenomena of pain is shaped by their ability to communicate their experience to others. Piaget's theory of cognitive development classifies children of this age as preoperational thinkers (Piaget & Inhelder, 1969). That is, children this age do not appreciate the relationship between cause and effect, especially if they cannot experience it with their own eyes and ears. While they may realize that their arm hurts because the dog bit them, they do not see the relationship between pain medication and pain relief—especially if the delivery of the medication is also painful, such as with injections. Because they cannot see the inside of their bodies, surgery and its resulting pain may be disconnected. In an effort to make some sense of it, the pain experience may be viewed as a punishment, or children may attribute the pain to something that they did or thought (Di Maggio, 2002).

Young children relate best to concrete passive interventions for pain such as medication, application of a bandage or sticker, diversion, or physical affection from a parent (Thompson & Gustafson, 1996). Even brief cognitive behavioral interventions, such as distraction, for both the child and the parent can also be effective (Thompson & Gustafson, 1996). As in the case for infants, the importance of including the child's caregivers in the treatment plan cannot be underscored enough. Although children have been observed to react to painful procedures more intensely when a parent is present, presumably to elicit the sympathy of the parent, children unequivocally report that the most important pain intervention is having a parent present (Thompson & Gustafson, 1996).

## SCHOOL-AGED CHILDREN

Older school-aged children (ages 6 to 12 years) are starting to focus on achievement and recognition according to Erikson. In their struggle to complete tasks and abide by rules, they may exhibit feelings of inadequacy if they are unsuccessful due to pain. Piaget describes children in this age group as concrete operational thinkers. They have a basic understanding of bodily functions and are beginning to develop a sense of social awareness. Most children this age are able to fully participate in the self-report of their pain. The exception would be certain subpopulations, such as children with developmental disabilities, who still may not be able to fully communicate their pain (Oberlander, 2001).

Because school-aged children tend to be physically active and thus injury prone, acute pain such as bumps/bruises and broken bones is a common phenomenon for this age group. Chronic pain in children most often takes the form of headaches or abdominal pain (but can be as rare as sickle cell anemia or juvenile arthritis) (Bennett & Huntsman, 2000). Children may associate pain with bodily injury and therefore have a heightened emotional response. Some children this age may secretly worry that their pain signifies that there is something seriously wrong with their health (Rappaport & Frazer, 1995).

Diagnosing and treating pain syndromes in school-aged children is complicated because often the etiology of their pain is a combination of temperament, physiology, and environment (Rappaport & Frazer, 1995). These children need developmentally appropriate reassurance and explanations about the pain and its management. Complicating the treatment of pain in children is the real potential to indulge the child with special attention and benefits, therefore creating positive reinforcement for the child's pain behavior. As in the case of recurrent abdominal pain (RAP) without known cause, two-thirds of the children will go on to develop chronic abdominal pain or will develop other chronic syndromes such as headaches (Rappaport & Frazer, 1995). Instead of encouraging children to stay home from school or giving permission to circumvent household chores, health care providers should work with parents to develop a pain management plan that emphasizes and reinforces well behavior, active coping, and participation in daily activities (Thompson & Gustafson, 1996). Zeltzer (1995) encourages multidisciplinary pain management for young children to initiate a pattern of appropriate pain appraisal and the development of coping mechanisms for children to use over a lifetime.

Although the majority of children with pain will develop socially and academically quite normally, there is the potential for children with pain to develop problems at school or experience harmful changes in family dynamics (Bennett & Huntsman, 2000; Thompson & Gustafson, 1996). One study of 6-year-olds with chronic headaches indicates that these children have more problems at day care, have fewer hobbies, and even avoid some play situations for fear of hurting themselves (Aromaa, Sillanpaa, Rautava, & Helenius, 2000). Children with pain also more often miss school and miss participation in sports or extracurricular activities than do healthy children (Gil et al., 2000; Bennett & Huntsman, 2000). Decreased attendance in school may potentially affect academic performance, as well as limit the child's socialization with peers. Some even speculate that the missed opportunities that a child with chronic pain experiences may have lifelong implications (Bennett & Huntsman, 2000).

## ADOLESCENTS

As in adults, chronic pain can negatively impact the quality of life for adolescents (Hunfeld et al., 2001). Erikson describes this developmental stage as one of developing personal identity as well as peer acceptance, whereas Piaget emphasizes that adolescence is defined by abstract thinking and social awareness. Of all the pediatric populations, adolescents are the most concerned with their own body image as well as their ability to mesh with their peers. They might demonstrate anger, hostility, or withdrawal because the experience of pain makes them "different" from their friends. Pain management options that allow a sense of "normalcy" are important to all pediatric pain patients, especially adolescents.

Examples of pain syndromes common to adolescents include headache, abdominal or back pain, endometriosis, and reflex sympathetic dystrophy (Kemper et al., 2000; Hunfeld et al., 2001). Adolescent females have been observed to report higher pain levels and more frequent pain relative to their male counterparts (Hunfeld et al., 2001). However, there is also evidence that the severity of the pain or disease may not be as important in predicting outcomes as are the perceived stress, mood, and coping abilities of the pediatric client (Gil et al., 2000).

## THE ROLE OF FAMILY

When there is a change in the health of one family member, the entire family dynamic is affected. Parents often bear the weight of a child's suffering. Many parents of children with severe pain feel frustrated that they are not able to meet their own obligation to protect their child from harm. There is evidence that the daily stress of caring for a child with pain can negatively impact both the parental relationship as well as the atmosphere of the entire household (Aromaa et al., 2000). Some additional stressors for parents may include having to take time off from work to care for the child or to take the child to various appointments; the financial burden of paying for medications and therapies; and the guilt of stealing attention, time, and energy from the rest of the family and/or the marriage to care for the child in pain (Bennett & Huntsman, 2000; Hunfeld et al., 2001). There is evidence to suggest that levels of parental stress related to caring for a child with chronic pain may be directly related to the amount of pain the child typically has (Hunfeld et al., 2001). Watching one's own child writhe in pain can even be enough to leave parents questioning their faith in God (Ferrell, 1996).

The entire family unit contributes to the pain experience of a child or adolescent. Research suggests that the pain-coping strategies of a child with chronic pain are correlated with their parents' pain-coping strategies (Thastum, Zachariae, & Herlin, 2001). Likewise, Chambers and colleagues' (2002) laboratory research indicates that maternal behavior can have a direct impact on levels of pain intensity reported by their daughters. In this particular study, pain reports from the boys were not significantly related to the mothers' pain behavior, suggesting that social expectations may already influence the pain reports of 8- to 12-year-old boys.

Generally, parents and children agree on their perception of the child's pain intensity and pain response; however, sometimes there is discrepancy between the parents' and the child's appraisal of the pain (Gil et al., 2000). Specifically, one study indicated that parents tend to overestimate the number of pain sites and underestimate the child's ability to tolerate pain (Graumlich et al., 2001). With this in mind, treatment options and goals need to be determined with the child as well as the parents because they are often responsible not only for the emotional influence but also the practical concerns: finances, transportation, and even the administration of medications. Particularly interesting is Gil and colleagues' study of pediatric pain diaries (2000). The authors note that pain medication was often withheld until pain scores were exceedingly high in this population. In other words, children and adolescents were not taking medication when adults would traditionally be taking it. Pediatric patients have the same rights to effective pain management as adults do.

To best benefit from these rights, both the patient and the parents need to fully understand the pain management plan.

## Developmental Aspects of Pain— Adults

Adults with pain have the benefit of being the most researched and the most aggressively treated of any population. However, among adults, the experience of pain and its management varies with certain characteristics, including age, culture, and gender. Middle-aged adults (ages 45 to 64 years old) appear to demonstrate the highest levels of pain and the most emotional distress with pain (Burckhardt, Clark, & Bennett, 2001; Riley, Wade, Robinson, & Price, 2000). Developmentally, middle-aged adults have the heaviest work and social responsibilities in our culture. Many of these adults are looking after the welfare of their grown children, and some are the primary care providers for both their grandchildren and their elderly parents—truly a sandwich generation. At the same time, they are trying to secure their own retirement and may be facing the onset of health concerns for themselves, their spouses, and their peers.

There is also evidence to suggest that adult women may experience pain differently from adult men via higher levels of pain intensity, fear, frustration, and depression (Riley, Robinson, Wade, Myers, & Price, 2001). Despite this, women continue to be doubted more and medicated less for their pain. Likewise, there is evidence to suggest that minorities also receive less pain medication (Todd, Samaroo, & Hoffman, 1993; Cleeland et al., 1994). Luckily, women have been noted to discuss their pain more openly and may find support in other forms. One study reports that women expressed that the greatest benefit of group therapy is the chance to gain recognition of their pain from other group members and the group leaders (Steihaug, Ahlsen, & Malterud, 2002). Because adult pain patients tend to be in relationships, health care providers should be assessing what level of support the clients are getting from their spouse or partner. Clients in pain who have less support from their spouse report higher levels of depression, regardless of gender (Cano, Weisberg, & Gallagher, 2000). Both adult men and women need to have their pain addressed in an individualized manner.

## Developmental Aspects of Pain— Elders

The rapidly growing elderly (greater than 65 years old) population comprises a major proportion of the population presently living with pain. The prevalence of pain among elderly people varies from 25% to an alarming 80%, depending on the source, but is believed to occur at even higher rates and greater severity among nursing home residents (Miaskowski, 2000; Otis & McGeeney, 2000). Arthritis is the most common source of pain in the elderly, followed by back pain and neuropathies. Despite having the highest incidence of pain, this age group reports the lowest emotional distress and pain behaviors (Riley et al., 2000). There are many possibilities for why this is so. For example, the elderly may have more experience coping with loss and frustration, or they may also erroneously accept pain as a normal consequence of aging.

It is particularly important to assess for depression when a geriatric patient is living with pain. In elders with pain, depression appears to play a bigger role in predicting who will have difficulty with physical functioning than the pain itself (Mossey, Gallagher, & Tirumalasetti, 2000). Loss of functioning has major implications for the elder who wishes to maintain independence because many elders who can no longer physically care for themselves may have to leave their homes and enter an assisted-living environment.

Treating elderly people with pain presents a special challenge because of their multiple comorbidities. Because pain is often treated pharmacologically, the risk of polypharmacy with the geriatric population is real. When choosing medication for the elderly, the old principle "Start low, go slow" still applies, but may also contribute to the widespread undertreatment of pain in this age bracket. Certainly, the elderly are at increased risk of drug reactions or renal impairment but at the same time can tolerate and should be offered strong pain medications and periodic dose increases if needed on an individual basis (Otis & McGeeney, 2000). Most elderly people can tolerate the traditional pain medications recommended by the WHO stepped approach, mentioned earlier in this chapter, with the exception of certain pain medications such as mixed agonists–antagonists, propoxyphene, or meperidine. These agents should be avoided in the elderly because they can cause severe reactions such as delirium, confusion, agitation, and seizures (Mia-skowski, 2000; Otis & McGeeney, 2000).

Whereas health care providers may be reluctant to prescribe pain medication for the elderly, in return elders are sending the message that taking medication is among their least preferred pain management strategies (Lansbury, 2000; Davis, Hiemenz, & White 2002). In Lansbury's (2000) qualitative study of elder's preferred strategies for pain management, she notes that elders are also disinterested in physical therapy or exercise for treating pain because this population is fearful of falling or developing a new injury. Instead, elders prefer treating their pain with "home remedies," topical agents, and distraction or social involvement. These options should be considered when developing a plan of care that will be mutually acceptable to the patient and health care provider. Important principles related to pain in the elderly include assessing for depression, pain, or discomfort frequently; reinforcing that it is acceptable to admit to pain; offering pain medication in conjunction with thorough patient education and offering alternative pain treatments; and active listening (Lansbury, 2000).

# When Pain Becomes Chronic—Human Experience of Living with Pain

Caring for a person of any age who has chronic pain is especially complicated. Typically before anyone receives the vague diagnosis of "chronic pain," they have been subject to repeated diagnostic tests, consults, and failed treatments. On average, most people with chronic pain have been seen by three physicians, but some have been seen by as many as five or more, including a family physician, internist, orthopedic surgeon, neurologist, rheumatologist, chiropractor, or pain specialist (Lazarus & Neumann, 2001). In search of relief, many people with chronic pain have tried an assortment of treatments such as home remedies, prescription medications, surgery(s), complementary therapies, and even various fad gadgets purchased as a last grasp for hope from a magazine or infomercial. By the time chronic pain is finally diagnosed as such, the physical, social, and psychological consequences of the pain may have already emerged. As noted earlier in the chapter, living with chronic pain can affect all areas of life.

## Physical Consequences

The physical consequences of pain seem most obvious to the person experiencing the pain. A common theme among chronic pain sufferers is that they are ever conscious of every movement of the body (Hallberg & Carlsson, 2000). Each bend, lean, turn, or step becomes a very deliberate process in an attempt to anticipate and minimize the pain. It is difficult for people in pain to focus on where they are going, or why they are going, when all they can think of is how they are going to physically bear the pain of moving. Physical pain seems to be at the forefront of every thought. However, a most distressing component of chronic pain is its relative invisibility to other people (Thomas, 2000). Although a young woman may be too proud to use her walker or a businessman too embarrassed to wear his neck brace to a meeting, many people with chronic pain wish their pain was more readily observable and acknowledged by other people.

The physical consequences that are associated with chronic pain include deconditioning and the resulting loss of independence. In many cases the deterioration in strength and ability is directly related to the pain and not the disease process specifically. An example would be a woman with osteoarthitis of her thumbs who, despite the illness, has the ability to use the joints but chooses not to bend her thumbs because of the pain it causes. Eventually her thumbs become very weak, and manipulating a pen or a fork and knife becomes difficult or impossible. This deconditioning can occur on a larger scale, especially when the source of pain is a major support structure of the body such as the legs, back, or neck (see Figure 21.5). These areas are the most common sources of chronic pain, and loss of function here can impact almost all activities of daily living, from the ability to bathe to the ability to walk (Lazarus & Neuman, 2001; Adams et al., 2001). Research indicates that the number of people with chronic pain who have difficulty doing everyday tasks at home may be as high as 91% (McHugh & Thomas, 2001a, b).

## Psychological Consequences

Persons with chronic pain grieve the loss of physical independence. What they desire most is sim-

---

*Figure 21.5*   Common Sources of Chronic Pain

- Lumbar/low back pain
- Joint disease/arthritis
- Headache/migraine
- Neck/upper back pain
- Neuropathic pain
- Fibromyalgia
- Cancer

---

*(Lazarus, H., & C. J. Neumann, 2001; Adams et al., 2001).*

ply the ability to care for themselves and their families, continue with their work or hobbies, and be able to maneuver from one spot to the next without the constant companion of pain. The reality of physical disability related to pain is that the inability to work or participate in hobbies can lead to significant social isolation. The predominant perception among people with chronic pain is that other people do not really care to discuss pain and even may question its legitimacy. Many people purposely avoid talking about their pain to appear more normal and to try to be less of a burden on others (Hallberg & Carlsson, 2000). One quarter of chronic pain patients do not even feel comfortable discussing their pain with their families (Lazarus & Neuman, 2001).

Some people with pain become reluctant to leave the house for anything other than appointments with their physicians. Patient-to-doctor discussions about pain appear to be the most common and are sometimes the only source of support regarding pain (Lazarus & Neuman, 2001). Very few people with chronic pain report using any formal social services or group therapy for support (McHugh & Thomas, 2001b). It is difficult to conceive of the substantial loneliness that chronic pain can create.

Both the physical and social consequences of chronic pain couple with the pain itself to contribute to the substantial psychological impact of chronic pain. Reactions to chronic pain include anger, frustration, depression, anxiety, cognitive dysfunction, and low self-esteem.

## GRIEF

Feelings of denial, anger, bargaining, and depression in people with chronic pain mirror the stages Kubler-Ross (1969) describes for coping with death and dying (Ignatavicius, 1999). Much like a person mourns a loved one's death, people with chronic pain mourn the loss of their health as they once knew it. Chronic pain patients repeatedly report experiencing these stages of grief (Thomas, 2000; Riley et al., 2000, 2001).

## ANGER, FRUSTRATION, DEPRESSION

The anger and frustration most often stem from the uncertainty of chronic pain: unknown cause, unspecified treatment options, and indefinite prognosis. This is particularly problematic for people with chronic pain syndromes such as phantom pain, fibromyalgia, or chronic lower back pain, which are poorly explained by current medical diagnostic tests. Frustration starts early and returns often in chronic pain (Thomas, 2000; McHugh & Thomas, 2001b; Dudgeon et al., 2002; Peolsson, Hyden, & Larsson, 2000.). Questions that these people frequently ask are, "Why me?" "Why now?" "What is causing this?" "Why doesn't anyone believe me?" "Can anyone help my pain?" "Will I always be in pain?"

This frustration is usually shared with the people who are providing the care. Working with people with chronic pain is challenging. It is often difficult to see marked improvement, and the health care practitioner is ever conscious of the limits of modern medicine. All types of health care workers come into contact with people with chronic pain, either in the direct management of the pain or in dealing with a separate issue, such as preventative care or a cormorbid condition. It is important for health care providers to be conscious of their personal biases, especially regarding people who require chronic opioid therapy. Listening to the patient, believing the patient, and utilizing additional support resources will both decrease frustration for the client and the care provider.

Because anger and frustration are so common, there is little surprise that depression and anxiety occur in such high rates among people with chronic pain. Before 1990 there was uncertainty about which emerged first, depression or chronic pain. Originally, the assumption was that depression contributed to the development of the chronic pain. However, recently medical literature seems to support the idea that depression is indeed a consequence of and not a causative factor in the development of chronic pain (Breen, 2002).

Because pain carries a long history of being a psychologically induced entity, it has been a struggle to redefine pain. Unfortunately, people in chronic pain still face health care workers who doubt their reports of pain (McHugh & Thomas, 2001b).

## COGNITIVE ALTERATIONS

Depression, anger, and anxiety have frequently been associated with alterations in thinking. As expected, these cognitive disorders are more prevalent among people with chronic pain (Schnurr & MacDonald, 1995). Specifically, decreased concentration and memory, difficulty completing tasks, and minor accidents are some of the concerns that have been reported (Hallberg & Carlsson, 2000). Although the cause is still unclear, it may be a sum of many contributing factors including anxiety/depression, insomnia, and the pain itself.

One recent study suggested that use of opioids does not contribute to this cognitive impairment (McCracken & Iverson, 2001). Other research suggests opioids for chronic (nonmalignant) pain may actually help mental acuity (Haythornwaite, Menefee, Quartrano-Piacenti, & Pappagallo, 1998). Nonetheless, these cognitive complaints can be particularly disturbing in conjunction with the stressful circumstance of chronic pain.

## SENSE OF SELF

The person with chronic pain may also have poor self-esteem (Soderberg & Lundman, 2001). This self-perception is influenced predominantly by physical changes and/or the generalized feelings of being less productive. The body may actually look different because of surgical scars or the need to wear a brace or use a cane. Deconditioning may lead to weight gain or muscle loss. Modern culture emphasizes worth based on appearance and on one's contribution to society, which is often measured by profession. Many people are forced to leave their jobs because of their pain or its sequela (McHugh & Thomas, 2001a,b).

For example, an administrative worker may be unable to sit or type for prolonged periods because of chronic neck or shoulder pain. Or a truck driver may find himself out of work because his cancer pain requires an opioid. Even though he is physically able to drive despite his illness, U.S. interstate truck drivers may be prohibited from driving while taking this type of medication (Ross, 2001).

The inability to work has major implications. One study of people with chronic pain reports that despite workman's compensation and disability benefits, half of the study subjects had yearly incomes less than $15,000 (Gerstle et al., 2001). Financial assistance may help to pay the bills, but it does not foster the social support or self-esteem that an occupation does (Soderberg & Lundman, 2001). In fact, most pain clinics include the maintenance of or return to work as a major treatment goal in managing chronic pain because research suggests that people with chronic pain who are employed report significantly higher quality of life (Gerstle et al., 2001).

Living with chronic pain can be best described by the term "suffering" (Breen, 2002). Suffering has been defined as a largely unpredictable, personal experience that deeply impacts the way people view themselves (Kahn & Steeves, 1996). Pain and infirmity do not necessarily result in suffering. Rather, it is the individual perception of the meaning of pain that may impact the development of suffering.

Unless specifically directed otherwise, many chronic pain patients will describe life in very dismal terms (Thomas, 2000). Women from Hallberg and Carlsson's (2000) research describe their feelings regarding the experience of pain as follows:

> " *'there is no remedy for my pain . . . it's never going to get any better . . . will always be in pain'*
>
> *'. . . you just become sad and unhappy and you lose all desire to do things.'*
>
> *'I don't care about anything. I do nothing at all.'*" *(pp. 33–34, 2000)*

## The Stigma of Pain

Pain is unlike any other symptom or diagnosis. At its extreme, it may be the condition that people fear most in life. People with chronic pain are unlike people who have overcome disabilities or the people who are "cancer survivors." Instead of fighting a battle and winning, there is social stigma and hopelessness. Our society has not "mainstreamed" the diagnosis yet: there are no commercials, no publicized fundraisers or calendar days devoted to people in chronic pain. On the contrary, most people do not like to talk about chronic pain. Furthermore, a person who is open about experiencing chronic pain may be stigmatized as weak or as a burden. It is exceedingly rare for people entangled in chronic pain to identify any benefit of the pain experience. Especially for people with pain of unknown origin, positive thinking and hope are regretfully lost during the chronic pain journey. Life with chronic pain is often one of despair.

Ferrell (1996) writes that the widespread acceptance by health care providers of their patients' suffering is an outrage. The medical community has traditionally valued quantity of life over quality of life. Among health care providers there is a feeling of frustration, and even failure, when their patient's illness persists despite varied treatments. Ferrell stresses the importance of distinguishing pain from infirmity. Although there may be many diseases for which there is no known cure yet, the symptom of pain can and must be managed.

## Coping with Chronic Pain

How is it that some people are able to cope with chronic pain and disability quite well? Each person with chronic pain has a very unique experience and requires an individualized pain management program. One way to accomplish this is through a multidisciplinary approach. Most chronic pain patients have tried a wide array of medications and therapies. Interestingly enough, both prescription and OTC pharmacological interventions have been cited by a majority of people with chronic pain as ineffective in managing pain well (Lazarus & Neuman, 2001). Chronic pain defies the expectations of a "quick fix." Health care providers that attempt to treat

chronic pain in a 15-minute office visit or with medication alone do not understand or appreciate the phenomena of chronic pain.

### PAIN MANAGEMENT CLINICS

For this reason, our health care system has begun to see a surge of multidisciplinary pain management clinics. The purpose of these clinics is to provide intense, specialized care to people who have pain that has not been not well managed by conservative means. Often these clinics combine traditional pharmacological treatment with physical and behavioral therapies. These facilities have come under scrutiny, with third-party payers demanding evidence of efficacy and economic savings. The question of cost-effectiveness of this type of treatment is yet to be determined, because research to date has not fully considered the multiple outcome measures associated with chronic pain (Thomsen, Sorenson, Sjogren, & Eriksen, 2001).

However, there are many studies that seem to support the positive effects of specialized pain management centers on a number of outcomes including decrease in pain ratings, increase in functional performance, return to or maintenance of employment, and improved quality of life (Coughlin, Badura, Fleisher, & Guck, 2000; Guzman et al., 2002). One systematic review and meta-analysis revealed that cognitive behavioral interventions may work best for people with chronic fatigue syndrome and chronic back pain (Raine, Haines, & Sensky, 2002). Unfortunately many people, especially the elderly with chronic pain, are either referred much too late or indeed never referred to pain specialists at all (McHugh & Thomas, 2001a,b; Lansbury, 2000).

Chronic pain centers may influence the development of a more internal locus of control (Coughlin et al., 2000). An internal orientation facilitates the use of active coping strategies such as seeking help, fully participating in treatment, and taking ownership of the pain. Many people have difficulty understanding the importance of this concept for their health. Helping people cope with chronic pain directly involves addressing attitude and self-efficacy. Arnstein suggests that both the severity of chronic pain and one's attitude toward that pain directly influence both depression and disability (Arnstein, Caudill, Mandle, Norris, & Beasley, 1999; Arnstein, 2000). Thus, people with negative thoughts may be more likely to be depressed and have difficulty with their daily functional performance, perpetuating a cycle of hopelessness. Other thoughts that contribute to hopelessness include anger, blame, or a passive approach to pain management (Figure 21.6). With the high prevalence of pessimism among chronic pain patients, clearly the role of cognitive therapy in addition to treating the pain itself is paramount.

## OTHER WAYS OF COPING

Changing the way people perceive and respond to pain is difficult. Although pain management centers offer one means for doing this, clearly there are multiple avenues to reach this end. Because the experience of pain is so dynamic, even variable in the same person over the life span, people with pain have developed numerous strategies to adapt to everyday stressors. Many of these focus on remaining active and involved by utilizing periods of rest and moderation (Taylor, 2001). For instance, the mother with chronic lower back pain may choose to host the holiday meal but will ask her guests to bring the heaviest parts of the meal so that she will not have to expend so much effort and endure discomfort with lifting. Learning to adapt

to the limits of chronic pain is often an unconscious process of trial and error (Peolsson et al., 2000).

There are a number of clinics, programs, and books that are available for people with chronic pain to help adaptation become a more intentional process. A good program includes means for addressing attitude and encouraging characteristics such as stress hardiness, optimism, altruism, control, and forgiveness (Caudill, 1995). Repeatedly, the research suggests that what people with chronic pain want most are support and information (Lansbury, 2000; McHugh & Thomas, 2001a,b). Unfortunately, very few people actually utilize any formal support programs. Perhaps health care workers need to be more assertive and creative in their recommendations about obtaining additional support. To facilitate use of group support, health care personnel should provide written information regarding the format, expectations, and specifics, such as dates and locations of groups in the local vicinity. Some people are intimidated by a group and should therefore be referred for individual counseling or even encouraged to try a reputable Internet chat room to further discuss their pain in a format that protects their anonymity (see chapter Appendix).

# In Conclusion: Implications for Clinicians

Because pain is a unique and subjective experience, each person with pain must be assessed and managed on an individual basis. Developing a mutually acceptable pain treatment plan requires that the clinician be ever cognizant of the potential physical, psychological, economic, and social consequences of poorly treated pain. Society's tolerance for the undertreatment of pain is dissipating. In fact, to meet JCAHO certification requirements, all health care agencies have to demonstrate that they adhere to stringent pain control policies (Figure 21.7).

Living with pain, especially chronic pain, is a life-changing experience. Whereas acute pain is

---

*Figure 21.6*    Internal Locus/External Locus of Control

---

*Internal Locus of Control (active coping)*

"I take pain medicine when I need it."

"I can do that, I'll use my walker."

"I manage my chronic pain disorder."

*External Locus of Control (passive coping)*

"My doctor tells me when to take medicine."

"My pain is too bad, I can't do it."

"I am just destined to have bad health."

---

---

**Figure 21.7**    Selected JCAHO Pain Standards (2001)

- Recognize the rights of clients to appropriate assessment and management of pain.
- Identify clients with pain through an initial screening assessment.
- Perform a comprehensive assessment when pain is identified.
- Document assessment of the pain in such a way that it will facilitate ongoing assessment and follow-up.
- Educate health care providers regarding pain assessment and management.
- Determine and ensure staff competency in pain assessment and management.
- Address pain assessment and management in the orientation of new staff.
- Establish policies and procedures that support appropriate prescription of effective pain medications.
- Ensure that pain does not interfere with participation in rehabilitation.
- Educate clients and families about the importance of effective pain management.
- Address clients' needs for symptom management in discharge planning.
- Collect data to monitor the appropriateness and effectiveness of pain management.

---

eventually resolved, the pain will never go away for many people with chronic pain, but it can be managed. Our role as health care personnel is to recognize their feelings of frustration and depression, to acknowledge chronic pain as disabling, and to empower patients to manage their own pain without compromise. Our tools for treatment may sometimes seem inadequate, but our knowledge, empathy, and support are key.

# Appendix: Additional Resources for People with Chronic Pain

National Chronic Pain Outreach Association
P.O. Box 274
Millboro, VA 24460
540-997-5004

The National Foundation for the Treatment of Pain
1330 Skyline Drive #21
Monterey, CA 93910
831-655-8812
www.paincare.org

National Center for Complementary and Alternative Medicine
Bethesda, MD 20892
http://hccam.nih.gov

American Pain Foundation
111 South Calvert Street, Suite 2700
Baltimore, MD 21202
410-385-5276
www.painfoundation.org

# References

Agency for Health Care Policy and Research, Management of Cancer Pain Guideline Panel. (1994). *Management of cancer pain. Clinical practice guideline.* AHCPR Pub. No. 94-0592. Rockville, MD: Public Health Service, US Department of Health and Human Services.

Adams, N. J., Plane, M. B., Fleming, M. F., Mundt, M. P., Saunders, L. A., & Stauffacher, E. A. (2001). Opioids and the treatment of chronic pain in a primary care sample. *Journal of Pain and Symptom Management, 22,* 791–796.

Agency for Health Care Policy and Research, Acute Pain Management Guideline Panel. (1992). Acute pain management: Operative or Medical Procedures and Trauma. Clinical practice guideline. No. 92-0032. Rockville, MD: Public Health Service, U.S. Department of Health and Human Services.

American Academy of Pediatrics. (1999). News Release: *New AAP circumcision policy released.* Pediatrics. Retrieved December 14, 2002, from *http://www.aap.org/advocacy/archives/marcircum.htm.*

American Academy of Pediatrics. Committee on Psychosocial Aspects of Child and Family Health; American Pain Society. Taskforce on Pain in Infants, Children and Adolescents. (2001). The assessment and management of acute pain in infants, children, and adolescents. *Pediatrics, 108,* 793–797.

American Pain Society. (1999). *Principles of analgesic use in the treatment of acute pain and cancer pain* (4th ed.). Glenview, IL: American Pain Society.

Arnstein, P. (1997). The neuroplastic phenomenon: A physiologic link between chronic pain and learning. *Journal of Neuroscience Nursing, 29,* 179–186.

Arnstein, P. (2002). Theories of pain. In B. St. Marie (Ed.), *Core curriculum for pain management nursing* (pp. 107–116). Philadelphia: Saunders.

Arnstein, P. (2000). The mediation of disability by self efficacy in different samples of chronic pain patients. *Disability and Rehabilitation, 22,* 794–801.

Arnstein, P., Caudill, M., Mandle, C. L., Norris, A., & Beasley, R. (1999). Self-efficacy as a mediator of the relationship between pain intensity, disability, and depression in chronic pain patients. *Pain, 80,* 483–491.

Aromaa, M., Sillanpaa, M., Rautava, P., & Helenius, H. (2000). Pain experience of children with headache and their families: A controlled study. *Pediatrics, 106,* 270–275.

Bennett, P., & St. Marie, B. (2002). The epidemiology of pain. In B. St. Marie (Ed.), *Core curriculum for pain management nursing* (pp. 45–53). Philadelphia: Saunders.

Bennett, S., & Huntsman, E. (2000). Parent perceptions of the impact of chronic pain in children and adolescents. *Children's Health Care, 29,* 147–160.

Blacker, M. (2002). Meditation. In M. A. Bright (Ed.), *Holistic health and healing* (pp. 105–112). Philadelphia: F.A. Davis.

Breen, J. (2002). Transitions in the concept of chronic pain. *Advances in Nursing Science, 24* (4), 48–59.

Burckhardt, C. S., Clark, S. R., & Bennett, R. M. (2001). Pain coping strategies and quality of life in women with fibromyalgia: Does age make a difference? *Journal of Musculoskeletal Pain, 9*(2), 5–18.

Cano, A. C., Weisberg, J. N., & Gallagher, R. M. (2000). Martial satisfaction and pain severity mediate the association between negative spouse responses to pain and depressive symptoms in a chronic pain patient sample. *Pain Medicine, 1,* 35–43.

Carrieri-Kohlman, V., Lindsey, A. L., & West, C. M. (1993). *Pathophysiological phenomena in nursing.* Philadelphia: W.B. Saunders.

Caudill, M. (1995). *Managing pain before it manages you.* New York: Guilford Press.

Cleary-Guida, M. B., Okvat, H. A., Oz, M. C., & Ting, W. (2001). A regional survey of health insurance coverage for complementary and alternative medicine: CURRE. *Journal of Alternative and Complementary Medicine, 7,* 269–274.

Cleeland, C. S., Gonin, R., Hatfield, K., Edmonson, J. H., Blum, R. H., Steward, J. A., et al. (1994). Pain and its treatment in outpatients with metastatic cancer. *New England Journal of Medicine, 330,* 592–596.

Coderre, T. J., Katz, J., Vaccarino, A. L., & Melzack, R. (1993). Contribution of central neuroplasticity to pathologic pain: Review of clinical and experimental evidence. *Pain, 52,* 259–285.

Coughlin, A. M., Badura, A. S., Fleisher, T. D., & Guck, T. P. (2000). Multidisciplinary treatment of chronic pain patients: Its efficacy in changing patient locus of control. *Archives of Physical Medicine and Rehabilitation, 81,* 739–740.

Davies, H., Crombie, I., Brown, J., & Martin, C. (1997). Diminishing returns or appropriate treatment strategy? An analysis of short-term outcomes after pain clinic treatment. *Pain, 70,* 203–208.

Davis, G. C., Hiemendz, M. L., & White, T. L. (2002). Barriers to managing chronic pain of older adults with arthritis. *Journal of Nursing Scholarship, 34,* 121–126.

Di Maggio, T. J. (2002). Pediatric pain management. In B. St. Marie (Ed.), *Core curriculum for pain management nursing* (pp. 45–53). Philadelphia: Saunders.

Dubner, R., & Gold, M. (1999). The neurobiology of pain. *Proceedings of the National Academy of Sciences of The United States of America, 96,* 7627–7630.

Eisenberg, D. M., et al. (1998). Trends in alternative medicine use in the United States, 1990–1997: Results of a follow-up national survey. *Journal of the American Medical Association, 280*(18), 1569–1575.

Evans, P. J., Lloyd, J. W., & Jack, T. M. (1981). Cryoanalgesia for intractable perineal pain. *Journal of the Royal Society of Medicine, 74,* 804–809.

Ferrell, B. R. (1996). *Suffering.* Sudbury, MA: Jones and Bartlett.

Ferrell-Torry, A. T., & Glick, O. J. (1993). The use of therapeutic massage as a nursing intervention to modify anxiety and the perception of cancer pain. *Cancer Nursing, 16,* 93–101.

Furlan, A., Brosseau, L., Imamura, M., & Irvin, E. (2002). Massage for low back pain. *Cochrane Database System Review, 2,* CD001929.

Gerstle, D. All, A., & Wallace, D. C. (2001). Quality of life and chronic nonmalignant pain. *Pain Management Nursing, 2*(3), 98–109.

Gil, K. M., Porter, L., Ready, J., Workman, E., Sedway, J., & Anthony, K. K. (2000). Pain in children and adolescents with sickle cell disease: An analysis of daily pain diaries. *Children's Health Care, 29,* 225–242.

Goats, G. C. (1994). The scientific basis of an ancient art. Physiological and therapeutic effects. *British Journal of Sports Medicine, 28,* 153–156.

Graumlich, S. (2001). Multidimensional assessment of pain in pediatric sickle cell disease. *Journal of Pediatric Psychology, 26*(4), 203–214.

Green C. R., Wheeler, J. R. C., LaPort, F., Marchant, B., & Guerrero, E. (2002). How well is chronic pain managed? Who does it well? *Pain Medicine, 3,* 56–65.

Guzman, J., Esmail, R., Karjalainen, K, Malmivaara, A., Irvin, E., & Bombardier, C. (2002). *Multidisciplinary bio-psych-social rehabilitation for chronic low back pain.* The Cochraine Library (Oxford), 1 (CD000963).

Hallberg, L., & Carlsson, S. (2000). Coping with fibromyalgia. *Scandinavian Journal of Caring Sciences, 14*(1), 29–36.

Haythornwaite, J. A., Menefee, L. A., Quartrano-Piacenti, A. L., & Pappagallo, M. (1998). Outcome of chronic opioid therapy for non-cancer pain. *Journal of Pain and Symptom Management, 15,* 185–194.

Hemmila, H. M. (2002). Quality of life and cost of care of back pain patients in Finnish general practice. *Spine, 27,* 647–53.

Holmquist, G. L. (2001). Drug decisions for patients with chronic noncancer pain syndromes. *Drug Benefit Trends,* May, 1–12.

Hunfeld, J. (2001). Chronic pain and its impact on quality of life in adolescents and their families. *Pain, 94*(2), 205–213.

Ignatavicius, D. (1999). *Medical-surgical nursing across the health care continuum.* Philadelphia: Saunders.

Kabat-Zinn, J. (1982). An out-patient program in behavioral medicine for chronic-pain patients based on the practice of mindfulness meditation: Theoretical considerations and preliminary results. *General Hospital Psychiatry, 4,* 33.

Kabat-Zinn, J., Lipworth, L., & Burney, R. (1985). The clinical use of mindfulness meditation for the self-regulation of chronic pain. *Journal Behavioral Medicine 8,* 163.

Kabat-Zinn, J., Lipworth, L., Burney, R., & Sellers, W. (1986). Four year follow-up of a meditation-based program for the self regulation of chronic pain: treatment outcomes and compliance. *Clinical Journal of Pain, 2,* 159.

Kahn, D. L., & Steeves R. H. (1996). Chapter 1: An understanding of suffering grounded in clinical practice and research. In B. Ferrell (Ed.) *Suffering.* Sudbury, MA: Jones and Bartlett.

Kazanowski, M. K., & Laccetti, M. S. (2002). *Pain.* Thorofare, NJ: SLACK.

Keane, A., McMenamin, E. M., & Polomano, R. C. (2002). Pain: The fifth vital sign. In D. Ignatavicius & M. L. Workman (Eds.), *Medical-surgical nursing* (4th ed.) (pp. 61–94). Philadelphia: W.B. Saunders.

Kemper, K. J., Sarah, R., Silver-Highfield, E., Xiarhos, E., Barnes, L., and Berde, C. (2000). On pins and needles? Pediatric pain patients' experience with accupuncture. *Pediatrics, 105,* 941–947.

Kuhn, M. A. (1999). *Complementary therapies for health care providers.* Philadelphia: Lippincott.

Lansbury, G. (2000). Chronic pain management: A qualitative study of elderly people's preferred coping strategies and barriers to management. *Disability and Rehabilitation, 22*(1/2), 2–14.

Lazarus, H., & Neumann, C. J. (2001). Assessing undertreatment of pain: The patient's perspectives. *Journal of Pharmaceutical Care in Pain & Symptom Control, 9*(4), 5–34.

Martin, L. S. (1997). Neuropathic pain in cancer patients. *Journal of Pain and Symptom Management, 14*(2), 99–117.

McCaffery, M. (2002). *Pain: Assessment and use of analgesics syllabus.* Presented October 22, 2002, pp. 1–63.

McCaffery, M., & Pasero, C. (1999). *Pain: Clinical manual,* 2nd ed. St. Louis, MO: Moby.

McCracken, L. M., & G. L. Iverson. (2001). Predicting complaints of cognitive functioning in patients with chronic pain. *Journal of Pain and Symptom Management, 21,* 392–396.

McHugh, G., & Thomas G. (2001a). Living with chronic pain: The patient's perspective. *Nursing Standard, 15*(52), 33–37.

McHugh, G., & Thomas, G. (2001b). Patient satisfaction with chronic pain management. *Nursing Standard, 15*(51), 33–38.

McQuay, H. J. (2002). *Relief of chronic non-malignant pain.* University of Oxford. Retrieved from http://www.jr2.ox.ac.uk/bandolier/booth/painpag/ wisdom/493HJM.html.

Melzack, R., & Wall, P. D. (1983). *The challenge of pain.* New York: Basic Books.

Melzack, R., & Wall, P. D. (1965). Pain mechanisms: A new theory. *Science, 150,* 971–979.

Miaskowski, C. (2000). The impact of age on a patient's perception of pain and ways it can be managed. *Pain Management Nursing, 1*(3), 2–7.

Mossey, J. A., Gallagher, R. M., & Tirumalasetti, F. (2000). The effects of pain and depression on physical functioning in elderly residents of a continuing care retirement community. *Pain Medicine, 1,* 340–350.

National Center for Complementary and Alternative Medicine. (2000, December). NCCAM Clearinghouse Publication. No.: X-42. Silver Spring, MD: National Institutes of Health.

Oberlander, T. F. (2001). Pain assessment and management in infants and young children with developmental disabilities. *Infants and Young Children, 14*(2), 33–47.

Otis, J. A. D., & McGeeney, B. (2000). Managing pain in the elderly. *Clinical Geriatrics, 8,* 48, 51–52, 54, 60.

Paice, J. Pain. In C. H. Yarbro, M. H. Frogge, & Goodman, M. (Eds.), *Cancer symptom management* (2nd ed.) (pp. 118–147). Boston: Jones and Bartlett.

Peolsson, M., Hyden, L. C., & Satterlund Larsson, U. (2000). Living with chronic pain: A dynamic learning process. *Scandinavian Journal of Occupational Therapy, 7,* 114–125.

Peter, E., & Watt-Watson, J. (2002). Unrelieved pain: An ethical and epistemological analysis of distrust in patients. *The Canadian Journal of Nursing Research, 34*(2), 65–80.

Piaget, J., & Inhelder, B. (1969). *The psychology of the child.* New York: Basic Books.

Raine, R., Haines, A., & Sensky, T. (2002). Systematic review of mental health interventions for patients with common somatic symptoms: Can research evidence from secondary care be extrapolated to primary care? *BMJ, 325,* 1082–1093.

Rakel, B., & Barr, J. O. (2003). Physical modalities in chronic pain management. *The Nursing Clinics of North America, 38,* 477–494.

Rappaport, L., & Frazer, C. (1995). Comment. *Journal of Developmental and Behavioral Pediatrics, 16*(4), 278–279.

Riley, J. L., Robinson, M. E., Wade, J. B., Myers, C. D., & Price, D. D. (2001). Sex differences in negative emotional responses to chronic pain. *The Journal of Pain, 2,* 354–359.

Riley, J. L., Wade, J. B., Robinson, M. E., & Price, D. D. (2000). The stages of pain processing across the adult lifespan. *The Journal of Pain, 1,* 162–170.

Ross, E. (2001). Opioid management in pain relief: Promises and pitfalls. In B. Nicholson (Ed.), *Pain relief and opioids: Benefits, concerns, and prescribing issues* (pp. 13–27). London: Royal Society of Medicine Press Limited.

Schnurr R. F., & MacDonald, M. R. (1995). Memory complaints in chronic pain. *Clinical Journal of Pain, 11,* 103–111.

Soderberg, S., & Lundman, B. (2001). Transitions experienced by women with fibromyalgia. *Health Care for Women International, 22,* 617–631.

Steihaug, S., Ahlsen, B., & Malterud, K. (2002). "I am allowed to be myself": Women with chronic muscu-lar pain being recognized. *Scandinavian Journal of Public Health, 30,* 281–287.

Tasmouth, T., Estlanderb, A., & Kalso, E. (1996). Effect of present pain and mood on the memory of past postoperative pain in women treated surgically for breast cancer. *Pain, 68,* 343–347.

Taylor, B. (2001). Promoting self-help strategies by sharing the lived experience of arthritis. *Contemporary Nurse, 10,* 117–125.

Thomas, S. (2000.) A phenomenologic study of chronic pain. *Western Journal of Nursing Research, 22,* 683–706.

Thomsen, A. B., Sorensen, J., Sjogren, P., & Eriksen, J. (2001). Economic evaluation of multidisciplinary pain management in chronic pain patients: A qualitative systematic review. *Journal of Pain and Symptom Management, 22,* 688–698.

Todd, K. H., Samaroo, N., & Hoffman, J. R. (1993). Ethnicity as a risk factor for inadequate emergency department analgesia. *JAMA, 269,* 1537–1539.

Turk, D. C., Meichenbaum, D., & Genest, M. (1983). *Pain and behavioral medicine.* New York: The Guilford Press.

Urban, M. O., & Gebhart, G. F. (1999). Supraspinal contributions to hyperalgesia. *Proceedings of the National Academy of Sciences of the United States of America, 96,* 7687–7692.

Vasudevan, S., Hegmann, K., Moore, A., & Cerletty, S. (1992). Physical methods of pain management. In P. P. Ray (Ed.), *Practical management of pain* (2nd ed.) (pp. 669–679). Baltimore: Mosby Year Book Medical Publishers.

Vaughan, V. (2002). Therapeutic massage. In M. A. Bright (Ed.), *Holistic health and healing* (pp. 161–169.) Philadelphia: F.A. Davis.

Weinrich, S. P., & Weinrich, M. C. (1990). The effect of massage on pain in cancer patients. *Applied Nursing Research, 3*(4), 140–145.

Whitney, S. L. (1989). Physical agents: Heat and cold modalities. In R. Scully & M. Barnes (Eds.), *Physical therapy.* Philadelphia: J.B. Lippincott.

Wong, D. L. (1993). *Whaley & Wong's essentials of pediatric nursing* (4th ed.). St. Louis: Mosby.

Zeltzer, L. Recurrent abdominal pain. *Journal of Developmental and Behavioral Pediatrics, 16*(4), 279–281.

# Part Five

# PHILOSOPHICAL PERSPECTIVES ON HUMAN DEVELOPMENT

# Chapter 22

# Hope and Health in the Postmodern Age

Mary M. Brabeck

The terrorist attack on the World Trade Center and the death of thousands on September 11, 2001 shattered the blissful innocence and sense of invulnerability enjoyed by many United States citizens. Europeans noticed it immediately. The face of the U.S. tourist waiting to clear customs in international airports no longer was that of a fearless adolescent with a baseball cap turned backwards. What Europeans noticed in the wake of September 11th was the face of fear—traces of anxiety on American faces, suspicion as they looked at their fellow travelers. Of course, it had happened already in most of the world. Car bombs, suicide terrorists, and innocent bystanders as targets are part of the fabric of the lives of people who live in much of Central America, Africa, Northern Ireland, and The Mideast. With the incineration of the World Trade Center twin towers and four jumbo jet airplanes, belief in the ability of the U.S. government and its institutions to protect innocent citizens also was shaken.

Yet, faith in the U.S. intelligence systems was only the most recent of our cherished beliefs to be toppled. The philosophy of postmodernism that has dominated philosophical thought and academic discourse for the past two decades is de-

stroying our assumptions about the integrity of institutions, the possibility of objective truth, and existence of universal principles. The health care system has suffered the same fate, although physicians and nurses still enjoy the respect and admiration of most of the public, cynicism about a system that is broken is pervasive. Over 40 million U.S. citizens lack health care and are only "one illness" away from bankruptcy. Ironically, what we most need to energize us into solutions and the ability to dream of new alternatives to the problems our society faces is that which we are in danger of losing: Hope. Hope is the mental and motivational force that can bring us out of our pessimism and anxious distrust of the future. Hope offers a corrective to our postmodern malaise and provides an alternative for health care providers, parents, teachers, and community leaders as they try to guide youth into an uncertain future. Hope is what helps terminally ill patients and their caregivers face each day and what will sustain the work that is needed to design a health care system that works for all U.S. citizens (Salovey, Rothman, Detweiler, & Steward, 2000).

In this essay, I argue for hope, the forgotten virtue among the three theological virtues of faith, hope, and love. I suggest that psychologists and philosophers have viewed hope as different from optimism and a buffer against despair and other illnesses. Drawing from works of fiction and philosophers, I claim hope is the result of imagining possibilities even while facing dangerous memories of evil and wrongdoing. Drawing from theologians, I argue that hope is a motherly virtue that puts us in solidarity with the human community. Hope, I suggest, creates the bridge for health care providers to reach patients and accompany them on the difficult road of illness. And I claim that hope compels us to work for social justice. Thus, as an impulse for action, hope is both a path out of despair for individuals and a road to enhancing the human condition by making the institutions that affect health and well-being (schools, insurance companies, hospitals) more just.

# The Psychology of Hope

Many philosophers and some theologians claim that hope is a secular virtue, and some psychologists would agree. Martin Seligman (Seligman & Csikszentmihalyi, 2000), past president of the American Psychological Association, says that in the new millennium, we as a society face a critical choice: "The United States can continue to increase its material wealth while ignoring the human needs of its people and those of the rest of the planet . . . Such a course is likely to lead to increasing selfishness, to alienation between the more and the less fortunate, and eventually to chaos and despair" (Seligman & Csikszentmihalyi, 2000, p. 5).

Seligman and Csikszentmihalyi's words are surprising because mainstream psychology has not been particularly interested in the study of what makes life worth living, what leads to courage, wisdom, faith, love, and hope. It has not been interested in understanding the subjective life of humans. Constructs like virtue, spirituality, wisdom, hope, and even optimism have been

largely ignored. In part this is because psychology has been concerned primarily with relieving suffering by investigating psychological pathology or dysfunctional behaviors. In part it is because, since the early days of giants like Carl Jung and William James, psychology has been trying to move closer to science than to philosophy. The move to be closer to an objective science has led to methods of inquiry that are reductionistic, not emancipatory or aspirational. Rejecting the null hypothesis leads to greater degrees of probability but not necessarily greater understanding of what it means to be human, or greater insight into what humanity might aspire to become.

## Therapeutic Hope

Although most psychologists are not concerned with knowing what the "right thing" is, the best in psychology have always been committed to understanding what *is* and what *could be* (Seligman & Csikszentmihalyi, 2000, p. 7, emphasis in original). Psychiatry, more than psychology (i.e., the therapy room rather than the experimental lab), has been interested in hope at least since the 1950s. Jerome Frank (1961) called hope a necessary condition for therapeutic gain, and many theorists saw suicide and depression as the result, at least in part, of the loss of hope.

The association between hope and therapeutic gain has been noted as early as the 1950s (Beker, 1987; Frank & Frank, 1961; Frankl, 1966). In these early studies hope was operationalized as a level of expectation of goal achievement (Stotland, 1969, p. 3). Hope was believed to be a "mediating process" tying together antecedent events (probability based on previous events), an action (behavior), and consequent events (probability of future outcome).

More recently, Snyder (1994) claimed that "Hope is the sum of the mental will power and way power that you have for your goals." Thus, for Snyder hope is finding the will to persevere and finding the way to succeed. "Hope is more than distancing oneself from and delimiting the impact of failures; hope is the essential process of linking oneself to potential success" (Snyder, 1994, p. 18). This is the opposite of ruminating on what we don't have, can't do, or are not able to achieve. Rather, hope focuses attention on goals, objects of desire, outcomes we want, and problem solving to achieve our goals.

Prevention researchers also have found that there are many sources of strength that serve as buffers against both physical and psychological illness. These include courage, optimism, interpersonal skills, faith, a work ethic, honesty, perseverance, and, of course, hope (Seligman & Csikszentmihalyi, 2000, p. 7). Snyder (1994) showed that hope, as he defines it, is a buffer against depression. In fact, hopelessness is more powerful than depression in predicting suicidal tendencies in children (Snyder, 1994, p. 156). Building hope rather than attacking depression may be a proper therapeutic goal.

Hope is valuable for adults as well as children and adolescents. It serves as a buffer against depression when people face divorce, traumatic injury, or severe or prolonged illnesses (Snyder, 1994). Hope leads to less anxiety and to better problem solving. It minimizes negativity when we face adversities. Hope looks outward and prompts us to call on friends, laugh, exercise, eat more healthy foods, and take better care of our emotional, spiritual, and physical health. Clearly there are many benefits to hope as psychology has defined it. These benefits mark it as separate from something often confused with hope—optimism.

# Hope and Optimism

Hope correlates with optimism, but it is not the same thing. In *Optimism: The Biology of Hope,* Lionel Tiger (1979) located optimism in human nature and claimed it was selected throughout evolution along with our cognitive abilities. Because optimism is future oriented, Tiger argued, it is essential to our evolutionary history.

The argument goes like this: When humans became capable of imagining the future, we could imagine horrible possibilities in the future. We needed something to counteract this, and Tiger argued that optimism is that thing (Peterson, 2000, p. 46). This future orientation motivates us to solve problems and act to achieve goals. The opposite of future seeking—rumination on what we don't have/can't do/are not able to achieve—is associated with depression.

In *The Madwoman of Chaillot,* a play of hope in a state of madness, written by Jean Giraudoux (1947), a man is arrested for trying to commit suicide. The Madwoman (the Countess) intervenes to stop the arresting officer, who says he is "busy saving a drowning man" (p. 26). The Madwoman responds that that is not the way to save a life; you must give him a reason for living. "To be alive is to be fortunate," she says.

*"Of course, in the morning, when you first awake, it does not always seem so very gay. When you take your hair out of the drawer and your teeth out of the glass, you are apt to feel a little out of place in the world. Especially if you've just been dreaming that you're a little girl on a pony looking for strawberries in the woods. But all you need to feel the call of life once more is a letter in your mail giving you your schedule for the day—your mending, your shopping, that letter to your grandmother that you never seem to get around to. And so, when you've washed your face with rosewater and powdered it, and put on your pins, your rings, your brooches, bracelets, earrings and pearls—in short, when you have dressed for your morning coffee—and have had a good look at yourself—not in the glass naturally, it lies—but in the old brass gong that once belonged to Admiral Courbet . . . then you're armed, you're strong, you're ready—you can begin again" (pp. 26–27).*

Hope and optimism share a future orientation and a desire and longing for something that is not yet. Steindl-Rast (1983, p. 1310) says that hope is "poised between the already and the not-yet"—not-yet in both expectation and desire, between the story that we have constructed and the future that is not here (Capps, 1970, p. 2).

The object of hope, however, is different from the object of optimism. Hope is not just putting on a "good face," as Dale Carnegie or Norman Vincent Peale teach. In Donald Meyer's 1988 book, *The Positive Thinkers,* Meyer traces the roots of optimistic thought in America from Phineas Quimby and Dale Carnegie to Norman Vincent Peale and Ronald Reagan. He argues that the psychology of positive thinking flourishes among people who, from positions of comfort and security, have the luxury of seeing the only thing wrong with their lives within themselves. From their privileged perspectives, if they just make the right mental adjustment, if they have the right positive attitude, all things are possible, all goals achievable.

Optimism under this line of thinking means materialism, individualism, and a distortion of reality in order to secure one's own state of well-being. It is looking in the brass gong, denying one has a terminal illness. Of course, such positive thinking was always defined in opposition to what it was not: Namely, the optimists are not Catholics, not Jews, not women, not African Americans or Latinos, not the lower class, not homosexual, and so on. Those groups that the optimist defines as "not me" are, as Spiro Agnew saw them, "the nattering nabobs of negativism." Such optimism clouds one's ability to see real problems, such as the moral issues that result from lack of universal health care. Optimism, but not hope, is a Pollyanna view of the world.

Hope, however, connects us with others and makes us responsible to others, within families and communities. It does this, I argue, through narrative based on memory and a vision of future based on imagination. And it begins in childhood.

## Origins of Hope

Hope is not simple, but it has simple roots (Reed, 2000). And reflections on childhood are perhaps the quickest way to get in touch with hope.

Aristotle says, "The young . . . are full of passion, which excludes fear; and of hope, which inspires confidence." Hope is found in a child's face, and the radiance of childhood links hope to youthfulness. My understandings of church, religion, and hope are all rooted in the experiences of community that taught us children the responsibility we had to others. My mother had a ready solution for childhood complaints about boredom or feeling sad: "Go do something nice for someone else," she would say, and if we could shake off our slothful self-absorption and do what she suggested, the boredom did indeed melt away. *Self-efficacy* is what Bandura (1997) would call it 35 years later. *Hope building,* I now say.

Similarly, research done during the cold war, when we had regular reports that showed the doomsday clock was moving us ever closer to nuclear annihilation, showed that parents who do something in response to a threat (e.g., worked on arms control or reduction of nuclear weapons) have less-anxious children. When they see that adults are doing something together for the family, the community, or the world, children feel both security and hopefulness. Yet how many examples of courageous action do young people see these days? Perhaps postmodernism has driven it off our campuses and out of our homes.

## Postmodern Hopelessness and the Corrective of Hope

Postmodernism arose as a critique of modernity and modernity's belief in infinite progress. Postmodern philosophy and its methodology—*deconstruction*—stripped us of the illusion of progress that the modern era had promised. We have been to the moon, and we have unlocked the secrets of our genetic code, but 10-year-old girls are still being sold as sex slaves, and millions of children are still dying of neglect, abuse, and starvation. Millions more are illiterate. From genocide to school children shooting school children, instead of progress we have witnessed the rape of persons and the rape of our natural resources. We have watched on TV the horrors of the Vietnam war and the killing fields, Rwanda and Bosnia, Indonesia and East Timor and the Northern Ireland and the Middle East. The postmodern lens exposed humanity as capable of inhumane acts and revealed our American idealism as optimistic delusional thinking. Hannah Arendt (1973) called the last century the "cruelest century" of recorded history. Postmodern writers and artists have forced us to face that cruelty. They forced us to reckon with the trajectory of the abuse of power in our past and its prediction of abuses in the future.

The postmodern argument is that what has been called progress is really only domination and exploitation: "We have valued our Western culture over the Third World; we have privileged the affluent over the poor, white over all others, men over women. We have used our considerable advances in science, technology and education to impose our way of thinking on all others: Our values and our way of life, claiming our way, the way of the western elite, is universal, even as we wiped out entire indigenous cultural traditions." (Bauckham & Hart, 1999, p. 18). The modern era, it seems, changed everything but our generosity and our ability to get along with each other. And so, to escape exposed human condition, we retreat from history and from memory. The past rejected, the future too fearful to face, we live in the present, a bleak but seductive "now." Our Generation X has no burdens of the past because from the postmodern perspective, there is no knowledge of history, no history worth knowing. That knowledge has been replaced by what William Lynch (1965) called a "fascination with despair." And this despair, which drives out all hope, is derived in large measure from our alienation.

## Two Kinds of Alienation

We are, first of all, alienated from history. Each day is new and must be interrogated, examined, and questioned endlessly in a hermeneutic of suspicion. Reifying the immediate experience, the eternal now, both past and future are rejected, and we alienate ourselves from our (complicit) stories of times past and times to come. We are also alienated from each other. Autonomous and independent, we feel responsible only for self, because only the self exists.

Sadly, American youth, with all their independence, autonomy, and choice, are bored. Studies show that American youth are bored as much as 50% of the time, trapped in the present, waiting for someone to prove to them that life—which is always and only this moment—is worth living (Larson, 2000; Larson & Richards, 1991). It is not enough to answer Camus' questions, "Why *not* choose death?" with merely a therapy for depression (Seligman & Csikszentmihalyi, 2000). Can a transformative virtue of hope provide a moral light? Can it point directions to positive action that will pull our students—and ourselves—away from the grips of despair? Certainly both narrative and memory will be critical to finding that place where, in the poet Seamus Heaney's wonderful phrase, "Hope and history rhyme."

## Hope and Stories

When postmodernists rejected the myth of progress, exposing it as a story of domination and exploitation, they rejected all explanatory systems, all grand narratives, all the stories by which we make meaning of our lives—the stories of our culture, the stories of our faith. And yet, we live by stories, personal narrative, historical narrative, and fictional narrative. Personal narrative gives identity coherence and makes meaning of our individual lives. History both reveals our terrible errors and reminds us that we *can* build a better future. Fiction consoles, it humanizes the horrific, and it wards off the anxieties about the future. Narrative—historical, personal or fictional—can be interrogated and deconstructed, reconstructed and critiqued, but it cannot be replaced. Narrative can create the future that we desire. It can chart a new direction for us to take our lives. Narrative can make us the people that we want to be. Such narrative is not private nor accomplished in isolation. Rather, it is public and shared, and ultimately it is political because it can bridge the differences and varieties of culture and context that separate us as individuals. This is a hopeful narrative that can help build a future that makes us into the people we imagine we can be.

## Hope and Imagination

In his surprising and magical narrative, *Imagining Argentina,* Lawrence Thornton (1987) tells the story of a man caught in the horrors of the Dirty War in Argentina. The generals, members of the junta, ordered the disappearance, torture, and murder of thousands during those terrible years. Carlos Rueda, the protagonist of the story, has a gift through which he can imagine what happens to the people who have disappeared. And as he uses his gift to help frantic parents learn the whereabouts of their children and desperate wives locate their husbands, he is gradually able to imagine them out of prison, and in imagining their future he makes it happen. One day Carlos is walking down the street with his friend, Silvio, the narrator of the book, and he sees a green Falcon (green Falcons were the preferred car of the secret police). "Can you see the men sitting in the car?" Carlos says to his friend, "Do you know what they see?"

His friend answers,

*"I suppose you'll say nothing." But Carlos responds. "Sheep and terrorists. . . . They see sheep and terrorists because they imagine us that way. . . . So long as we accept what the men in the car imagine, we're finished. All I've been trying to tell you is that there are two Argentina's, Silvio, the regime's travesty of it, and the one we have in our hearts. . . . Last week I went to the Riachuelo to find a leather bag for Teresa's birthday. In one stall I discovered a lacquered bamboo cage in which two Amazon parrots perched lifelessly. Just then the woman who kept the stall unlatched the door and the parrots flew out. I don't know why she did it but that's what imagina-*

*tion can do, Silvio, fly like the parrots as they arched into the sky where they caught the scent of the jungle and rode the free air back to where they belonged. We have to believe in the power of imagination because it is all we have, and ours is stronger than theirs." (Thornton, 1987, p. 65).*

And we have the power to imagine a better, more hopeful future. Hope imagines constantly, ceaselessly exploring the possible, seeing what is not yet seen, seeking solutions. It tests, reflects, rehypothesizes, and tries again when what one tries doesn't work. Hope helps the patient with terminal cancer face the next radiation treatment and inspires the nurse and physician to work to achieve a single-payer insurance system.

## Hope and Dangerous Memories

A hopeful imagination does not mean creating stories that deny what is ugly in the past or what has been painful or shameful. In fact, transformative hope, hope that creates a future worth struggling to achieve, requires that we recall the dangerous memories, memories of suffering we have experienced and suffering that we have caused, the memories of exploitation and the memories of resistance. These are dangerous memories because they can detach people from a given interpretation, often from the "official story," and bring to light new possibilities for a *different* future. Hope allows us to confront the terrible task of remembering precisely because of its insistence that we imagine a different future (Agosin, 1999; Golden & Collins, 1982).

Eli Wiesel, the Jewish writer and Auschwitz survivor, is the living voice of the Holocaust, the dangerous memory of humanity's most shameful moment. In all his books, stories, and essays Wiesel says the same thing over and over: We are obliged to remember, even when it is painful, even when it is shameful. In return for honest engagement, dangerous memories *give back* by informing the future. Insisting that we do not succumb to *amnesia*, by forgetting and avoiding, or to *nostalgia*, through optimistic daydreaming, dangerous memories create narratives that bind us to each other in a shared experience and a shared desire for a better, hopeful, and hope-inspiring future. Such memories are both from a community and inform a community. They shape the community's story and bind us together as humanity, past, present, and future. And we cannot live with our dangerous memories alone. We cannot imagine a better future, one without assassinations and torture, one that is built on hope without others.

But building these connections, these communities of memory, requires that we first acknowledge our own neediness, our dependence on each other. In our postmodern alienated culture we have denied the need for help. In our love affair with autonomy we dodge the fact that neediness is part of the human experience (Lynch, 1965, p. 42). Hope depends on others and acknowledges our dependencies. Hospice workers know that by tenaciously connecting with their patients, they give both love and hope and receive them in return.

# A Story about Hope and Interdependence

A few Christmases ago, I received a note from a dear friend, Dr. Eoin McKiernan, founder of the Irish American Cultural Institute, whose wife of 50 years has been lost to Alzheimer's disease. He wrote about a spirituality in Ireland that has diminished, disappeared, or been transformed—altered, perhaps, by failures in charity. This spiritual attitude was summed up in the phrase his county-Clare–born mother taught him, "God bless the mark," a text that is profoundly charitable in itself. The theology of this statement personally challenged everyone by the presence of a God-given blemish, an imperfection, a failing: a terminally ill cancer patient, a lame child, a blind woman, a student unable to master a passage, or an adolescent paralyzed with self-doubt or depression. Such behavior called forth not malice, irritation or condescension, but the supremely charitable exclamation, "God bless the mark."

This, Dr. McKiernan said, was the spiritual aspect of the old Irish folk proverb, *"Are scath a cheile a mhaireas na daoine,"* which translates as, "It is in the shadow of one another that we live." This spiritual and proverbial statement draws attention to our enormous interdependence. We live in the shadow of each other, we are profoundly and always affected by and affect the lives of others. Each of us carries the mark—deficiencies, inadequacies, lapses—within each of us that can only be remedied by the help of others. To the extent that we can acknowledge, know, and accept the mark in ourselves, we will be able to bridge the chasm of human separation and will be able to reach another human being who also shares the mark. As we build a bridge to another's suffering, from "the mark" in ourselves and the mark in others, to a better future, we build a community. Despair is the individual act; hope is the act of community. Whether the community is a church, a synagogue, a mosque, a university, a profession, or a nation, hope happens in relationship between persons, and between an individual and God.

"If optimists and pessimists are politicians, hope is a mother." says Steindl Rast, not pretending things will be all right, but continuing to do her thing, like a spider rebuilding her web. Hope, the theological virtue, is a gift from a motherly god, who will take care, will heal, and will protect and nourish always. Even in a world of cruelty and injustice, even here, with *this* flawed humanity, even *now,* in our moment of distress and inadequacy. Hope is the gift that calls us back into relationships and community that is strong as mother love (Johnson, 1998). Emily Dickinson captured the same tenacity of hope that Johnson describes in a stanza of her poem:

*Hope is the thing with feathers*
*That perches in the soul,*
*And sings the tune without the words*
*And never stops at all.*

Hope, like a mother's love, never stops at all. Hope gets up each time it is knocked down, each time with a new "as if," a new imagined possibility. This is not a placid hope, a languid, optimistic feel-good hope. It is a hope that is born out of a fearless facing of the despairing finality of death, of the dangerous memories of rapes and wars, of facing the fact that, as George Santyana says, "we are all more human than otherwise." God bless the mark. This hope *is both gift* and burden and it requires us, even as it *propels* us, into action. This hope, born out of stories with dangerous memories and loving imagination, is a restless searching hope that never stops at all.

As Christian theologian and architect of the theology of hope, Jurgen Moltmann (1967), writes, ". . . hope causes not rest but unrest, not patience but impatience. Those who hope in Christ can no longer put up with reality as it is, but begin to suffer under it, to contradict it." Moltmann's theology of hope describes a world not yet redeemed; a world closer to the Jewish view of a world that exists, "as only a promise of redemption, a future yet to come" (Fackenheim, 1970). A world, in other words, that needs some work but can be redeemed through hope.

But changing from a hermeneutic of doubt and suspicion to one of transformative hope is not easy. One can imagine the virtues of courage, patience, generosity, and wisdom it would take to engage in a hermeneutic of hope. And engagement is what it requires. Of course action requires hope. We don't move if we think movement is hopeless. But I suggest that transformative hope *requires* action. When Nelson Mandela was released from prison, he appeared on the David Frost show: Frost asked him, "Aren't you bitter?" "Bitter?" the post Apartheid leader of South Africa said. "I would like to be bitter, but there is too much work to do."

I believe that it is in the *doing*, the hopeful and hope-filling *act*, where transformative hope resides. This is not an 'other world' escape theology of hope. Both poverty and human alienation are overcome *by work*, not by daydreaming (so says

Feurbach, and my mom). In the doing, the action, the future is brought into the present, Metz and Moltman and Bloch and other hope theologians and philosophers argue. The future is a reality that does not yet exist. We don't and can't in any real sense know the future. However, we can get a glimpse at the future from "being for others" (Bonhoffer, 1996; Schuster & Boschert-Kimming, 1999).

Again and again the Bible, the grand narrative of Christianity, the Koran of the Muslim world, and the Torah of the Jewish religion, challenge us to be responsible toward society, toward our human community, toward one another, and toward those who are yet to come. Hope requires no less than that we change the world, that we bring justice and loving peace to the broken and alienated world.

When Elie Weisel was interviewed by Bill Clinton ("Millennium Evening at the White House," April 12, 1999), Clinton asked the survivor of the Nazi Holocaust, "From whence comes your extraordinary hope?" Weisel replied: "It comes from hopelessness," and then he told a story:

*There once was an emperor who was very powerful. In his empire, a wise man with occult powers lived peacefully. He knew the language of the wind and understood the song of the birds. The emperor heard of the man and sent for him because he wanted to set a test. He took a baby robin and held it behind his back in one of his hands. He then said to the wise man, "Tell me, if you can, is the bird alive or is it dead." The wise man of course, knew the stakes. If he said the bird was alive, the emperor would kill it. If he said dead, the emperor would show him the bird and prove his power by killing it. The man paused and thought and then said, "Mightiness, the answer is in your hands."*

Hope, said Elie Weisel from whom all was taken in a Nazi concentration camp, is in our hands. "When there is no hope," he told President Clinton, "I assume it and take it as something that belongs to me." This was Eli Weisel's answer to Clinton's question about the origin of hope, and my last story.

Out of our dangerous memories, and through the power of our imaginations, I believe, we can build a narrative that draws from our tradition and directs action to build a future that is worth hoping for; a future worth working toward; and worth building with and for our families, our communities, our world. United as a community, we can solve the health care crisis and accompany with hope the individual patient on the road of illness. This, I believe, is what we must do to live through the dangerous memories of September 11, 2001, into a better future.

# References

Agosin, M. (1999). *A map of hope: Women's writing on human rights—an international literary anthology.* New Brunswick, NJ: Rutgers University Press.

Arendt, H. (1973). The origins of totalitarianism. New York: Harcourt, Brace, Jovanovich.

Bandura, A. (1997). *Self-efficacy: The exercise of control.* New York: Freeman.

Bauckham, R., & Hart, T. (1999). *Hope against hope: Christian eschatology at the turn of the millennium.* Grand Rapids, MI: William B. Eerdmans Publishing.

Beker, J. C. (1987). *Suffering and hope.* Philadelphia: Fortress Press.

Bloch, E. (1970). Man as possibility. In Capps, W. H. (Ed.), *The future of hope,* (pp. 50–67). Philadelphia: Fortress Press.

Bonhoffer, A. (1996). *The ethics of the stoic Epictetus.* New York: Peter Lang.

Capps, W. H. (1970). Mapping the hope movement. In Capps, W. H. (Ed.), *The future of hope* (pp. 1–49). Philadelphia: Fortress Press.

Fackenheim, E. L. (1970). The commandment to hope: A response to contemporary Jewish experience. In Capps, W. H. (Ed.), *The future of hope* (pp. 68–91). Philadelphia: Fortress Press.

Fackenheim, E. L., Metz, J. B., & Moltman, J. (1970). Hope—After Auschwitz and Hiroshima? In Capps, W. H. (Ed.), *The future of hope* (pp. 92–101). Philadelphia: Fortress Press.

Frank, J. D., & Frank, J. B. (1961). *Persuasion and healing: A comparative study of psychotherapy.* Baltimore: Johns Hopkins University Press.

Frankl, V. E. (1966). *The Doctor and the soul: From psychotherapy to logotherapy.* New York: Alfred A. Knopf.

Giraudoux, J. (1947). *The Madwoman of Chaillot.* New York: Random House.

Golden, R., & Collins, S. (1982). *Struggle: Is a name for hope.* Minneapolis: West End Press.

Johnson, E. A. (1998). *Friends of God and prophets: A feminist theological reading of the Communion of Saints.* New York: Continuum Publishing.

Larson, R. W. (2000). Toward a psychology of positive youth development. *American Psychologist, 55,* 170–183.

Larson, R. W., & Richards, M. H. (1991). Boredom in the middle school years: Blaming schools versus blaming students. *American Journal of Education, 99,* 418–443.

Lynch, W. F. (1965). *Images of hope.* Baltimore, MD: Helicon Press.

Meyer, D. (1988). *The Positive Thinkers.* Scranton, PA: Wesleyan University Press.

Peterson, C. (2000). The future of optimism. *American Psychologist, 55,* 44–55.

Reed, W. (2000). Toward a psychology of positive youth development. *American Psychologist, 55,* 170–183.

Ryan, R. M., & Deci, E. L. (2000). Self-determination theory and the facilitation of intrinsic motivation, social development, and well-being. *American Psychological Association, 55,* 68–78.

Salovey, P., Rothman, A. J., Detweiler, J. B., & Steward, W. T. (2000). Emotional states and physical health. *American Psychological Association, 55,* 110–121.

Schuster, E. & Boschert-Kimming, R. (1999). *Hope against hope: Johann Baptist Metz and Elie Wiesel speak out on the Holocaust.* New York: Paulist Press.

Selgiman, M. E. P., & Csikszentmihalyi, M. (2000). Positive psychology: An introduction. *American Psychologist, 55,* 5–14.

Snyder, C. R. (1994). *The psychology of hope: You can get there from here.* New York: The Free Press.

Steindl-Rast, D. (1983). *A listening heart.* New York: Crossroad.

Stotland, E. (1969). *The psychology of hope.* New York: Jossey Bass.

Thornton, L. (1987). *Imagining Argentina.* New York: Doubleday.

Tiger, L. (1979). *Optimism: The Biology of Hope.* New York: Harper & Row.

# Index